*16th Edition*

# HARRISON'S
## PRINCIPLES OF
# Internal
# Medicine

## SELF-ASSESSMENT
## AND BOARD REVIEW

D1219405

*16th Edition*

# HARRISON'S
## PRINCIPLES OF
# Internal Medicine
## SELF-ASSESSMENT
## AND BOARD REVIEW

*For use with the 16th edition of HARRISON'S PRINCIPLES OF INTERNAL MEDICINE*

**EDITED BY**

**CHARLES WIENER, MD**
Vice Chair, Department of Medicine
The Johns Hopkins University School of Medicine
Baltimore, Maryland

**Contributing Editors**

**Cynthia D. Brown, MD**

**Anna R. Hemnes, MD**

**Philip J. Nivatpumin, MD**

Department of Internal Medicine
The Johns Hopkins University School of Medicine
Baltimore, Maryland

*McGraw-Hill*
MEDICAL PUBLISHING DIVISION

New York     Chicago     San Francisco     Lisbon     London     Madrid     Mexico City
Milan     New Delhi     San Juan     Seoul     Singapore     Sydney     Toronto

Harrison's
**PRINCIPLES OF INTERNAL MEDICINE, 16e**
**Self-Assessment and Board Review**

1 2 3 4 5 6 7 8 9 0    WCTWCT    0 9 8 7 6 5 4

ISBN     0-07-143534-4

---

**Notice**

This book was set in Times Roman by Progressive Information Technologies.
The editors were James Shanahan and Mariapaz Ramos Englis.
The production supervisor was Catherine H. Saggese.
Quebecor World was printer and binder.

This book is printed on acid-free paper.

**Library of Congress Cataloging-in-Publication Data**

Harrison's principles of internal medicine: self-assessment and board review/edited by Charles M. Wiener.-- 16th ed.
   p.; cm.
"For use with the 16th edition of Harrison's principles of internal medicine."
Includes bibliographical references.
ISBN 0-07-143534-4
  1. Internal medicine--Examinations, questions, etc. I. Title: Principles of internal medicine. II. Wiener, Charles M. III. Tinsley Randolph, 1900- Principles of internal medicine.
  [DNLM: 1. Internal Medicine--Examination Questions. WB 18.2 H323 2004 Suppl.]
RC46 .H333 2005 Suppl.
616--dc22                      2004050951

# CONTENTS

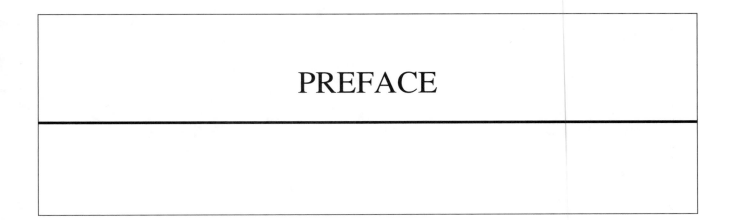

# PREFACE

People who pursue careers in Internal Medicine are drawn to the specialty by a love of patients, mechanisms, problems, and therapeutics. We love hearing the stories told to us by our patients, linking signs and symptoms to pathophysiology, solving the diagnostic dilemmas, and proposing strategies to prevent and treat diseases. It is not surprising given these tendencies that internists prefer to review past information or learn new material through problem solving.

This book is offered as a companion to the amazing accomplishment of the 16th edition of *Harrison's Principles of Internal Medicine*. It is designed for the student of medicine to reinforce the knowledge contained in the parent book in a format that is active rather than passive. This book contains over 800 questions, almost all centered around a patient presentation. Answering the questions requires an understanding of pathophysiology, epidemiology, differential diagnosis, diagnostic strategy, and therapeutics. We have tried to make the questions and the discussion of the answers timely and relevant to clinicians. We recommend this book for those preparing for the Internal Medicine boards and for those looking for an active method of life long learning.

Approximately 80% of the questions and answers in this book are original to this edition. We acknowledge Dr. Stone and Dr. DeAngelo, the editors of the 15th edition of the Self Assessment and Board Review, for their contributions to this edition. We also thank our colleagues Kerri Cavanaugh, MD, and Franco D'Alessio, MD, for contributing questions. The dedicated physicians of The Johns Hopkins Osler Medical Housestaff inspire us daily with their devotion to patient care and to learning. Many of the patient presentations included in this book derive from cases they've presented and the discussions they've stimulated.

# I. INTRODUCTION TO CLINICAL MEDICINE: GENERAL CONCEPTS AND CARDINAL MANIFESTATIONS OF DISEASE

## *QUESTIONS*

**DIRECTIONS:** Each question below contains four or five suggested responses. Choose the **one best** response to each question.

**I-1.** A physician is deciding whether to use a new test to screen for disease X in his practice. The prevalence of disease X is 5%. The sensitivity of the test is 85%, and the specificity is 75%. In a population of 1000, how many patients will have the diagnosis of disease X missed by this test?

A. 50
B. 42
C. 8
D. 4
E. 0

**I-2.** How many patients will be erroneously told they have diagnosis X on the basis of the results of this test?

A. 713
B. 505
C. 237
D. 42
E. 8

**I-3.** A patient is seen in the clinic for evaluation of chest pain. The patient is 35 years old and has no medical illnesses. She reports occasional intermittent chest pain that is unrelated to exercise but is related to eating spicy food. The physician's pretest probability for coronary artery disease causing these symptoms is low; however, the patient is referred for an exercise treadmill test, which shows ST depression after moderate exercise. Using Bayes' theorem, how does one interpret these test results?

A. The pretest probability is low, and the sensitivity and specificity of exercise treadmill testing in females are poor; therefore, the exercise treadmill test is not helpful in clinical decision making in this case.
B. Regardless of the pretest probability, the abnormal result of this exercise treadmill testing requires further evaluation.
C. Because the pretest probability for coronary artery disease is low, the patient should be referred for further testing to rule out this diagnosis.

**I-3.** *(Continued)*
D. Because the pretest probability was low in this case, a diagnostic test with a low sensitivity and specificity is sufficient to rule out the diagnosis of coronary artery disease.
E. The testing results suggest that the patient has a very high likelihood of having coronary artery disease and should undergo cardiac catheterization.

**I-4.** Drug X is investigated in a meta-analysis for its effect on mortality after a myocardial infarction. It is found that mortality drops from 10 to 2% when this drug is administered. What is the absolute risk reduction conferred by drug X?

A. 2%
B. 8%
C. 20%
D. 200%
E. None of the above

**I-5.** How many patients will have to be treated with drug X to prevent one death?

A. 2
B. 8
C. 12.5
D. 50
E. 93

**I-6.** Which of the following statements regarding coronary heart disease in females is true?

A. Death rates for coronary heart disease in females have been increasing over the last 30 years.
B. The most common initial symptom of coronary heart disease in females is angina.
C. Females are more likely to die of breast cancer than from coronary heart disease.
D. Females in all age groups have lower mortality from acute myocardial infarction than do males.
E. Females with myocardial infarction are more likely than males to present with ventricular tachycardia.

**I-7.** The leading cause of cancer death in females is

A. breast cancer
B. colon cancer
C. lung cancer
D. malignant melanoma
E. pancreatic cancer

**I-8.** What is the main contributor to the resting energy expenditure of an individual?

A. Adipose tissue
B. Exercise level
C. Lean body mass
D. Resting heart rate
E. None of the above

**I-9.** A 45-year-old male with a long history of alcohol abuse is admitted to the intensive care unit with severe pancreatitis, requiring intubation and mechanical ventilation. On the third day after admission, fever develops and imipenem-cilastatin is started for a possibly infected necrotic pancreas. The patient defervesces and is extubated. However, on the tenth day of hospitalization the patient becomes febrile again to 39.5°C (103.1°F), and fever persists for the next 4 days with no positive culture data, including samples of blood, urine, and sputum. On examination the patient is hemodynamically stable and has an erythematous rash over the trunk. He has no central venous catheter. Laboratories show a white blood cell count of 15,000 and a newly elevated creatinine of 3.2 mg/dL. Computed tomography (CT) of the abdomen and thorax shows no pseudocyst or other source of infection. Which of the following is the most appropriate next step in the management of this patient?

A. Obtain an [111]In-labeled white blood cell scan.
B. Discontinue imipenem-cilastatin.
C. Add amphotericin B.
D. Initiate hemodialysis.
E. Add vancomycin.

**I-10.** A 35-year-old pest service employee presents to the emergency department with complaints of nausea, vomiting, and abdominal pain. The examination is notable for normal vital signs, mild diffuse abdominal pain, a garlicky odor to his breath, and the following fingernail changes (see Fig. I-10, Color Atlas):
What is the underlying disorder?

A. Arsenic poisoning
B. Cadmium ingestion
C. Ethylenediaminetetraacetic acid (EDTA) exposure
D. Lead poisoning
E. Mercury poisoning

**I-11.** A 19-year-old female is brought to the emergency department after ingesting a large napkin filled with co-

**I-11.** *(Continued)*
caine to hide it from the police. The ingestion occurred 3 h ago, and she is now complaining of palpitations, chest pains, and anxiety. She has no other medical conditions and takes no medications. The patient drinks approximately two beers per day and occasionally uses intravenous cocaine. The examination is notable for a heart rate of 155, blood pressure of 180/95, temperature of 38.1°C (100.6°F), and respiratory rate of 24. The remainder of the examination is normal except for moderate agitation. An electrocardiogram (ECG) shows left ventricular hypertrophy but no acute ischemic changes. Which of the following would be the most appropriate initial management of the patient's cocaine ingestion?

A. Metoprolol
B. Verapamil
C. Intravenous nitroglycerine
D. Lorazepam
E. Heparin

**I-12.** An 82-year-old male with a long history of Parkinson's disease managed with carbidopa-levodopa is admitted to the medical service for evaluation of a temperature of 40°C (104°F), mental status changes, and worsening of baseline rigidity. His wife reports several episodes of vomiting for 3 days before admission. On admission, vital signs are normal except for the temperature. The remainder of his examination shows lead pipe rigidity in the extremities and moderate confusion. Blood work is obtained, and the chemistries are normal, with a white blood cell count of 8560 mm³ and a normal hematocrit and platelets. The most likely diagnosis is

A. bacterial meningitis
B. neuroleptic malignant syndrome
C. salmonellosis
D. tetanus
E. viral gastroenteritis

**I-13.** You are seeing a 19-year-old female in the university health clinic who returned 1 week ago from spring break, during which she went to the Caribbean with friends. She reports persistent redness over the face, shoulders, and arms without itching. Past medical history is notable for systemic lupus erythematosus and acne. Examination confirms the patient's report. There are no papules, and the rash spares the underarms and buttocks. Her current medications are ciprofloxacin, which was recently prescribed for a urinary tract infection, hydroxychloroquine, and minocycline. Which of the following is the likely cause of the skin eruption?

A. Ciprofloxacin
B. Hydroxychloroquine
C. Minocycline
D. A and B
E. A and C

**I-14.** A 28-year-old female presents to your clinic with complaints of episodic chest pain and palpitations for the last 2 months. The episodes can occur at rest or while she is walking. They are characterized by nonradiating chest discomfort, shortness of breath, dizziness, diaphoresis, and numbness in the hands bilaterally. The episodes last 5 to 15 min and are accompanied by feelings of dread. They typically occur once or twice a day. Past medical history is unremarkable. She is on no medications. She works as a paralegal. The patient is married but has been separated for 6 months. She has no children. She denies tobacco or illicit drug use and drinks two mixed drinks a day. The patient denies withdrawal symptoms and feelings of guilt or anger related to drinking. The examination is notable for stable vital signs, no jugular venous distention, normal heart sounds, and clear lungs. There is no edema. What is the most likely diagnosis?

A. Hyperthyroidism
B. Hypoglycemia
C. Panic disorder
D. Paroxysmal atrial tachycardia
E. Pheochromocytoma

**I-15.** A homeless male is evaluated in the emergency department. He has noted that after he slept outside during a particularly cold night his left foot has become clumsy and feels "dead." On examination, the foot has hemorrhagic vesicles distributed throughout the foot distal to the ankle. The foot is cool and has no sensation to pain or temperature. The right foot is hyperemic but does not have vesicles and has normal sensation. The remainder of the physical examination is normal. Which of the following statements regarding the management of this disorder is true?

A. Active foot rewarming should not be attempted.
B. During the period of rewarming, intense pain can be anticipated.
C. Heparin has been shown to improve outcomes in this disorder.
D. Immediate amputation is indicated.
E. Normal sensation is likely to return with rewarming.

**I-16.** A 30-year-old female who recently underwent renal transplantation is brought to the emergency department because of shortness of breath. She reports that the symptoms have begun slowly over the last 4 days since her discharge from the hospital. In addition, she has noted a progressive bilateral headache. The patient has been compliant with all her medications, which include prednisone, cyclosporine, mycophenolate mofetil, dapsone, acyclovir, and ranitidine. Past medical history includes focal segmental glomerular sclerosis and hypertension. Physical examination is notable for a normal temperature, a pulse of 123 beats/min, a respiratory rate of 26 breaths/min, and

**I-16.** *(Continued)*
normal blood pressure. Oxygen saturation is 83% on room air. Her mucous membranes have a brown discoloration. The cardiac examination, besides tachycardia, is normal. The lungs are clear bilaterally. Which of the following tests is likely to yield the diagnosis?

A. Arterial blood gas sample for $P_{O_2}$ and $P_{CO_2}$
B. Carboxyhemoglobin level
C. Helical contrast-enhanced computed tomogram of the chest
D. Lower extremity Doppler examination
E. Methemoglobin level

**I-17.** A 23-year-old female is brought to the emergency department after a witnessed suicide attempt involving the ingestion of approximately 30 sertraline tablets that were prescribed for depression. She has no other medical conditions. Which of the following statements is true?

A. Appropriate therapy for toxic ingestion of sertraline includes benzodiazepines.
B. Autonomic dysfunction is rare with overdosage with sertraline.
C. Complications of overdosage with sertraline include hypothermia, constipation, and liver failure.
D. She is likely to have decreased tone in her muscles with a depressed sensorium.
E. Similar signs and symptoms have been described with toxic ingestions of tramadol.

**I-18.** A 78-year-old female is seen in the clinic with complaints of urinary incontinence for several months. She finds that she is unable to hold her urine at random times throughout the day; this is not related to coughing or sneezing. The leakage is preceded by an intense need to empty the bladder. She has no pain associated with these episodes, though she finds them very distressing. The patient is otherwise independent in the activities of daily living, with continued ability to cook and clean for herself. Which of the following statements is true?

A. The abrupt onset of similar symptoms should prompt cystoscopy.
B. First-line therapy for this condition consists of desmopressin.
C. Indwelling catheters are rarely indicated for this disorder.
D. Referral to a genitourinary surgeon is indicated for surgical correction.
E. Urodynamic testing must be performed before the prescription of antispasmodic medications.

**I-19.** All but which of the following statements regarding medications in the geriatric population are true?

A. Falling albumin levels in the elderly lead to increased free (active) levels of some medications, including warfarin.

**I-19.** *(Continued)*

   B. Fat-soluble drugs have a shorter half-life in geriatric patients.

   C. Hepatic clearance decreases with age.

   D. The elderly have a decreased volume of distribution for many medications because of a decrease in total body water.

   E. Older patients are two to three times more likely to have an adverse drug reaction.

**I-20.** A 50-year-old male is seen in the clinic for atrial fibrillation. He was diagnosed with this condition several months ago. Past medical history includes hypertension and ischemic heart disease. Current medications include atenolol, aspirin, losartan, warfarin, and simvastatin. It is recommended that the patient begin therapy with amiodarone. Amiodarone can be expected to interfere with the metabolism of which of his current medications?

   A. Warfarin

   B. Warfarin and losartan

   C. Losartan and simvastatin

   D. Warfarin and simvastatin

   E. Warfarin, losartan, and simvastatin

**I-21.** You are a physician working in an urban emergency department when several patients are brought in after the release of an unknown gas at the performance of a symphony. You are evaluating a 52-year-old female who is not able to talk clearly because of excessive salivation and rhinorrhea, although she is able to tell you that she feels as if she lost her sight immediately upon exposure. At present, she also has nausea, vomiting, diarrhea, and muscle twitching. On physical examination the patient has a blood pressure of 156/92, a heart rate of 92, a respiratory rate of 30, and a temperature of 37.4°C (99.3°F). She has pinpoint pupils with profuse rhinorrhea and salivation. She also is coughing profusely, with production of copious amounts of clear secretions. A lung examination reveals wheezing on expiration in bilateral lung fields. The patient has a regular rate and rhythm with normal heart sounds. Bowel sounds are hyperactive, but the abdomen is not tender. She is having diffuse fasciculations. At the end of your examination, the patient abruptly develops tonic-clonic seizures. Which of the following agents is most likely to cause this patient's symptoms?

   A. Arsine

   B. Cyanogen chloride

   C. Nitrogen mustard

   D. Sarin

   E. VX

**I-22.** All the following should be used in the treatment of this patient *except*

   A. atropine

   B. decontamination

**I-22.** *(Continued)*

   C. diazepam

   D. phenytoin

   E. 2-pralidoxime chloride

**I-23.** A 24-year-old male is brought to the emergency department after taking cyanide in a suicide attempt. He is unconscious on presentation. What drug should be used as an antidote?

   A. Atropine

   B. Methylene blue

   C. 2-Pralidoxime

   D. Sodium nitrite alone

   E. Sodium nitrite with sodium thiosulfate

**I-24.** A 40-year-old female is exposed to mustard gas during a terrorist bombing of her office building. She presents to the emergency department immediately after exposure without complaint. The physical examination is normal. What is the next step?

   A. Admit the patient for observation because symptoms are delayed 2 h to 2 days after exposure and treat supportively as needed.

   B. Administer 2-pralidoxime as an antidote and observe for symptoms.

   C. Irrigate the patient's eyes and apply ocular glucocorticoids to prevent symptoms from developing.

   D. Discharge the patient to home as she is unlikely to develop symptoms later.

   E. Discharge the patient to home but ask that she return in 7 days for monitoring of the white blood cell count.

**I-25.** Which type of radiation exposure is most likely to cause penetrating tissue damage?

   A. Alpha radiation

   B. Beta radiation

   C. Gamma radiation

   D. X-rays

   E. C and D

**I-26.** In the event of a radioactive terrorist event, which of the following would result in the greatest amount of radiation exposure?

   A. Fallout of radioactive particles

   B. Internal contamination

   C. Localized exposure

   D. Whole-body exposure

**I-27.** A 42-year-old male presents to the emergency department after an accident at the nuclear power plant where he works. He reports that his total radiation exposure was approximately 6 gray (Gy) and occurred approximately 2 h ago. He underwent decontamination at the power plant that included removal of his clothing and

**I-27.** *(Continued)*

shoes and showering. The patient's right forearm has a burn that extends along the entire extensor surface. The wound was decontaminated and flushed. A radiation detector demonstrated no residual radiation. On arrival at the emergency department, the patient complains of nausea and has had two episodes of vomiting. On physical examination, the patient appears uncomfortable, with repeated emesis of bilious material. Vital signs are unremarkable. Head, eyes, ears, nose, and throat (HEENT), cardiac, pulmonary, and abdominal examinations are normal. There is a full-thickness burn on the right forearm as well as mild skin erythema on the right side of the face. Which of the following symptoms would be expected to follow in this patient?

- A. Bone marrow depression often lasting several weeks
- B. Cardiovascular collapse
- C. Gastrointestinal symptoms, including diarrhea and malabsorption
- D. Neurologic symptoms, including seizures
- E. A and C

**I-28.** Which of the following is not a key feature of biologic agents that can be used as bioweapons?

- A. Lack of effective therapy
- B. Lack of rapid diagnostic capability
- C. Lack of universally available vaccine
- D. Potential for person-to-person spread
- E. Potential to cause anxiety

**I-29.** The Centers for Disease Control and Prevention (CDC) has designated several biologic agents as category A in their ability to be used as bioweapons. Category A agents include agents that can be easily disseminated or transmitted, result in high mortality, can cause public panic, and require special action for public health preparedness. All the following agents are considered category A *except*

- A. *Bacillus anthracis*
- B. *Francisella tularensis*
- C. Ricin toxin from *Ricinus communis*
- D. Smallpox
- E. *Yersinia pestis*

**I-30.** A 58-year-old male presents to the emergency department complaining of fever, malaise, and chest pain. He is given the diagnosis of viral syndrome and sent home. Within 24 h, the patient is brought back to the emergency department by the emergency medical service; he is in a comatose state with sepsis syndrome. The patient rapidly succumbs to the illness. Chest radiography shows mediastinal widening and bilateral pleural effusions. The patient's illness began 4 days after he attended a national conference on global warming. Shortly afterward, 20 ad-

**I-30.** *(Continued)*

ditional people who stayed in the same hotel develop a similar illness, and 10 of those patients die. A biologic terrorist attempt is suspected. Which of the following would be the agent most likely to have caused this illness?

- A. *Bacillus anthracis*
- B. *Clostridium botulinum*
- C. *Escherichia coli* O157:H7
- D. *Francisella tularensis*
- E. *Yersinia pestis*

**I-31.** What would be the most appropriate therapy for the other patrons of the hotel who also have potential exposure without evidence of active disease?

- A. Adminstration of an attenuated vaccine and initiation of antibiotic therapy if the patient develops symptoms of active disease
- B. Amoxicillin 500 mg orally three times daily for 60 days
- C. Ciprofloxacin 500 mg orally twice daily for 30 days
- D. Doxycycline 100 mg orally twice daily for 60 days
- E. Doxycycline 100 mg intravenously twice daily plus rifampin 300 mg intravenously twice daily; switch to oral medications when clinically stable

**I-32.** Smallpox vaccination is no longer routinely given to the population of the United States because smallpox was eradicated as a sporadic disease more than 25 years ago. Smallpox has potential use as an agent of bioterrorism as a result of the highly infectious nature of the organism as well as the current vulnerability of the American population. Smallpox vaccination effectively protects against the dissemination of the disease even when given after the onset of an outbreak. For which of the following persons is smallpox vaccine recommended?

- A. A 48-year-old nurse who routinely works in a bone marrow transplant ward who has volunteered as a first responder in an outbreak
- B. A 24-year-old army recruit with history of severe eczema
- C. A 32-year-old physician in an emergency department who is designated as part of a smallpox-response team
- D. A 48-year-old male who previously received the vaccine in childhood who works in the public health department of a large metropolitan area
- E. A 28-year-old woman who is employed as a translator at a U.S. Embassy in the Middle East. She received a renal transplant 5 years ago and has a normal serum creatinine.

**I-33.** Several patients present to hospitals in a large metropolitan area with fever, myalgia, and disseminated intravascular coagulation. Ebola virus is isolated as part of

**I-33.** *(Continued)*

a bioterrorist strike. Treatment of the victims and prevention of dissemination include all the following *except*

A.  full barrier precautions
B.  negative-pressure isolation
C.  powered air-purifying respirators
D.  ribavirin
E.  support with blood products and vasopressors as needed

**I-34.** A 24-year-old female is diagnosed with anorexia nervosa. Which of the following criteria would identify the patient as being at risk for malnutrition?

A.  Body mass index less than 18.5
B.  Body weight less than 90% of ideal for height
C.  Unintentional weight loss of more than 10% of usual body weight in the preceding 3 months
D.  A and B
E.  All of the above

**I-35.** In the evaluation of malnutrition, which of the following proteins has the shortest half-life and thus is most predictive of recent nutritional status?

A.  Albumin
B.  Fibronectin
C.  Retinol-binding protein complex
D.  Prealbumin
E.  Transferrin

**I-36.** A 56-year-old female is hospitalized in the medical intensive care unit with pneumococcal sepsis. She is intubated and put on two vasopressors. On hospital day 3, the patient continues to have evidence of multisystem organ dysfunction. The patient has not yet started receiving nutritional support. All but which of the following statements regarding enteral nutritional support are true?

A.  The bowel obtains 70% of the required nutrition from food in the lumen of the intestine.
B.  Enteral feeding improves splanchnic blood flow.
C.  Enteral nutritional support is appropriate for use in cases of severe hemorrhagic pancreatitis and necrotizing enterocolitis.
D.  Enteral nutrition stimulates the secretion of gastrointestinal (GI) hormones, helping to maintain the integrity of the GI lining.
E.  Immunoglobulin A is released into the GI lumen when it is stimulated by enteral feeding.

**I-37.** Which of the following provides the largest percentage of calories in standard enteral and parenteral nutritional support in hospitalized patients?

A.  Carbohydrates
B.  Medium-chain triglycerides

**I-37.** *(Continued)*

C.  Polyunsaturated vegetable oils
D.  Protein

**I-38.** A 45-year-old alcoholic is brought to the emergency department after a fall. He is homeless and drinks 1 pint of liquor every day. He appears disheveled and malnourished. The initial physical examination is normal except for mild somnolence. Laboratory studies reveal a serum alcohol level of 175 mg/dL, and a head CT scan is normal. Intravenous fluids are begun. An hour later, repeat physical examination shows that his mental status is worse: The patient responds only with movement to noxious stimuli and has horizontal nystagmus, and there is no eye movement when he turns his head. Administration of which of the following is most likely to improve his symptoms?

A.  Niacin (vitamin $B_3$)
B.  Pyridoxine (vitamin $B_6$)
C.  Riboflavin (vitamin $B_2$)
D.  Thiamine (vitamin $B_1$)
E.  Vitamin C

**I-39.** One of your patients brings her father to see you for altered mental status. The patient is originally from China, and her parents are visiting from there. The patient's mother has noted over the last year that her husband's memory has deteriorated and that he has become more irritable. He now spends most of the day around the house and seems weak and fatigued. He has lost approximately 10 lb over the last 6 months as a result of anorexia and diarrhea. The parents live in a poor rural part of China and eat a predominantly corn-based diet. On physical examination, vital signs are normal. The tongue is bright red, and the skin examination reveals a pigmented scaling rash around the neck in sun-exposed areas. The neurologic examination is normal except for poor recall. Which of the following should be prescribed?

A.  Nicotinamide
B.  Pyridoxine
C.  Thiamine
D.  Vitamin A
E.  Vitamin C

**I-40.** A 74-year-old female is brought to your office by her son for evaluation of weight loss and alopecia. The female reports that she has been taking ultrahigh doses of nutritional supplements to prevent cancer for the last 9 months. She has noted that her skin has become dryer and that she frequently gets sores at the corners of the mouth. Over the last month the patient has begun to lose her hair and has diffuse bone pains. The physical examination is notable for red, scaly lips and a red, friable tongue. The patient's joints have no inflammation, effusion, or synovitis. The long bones are diffusely tender to touch. Her skin is dry,

**I-40.** *(Continued)*

but there are no rashes, petechiae, or echymoses. Which of the following is the most likely diagnosis?

A.  Copper toxicity
B.  Vitamin A toxicity
C.  Vitamin $B_1$ toxicity
D.  Vitamin C toxicity
E.  Zinc toxicity

**I-41.** A 54-year-old female complains of hair loss over the last 2 months. A close examination of her scalp reveals that hair follicles are present, but the hair shafts are missing. All the following drugs may be responsible for this finding *except*

A.  daunorubicin
B.  isotretinoin
C.  lithium
D.  propranolol
E.  warfarin

**I-42.** A 54-year-old homeless male is brought to the hospital by friends because of a rapidly worsening rash and blisters. Past medical history is notable for head trauma that left him with reduced mental function and a seizure disorder. He also has degenerative joint disease and hypercholesterolemia. Ten days ago the patient was seen in a medical clinic at the homeless shelter, where he was started on a variety of medications for health maintenance and a possible skin infection. Physical examination is notable for a temperature of 38.8°C (101.8°F) and diffuse erythema of the trunk, face, arms, and legs. There are fluid-filled bullae over many of the areas with erythema, and some of those areas have ecchymoses. The mucous membranes of the mouth are involved. All the following medications may cause this disorder *except*

A.  dilantin
B.  naprosyn
C.  phenobarbital
D.  simvastatin
E.  trimethoprim-sulfamethoxazole

**I-43.** A 33-year-old female is seen in the clinic for shortness of breath. She is 30 weeks pregnant and has noted 2 weeks of increasing peripheral edema, orthopnea, and paroxysmal nocturnal dyspnea. This is the patient's first pregnancy, and she has no other medical problems. Her only medication is a prenatal vitamin. She recently immigrated to the United States from Guatemala. On physical examination, the patient is afebrile, pulse is 112 beats/min, blood pressure is 125/80 mmHg, respiratory rate is 24, and oxygen saturation is 93% on room air. Jugular venous pressure is visible at the angle of the jaw, and there is +++ peripheral edema. Cardiac examination shows a normal point of maximal impulse, tachycardia with a reg-

**I-43.** *(Continued)*

ular rhythm, an opening snap, and a diastolic rumble. Which of the following statements regarding her condition is correct?

A.  Balloon valvulotomy is contraindicated.
B.  Management should include emergent delivery of the fetus.
C.  Medical management should include furosemide and beta blockers.
D.  Medical management should include furosemide and lisinopril.
E.  Pulmonary hypertension rarely develops in patients with this valvular lesion.

**I-44.** This patient develops hemodynamically stable atrial fibrillation. What is the best first step in management?

A.  Amiodarone
B.  Digoxin
C.  Flecainide
D.  Electrical cardioversion
E.  Ibutilide

**I-45.** A 30-year-old female with essential hypertension is evaluated in the clinic for preconception counseling. She is concerned about the effects of her hypertension on her desired pregnancy. Her current medications are lisinopril and amlodipine. Which of the following statements regarding pregnancy and hypertension is false?

A.  The patient's child would be at increased risk of intrauterine growth restriction.
B.  The child would be at increased risk of perinatal mortality.
C.  The patient is at no increased risk of placental abruption.
D.  The patient can no longer take lisinopril when she becomes pregnant.
E.  The patient will need to have her renal function measured regularly, and a creatinine of 1.5 mg/dL or higher is associated with a poorer prognosis.

**I-46.** A 43-year-old female is admitted to the hospital with 2 days of painful swelling of the left leg. Past medical history is notable for hypertension and hypercholesterolemia. Medications include atenolol, hydrochlorothiazide, aspirin, and simvastatin. Physical examination is notable for normal vital signs, clear lungs, an $S_4$, and a warm, erythematous tender left thigh. The neurologic examination is normal. A lower extremity Doppler study reveals a left deep venous thrombosis. She is begun on enoxaparin and coumadin. Three days later the patient develops macular lesions on the breast and buttock that over the course of hours develop the appearance seen in Figure I-46 (in Color Atlas). Which of the following was most likely the underlying reason for the development of the skin lesions?

**I-46.** *(Continued)*

A. Calciphylaxis
B. Cholesterol emboli
C. Occult breast cancer
D. Paroxysmal atrial fibrillation
E. Protein C deficiency

**I-47.** A 32-year-old male sees his physican because of "spots" on his tongue. He has a history of HIV infection and is receiving highly active antiretroviral therapy (HAART). The lesion shown in Fig. I-46 (in Color Atlas) has been present for about 5 days. It is not tender or painful. The remainder of the physical examination is unremarkable. Which of the following medications should be prescribed?

A. Acyclovir
B. Fluconazole
C. Ganciclovir
D. Prednisone
E. Trimethoprim-sulfamethoxazole

**I-48.** A 55-year-old male is seen in the clinic to discuss treatment options for alcohol dependence. He recently completed an inpatient detoxification program and is regularly attending Alcoholics Anonymous (AA) meetings but is interested in pharmacotherapy to maintain abstinence in addition to continuing the AA program. Which of the following statements is true?

A. A prolonged benzodiazepine taper should be prescribed.
B. Disulfuram will decrease the relapse rate in patients like this one.
C. If insomnia is a major complaint, sedative-hypnotic medications should be used.
D. Naltrexone may decrease the relapse rate.
E. No medical therapy has been shown to be superior to placebo in reducing the relapse rate in this population.

**I-49.** You are a physician in an urban health clinic in which approximately 20% of your patients use intravenous heroin regularly. You would like to incorporate drug rehabilitation into your practice. Which of the following options is the most effective therapy for use in the primary care setting?

A. Buprenorphine intramuscularly three times weekly
B. Buprenorphine orally or sublingually three to seven times weekly
C. Heroin maintenance
D. Methadone maintenance
E. Naltrexone orally daily

**I-50.** Monoamine oxidase inhibitors can be used safely with which of the following medications or foods?

**I-50.** *(Continued)*

A. Amitriptyline
B. Fluoxetine
C. Oxycodone
D. Sharp cheddar cheese
E. Red wine

**I-51.** A 33-year-old male has heroin dependence. He has been using intravenous heroin since age 17 and has never maintained sobriety for more than 6 months. He is hospitalized for mitral valve endocarditis with methicillin-sensitive *Staphylococcus aureus*. Approximately 8 h after admission, you are called to evaluate the patient for profuse sweating, nausea, vomiting, abdominal pain, and shortness of breath. On evaluation, the patient has a heart rate of 112, a blood pressure of 134/89, a respiratory rate of 22, and a temperature of 38.3°C (100.9°F). The patient has profuse sweating, soaking his sheets. He is continuously retching and is writhing in pain. Piloerection is noted. The cardiovascular examination reveals a regular tachycardia with a grade III/VI holosystolic murmur at the apex radiating to the axilla. The lungs are clear. No crackles are appreciated. The abdominal examination shows diffuse mild tenderness with hyperactive bowel sounds. No rebound, guarding, or masses are noted. What is the most likely diagnosis?

A. Acute mitral valve regurgitation
B. Arterial embolus to the superior mesenteric artery
C. Opiate withdrawal
D. Sepsis syndrome
E. Surreptitious use of heroin while hospitalized

**I-52.** A 32-year-old male presents to the emergency department complaining of a painful red eye. The redness began abruptly with pain that the patient first noticed upon awakening from bed. He wears contact lenses and occasionally sleeps in them. He has not had any fevers, chills, viral symptoms, joint pain, rashes, or bowel symptoms. An ophthalmologic examination reveals the following as shown in Fig. I-52. How should the patient be treated?

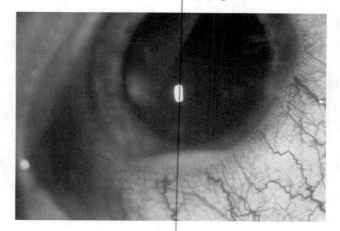

**I-52.** *(Continued)*

    A. Intraocular gentamicin

    B. Oral clindamycin

    C. Oral corticosteroids

    D. Topical ciprofloxacin

    E. Topical clotrimazole

**I-53.** A 27-year-old female presents to the emergency department for evaluation of a painful red left eye. The redness began late in the afternoon. She notes pain when looking at bright lights. The patient has had no viral symptoms or fevers but recently has noticed dyspnea with exertion and a dry cough. She was treated for a single episode of acute cystitis 10 weeks ago. Slit-lamp examination of the eye shows inflammation in the aqueous humor and inflammatory deposits on the corneal epithelium. Head and neck examination shows lymphadenopathy. There are a few dry crackles at the bases. Occasional wheezes are heard. There is no joint inflammation. Pulmonary function tests show a combined obstructive and restrictive defect. What is the diagnosis of this patient's eye disease?

    A. Conjunctivitis

    B. Episcleritis

    C. Keratitis

    D. Keratoconjunctivitis sicca

    E. Uveitis

**I-54.** What is the most likely underlying disorder?

    A. Ankylosing spondylitis

    B. Inflammatory bowel disease

    C. Reiter's syndrome

    D. Sarcoidosis

    E. Sjögren's syndrome

**I-55.** A 62-year-old female presents to her primary care doctor complaining of gradual visual loss. She feels as if she has to turn her head slightly to one side to get a full field of view. There is a past history of diabetes mellitus. She currently takes insulin glargine 16 units at night, with an insulin aspartate sliding scale. The last hemoglobin $A_{1C}$ was 7.4%. The most recent eye examination was 1 year ago. She wears bifocal lenses for presbyopia and myopia with astigmatism. Currently, intraocular pressure is 14 mmHg. The red reflex to light is normal. She has several discrete yellow lesions that are irregularly shaped, as shown in Fig. I-55 (Color Atlas). No vitreal hemorrhage or vascular proliferation is seen. There is a normal disc-to-cup ratio. What is the most likely diagnosis?

    A. Age-related macular degeneration

    B. Cataracts

    C. Diabetic retinopathy

    D. Glaucoma

    E. Orbital pseudotumor

**I-56.** A 46-year-old female presents to her primary care doctor complaining of a feeling of anxiety. She notes that she always had been what she describes as a "worrier," even in grade school. The patient has always avoided speaking in public and recently is becoming anxious to the extent where she is having difficulty functioning at work and in social situations. She has difficulty falling asleep at night and finds that she is always "fidgety" and has a compulsive urge to move. The patient owns a real estate company that has been in decline since a downturn in the local economy. She recently has been avoiding showing homes for sale. Instead, she defers to her partners because she finds that she is nervous to the point of being unable to speak to her clients. She has two children, ages 16 and 12, who are very active in sports. She feels overwhelmed with worry over the possibility of injury to her children and will not attend their sports events. You suspect that the patient has a generalized anxiety disorder. All but which of the following statements regarding this diagnosis are true?

    A. The age at onset of symptoms is usually before 20 years, although the diagnosis usually occurs much later in life.

    B. Over 80% of these patients will have concomitant mood disorders such as major depression, dysthymia, or social phobia.

    C. As in panic disorder, shortness of breath, tachycardia, and palpitations are common.

    D. Experimental work suggests that the pathophysiology of generalized anxiety disorder involves impaired binding of benzodiazepines at the $\gamma$-aminobutyric acid (GABA) receptor.

    E. The therapeutic approach to patients with generalized anxiety disorder should include both pharmacologic agents and psychotherapy, although complete relief of symptoms is rare.

**I-57.** A 30-year-old Hispanic female in the second trimester of pregnancy receives a 100-g oral glucose challenge. She has elevated values of serum glucose at each of the 1-, 2-, and 3-h time points. Which of the following statements concerning this clinical situation is correct?

    A. A trial of caloric restriction and minimal intake of concentrated sweets should be undertaken.

    B. The patient should be given subcutaneous insulin therapy.

    C. The patient should be treated with oral hypoglycemic agents.

    D. The patient should be treated with magnesium sulfate.

    E. The patient should receive insulin by continuous intravenous infusion.

**I-58.** Which of the following strategies will best minimize the risk of mother-to-child transmission of HIV?

**I-58.** *(Continued)*
  A.  Induction of delivery as early as possible in pregnancy consistent with maintaining good fetal maturity
  B.  Cesarean section
  C.  Use of zidovudine
  D.  Elective cesarean section at term plus zidovudine
  E.  Zidovudine plus protease inhibitor therapy

**I-59.**  A 75-year-old widower who lives alone is brought to his primary care physician by his daughter because she feels that he has been confused over the last few days. Before this he was quite independent and cognitively intact. The patient has a history of hypertension and is on hydrochlorothiazide. He is due for bilateral cataract extraction in 2 months. Of note, the patient reports a fall in his living room about 2 weeks ago, at which time he sustained a hip bruise and bumped his head.

  At this time the general physical examination is unremarkable; the neurologic examination is normal except for the mental status component, which discloses defects in short-term memory. Which of the following diagnostic studies is most likely to explain this patient's condition?

  A.  Neuropsychiatric battery
  B.  CT scan of head
  C.  Electroencephalogram
  D.  Serum chemistry panel
  E.  Urinary screen for toxic substances

**I-60.**  For which of the following herbal remedies is there the best evidence for efficacy in treating the symptoms of benign prostatic hypertrophy?

  A.  Saint John's wort
  B.  Gingko
  C.  Kava
  D.  Saw palmetto
  E.  No herbal therapy is effective

**I-61.**  A 25-year-old male who was recently admitted to a psychiatric hospital with a diagnosis of severe depression complicated by psychosis is brought to the emergency room because of worsening mental status and fever. The patient is unable to give a history because he is profoundly confused and claims to be on Mars. The psychiatrist informs you that the patient has been started recently on haloperidol and amitriptyline. Physical findings include a rectal temperature of 40.6°C (105°F), muscle rigidity, and dry skin. A cooling blanket is ordered, and you administer acetaminophen. Which of the following agents would it be most appropriate to order at this time?

**I-61.** *(Continued)*
  A.  Bromocriptine
  B.  Atropine
  C.  Levarterenol
  D.  Chlorpheniramine
  E.  Methylprednisolone

**I-62.**  Which of the following personality traits is most likely to describe a young female with anorexia nervosa?

  A.  Depressive
  B.  Borderline
  C.  Anxious
  D.  Perfectionist
  E.  Impulsive

**I-63.**  Which of the following therapies is most effective for a patient with anorexia nervosa who is 70% of ideal body weight?

  A.  Tricyclic antidepressant
  B.  Serotonin uptake antagonist antidepressant
  C.  Supervised oral refeeding in the hospital
  D.  Total parenteral nutrition
  E.  Oral refeeding with outpatient psychiatric treatment

**I-64.**  Why is it necessary to coadminister vitamin $B_6$ (pyridoxine) with isoniazid?

  A.  Vitamin $B_6$ requirements are higher in tuberculosis patients.
  B.  Isoniazid causes decarboxylation of $\gamma$-carboxyl groups in vitamin K–dependent enzymes.
  C.  Isoniazid interacts with pyridoxal phosphate.
  D.  Isoniazid causes malabsorption of vitamin $B_6$.
  E.  Isoniazid causes a conversion of homocysteine to cystathionine.

**I-65.**  Which of the following patients is least likely to benefit from nutritional support?

  A.  A 50-year-old female malnourished alcoholic about to undergo lumpectomy for lung cancer
  B.  A 23-year-old patient hospitalized for management of a severe burn injury
  C.  A 50-year-old male with malnourishment resulting from pancreatic cancer
  D.  A 38-year-old female undergoing allogeneic bone marrow transplantation
  E.  A 45-year-old male with advanced liver failure caused by autoimmune hepatitis who is awaiting liver transplantation

# I. INTRODUCTION TO CLINICAL MEDICINE: GENERAL CONCEPTS AND CARDINAL MANIFESTATIONS OF DISEASE

## ANSWERS

**I-1 and I-2.  The answers are C and C.**  *(Chap. 2)*  In evaluating the usefulness of a test, it is imperative to understand the clinical implications of the sensitivity and specificity of that test. By obtaining information about the prevalence of the disease in the population—the specificity and sensitivity—one can generate a two-by-two table, as shown below. This table is used to generate the total number of patients in each group of the population.

|  | Disease Status | |
|---|---|---|
| Test Result | Present | Absent |
| Positive | True-positive | False-positive |
| Negative | False-negative | True-negative |
|  | Total number of patients with disease | Total number of patients without disease |

The sensitivity of the test is $TP/(TP + FN)$. The specificity is $TN/(TN + FP)$. In this case the table is filled in as follows:

|  | Disease Status | |
|---|---|---|
| Test Result | Present | Absent |
| Positive | 42 | 237 |
| Negative | 8 | 713 |
|  | Total number of patients with disease = 50 | Total number of patients without disease = 950 |

**I-3.  The answer is A.**  *(Chap. 2)*  Bayes' theorem is used in an attempt to quantify uncertainty by employing an equation that combines pretest probability with the testing characteristics of specificity and sensitivity. The pretest probability quantitatively describes the clinician's certainty of a diagnosis after doing a history and physical examination. The equation is

$$\text{Posttest probability} = \frac{\text{Pretest probability} \times \text{test sensitivity}}{\begin{array}{c}\text{Pretest probability} \times \text{test sensitivity} + \\ (1 - \text{disease prevalence}) \times \text{test false-positive rate}\end{array}}$$

In this manner, the uncertainty one faces in clinical decision making is quantified. By inserting numbers into the equation, one can see that a low pretest probability combined with a poorly sensitive and specific test will yield a low posttest probability. However, the same test result, when combined with a high pretest probability, will yield a high posttest probability. There have been criticisms of this theorem. Unfortunately, few tests have only two outcomes: positive and negative. This theorem does not take into account the useful information that is gained from nonbinary test results. Further, it is cumbersome to calculate the posttest probability for each individual circumstance and patient. Perhaps the most useful lesson from Bayes' theorem is to take into account pretest probability when ordering tests or interpreting test results. To be clinically useful, a clinical scenario with a low pretest probability will require a test with high sensitivity and specificity. Conversely, a high pretest probability presentation can be confirmed by a test with only average sensitivity and specificity.

**I-4 and I-5.   The answers are B and C.**   *(Chap. 2)*   The goal of a meta-analysis is often to summarize the treatment benefit conferred by an intervention. Risk reduction is frequently expressed by relative risk or odds ratios; however, clinicians also find it useful to be familiar with the absolute risk reduction (ARR). This is the difference in mortality (or another endpoint) between the treatment and the placebo arms. In this case, the absolute risk reduction is 10% − 2% = 8%. From this number, one can calculate the number needed to treat (NNT), which is 1/ARR. The NNT is the number of patients who must receive the intervention to prevent one death (or another outcome assessed in the study). In this case the NNT is 1/8% = 12.5 patients.

**I-6.   The answer is B.**   *(Chap. 5)*   It is a common misconception that females are more likely to die of breast cancer than from any other cause. In fact, the most common cause of death in females is coronary heart disease, followed by lung cancer, breast cancer, and cerebrovascular disease. Unfortunately, these popular misconceptions often lead to a lack of attention on the part of both physicians and patients to discussions about common lifestyle and disease modifications to reduce the risk of mortality from coronary heart disease. Indeed, mortality from coronary heart disease has been increasing among females for the last 30 years, whereas mortality among males has been decreasing. According to the Framingham study, angina is the most common presentation of coronary heart disease in females; in males it is myocardial infarction. Interestingly, females with myocardial infarction are more likely to present with cardiac arrest and cardiogenic shock, whereas males are more likely to present with ventricular tachycardia. Once they are diagnosed, females are more likely to die of myocardial infarction than are males and are less likely to receive therapies such as angioplasty, thrombolysis, and coronary artery bypass grafting. Even when females do receive these therapies, they often have worse outcomes. These disparities in statistics between males and females have spurred many investigations into the differences in pathophysiology and treatment options in females versus males with coronary heart disease.

**I-7.   The answer is C.**   *(Chap. 5)*   Lung cancer is the leading cause of cancer death among females and males alike. Although females fear breast cancer the most, lung cancer remains the leading killer. Because of this misperception, concerns arise that insufficient time and discussion are given to tobacco use cessation among females and physicians. Females should be educated about the most common causes of death—coronary heart disease and lung cancer—to serve as a springboard for discussions of modifiable risk factors, especially diet, exercise, dyslipidemia, hypertension, and tobacco abuse, to name a few.

**I-8.   The answer is C.**   *(Chap. 60)*   To keep body weight stable, energy intake must match energy output. Energy output has two main determinants: resting energy expenditure and physical activity. Other, less clinically important determinants include energy expenditure to digest food and thermogenesis from shivering. Resting energy expenditure can be calculated and is $900 + 10w$ (where $w$ = weight) in males and $700 + 7w$ in females. This calculation is then modified for physical activity level. The main determinant of resting energy expenditure is lean body mass.

**I-9.   The answer is B.**   *(Chap. 18)*   Newly refined criteria for classifying fever of unknown origin (FUO) subdivide FUO into four subcategories: classic, nosocomial, neutropenic, and HIV-associated. This patient has nosocomial FUO, which is defined by a temperature >38.2°C (100.7°F) on several occasions in a hospitalized patient receiving acute care in whom infection was not evident at admission. Further, a specific etiology is not identified after 3 days of evaluation and at least 48 h of culture incubation. More than 50% of cases of nosocomial FUO have an infectious etiology; suspect sources include intravascular catheterization, urinary tract infections, *Clostridium difficile* colitis, and septic phlebitis. However, approximately 25% of these patients have a noninfectious etiology, examples of which include alcohol withdrawal, drug fever, pancreatitis, and adrenal insufficiency.

In this case, the patient has been hospitalized and on broad-spectrum antibiotics for over 1 week with new development of an erythematous truncal rash and acute renal failure. Standard cultures are unrevealing. The presence of a rash and the development of fever 1 week into antibiotic therapy suggest drug fever. The acute renal failure probably is secondary to allergic interstitial nephritis, and the white blood cell count may indicate significant eosinophilia. In light of the absence of positive culture data and the patient's clinical stability and lack of underlying immunodeficiency, it is not necessary at this time to add either amphotericin B or vancomycin. Hemodialysis is unlikely to address the patient's fevers. An $^{111}$In-labeled white blood cell scan would be indicated if no source of fever could be localized, but a drug fever is a fitting hypothesis. The most appropriate treatment would be to discontinue the most likely offending drug: imipenem-cilastatin. In the case of drug fever, the fevers should cease after 2 to 3 days.

**I-10.**   **The answer is A.**  *(Chap. 376)*  Arsenic exposure generally occurs in the setting of occupational exposure or the ingestion of deep well water. Primary sources of arsenic include wood preservatives, pesticides, fungicides, herbicides, smelting, and microelectronics. Poisoning from arsenic can be acute or chronic. Acute toxicity results in necrosis of intestinal mucosa with hemorrhagic gastroenteritis, nausea, vomiting, renal failure, cardiomyopathy, and hemolysis. Classically, these patients have a garlicky odor to their breath. Mee's lines, which are shown in the picture, are transverse white striae of the fingernails and have also been described in cases of arsenic toxicity. Chronic arsenic toxicity can cause many disorders, notably diabetes, peripheral vascular disease, and neuropathy. A diagnosis can be made by elevated arsenic levels in the hair or on a 24-h urine sample. Treatment for ingestion consists of ipecac syrup, charcoal, and supportive care. Chronic arsenic toxicity is treated with chelating agents. Cadmium poisoning generally presents with pulmonary symptoms from inhalation, anosmia, and yellow teeth. Lead poisoning classically presents in adults with anemia, peripheral neuropathy, and hypertension. Mercury poisoning has many manifestations, primarily in the central nervous system. EDTA is one of the chelating agents used to treat heavy metal toxicity.

**I-11.**   **The answer is D.**  *(Chap. 374)*  Cocaine is an illegal drug that exerts a euphoric effect by blocking reuptake of norepinephrine, serotonin, and dopamine at the neuronal synapse. Cocaine use can acutely cause hyperthermia, tachycardia, hypertension, and, most seriously, myocardial infarction, malignant arrhythmia, and stroke. Chronic use can result in a number of psychiatric symptoms, including hallucinations and paranoia. In this case, the patient presents with acute cocaine intoxication. Because the drug was absorbed via the gastrointestinal tract, the onset of symptoms was later than it would be for inhaled, smoked, or injected cocaine. Initial therapy should be aimed at decreasing anxiety, which frequently results in decreased blood pressure and heart rate. Therefore, lorazepam is the correct therapy. Additional therapy should include oral charcoal to prevent further absorption of the drug from the gastrointestinal tract. Beta blockers are relatively contraindicated in this situation because of concern for unopposed alpha constriction stimulated by the cocaine. Verapamil, nitroglycerine, and heparin may be appropriate choices when there is evidence of myocardial ischemia or infarction.

**I-12.**   **The answer is B.**  *(Chap. 16)*  This patient has not been able to absorb his dopaminergic agonists for several days because of his gastrointestinal illness. The sudden withdrawal of these agents puts him at risk for neuroleptic malignant syndrome. This syndrome classically presents with muscular rigidity, extrapyramidal side effects, autonomic dysregulation, and hyperthermia. In this disorder, heat production is increased and dissipation is decreased, driven by inhibition of central dopamine receptors in the hypothalamus. Although meningitis, salmonellosis, and viral gastroenteritis are all possible sources of fever and altered mental status, none are associated with rigidity. Tetanus generally causes increased muscle tone, but more commonly that occurs in the axial muscles.

**I-13.** **The answer is E.** *(Chap. 51)* This patient presents with classic photosensitivity with erythema in sun-exposed areas. Although the patient is at risk for photoaggravation with classic malar rash from her systemic lupus erythematosis, the current eruption is in a larger distribution of sun-exposed skin, including the arms and shoulders, and suggests photosensitivity. Her most likely risk factor for photosensitivity is medications. Medications commonly associated with this disorder are flouroquinolones, furosemide, phenothiazines, sulfonamides, retinoids, tetracyclines, and amiodarone. A more extensive list can be found in the table. Hydroxychloroquine has not been associated with light eruptions.

| | Topical | Systemic |
|---|---|---|
| Amiodarone | | + |
| Dacarbazine | | + |
| Fluoroquinolones | | + |
| 5-Fluorouracil | + | + |
| Furosemide | | + |
| Nalidixic acid | | + |
| Phenothiazines | | + |
| Psoralens | + | + |
| Retinoids | +/− | + |
| Sulfonamides | | + |
| Sulfonylureas | | + |
| Tetracyclines | | + |
| Thiazides | | + |
| Vinblastine | | + |

**I-14.** **The answer is C.** *(Chap. 371)* Panic disorder is defined by the presence of recurrent and unpredictable panic attacks. Panic attacks are episodes of intense fear and discomfort associated with a variety of symptoms. These patients may complain of chest pain, shortness of breath, palpitations, sweating, trembling, dizziness, paresthesias, gastrointestinal distress, and feelings of doom. The attacks continue for at least a month and may cause a change in behavior in response to them. Panic disorder occurs in up to 3% of individuals over the course of a lifetime. The symptoms arise suddenly and may last from a few minutes to an hour. With progressive concern about recurrent attacks, these patients may fear going to places where they may feel trapped; this is known as agoraphobia. The differential diagnosis includes a variety of medical conditions. Cardiac causes include arrhythmias. Other considerations include thyrotoxicosis, hypoglycemia, pheochromocytoma, and mitral valve prolapse. This patient's age and normal physical examination make panic disorder the overwhelmingly most likely diagnosis. Treatment is centered on antidepressant therapy, including tricyclic antidepressants and selective serotonin reuptake inhibitors. Benzodiazepines may be useful in the initial course of treatment, but patients must be monitored closely for dependence.

**I-15.** **The answer is B.** *(Chap. 19)* This patient presents with frostbite of the left foot. The most common presenting symptom of this disorder is sensory changes that affect pain and temperature. Physical examination can have a multitude of findings, depending on the degree of tissue damage. Mild frostbite will show erythema and anesthesia. With more extensive damage, bullae and vesicles will develop. Hemorrhagic vesicles are due to injury to the microvasculature. The prognosis is most favorable when the presenting area is warm and has a normal color. Treatment is with rapid rewarming, which usually is accomplished with a 37 to 40°C (98.6 to 104°F) water bath. The period of rewarming can be intensely painful for the patient, and often narcotic analgesia is warranted. If the pain is intolerable, the temperature of the water bath can be dropped slightly. Compartment syndrome can develop with rewarming and should be investigated if cyanosis persists after rewarming. No medications have been shown to improve outcomes, including heparin, steroids, calcium channel blockers, and hyperbaric oxygen. In the absence of wet gangrene or another emergent surgical indication, decisions about the need for amputation or debridement should be deferred until the boundaries of the tissue injury are well demarcated. After recovery from the initial insult, these patients often have neuronal injury with abnormal sympathetic tone in the extremity. Other remote complications include cutaneous carcinomas, nail deformities, and, in children, epiphyseal damage.

**I-16.** **The answer is E.** *(Chaps. 31 and 91)* This patient has a classic presentation for methemoglobinemia with dyspnea, headache, gray-brown discoloration of the skin, and abnormal oxygen saturation. Her risk factor for the induction of this disorder is dapsone, but other causes include aniline derivatives, local anesthetics, nitrates, nitrosohydrocarbons, sulfonamides, and primaquine-type antimalarials, among others. Methemoglobin occurs when oxidation of hemoglobin iron from ferrous ($Fe^{2+}$) to ferric ($Fe^{3+}$) inhibits oxygen binding, transport, and tissue uptake as the oxyhemoglobin dissocation curve is shifted to the left. In addition, oxidized hemoglobin will precipitate and cause hemolytic anemia. Heinz bodies and bite cells can be seen on the peripheral smear. The diagnosis is confirmed by detection of elevated methemoglobin levels in the blood. At levels above 15 to 20%, the gray-brown cyanosis can be seen along with headache, and often lactic acidosis is found at levels >45%. Of note, the $P_{o_2}$ is normal in arterial blood gas analysis because it reflects only dissolved oxygen in blood, not the percentage of hemoglobin bound to oxygen or methemoglobin. Oxygen saturation by pulse oximetry can be either normal or decreased in patients with this disorder. Treatment is with high-dose oxygen in all cases. Intravenous methylene blue is used in patients with methemoglobin levels >30%, symptomatic cases, and patients with evidence of ischemia. In refractory cases, exchange transfusion and hyperbaric oxygen can be used.

**I-17.** **The answer is E.** *(Chap. 377)* Ingestion of a number of different compounds, including selective serotonin reuptake inhibitors, amphetamines, cocaine, dextromethorphan, meperidine, tricyclic antidepressants, tramodol, and monoamine oxidase (MAO) inhibitors, can result in the serotonin syndrome. This syndrome results from several possible mechanisms, depending on the compound ingested; it can result from promotion of release of serotonin, inhibition of serotonin reuptake, or direct stimulation of serotonin receptors in either the central or the peripheral nervous system. Often multiple mechanisms are present simultaneously. These patients generally present with altered mental status ranging from agitation to coma, neuromuscular hyperactivity with hyperreflexia, myoclonus, rigidity and tremors, and autonomic dysfunction with diarrhea, diaphoresis, fever, mydriasis, salivation, tachycardia, and labile hypertension. Complications of the syndrome include lactic acidosis, hyperthermia, and multisystem organ failure. Treatment, aside from gastrointestinal decontamination when appropriate, includes serotonin receptor antagonists, cyproheptadine, or chlorpromazine.

**I-18.** **The answer is C.** *(Chap. 8)* Urinary incontinence occurring randomly without associated Valsalva or other stress is most likely detrussor overactivity. This disorder is the most common type of incontinence in the elderly, both males and females. In females there is no need to do further testing in a patient with long-standing incontinence; however, in males urethral obstruction is often coexistent, and urodynamic testing is indicated to investigate this possibility. An abrupt onset of symptoms or associated suprapubic pain in either sex should prompt cystoscopy and urine cytologic testing to evaluate for bladder stones, tumor, or infection. First-line therapy is behavioral therapy with or without biofeedback. Frequent timed voiding is often successful. If drugs are imperative, oxybutynin or tolterodine can be tried with close follow-up to ensure that urinary retention does not occur. Desmopressin must be used with extreme caution in this population. Indeed, patients with heart failure, chronic kidney disease, or hyponatremia should not take this medication. Indwelling catheters are rarely indicated for this disorder; instead, external collection devices or protective pads or undergarments are favored.

**I-19.** **The answer is B.** *(Chaps. 3 and 8)* Adverse drug reactions in the geriatric population are common, occurring two to three times more frequently than they do in younger patients. This change is due to several factors. Drug clearance is altered because of decreased renal plasma flow and glomerular filtration as well as decreased hepatic clearance. Furthermore, the volume of distribution of many drugs is decreased with a drop in total body water. However, in older persons there is a relative increase in fat, which will lengthen the half-life of fat-soluble medications. Serum albumin levels decline in general in the elderly, particularly in the hospitalized and sick population. As a result, drugs that are primarily protein-bound, such as warfarin and phenytoin, will have higher free or active levels at similar doses. Care must be taken in interpreting total serum levels for these drugs because a low total level may be accompanied by a normal free level and thus be appropriately therapeutic.

**I-20.** **The answer is E.** *(Chap. 3)* Medication interactions and errors are increasingly being recognized as a serious source of morbidity and even mortality not only in hospital inpatients but also in the outpatient population. A handful of drugs account for the majority of the adverse events, including nonsteroidal anti-inflammatory drugs (NSAIDs), analgesics, digoxin, anticoagulants, diuretics, antimicrobials, glucocorticoids, antineoplastics, and hypoglycemics. When prescribing new medications to patients, physicians must review the preexisting drug list and evaluate any potential interactions. A common offender for changes in drug metabolism is amiodarone. This medication inhibits CYP3A and CYP2C9. CYP3A is important in the degradation of calcium channel blockers, antiarrhythmics, HMG-CoA reductase inhibitors, cyclosporine, tacrolimus, indinavir, saquinavir, and ritonavir. In this patient amiodarone would inhibit the metabolism of simvastatin by this mechanism. CYP2C9 degrades warfarin, phenytoin, glipizide, and losartan. Subsequently, losartan and warfarin levels would be altered (see Table 3-1 in Harrison's, page 17, for further information regarding molecular pathways affecting drug metabolism). Additional information regarding drug-drug interactions and adverse drug reactions can be obtained from a number of websites, including *http://www.hc-sc.ca/hpb-dgps/therapeut/htmleng/cadrnwsletter.html*.

**I-21 and I-22.** **The answers are D and D.** *(Chap. 206)* This patient has symptoms of an acute cholinergic crisis as seen in cases of organophosphate poisoning. Organophosphates are the "classic" nerve agents, and several different compounds may act in this manner, including sarin, tabun, soman, and cyclosarin. Except for agent VX, all the organophosphates are liquid at standard room temperature and pressure and are highly volatile, with the onset of symptoms occurring within minutes to hours after exposure. VX is an oily liquid with a low vapor pressure; therefore, it does not acutely cause symptoms. However, it is an environmental hazard because it can persist in the environment for a longer period. Organophosphates act by inhibiting tissue synaptic acetylcholinesterase. Symptoms differ between vapor exposure and liquid exposure because the organophosphate acts in the tissue upon contact. The first organ exposed with vapor exposure is the eyes, causing rapid and persistent pupillary constriction. After the sarin gas attacks in the Tokyo subway in 1994 and 1995, survivors frequently complained that their "world went black" as the first symptom of exposure. This is rapidly followed by rhinorrhea, excessive salivation, and lacrimation. In the airways, organophosphates cause bronchorrhea and bronchospasm. It is in the alveoli that organophosphates gain the greatest extent of entry into the blood. As organophosphates circulate, other symptoms appear, including nausea, vomiting, diarrhea, and muscle fasciculations. Death occurs with central nervous system penetration causing central apnea and status epilepticus. The effects on the heart rate and blood pressure are unpredictable.

Treatment requires a multifocal approach. Initially, decontamination of clothing and wounds is important for both the patient and the caregiver. Clothing should be removed before contact with the health care provider. In Tokyo, 10% of emergency personnel developed miosis related to contact with patients' clothing. Three classes of medication are important in treating organophosphate poisoning: anticholinergics, oximes, and anticonvulsant agents. Initially, atropine at doses of 2 to 6 mg should be given intravenously or intramuscularly to reverse the effects of organophosphates at muscarinic receptors; it has no effect on nicotinic receptors. Thus, atropine rapidly treats life-threatening respiratory depression but does not affect neuromuscular or sympathetic effects. This should be followed by the administration of an oxime, which is a nucleophile compound that reactivates the cholinesterase whose active site has been bound to a nerve agent. Depending on the nerve agent used, oxime may not be helpful because it is unable to bind to "aged" complexes that have undergone degradation of a side chain of the nerve agent, making it negatively charged. Soman undergoes aging within 2 min, thus rendering oxime therapy useless. The currently approved oxime in the United States is 2-pralidoxime. Finally, the only anticonvulsant class of drugs that is effective in seizures caused by organophosphate poisoning is benzodiazepines. The dose required is frequently higher than that used for epileptic seizures, requiring the equivalent of 40 mg of diazepam given in frequent doses. All other classes of anticonvulsant medications, including phenytoin, barbiturates, carbamazepine, and valproic acid, will not improve seizures related to organophosphate poisoning.

**I-23.**    **The answer is E.**   *(Chap. 206)*    Cyanide is an asphyxiant that causes death by inhibiting cellular respiration. It is a colorless liquid or gas that has a typical smell of almonds. The onset of symptoms after cyanide exposure is rapid and usually begins with eye irritation. The skin is flushed. The patient rapidly develops confusion, tachypnea, and tachycardia. With severe poisoning, death results from acute respiratory distress syndrome (ARDS) and hypoxemia with lactic acidosis. The antidote for cyanide poisoning is a combination of sodium nitrite and sodium thiosulfate.

**I-24.**    **The answer is A.**   *(Chap. 206)*    Sulfur mustard was the first weaponized chemical and was first used in World War I, accounting for 70% of the estimated 1.3 million chemical casualties in that war. It remains a significant terrorist threat today because of simplicity of manufacture and effectiveness. Sulfur mustard constitutes both a vapor and a liquid chemical threat. It acts as a DNA-alkylating agent and affects rapidly dividing cells. The effects of sulfur mustard are delayed 2 h to 2 days, depending on the severity of exposure. The organs most commonly affected are the skin, eyes, and airways. Late bone marrow suppression also occurs 7 to 21 days after exposure. Erythema resembling a sunburn is the mildest form of injury. This progresses to large flaccid bullae containing sterile serous fluid. Large portions of body-surface area may be affected, similar to the situation in burn victims. The primary airway lesion is necrosis of the mucosa. Clinically, this causes pseudomembrane formation and, in the most severe cases, airway obstruction. Laryngospasm may also occur. The effects on the eyes include conjunctivitis, blepharospasm, pain, and corneal damage. Death results from airway obstruction, pneumonia, secondary skin infections, or sepsis with neutropenia. There is no antidote to mustard gas or liquid exposure. Treatment is supportive, ensuring adequate analgesia and hydration. Application of topical glucocorticoids before denudation of skin may be useful. Small blisters should be left intact, but large bullae should be unroofed. The fluid is sterile and does not contain mustard derivatives. Silver sulfadiazine or other topical antibiotics should be used to prevent secondary skin infections. Conjunctival irritation should be treated with topical solutions, including antibiotics. Petroleum jelly should be applied to the eyelids to prevent them from sticking together. Intubation may be necessary for protection against airway obstruction. Repeated bronchoscopy may also be needed to remove pseudomembranes. Finally, careful follow-up for the development of marrow suppression is needed.

**I-25.**    **The answer is E.**   *(Chap. 207)*    Radiation is the emission of particles or energy to matter from unstable isotopes with uneven numbers of protons and/or neutrons. There are several types of radiation, but the ability to cause tissue damage is related to the ability of the particles to penetrate tissue. Alpha radiation consists of heavy positively charged particles that contain two protons and two neutrons. Alpha particles are emitted from large molecules, usually those with an atomic number higher than 82. Thus, these particles are quite large and do not penetrate tissue if skin is intact. Beta radiation consists of electrons that are small and light. These particles have limited energy and can travel only a small distance in tissue. Clothing and plastic barriers can prevent tissue penetration. With large exposures, a thermal burn may result. Most tissue damage in radiation exposure is related to exposure to gamma radiation or x-rays. Both gamma radiation and x-rays are photons and can travel easily through matter. These types of radiation have no mass and consist primarily of energy. Neutrons may also be present in radiation exposure and possess a wide range of energy. Their ability to penetrate tissue is thus variable, depending on the energy they possess.

**I-26.    The answer is A.**    *(Chap. 207)*    External contamination is a result of the fallout of radioactive particles that land on the body surface and clothing. This is the dominant element after a radiation terrorist strike. The common contaminants emit primarily alpha and beta radiation. The alpha particles do not penetrate, but the beta particles can cause extensive burns. Gamma particles are the most dangerous because they cause local tissue injury and also penetrate, causing whole-body radiation exposures. The medical treatment of external exposure consists primarily of decontamination and treatment of wounds. Generally, health care providers are not at risk from exposure to contaminated clothing and patients. Health care should not be delayed for fear of secondary contamination.

Whole-body exposure is the most damaging type of exposure and results from exposure to x-rays, gamma radiation, and neutrons. However, tissue damage occurs only in those with a high degree of exposure and thus would be limited to those in the immediate area of a blast. Internal contamination can also cause extensive tissue injury and results from inhalation, translocation, or ingestion of radioactive material. The respiratory system is the primary portal of injury, and bronchial lavage is sometimes employed for decontamination. Localized exposures occur when a part of the body is in close contact with a source of radiation. This usually results in localized burns that resemble thermal burns, but those burns do not pose a significant threat to tissues.

**I-27.    The answer is E.**    *(Chap. 207)*    Acute radiation sickness manifests in various ways, depending on the dose and duration of exposure. The major organ systems affected are the hematopoietic, gastrointestinal, neurologic, and cardiovascular. After exposure, these patients progress through four stages that are quite variable in onset, again depending on dose and duration of exposure. The prodrome appears within a few hours to 4 days after exposure. The primary symptoms during this stage are nausea, vomiting, and diarrhea. This progresses to the latent phase, with minimal or no symptoms, which can last from 2 to 6 weeks. After the latent phase, the patient will experience various symptoms of illness with either recovery or death to follow. At doses less than 1 Gy, acute radiation sickness is generally mild. The main clinical manifestation at this dose is bone marrow suppression that lasts 2 to 3 weeks. Doses up to 4 Gy results in more persistent bone marrow suppression from which it takes longer to recover. Gastrointestinal symptoms develop with radiation exposure of 6 to 8 Gy. This manifests as loss of absorptive membranes with malnutrition, diarrhea, and occasionally hemorrhage and sepsis. Doses >9 Gy are almost always fatal, with hypotension, seizures, and death.

**I-28.    The answer is A.**    *(Chap. 205)*    The Working Group for Civilian Biodefense created a list of several features of biologic agents that make them effective bioweapons. Chief among these features is the ease of spread of an agent with high morbidity and mortality. However, many of the agents that are used, including *Bacillus anthracis,* have effective antibiotic therapy when the disease is diagnosed early in its course. Another characteristic of an effective bioweapon is lack of rapid diagnostic capability, particularly early in the course of disease, when a patient with limited or no symptoms may be able to spread the disease. Other features include lack of a readily available vaccine, ease of weaponization, potential for person-to-person spread, potential to cause anxiety, low infectious dose, environmental stability, and availability of the pathogen with a database of prior research on the feasibility of production.

**I-29.    The answer is C.**    *(Chap. 205)*    Using the characteristics listed in the question, the CDC developed classifications of biologic agents that are based on their potential to be used as bioweapons. Six types of agents have been designated as category A: *Bacillus anthracis,* botulinum toxin, *Yersinia pestis,* smallpox, tularemia, and the many viruses that cause viral hemorrhagic fever. Those viruses include Lassa virus, Rift Valley fever virus, Ebola virus, and yellow fever virus.

**I-30 and I-31.    The answers are A and D.**    *(Chap. 205)*    As evidenced by the September–October 2001 anthrax attacks in the United States, anthrax is capable of causing death when manufactured in weapons-grade spores and also can cause widespread panic and disruption of social activities, including disruption of the legislative branch of the government and the postal system. Anthrax is caused by the bacteria *Bacillus anthracis,* a gram-positive spore-forming anaerobic rod. The long-lived spores are found naturally in the soil and infrequently cause disease in humans in their natural state. When they occur naturally, the most common manifestation of disease is cutaneous anthrax, which causes a black necrotic eschar at the site of introduction. Without antibiotics, cutaneous anthrax has a 20% mortality rate. When used as a bioweapon, anthrax can be manufactured in smaller spores and can cause inhalational anthrax, which is most likely to cause death in the setting of a bioterrorist attack. Inhalation of small spores allows the bacteria to become deposited in the alveolar spaces, where they are phagocytosed by macrophages. The organisms then travel by the lymphatics to the peribronchial and mediastinal lymph nodes, where they proliferate. The initial symptoms are those of a viral illness, with fever, malaise, and chest or abdominal pain. If they are not recognized early, these symptoms will progress to sepsis and cardiovascular collapse within 24 to 48 h. Chest radiography may be helpful in early diagnosis because of frequent findings of mediastinal widening, pulmonary infiltrates, and bilateral pleural effusions that are hemorrhagic on thoracentesis. In the 2001 attack, fatality was 55% at 7 days, and rapid diagnosis and treatment were key in the patients who survived.

Multiple antibiotics are successful in treating anthrax when the disease is recognized early. Traditionally, penicillins have been the mainstay of therapy, but there is the potential for creating a penicillin-resistant bioweapon. Therefore, until sensitivities are known, the recommended treatment for anthrax is ciprofloxacin or doxycycline plus rifampin or clindamycin. In cases of likely exposure, extended courses of antibiotics are needed because of the long half-life of the anthrax spores. Among the options listed, only doxycycline 100 mg twice daily orally for 60 days is a regimen for postexposure treatment. The efficacy of the anthrax vaccine has not been established in postexposure prophylaxis.

**I-32.   The answer is C.**   *(Chap. 205)*   Smallpox is a preventable disease after immunization, which can confer immunity even when given after the onset of an outbreak. Large-scale vaccination has not been undertaken because of the known side effects of vaccination and the increased population of immunocompromised patients. Currently, the recommendations for smallpox vaccination include virtually all patients in the armed services and civilian health care workers who might compromise smallpox-response teams. Contraindications to the vaccination are underlying skin disease, including eczema; an immunocompromised state; and close contact with someone who is immunocompromised. Vaccination is voluntary for persons who are part of first-response teams after a smallpox outbreak.

**I-33.   The answer is D.**   *(Chap. 205)*   Viral hemorrhagic fevers have no approved or effective antiviral therapies. If a patient is suspected of having viral hemorrhagic fever, care should be primarily supportive with blood products and the usual critical care modalities. Prevention of further dissemination of disease is of paramount importance. Full barrier precautions with use of an N95 or powered air-purifying respirator should be used. Unprotected skin contact with cadavers has been implicated in disease spread in Ebola outbreaks. In addition, negative-pressure rooms should be used. There are anecdotal reports of the use of hyperimmune globulin, interferon $\alpha$, and ribavirin. The only data to support the use of these agents are for the use of ribavirin in the treatment of the arenaviruses that cause Lassa fever and New World fever.

**I-34.   The answer is E.**   *(Chap. 62)*   Both inpatients and outpatients can be considered to be at risk for malnutrition if they meet one or more of the criteria listed in the question. The criteria for diagnosing a patient at risk for malnutrition are (1) unintentional weight loss of >10% of usual body weight in the preceding 3 months, (2) body weight <90% of ideal for height, and (3) body mass index <18.5. When body weight is <85% of ideal for height, a patient is considered malnourished. If a patient is <70% of ideal for height, that patient is described as severely malnourished, and <60% of ideal for height is incompatible with survival.

**I-35. The answer is B.** *(Chap. 62)*    Albumin has a half-life of 2 to 3 weeks and is a sensitive but nonspecific measure of protein-calorie malnutrition. Other situations in which albumin is low include sepsis, surgery, overhydration, and increased plasma volume, including congestive heart failure, renal failure, and chronic liver disease. Among the other markers of nutritional state, transferrin has a half-life of 1 week. Prealbumin and retinol-binding protein complex have the same half-life of 2 days. Fibronectin has the shortest half-life: 1 day.

**I-36. The answer is C.** *(Chap. 63)*    Enteral nutrition is the preferred route of nutrition except in cases of severe gastrointestinal illness, including severe hemorrhagic pancreatitis, necrotizing enterocolitis, prolonged ileus, and bowel obstruction. The benefits of enteral nutrition are numerous. The bowel and the associated digestive organs receive 70% of their nutrition directly from food in the lumen. Also, continued stimulation of the gut through enteral nutrition promotes the immunologic function of the gut by improving splanchnic blood flow, stimulating the secretion of IgA, and stimulating the ongoing production of growth hormones needed to maintain the integrity of the GI lumen.

**I-37. The answer is A.** *(Chap. 63)*    Sixty to 70% of caloric intake in both parenteral and enteral nutritional support is supplied by carbohydrate formulas. In parenteral nutrition, glucose is the carbohydrate source; in enteral nutrition, disaccharides and oligosaccharides provide the same carbohydrates. However, oxidation of exogenous glucose plateaus at 25 kcal/kg daily, and higher glucose loads will produce hepatic steatosis. Thus, caloric intake is supplemented with lipid solutions. Polyunsaturated vegetable oils provide most of the lipids in enteral solutions because they are better digested than are animal fats. In patients who have ongoing impairment of digestion with these formulas, medium-chain triglycerides are used because they are simpler to digest. Protein is provided at allowances of 0.8 to 1.5 g/kg body weight daily, depending on the patient's predicted requirements. Patients who are in highly catabolic states, for example, those with burns or sepsis, have higher protein requirements.

**I-38. The answer is D.** *(Chap. 61)*    Thiamine functions in energy generation by participating in the decarboxylation of α-ketoacids and branched-chain amino acids. It also acts as a coenzyme in the reaction that mediates the conversion of hexose and pentose phosphates. The primary food sources of thiamine include yeast, pork, beef, legumes, whole grains, and nuts. Tea and coffee contain thiaminases that can destroy the vitamin. In Western countries, most cases of thiamine deficiency are caused by poor dietary intake. Most patients with thiamine deficiency have cancer or alcoholism. Chronic thiamine deficiency causes dry or wet beriberi. Alcoholic patients with chronic thiamine deficiency may develop acute Wernicke's encephalopathy when administered a carbohydrate load (in this case, intravenous fluids containing glucose). Wernicke's encephalopathy is manifest by horizontal nystagmus, ophthalmoplegia (caused by extraocular muscle weakness), cerebellar ataxia, and mental impairment. Wernicke-Korsakoff syndrome consists of Wernicke's encephalopathy plus loss of memory and confabulatory psychosis. Thiamine should be administered prophylactically to all patients with a history of alcoholism before the administration of glucose-containing fluids. Riboflavin deficiency manifests mostly with mucous membrane and skin findings. Niacin deficiency causes pellagra. Pyridoxine deficiency causes glossitis and neurologic changes. Vitamin C deficiency causes scurvy.

**I-39. The answer is A.** *(Chap. 61)*    This patient presents with pellagra caused by niacin deficiency. The four D's classically describe the pellagra syndrome: dermatitis, diarrhea, dementia, and death. Niacin deficiency is rare in North America because of the presence of niacin in beans, milk, meat, eggs, and fortified flour. Tryptophan may also be converted to niacin. Cases usually occur in parts of China, India, and Africa where people eat predominantly corn-based diets that are low in niacin and tryptophan. Niacin consists of nicotinamide and nicotinic acid, precursors of the coenzymes nicotinamide adeninine dinucleotide (NAD) and NAD phosphate (NADP), which participate in a variety of metabolic reactions. High doses of nicotinic acid may be used for therapy for hypercholesterolemia and hypertriglyceridemia. Supplemental niacin may cause flushing when taken for these indications.

I-40. **The answer is B.** *(Chap. 61)* Vitamin A toxicity can occur acutely or chronically. Vitamin A is retinol; however, the oxidative metabolites retinoic acid and retinaldehyde are also biologically active. Retinoids are synthetic compounds similar to retinol. Carotenoids (most commonly β-carotene) exist in nature and may be converted to vitamin A. Vitamin A participates in vision, morphogenesis, growth, cell division, iron utilization, humoral and cellular immunity, and phagocytosis. Acute vitamin A toxicity was first described in Arctic explorers who consumed polar bear liver, which contains high levels of vitamin A. Acute toxicity presents with neurologic findings, including increased intracranial pressure, seizures, vertigo, diplopia, exfoliative dermatitis, and death. Chronic vitamin A toxicity in adults may occur with the ingestion of >15 mg/d for several months. The signs and symptoms are as described in this patient as well as lymphadenopathy, pseudotumor cerebri, hepatic fibrosis, and bone demineralization. In pregnant females, vitamin A excess may cause congenital malformations and spontaneous abortion. No adverse effects of thiamine have been recorded in chronic use. Anaphylaxis has been described with high doses. Chronic ingestion of vitamin C theoretically could promote nephrolithiasis, but that has not been found in several trials. Vitamin C may provoke hemolysis in patients with glucose-6-phosphate dehydrogenase deficiency. There is also an unproven risk of iron overload in patients who ingest high doses of vitamin C. Zinc toxicity acutely causes nausea, vomiting, and fever. Chronic excessive zinc ingestion may depress immune function and cause hypochromic anemia as a result of copper deficiency. Copper toxicity is usually accidental and acute, leading to fulminant hepatic toxicity. Chronically, it may manifest with the hepatic and neurologic complications of Wilson's disease.

I-41. **The answer is A.** *(Chap. 48)* Alopecia occurs as a scarring or a nonscarring process. In nonscarring alopecia, the hair follicles are not damaged but the hair shafts are missing. In scarring alopecia, the damage to the follicle results in a smooth scalp with a decreased number of follicular openings. Microscopically, there is fibrosis and inflammation. Only nonscarring alopecia is reversible. It is usually caused by telogen effluvium, androgenetic alopecia, alopecia areata, tinea capitis, and traumatic alopecia (see Table 48-5 in Harrison's, page 299). Many drugs may cause nonscarring alopecia, included those listed in the question plus heparin, propylthiouracil, vitamin A, colchicines, and amphetamines. Hair loss caused by these drugs is reversible with discontinuation of the drugs. Scarring alopecia is usually caused by primary skin disorders such as lichen planus, cutaneous lupus, and linear scleroderma. Antimitotic agents such as daunorubicin may also cause scarring alopecia.

I-42. **The answer is D.** *(Chap. 48)* Toxic epidermal necrolysis (TEN) is characterized by sloughing bullae that develop after widespread mucocutaneous erythema. TEN and Stevens-Johnson syndrome (SJS) are similar clinically and probably represent a continuum of disease, with SJS involving 10 to 15% of the epidermis and TEN involving >25%. These patients often have a flulike syndrome before the development of the erythema. Most cases of TEN are caused by drugs started 1 to 3 weeks before the presentation. The most common among these drugs are phenytoin, barbiturates, sulfonamides, penicillins, and nonsteroidal anti-inflammatory drugs. TEN may be distinguished from staphylococcal scalded skin syndrome histologically or by the absence of oral lesions. Simvastatin is not associated with TEN but may cause rhabdomyolysis.

I-43 and I-44. **The answers are C and B.** *(Chaps. 209, 214, and 219)* This patient probably has long-standing mitral stenosis that has become clinically significant with the increase in cardiac output and blood volume needed in pregnancy. Mitral stenosis is the valvular disease that is most likely to cause death during pregnancy. Patients with mitral stenosis may develop pulmonary hypertension during pregnancy. In addition, because preload is an important factor in left ventricular filling in these patients, hypovolemia has been associated with sudden death. Medical management of mitral stenosis and associated heart failure during pregnancy necessitates diuretics for symptom management and beta blockers to decrease heart rate and improve left ventricular filling. Balloon valvulotomy is an option for medically refractory cases. Atrial fibrillation may ensue, with increased left ventricular filling pressures. First-line therapy includes digoxin and beta blockers. Ibutilide is class C in pregnancy, and amiodarone is class D and should be reserved for arrhythmias refractory to other measures. Flecanide, which is suitable for the treatment of ventricular tachycardia, is not indicated for the management of atrial fibrillation. Electrical cardioversion is generally well tolerated during pregnancy and may be an appropriate management option if medications fail.

**I-45.  The answer is C.**  *(Chap. 6)*  Pregnancy is relatively commonly complicated by medical conditions; perhaps the most frequently seen is hypertension. Pregnancy complicated by hypertension is associated with intrauterine growth restriction, increased perinatal mortality, and an increased risk of preeclampsia and placental abruption. It is important to note that certain blood pressure medications are contraindicated by pregnancy, notably, the angiotensin-converting enzme (ACE) inhibitors and angiotensin receptor blockers, which increase the risk of oligohydramnios and have adverse effects on fetal renal function. Most practitioners use α-methyldopa and labetalol during pregnancy. Baseline renal function should be measured so that abnormal function noted later in pregnancy will be appropriately interpreted. Pregnancies in females with a creatinine less than 1.5 mg/dL are associated with a favorable prognosis.

**I-46.  The answer is E.**  *(Chap. 50)*  Warfarin-induced skin necrosis occurs 3 to 10 days after the initiation of warfarin or its derivatives. The lesions begin as erythematous macules and progress to indurated, pupuric, hemorrhagic bullous, or necrotic lesions. The lesions typically appear on fatty tissues such as the breast, buttocks, thighs, and trunk. These reactions are not related to the underlying disease. The necrosis is related to the early rapid reduction in protein C concentration and the resultant hypercoagulability early in warfarin therapy. Warfarin-induced skin necrosis is associated with heterozygous protein C deficiency. These patients should receive vitamin K to reverse the effects of warfarin and should be maintained on heparin-based anticoagulation. Calciphylaxis causes necrotic skin lesions in similar areas; however, it is unlikely in the absence of renal failure, hyperparathyroidism, or altered calcium and phosphate metabolism. Cholesterol emboli typically present in distal extremities with livedo reticularis in the distal lower extremities. Paroxysmal atrial fibrillation is a risk factor for stroke and other systemic thromboembolic events, but skin necrosis is unusual. Occult breast cancer may predispose to a hypercoagulable state and venous thromboemboli (Trousseau syndrome); however, skin necrosis is unusual.

**I-47.  The answer is A.**  *(Chap. 28)*  The lesion shown is hairy leukoplakia. These lesions usually arise on the lateral tongue and rarely involve other sites of the oral mucosa. They appear as white areas ranging from small and flat to extensive accentuation of the vertical folds. The lesions are due to Epstein-Barr virus infection and respond to high-dose acyclovir, but they may recur. Patients with HIV infection or risk factors are at increased risk. Painful lesions should raise the suspicion of candidal secondary infection. Other white lesions (Table 28-3, Harrison's, page 199) in the mouth include smoker's leukoplakia, erythroplakia (squamous cell carcinoma), candidal infection, and warts.

**I-48.  The answer is D.**  *(Chap. 372)*  Physicians often see patients with alcohol abuse or alcohol dependence in the clinic, and by some estimates approximately 20% of patients in affluent communities fall into one of these categories. After identifying such patients, physicians should make referrals for detoxification, counseling, and rehabilitation programs. Physicians often are involved in the selection of appropriate medications for the acute detoxification and for long-term abstinence when appropriate. The initial detoxification is generally accomplished by using a taper of benzodiazepines and occasionally beta blockers and carbamazepine as appropriate. The long-term maintenance of abstinence remains a challenge for many patients and the physicians who care for them. Referrals to a support group or counseling are essential. These patients often have difficulty with anxiety and insomnia, which should be treated with behavior modification, including reassurance that this is a common phenomenon after acute withdrawal is complete and will resolve spontaneously in a few weeks. Caffeine and naps should be avoided, and a strict bedtime and awakening schedule should be followed. Sedatives and hypnotics should be avoided during this period in the majority of cases. Several medications have been studied to lower the relapse rate. Disulfuram, an aldehyde dehydrogenase (ALDH) inhibitor, produces an unpleasant reaction to alcohol as a result of rapidly rising levels of acetaldehyde. This drug has many side effects and should be used with caution in patients with heart disease, hypertension, stroke, and diabetes mellitus. Furthermore, it has not been consistently shown to be superior to placebo in clinical trials. The opioid antagonist naltrexone has been used in this population, and several small studies have suggested a decreased probability of relapse and shortened periods of relapse. Larger trials have questioned this finding, and definitive data are lacking. Acamprosate has been tested in Europe and has been found to have efficacy similar to that of naltrexone. Benzodiazepine tapers should be reserved for the management of acute alcohol withdrawal.

**I-49. The answer is B.** *(Chap. 373; Fudala et al, Buprenorphine/Neloxone Collaborative Study Group, N Engl J Med 349:949–958, 2003.)* Oral or sublingual buprenorphine maintenance therapy has recently been proposed as a new office-based therapy for opiate dependence. Buprenorphine is a drug with mixed properties, acting as an agonist at the $\mu$ receptor and an antagonist at the $\kappa$ receptor. It is usually administered at a dose of 8 to 32 mg daily for 3 to 7 days a week. The advantages of buprenorphine over other maintenance options include a low potential for overdose, easier detoxification, and a ceiling threshold that limits its ability to cause a feeling of euphoria. In a recent placebo-controlled trial, buprenorphine with or without naloxone was shown to lead to a significant decrease in the proportion of urine samples positive for opiates and a decrease in opiate cravings. In contrast to methadone, buprenorphine is the first drug approved for the office-based treatment of opiate addiction. Primary care physicians in the community can prescribe buprenorphine if they are designated as addiction specialists by completing training programs through the American Society for Addiction Medicine, the American Psychiatric Association, and the American Osteopathic Association, among others (*www.fda.gov*).

Methadone has long been the standard for drug treatment for heroin addiction. However, methadone can be given only within the structure of a drug treatment program and is not available for primary care physicians in the office. Methadone is a long-acting opioid that blocks the euphoria of heroin and decreases craving. In Great Britain, heroin maintenance has been used in a similar fashion, although heroin has a higher street value and a greater potential for misuse. Naltrexone is an opioid antagonist that is used in conjunction with psychological support because it too blocks the euphoria from heroin. However, patients must be free from narcotics for 5 days before the initiation of therapy because it will precipitate acute narcotic withdrawal.

**I-50. The answer is A.** *(Chap. 371)* Monoamine oxidase inhibitors (MAOIs) were among the earliest antidepressants used. However, they have fallen out of favor because of their serious and common side effects. MAOIs may potentiate hypertensive crises in patients with sympathetic overload such as pheochromocytoma. In addition, MAOIs cannot be used with sympathomimetic drugs, including cocaine, amphetamines, dopamine, and epinephrine. In addition, drugs such as L-dopa, phenylalanine, and methyldopa are structurally similar to many sympathomimetic drugs and can stimulate a hypertensive crisis. Foods that contain tyramine are also dangerous in combination with MAOIs. Some of these foods are aged cheeses, beer, wine, liver, dry sausage, fava beans, and yogurt. Narcotics and other central nervous system (CNS) depressants may precipitate seizures, delirium, hyperpyrexia, and coma or death. Finally, serotonin syndrome may be life-threatening and occurs in association with selective serotonin reuptake inhibitors.

**I-51.   The answer is C.**   *(Chap. 373)*   Opioids are highly addictive, with a high prevalence of misuse. In 2002, a national survey revealed that 10% of twelfth-graders had tried opioids without a doctor's prescription and 2% had tried heroin. Opioid dependence is defined by repeated use of narcotic medications to the extent that it interferes with normal psychosocial functioning and causes tolerance and withdrawal. Patients who have opioid dependence become both physically and psychologically addicted to the drugs. Heroin has a shorter half-life compared with other narcotics, and symptoms of withdrawal appear within 8 to 16 h of the last dose. The symptoms are in general opposite to those of opiate intoxication and include nausea, diarrhea, sweating, piloerection, mydriasis, and muscle fasciculations. In addition, mild elevations in heart rate, temperature, respiratory rate, and blood pressure may be seen. Symptoms peak within 36 to 72 h and persist for up to 5 days. Mood disturbance and changes in pain threshold and sleep pattern may persist for up to 6 months.

**I-52.   The answer is D.**   *(Chap. 25)*   The photo shows a hypopyon, which is diagnostic of keratitis. A hypopyon is a collection of pus that is seen layering in the bottom portion of the anterior chamber of the eye. Keratitis can cause blindness if it is not treated properly and promptly. Worldwide, the most common causes of keratitis are vitamin A deficiency and trachoma, a chlamydial infection. In the United States, contact lens wear is associated with an increased risk of keratitis. A superficial infection is called keratoconjunctivitis and must be distinguished from keratitis, which is accompanied by greater visual loss, increased pain, photophobia, and discharge. Slit-lamp examination is helpful in the diagnosis, showing disruption of corneal epithelium, a cloudy infiltrate, and an inflammatory cellular reaction in the anterior chamber. At its most serious, hypopyon will appear. Empirical antibiotics should be started while one awaits the results of cultures from corneal scrapings. Fortified topical antibiotics are the treatment of choice. Fluoroquinolones have a broad spectrum of activity and are considered first-line therapy. They may be combined with aminoglycosides. Occasionally, they have to be supplemented with subconjunctival antibiotics. Fungal infection should be considered if there is failure to improve.

**I-53 and I-54.   The answers are E and D.**   *(Chap. 25)*   This patient has evidence of anterior uveitis that is associated with sarcoidosis. Anterior uveitis is usually marked by the abrupt onset of pain and photophobia. Specifically anterior uveitis causes iritis and iridocyclitis. Constriction of the pupil causes increased pain. Slit-lamp examination is diagnostic, showing inflammatory cells in the aqueous humor or deposited along the corneal endothelium. These deposits on the corneal endothelium are called keratic precipitates. Many diseases are associated with anterior uveitis, including sarcoidosis and the seronegative spondyloarthropathies, including ankylosing spondylitis, psoriasis, inflammatory bowel disease, and Behçet's disease. Infectious disease may also cause uveitis. Some of the associated infections include herpesviruses, tuberculosis, onchocerciasis, and leprosy. In the majority of cases, uveitis is idiopathic. Treatment should include topical corticosteroids to decrease inflammation and mydriatics because dilation of the pupil decreases pain and the formation of synechiae.

**I-55.   The answer is A.**   *(Chap. 25)*   Age-related macular degeneraton is a common cause of blindness in older individuals. Visual loss is gradual and affects central vision. The most common form of macular degeneration is dry, or nonexudative. The hallmark of macular degeneration is the finding of drusen around the maculae. Drusen is the accumulation of pleomorphic extracellular deposits underneath the retinal pigment epithelium. These yellow deposits are initially small and are seen clustered around the maculae. Over time, they coalesce into large deposits. The retinal pigment epithelium becomes focally detached and atrophic, interfering with photoreceptor function. Treatment with multivitamin therapy may retard visual loss. In the exudative form of macular degeneration, neovascularization is prominent and starts at the choroid plexus. This neovascularization leaks into the potential space beneath the retinal pigment epithelium, causing blurring of vision.

**I-56.   The answer is C.**   *(Chap. 371)*   Generalized anxiety disorder is common, with a lifetime prevalence of approximately 5% and with the onset of symptoms often occurring before age 20. These patients frequently report having feelings of anxiety and social phobia that date back to childhood. Clinically, these patients report persistent, excessive, and unrealistic worries that prevent normal functioning. In addition, there is often the complaint of feeling "on edge" with nervousness, arousal, and insomnia. However, unlike panic disorder, palpitations, tachycardia, and shortness of breath are rare. Pathophysiologically, there is likely to be impaired function of the GABA receptor with decreased binding of benzodiazepines at that receptor. Therapy should include a combination of drugs and psychotherapy. Drugs that may be used include benzodiazepines, buspirone, and anticonvulsants with GABAergic properties, such as gabapentin, tiagabine, and divalproex.

**I-57.   The answer is A.**   *(Chap. 6)*   Unless a person is a member of a low-risk group, screening for gestational diabetes should be carried out in all pregnant females. Patients at low risk for gestational diabetes include those <25 years of age, with a body mass index <25 kg/m$^2$, no maternal history of macrosomia or gestational diabetes, no diabetes in a first-degree relative, and not members of a high-risk ethnic group (African American, Hispanic, or native American). If a patient has an elevated 1-h glucose level after taking 50 g of oral glucose, a 100-g challenge should follow. If elevated values of serum glucose are noted at the 1-, 2-, or 3-h time point, measures to control the gestational diabetes should be undertaken. Those with gestational diabetes are at an increased risk of preeclampsia, delivery of infants who are large for gestational age, and birth lacerations. Dietary measures are usually sufficient to control most patients with mild gestational diabetes. However, those who cannot maintain fasting serum glucose concentrations <5.8 mmol/L (<105 mg/dL) or 2-h postprandial glucose concentrations <6.7 mmol/L (<120 mg/dL) should be treated with insulin. Oral hypoglycemic agents are contraindicated in the treatment of gestational diabetes. Importantly, females in whom the diagnosis of gestational diabetes is made should be followed in the postpartum period for the development of type 2 diabetes, which is common in such patients.

**I-58.   The answer is D.**   *(Chap. 6; International Perinatal HIV Group, N Engl J Med 325: 1371, 1999.)*   Recent studies have shown that zidovudine treatment of both the mother during the prenatal and intrapartum periods and the neonate at birth can reduce the risk of vertical transmission to 7.3%. When such therapy is combined with elective cesarean section, the risk of vertical transmission drops to 2%. The benefit of multiple drug therapy has not been established. Risk factors for the transmission of HIV infection in the perinatal period include vaginal delivery, preterm delivery, trauma to the fetal skin, and maternal bleeding.

**I-59.   The answer is B.**   *(Chap. 8)*   Falls are a common problem in the elderly, occurring in about 30% of community-dwelling older individuals annually. The cause of a fall is usually multifactorial and may include (1) reduced visual acuity, (2) reduced hearing, (3) proprioceptive dysfunction, (4) dementia, (5) foot and other musculoskeletal disorders, (6) postural hypotension, and (7) use of medicines such as sedatives, antidepressants, and anticonvulsants. The most common complication of falls in the elderly is fracture, with hip fractures being particularly ominous; dehydration, electrolyte imbalance, pressure sores, hypothermia, and rhabdomyolysis may also occur. One insidious late complication is subdural hematoma, which may present with a new neurologic sign, such as confusion, even in the absence of headache and focal findings. A CT or magnetic resonance image of the brain is the best way to make the diagnosis of subdural hematoma, which may require surgery for optimal management.

**I-60.** **The answer is D.** *(Chap. 10; Wilt et al, JAMA 280:1604–1609, 1998.)* Because plant products are in widespread use in the well-accepted therapeutic armamentarium of Western medicine (e.g., digoxin, taxol, penicillin), it should not be surprising that several "herbal remedies" have been demonstrated in prospective clinical trials to be beneficial. For example, Saint John's wort is more effective than placebo for mild to moderate depression; the mechanism is not known, although the metabolism of several neurotransmitters is inhibited by this substance. Kava products have antianxiolytic activity. Extracts of the fruit of the saw palmetto, *Serona repens*, have been shown to decrease nocturia and improve peak urinary flow compared with placebo in males with benign prostatic hypertrophy. Saw palmetto extracts affect the metabolism of androgens, including the inhibition of dihydro-testosterone binding to androgen receptors.

**I-61.** **The answer is A.** *(Chaps. 16 and 371; Caroff, Med Clin North Am 77:185–202, 1993.)* This patient is suffering from the neuroleptic malignant syndrome, which is characterized by muscle rigidity, autonomic dysregulation, and hyperthermia. The patient probably has been exposed to phenothiazines for the first time, considering his relatively recent admission to the psychiatric facility. This syndrome represents an idiosyncratic reaction to inhibition of central dopamine receptors that results in increased heat production and failure of heat dissipation. In addition to rapid physical cooling and the administration of an antipyretic or acetaminophen (but not aspirin), the use of the dopamine agonist bromocriptine or dantrolene should be strongly considered. Dantrolene reverses the hypothalamic dysfunction caused by major tranquilizers.

**I-62.** **The answer is D.** *(Chap. 65)* The most important feature of patients with anorexia nervosa is refusal to maintain even a low-normal body weight. The full syndrome of anorexia nervosa occurs in about 1 in 200 individuals. These patients are always markedly underweight, hardly ever menstruate, and often engage in binge eating. The mortality rate is 5% per decade. The etiology of this serious eating disorder is unknown but probably involves a combination of psychological, biologic, and cultural risk factors. This illness often begins in an obsessive or perfectionist patient who starts a diet. As weight loss progresses, the patient has increasing fears of gaining weight and engages in stricter dieting practices. This disorder essentially occurs only in cultures in which thinness is valued, suggesting a strong cultural influence. Bulimia nervosa, in which patients continue to maintain a normal body weight but typically engage in overeating with binges followed by compensatory purging or purging behavior, has a higher than expected prevalence in patients with childhood or parental obesity. It is unclear whether anorexia nervosa is hereditary in nature.

**I-63.** **The answer is C.** *(Chap. 65)* Treating patients with severe anorexia nervosa (<75% of expected body weight) requires careful medical and psychiatric care. Patients with such severe weight deficits should be hospitalized, at which time a program of nutritional restoration with oral feeding with food or liquid supplements can be undertaken. However, much support and education are required to reassure the patient that the weight gain will not be permitted to get "out of control." Psychiatric treatment focuses on emotional support and improving self-esteem. Complications of refeeding can be as severe as congestive heart failure; abnormal liver function tests and low levels of magnesium and phosphate have been reported. Tricyclic antidepressants are contraindicated because of the possibility of prolongation of the QT interval in the setting of abnormal electrolyte levels. No psychotropic medicine has been shown to be beneficial in patients with this disorder.

**I-64.** **The answer is C.** *(Chap. 61)* Certain medications, including isoniazid used for tuberculosis, L-dopa used for Parkinson's disease, and penicillamine used for scleroderma, promote vitamin $B_6$ (pyridoxine) deficiency by reacting with a carbonyl group on 5-pyridoxal phosphate, which is a cofactor for a host of enzymes involved in amino acid metabolism. Foods that contain vitamin $B_6$ include legumes, nuts, wheat bran, and meat. Vitamin $B_6$ deficiency produces seborrheic dermatitis, glossitis, stomatitis, and cheliosis (also seen in other vitamin B deficiencies). A microcytic, hypochromic anemia may result from the fact that the first enzyme in heme synthesis (aminolevulonic synthetase) requires pyridoxal phosphate as a cofactor. However, vitamin $B_6$ is also necessary for the conversion of homocysteine to cystathionine. Consequently, a deficiency of this vitamin could produce an increased risk of cardiovascular disease caused by the resultant hyperhomocystinemia.

**I-65.** **The answer is C.** *(Chap. 63; Heyland et al, JAMA 280:2013–2019, 1998.)* Nutritional support is risky, depending on the route used, and expensive. Although nutritional support has been proposed in many situations, it has been proved beneficial in prospective, randomized clinical trials in a subset. Compared with other preoperative patients, only presurgical patients who have severe protein-calorie malnutrition benefit from parenteral nutrition. Critically ill patients, patients undergoing bone marrow transplantation, and those with liver failure, pancreatitis, and severe inflammatory bowel disease have all been shown to benefit from nutritional support. Patients with cancer cachexia probably get no net benefit except for those about to undergo cancer surgery who have severe protein-calorie malnutrition.

# II. GENETICS

## QUESTIONS

**DIRECTIONS:** Each question below contains four or five suggested responses. Choose the **one best** response to each question.

**II-1.** All the following disorders can cause ambiguous sexual differentiation *except*

A. 21-hydroxylase deficiency
B. androgen insensitivity syndrome
C. Klinefelter syndrome
D. mixed gonadal dysgenesis
E. testicular dysgenesis

**II-2.** An 18-year-old female is evaluated in an outpatient clinic for a complaint of amenorrhea. She reports that she feels as if she never developed normally compared with other girls her age. She has never had a menstrual period and complains that she has had only minimal breast growth. Past medical history is significant for a diagnosis of borderline hypertension. In childhood the patient frequently had otitis media and varicella infections. She received the standard vaccinations. She recently graduated from high school and has no learning difficulties. She is on no medications. On physical examination, the patient is of short stature with a height of 56 in. Blood pressure is 142/88. The posterior hairline is low. The nipples appear widely spaced, with only breast buds present. The patient has minimal escutcheon consistent with Tanner stage 2 development. Her external genitalia appear normal. Bimanual vaginal examination reveals an anteverted, anteflexed uterus. The ovaries are not palpable. What is the most likely diagnosis?

A. Hypothyroidism
B. Hyperthyroidism
C. Malnutrition
D. Testicular feminization
E. Turner syndrome (gonadal dysgenesis)

**II-3.** A 30-year-old male is seen for a physical examination when obtaining life insurance. The last time he saw a physician was 15 years ago. He has no complaints. Past medical history is notable for scoliosis that was surgically corrected when the patient was a teenager and a recent shoulder dislocation. He takes no medications and does not smoke, drink, or use illicit drugs. Family history is

**II-3.** *(Continued)*
notable for a father and a brother with colon cancer at ages 45 and 50 years, respectively. Physical examination is notable for normal vital signs, a tall habitus with hypermobile joints, normal skin, and ectopia lentis. Rectal examination is normal, and stool is guaiac-negative. The remainder of the examination is normal. Appropriate recommendations for follow-up should include which of the following annual studies?

A. Colonoscopy
B. Echocardiography
C. Fecal occult blood testing
D. Serum periodic acid–Schiff (PSA) measurement
E. Serum thyroid-stimulating hormone (TSH)

**II-4.** During meiosis, a single germ cell will divide and eventually result in

A. two gametes in a haploid state
B. two gametes in a diploid state
C. four gametes in a haploid state
D. four gametes in a diploid state

**II-5.** Proximal (5′) *cis*-acting regulatory regions that control gene expression are called

A. enhancers
B. exons
C. promoters
D. splice sites
E. transcription factors

**II-6.** All the following diseases are caused by errors in DNA repair *except*

A. ataxia-telangiectasia (AT)
B. Fanconi's anemia (FA)
C. fragile X (FX) syndrome
D. hereditary nonpolyposis colorectal cancer (HNPCC)
E. xeroderma pigmentosum (XP)

**II-7.** A 45-year-old male is evaluated for weakness and a progressive change in mental status. After extensive eval-

**II-7.** *(Continued)*

uation, he is diagnosed with a mitochondrial disorder. All but which of the following statements about mitochondrial disorders are true?

A. The mitochondrial genome does not recombine.
B. Inheritance is maternal.
C. The proportion of wild-type and mutant mitochondria in different tissues is identical.
D. Cardiomyopathy is a feature of many mitochondrial disorders.
E. Acquired somatic mitochondrial mutations may play a role in age-related degenerative disorders.

**II-8.** Prader-Willi syndrome (PWS) is a rare disorder that is characterized by diminished fetal activity, obesity, mental retardation, and short stature. A deletion on the paternal copy of chromosome 15 is the cause. A deletion on the same site on chromosome 15, but on the maternal copy, results in a different syndrome: Angelman's syndrome. This syndrome is characterized by mental retardation, seizures, ataxia, and hypotonia. What is the name of the genetic mechanism that results in this phenomenon?

A. Genetic anticipation
B. Genetic imprinting
C. Lyonization
D. Somatic mosaicism
E. Uniparental disomy

**II-9.** All the following are inherited disorders of connective tissue *except*

A. Alport syndrome (AS)
B. Ehlers-Danlos syndrome (EDS)
C. Marfan syndrome (MFS)
D. McArdle's disease
E. osteogenesis imperfecta (OI)

**II-10.** A 30-year-old male comes to your office for genetic counseling. His brother died at age 13 years with Tay-Sachs disease. His sister is unaffected. The patient and his wife wish to have children. Which of the following statements concerning Tay-Sachs disease is true?

A. It is seen most commonly in Scandinavian populations.
B. It is caused by mutations in the galactosidase gene.
C. Most patients die in the third or fourth decade of life.
D. Death occurs as a result of progressive neurologic decline.
E. Splenomegaly is common in these patients.

**II-11.** All but which of the following statements about Gaucher disease are true?

**II-11.** *(Continued)*

A. Bone pain is common.
B. Disease frequency is highest in Ashkenazi Jews.
C. Inheritance is autosomal recessive.
D. Splenomegaly is rare.
E. The disease is caused by mutations in the gene for acid $\beta$-glucosidase.

**II-12.** All but which of the following statements about chromosomal abnormalities are true?

A. Monosomic conditions are typically undetected in adulthood.
B. Trisomy 21 is the most common chromosome abnormality in live-born individuals.
C. Maternal age is the most important etiologic factor in congenital chromosomal disorders.
D. Up to 25% of all pregnancies involve chromosomally abnormal conceptions.
E. One-third of trisomy 21 cases occur as a result of errors in meiosis II.

**II-13.** A 4-year-old boy is evaluated for mental retardation, choreoathetosis, spasticity, and self-mutilative behavior. He is also noted to have marked hyperuricemia with episodes of urate nephropathy and gouty arthritis. The patient has an 8-year-old brother and a 12-year-old sister who are normal. Of note, his maternal grandmother described a brother who died at age 7 years with similar behavioral and clinical symptoms. Also, the boy's mother noted that when she was a child, she had a brother with similar symptoms who also died at a young age. The patient's serum uric acid is 15 mg/dL. Which of the following statements about this disease is true?

A. The boy's brother is a carrier for the disease.
B. The mother has a 50% chance of having another male child with the disorder.
C. Allopurinol will improve the neurologic symptoms of this disorder.
D. The disease is caused by an error in pyrimidine metabolism.
E. Female carriers have less severe neurologic symptoms.

**II-14.** Stem cell gene therapy has been attempted in patients with a variety of medical conditions. To date, this technique has had the most clinical success in which of the following conditions?

A. $\beta$ Thalassemia
B. Gaucher disease
C. Fanconi's anemia
D. Severe combined immune deficiency (SCID)
E. Wiscott-Aldrich syndrome (WAS)

**II-15.** The following pedigree is an example of what pattern of inheritance?

**II-15.** *(Continued)*

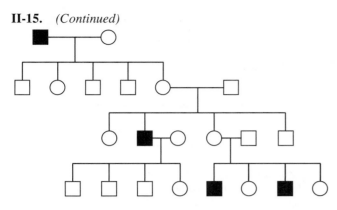

Solid figure = Affected individual
Open figure = Unaffected individuals

   A.   X-linked recessive inheritance
   B.   X-linked dominant inheritance
   C.   Autosomal recessive inheritance
   D.   Autosomal dominant inheritance
   E.   Cannot be determined by the limited information provided in this pedigree

**II-16.** The pedigree described below is an example of what pattern of inheritance?

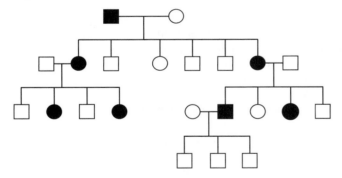

Solid figure = Affected individuals
Open figure = Unaffected individuals

   A.   X-linked recessive inheritance
   B.   X-linked dominant inheritance
   C.   Autosomal recessive inheritance
   D.   Autosomal dominant inheritance
   E.   Cannot be determined by the limited information provided in this pedigree

**II-17.** A 35-year-old female comes to your clinic for a consultation. She is 17 weeks pregnant with her second child. She is G2 P1. Her prior pregnancy was complicated by neonatal alloimmune thrombocytopenia (NATP). Analysis of the patient's serum reveals circulating anti-PI$^{A1}$ an-

**II-17.** *(Continued)*
tibodies. Which of the following statements concerning NATP is true?

   A.   If the gene frequency of PI$^{A2}$ is 0.02, the likelihood of the patient's second child having NATP is low.
   B.   Given the gene frequency of PI$^{A2}$ of 0.02, the likelihood of the patient's second child having NATP approaches 100%.
   C.   The incidence of NATP is approximately 1 in 20,000 neonates.
   D.   NATP is unrelated to the circulating anti-PI$^{A1}$ antibodies because IgG antibodies do not cross the placental barrier.
   E.   NATP is unrelated to the entity referred to as posttransfusion purpura.

**II-18.** A 42-year-old male (indicated by the star in the family history below) has renal failure as a result of Alport syndrome, which consists of nephritis associated with sensorineural deafness and is inherited as an autosomal dominant defect. He is being evaluated for a renal transplant from a living related donor. The best candidate for evaluation as a potential kidney donor for this patient would be his

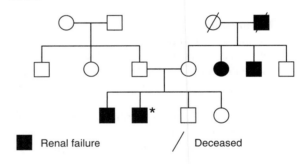

   ⬛ Renal failure      / Deceased

   A.   mother
   B.   father
   C.   unaffected brother
   D.   sister

**II-19.** Diseases that are inherited in a multifactorial genetic fashion (i.e., not autosomal dominant, autosomal recessive, or X- linked) and are seen more frequently in persons bearing certain histocompatibility antigens include

   A.   gluten-sensitive enteropathy
   B.   neurofibromatosis
   C.   adult polycystic kidney disease
   D.   Wilson's disease
   E.   cystic fibrosis

# II. GENETICS

## ANSWERS

**II-1. The answer is C.** *(Chap. 328)* This group of genetic disorders often presents with disorders of sexual differentiation. Genetically, Klinefelter syndrome results from a meiotic nondysjunction of sex chromosomes during gametogenesis, producing a 47,XXY individual. Phenotypically, these individuals are male but have eunochoid features, small testes, decreased virilization, and gynecomastia. The other disorders listed in the question may result in sexual ambiguity, more commonly in males. In mixed gonadal dysgenesis, there is mosaicism resulting from the genotype 46,XY/45,X. Depending on the proportion of cells with the 46,XY genotype, the phenotype can be either male or female. Testicular dysgenesis results from the absence of müllerian inhibiting substance during embryonic development and may be caused by multiple genetic mutations and may be associated with the absence of mullerian-inhibiting substance and reduced testosterone production. Feminization may also occur through androgen insensitivity and mutations in the androgen receptor. Virilization of females with resultant ambiguous sexual differentiation most commonly occurs in patients with congenital adrenal hyperplasia (CAH). The most common cause of CAH is 21-hydroxylase deficiency, which results in ambiguous female genitalia, hypotension, and salt wasting.

**II-2. The answer is E.** *(Chap. 328)* Turner syndrome, or gonadal dysgenesis, is a common chromosomal disorder that affects 1 in 2500 female births. The most common genetic defect is the 45,XO karyotype, which causes half of all phenotypic cases of this syndrome. Age at diagnosis is variable, based on the clinical manifestations. Most cases are diagnosed perinatally on the basis of reduced fetal growth or lymphedema at birth with nuchal folds, a low posterior hairline, or left-sided cardiac defects. Some girls may not be diagnosed in childhood and come to attention much later in life because of delayed growth and lack of sexual maturation. Limited pubertal development occurs in up to 30% of girls with Turner syndrome, with approximately 2% reaching menarche. Owing to the frequency of congenital heart and genitourinary defects, a thorough workup should be done after the diagnosis, including an echocardiogram and renal imaging. Long-term management includes growth hormone replacement during childhood and estrogen replacement to maintain bone mineralization and feminization.

**II-3. The answer is B.** *(Chap. 342)* This patient presents with the classic findings of an inherited disorder of connective tissue, particularly Marfan syndrome. The presentation is not consistent with the bony deformities or blue sclera seen in patients with osteogenesis imperfecta, and he is tall with long extremities, which makes chondroplasia very unlikely. However, his hypermobility and lens disorders suggest Marfan syndrome or, less commonly, Ehlers-Danlos syndrome.

**II-4. The answer is C.** *(Chap. 56)* Meiosis occurs only in the germ cells of the gonads. The final result is to reduce the number of chromosomes in a diploid ($2n$) cell to a haploid ($n$) state. When the egg is eventually fertilized by the sperm, the two haploid ($n$) sets combine to form the diploid ($2n$) state in the zygote. There are two distinct steps in cell division in meiosis. In the first step, two sister chromatids ($2n \rightarrow 4n$) are formed for each chromosome pair and there is recombination between maternal and parental DNA homologues. These chromosomes segregate randomly, generating up to $2^{23}$ possible combinations of chromosomes. This meiotic division results in two daughter cells ($2n$). In the second meiotic division, the two chromatids in each chromosome separate to yield four gametes in a haploid state (*n*).

**II-5.   The answer is C.**   *(Chap. 56)*   A gene locus includes both the regions of DNA that are transcribed and the regions that are necessary to control transcription. Exons are the portions of genes that are eventually spliced together to form mRNA. Introns are the spacing regions between exons that are eventually spliced out of the precursor RNAs to form mRNA. *Cis*-acting sequences that are upstream of the gene are called promoters. They typically contain specified sequences of nucleotides (e.g., TATA) that provide recognition and binding sites for *trans*-activating proteins called transcription factors. Transcription factors are proteins that bind to the regulatory regions of genes and initiate or repress transcription. Enhancers are regions of the genome that affect transcription but are not necessarily continuous with the affected gene.

**II-6.   The answer is C.**   *(Chap. 56)*   Neoplastic disorders may arise from mutations in DNA that affect oncogenes, tumor suppressor genes, apoptotic genes, and DNA repair genes. Several genetic disorders involving DNA repair enzymes underscore the importance of these mutations. Patients with xeroderma pigmentosum have defects in DNA damage recognition and in nucleotide excision and repair. These patients often have skin cancers as a result of the mutagenic effects of ultraviolet light. Ataxia-telangiectasia is characterized by large telangiectatic lesions on the face, cerebellar ataxia, immunologic defects, and hypersensitivity to ionizing radiation. Mutation in the ATM gene that causes AT gives rise to defects in meiosis and increasing damage from ionizing radiation. Fanconi's anemia is caused by mutations in multiple complementation groups that are characterized by various congenital anomalies and a marked predisposition to aplastic anemia and acute myeloid leukemia. HNPCC is caused by mutations in one of several mismatch repair genes that result in microsatellite instability and a high incidence of colon, ovarian, and uterine cancers. Fragile X syndrome is caused by unstable trinucleotide repeats that destabilize DNA. It is characterized by X-linked inheritance and typical large ears, macroorchidism, and mental retardation.

**II-7.   The answer is C.**   *(Chap. 56)*   Mendelian inheritance patterns do not apply to mitochondrial genetics. Mitochondrial DNA (mtDNA) consists of small encoding transfer and ribosomal RNAs and various proteins that are involved in oxidative phosphorylation and adenosine triphosphate (ATP) generation. mtDNA exists as a circular chromosome within cells. The mitochondrial genome does not recombine. The genetic material that is introduced into the egg by the sperm does not contain mitochondrial DNA, therefore, inheritance is maternal. All the children of an affected mother will inherit the disorder. An affected father will not transmit the disorder. The clinical manifestations of the various disorders in mitochondrial genetics are characterized by alterations in oxidative phosphorylation that lead to reductions in the ATP supply and apoptosis. Areas of high dependence on oxidative phosphorylation include skeletal and cardiac muscle and the brain. During replication, the number of mitochondria can drift among various cells and tissues, resulting in heterogeneity, or heteroplasmy. This results in further variation in the clinical phenotype. Acquired mutations in the mitochondrial genome are thought to play a significant role in age-related degenerative disorders such as Alzheimer's disease and Parkinson's disease.

**II-8.   The answer is B.**   *(Chap. 56)*   Genetic imprinting is gene inactivation that results in preferential expression of an allele depending on its parental origin. It has an important role in a number of diseases, including malignancies. Abnormal expression in the paternally derived copy of the insulin-like growth factor II (IGF-II) gene results in the cancer-predisposing Beckwith-Wiedemann syndrome. Uniparental disomy is the inheritance of dual copies of either maternal or paternal chromosomes. This may result in similar phenotypes, as in the case of imprinting. The Prader-Willi and Angelman's syndromes may result from uniparental disomy involving inheritance of defective maternal or paternal chromosomes, respectively. Similarly, hydatidiform moles may contain normal numbers of diplid chromosomes, all of which are of paternal origin. The opposite occurs in ovarian teratomas. Lyonization is epigenetic inactivation of one of the two X chromosomes in every cell of the female. Somatic mosaicism is the presence of two or more genetically distinct cell lines in the tissue of an individual. The term *anticipation* is often used to refer to diseases caused by trinucleotide repeats that are often characterized by worsening of clinical phenotypes in successive generations. These diseases, such as Huntington's disease and fragile X syndrome, are characterized by expansion of these repeats in subsequent generations of individuals, resulting in earlier and often more severe clinical phenotypes.

**II-9.   The answer is D.**   *(Chap. 342)*   Connective tissue is composed of macromolecules (collagen, elastin, fibrillin, proteoglycans, etc.) that are assembled into an insoluble extracellular matrix. Disorders of any of these macromolecules may result in a disorder of connective tissue. Osteogenesis imperfecta is caused by mutations in type I procollagen. Over 400 mutations have been found in patients with OI. Clinically, it is characterized by decreased bone mass, brittle bones, blue sclerae, dental abnormalities, joint laxity, and progressive hearing loss. The phenotype may range from severe disease with in utero death to milder forms with lesser severity and survival into adulthood. Ehlers-Danlos syndrome is a heterogenous set of disorders characterized by joint laxity, hyperelasticity of the skin, and other defects in collagen synthesis. A variety of defects have been identified in different types of collagen as well as enzymes that facilitate collagen cross-linking. Marfan syndrome is characterized by a triad of features: long, thin extremities (with arachnodactyly and loose joints), reduced vision as a result of ectopia lentis, and aortic aneurysms. Defects in the fibrillin gene are responsible for this syndrome. Alport syndrome is caused by mutations in type IV collagen, resulting in the most common phenotype of X-linked inheritance, hematuria, sensorineural deafness, and lenticonus. McArdle's disease is a defect in glycogenolysis that results from myophosphorylase deficiency.

**II-10.   The answer is D.**   *(Chap. 340)*   Lysosomes are subcellular organelles that contain specific hydrolyases that allow the processing and degradation of proteins, nucleic acids, carbohydrates, and lipids. Lysosomal storage diseases result from mutations in various genes for these hydrolyases. Clinical symptoms result from the accumulation of the undegraded macromolecule. Tay-Sachs disease is caused by a deficiency of hexosaminidase A. Buildup of $G_{M2}$ gangliosides results in a phenotype that is characterized by a fatal progressive neurodegenerative disease. In the infantile form, these patients have macrocephaly, loss of motor skills, an increased startle reaction, and a macular cherry red spot. The juvenile-onset form presents with ataxia and progressive dementia that result in death by age 15. The adult-onset form is characterized by clumsiness in childhood, progressive motor weakness in adolescence, and neurocognitive decline. Death occurs in early adulthood. Survival to the third or fourth decade is rare. Splenomegaly is uncommon. The disease is seen most commonly in Ashkenazi Jews, with a carrier frequency of about 1 in 30. Inheritance is autosomal recessive.

**II-11.   The answer is D.**   *(Chap. 340)*   Gaucher disease is an autosomal recessive lysosomal storage disorder caused by decreased activity of acid $\beta$-glucosidase. Nearly 200 mutations have been described. Type 1 Gaucher disease presents in childhood to adulthood. The average age at diagnosis is 20 years in white people. Clinical features result from an accumulation of lipid-laden macrophages, termed Gaucher cells, throughout the body. Hepatosplenomegaly is present in virtually all symptomatic patients. Bone marrow involvement is common, with subsequent infarction, ischemia, and necrosis. Anemia and thrombocytopenias may occur. Bone pain is common. Although the liver and spleen may become massive, severe liver dysfunction is very rare. The disease is most common in Ashkenazi Jewish populations. The diagnosis is made by measuring enzyme activity. Enzyme therapy is currently the treatment of choice in significantly affected patients. Other therapies include symptomatic management of the blood cytopenias and joint replacement surgery for bone injury. Type 2 Gaucher disease is a rare, severe central nervous system (CNS) disease that leads to death in infancy. Type 3 disease is nearly identical to type 1 disease except that the course is more rapidly progressive.

**II-12. The answer is A.** *(Chap. 57)*  Chromosomal abnormalities are extremely common in pregnancy. Up to 25% of pregnancies involve some type of chromosomal abnormality. Most go undetected, and the conceptus is spontaneously aborted. However, up to 10% of fetuses are chromosomally imbalanced. Most chromosomal numerical abnormalities occur in meiosis. Meiosis I involves the formation of two pairs of chromosomes, each with two chromatids ($2n \rightarrow 4n$). Each daughter cell gets one set of 23 chromosomes, each with two chromatids. In meiosis II, the two chromatids separate to generate four gametes with 23 chromosomes, each with one chromatid. By far the most common chromosomal abnormality is trisomy 21, which results in Down's syndrome. One-third of Down's cases are due to errors in meiosis II. In the case of trisomy 16, most of the errors occur in meiosis I. Although the precise mechanism is unknown, numerous observational studies have shown a strong correlation between maternal age and the presence of chromosomal abnormalities. These abnormalities range from less than 2% in females under age 25 to up to 33% in those over age 40. In contrast to trisomies, most monosomies are incompatible with life. Only 45,X, which causes Turner syndrome, is compatible with live birth. It occurs in up to 1% of all pregnancies.

**II-13. The answer is B.** *(Chap. 338)*  This patient has Lesch-Nyhan syndrome, which is characterized clinically by hyperuricemia, self-mutilative behavior, choreoathetosis, spasticity, and mental retardation. It is caused by a complete deficiency of hypoxanthine-guanine phosphoribosyltransferase (HPRT), a critical enzyme in the salvage pathway for purine bases. HPRT catalyzes the combination of the purine bases hypoxanthine and guanine with phosphoribosylpyrophosphate (PRPP). Loss of HPRT promotes increased uric acid production from the breakdown of purines. The disorder is X-linked recessive in inheritance. Affected males are hemizygous for the mutant gene. Carrier females are completely asymptomatic. The mother has a 50% chance of passing the affected X chromosome on to a male child. Allopurinol, although it improves the rheumatologic and renal complications of hyperuricemia, does not affect the neurologic decline. A partial deficiency in HPRT results in hyperuricemia but no neurologic decline. This is called the Kelley-Seegmiller syndrome.

**II-14. The answer is D.** *(Chap. 59)*  Stem cell therapy has held enormous promise for the last two decades. Stem cells are undifferentiated progenitors that can develop into highly specialized cells that form the various organs. Totipotent stem cells can form a placenta and can develop into a complete embryo. Pluripotent stem cells are capable of forming tissues derived from the three major germ-line layers: endoderm, mesoderm, and ectoderm. Multipotent stem cells are the progenitors of cells in particular tissues. Stem cells are self-renewing and may differentiate. The concept of correcting inborn genetic defects in stem cells has been the central theme in most gene therapy strategies for correcting congenital disorders. The success of bone marrow transplantation in the treatment of many congenital and acquired hematopoietic disorders has stimulated numerous attempts at gene therapy for those disorders. A variety of methods have been developed to transfer new genetic material into cells. Direct injection of DNA and gene transfer using viruses are two of the main methods. Adenoviral and adenovirus-associated viruses are effective vectors but do not integrate into the genome and do not often produce continued transcription. Retroviral and lentiviral vectors have been modified to remove the pathogenic sequences, leaving only the sequences that are important for integration. In 2000, the first successful stem cell gene therapy was reported. Cord blood CD34+ stem cells from X-SCID newborns were transduced with a γc retrovirus vector. Approximately 98% of circulating T lymphocytes contained the vector in transduced patients, compared with less than 0.1% in myeloid cells, representing selective expression. Many of the patients responded to clinical vaccinations and have remained healthy. However, two recipients developed acute hematologic disorders resembling leukemia, indicating aberrant integration of the vector into the patient's genome. Further studies have been suspended as researchers attempt to discover ways to avoid random integration of vectors into sites that are oncogenic.

**II-15.   The answer is A.**   *(Chap. 56)*   The information provided in the pedigree is adequate to determine the mode of a single-gene inheritance pattern. The example provided is typical of patients with hemophilia A or Duchenne's muscular dystrophy. Other examples exist. X-linked recessive inheritance is marked by the fact that the incidence of the trait is much higher in males than in females. The genetic trait is passed from an affected male through all his daughters to, on average, half their sons. The trait is never transmitted directly from father to son. The trait may be transmitted through a series of carrier females; if that occurs, the affected males are related to each other through the female, as in this case.

**II-16.   The answer is B.**   *(Chap. 56)*   The information provided in the pedigree is adequate to determine the mode of a single-gene inheritance pattern. The example given is character-istic of an X-linked dominant single-gene inheritance, as is common in the X-linked blood group system Xg. The Xg system is governed by a pair of alleles, $Xg^a$ and Xg. These alleles produce only two phenotypes, Xg (A+) and Xg (A−), respectively. Another ex-ample of X-linked dominant inheritance pattern is vitamin D−resistant rickets. The X-linked dominant inheritance pattern is characterized by the fact that affected females exist in the heterozygote state. Affected females are twice as common as affected males, and the affected males are hemizygotes. In vitamin D−resistant rickets, both sexes are affected. However, the serum phosphate level is less depressed; hence, the rickets is less severe in the heterozygous female than in the hemizygous male.

**II-17.   The answer is B.**   *(Chap. 56)*   Neonatal alloimmune thrombocytopenia (NATP) is a potentially life-threatening disorder that is limited to fetuses and neonates. It is immuno-logically mediated as a result of the genetic predisposition of the mother. Maternal IgG alloantibodies cross the placenta, resulting in immune destruction of platelets that bear paternal alloantigens. Firstborn offspring constitute about 50% of NATP cases, and sub-sequent affected siblings usually develop worsening degrees of thrombocytopenia. The GPIIb/IIIa receptor complex is the site of the polymorphism. The majority of cases of NATP are caused by anti-$PI^{A1}$ antibodies; <5% are due to less common polymorphisms. Mothers who are $PI^{A1-}$ (i.e., $PI^{A2}/PI^{A2}$) account for the vast majority of cases of NATP. The gene frequency of $PI^{A2}$ is 0.02; therefore, approximately 1 in 2500 neonates is born with NATP as a direct manifestation of the $PI^{A1}$ polymorphism. This entity is pathophy-siologically related to posttransfusion purpura in that both diseases involve the develop-ment of platelet-specific antibodies directed against the naturally occurring platelet receptor GPIIb/IIIa.

**II-18.   The answer is B.**   *(Chaps. 56, 264, and 265)*   Many autosomal dominant disorders vary in the time of onset and the severity of expression. Therefore, persons, such as the two apparently unaffected siblings, who are at risk for the development of hereditary nephritis, even in the absence of overt evidence of renal impairment, are poor renal donor candidates. In addition, the mother is clearly a carrier and a poor candidate. The father is the best close relative to evaluate as a potential donor.

**II-19.   The answer is A.**   *(Chap. 56)*   Many common diseases are known to "run in families" yet are not inherited in a simple Mendelian fashion. It is likely that the expression of these disorders depends on a family of genes that can impart a certain degree of risk and then be modified by subsequent environmental factors. The risk of the development of disease in a relative of an affected person varies with the degree of relationship; first-degree rel-atives (parents, siblings, and offspring) have the highest risk, which in itself varies with the specific disease. Many of these multifactorial genetic diseases are inherited in a greater frequency in persons with certain HLA (major histocompatibility system) types. For ex-ample, there is a tenfold increased risk of celiac sprue (gluten-sensitive enteropathy) in persons who have HLA-B8. This genotype also imparts an increased risk for chronic active hepatitis, myasthenia gravis, and Addison's disease. The incidence of diabetes mellitus is much higher in those expressing HLA-D3 and HLA-D4. Spondyloarthropathies, psoriatic arthritis (HLA-B27), hyperthyroidism (HLA-DR3), and multiple sclerosis (HLA-DR2) are other examples of diseases with histocompatibility predispositions. By contrast, Wilson's disease and cystic fibrosis are inherited in an autosomal recessive fashion, and adult poly-cystic kidney disease and neurofibromatosis are among the disorders inherited in an au-tosomal dominant manner.

# III. ONCOLOGY AND HEMATOLOGY

## QUESTIONS

**DIRECTIONS:** Each question below contains four or five suggested responses. Choose the **one best** response to each question.

**III-1.** A 44-year-old male was diagnosed with stage II colon cancer 2 years ago and was treated with complete resection and adjuvant chemotherapy. He presents with 2 weeks of anorexia, right upper quadrant pain, and elevated serum alkaline phosphatase. An abdominal CT scan demonstrates a solitary 4-cm mass in the liver. A biopsy reveals adenocarcinoma negative for hepatic markers and histologically identical to the patient's original colon cancer. Additional evaluation reveals no other evidence of metastatic or recurrent disease. Performance status is normal. Which of the following statements regarding subsequent therapy is true?

A. Chemotherapy with 5-fluorouracil, leucovorin, and irinotecan has a 25% chance of producing long-term disease-free survival.

B. Hepatic lobectomy has a 25% chance of producing long-term disease-free survival.

C. Immunotherapy with bacillus Calmette-Guerin (BCG) vaccine has a 25% chance of producing long-term disease-free survival.

D. There is no effective therapeutic option that offers a chance of long-term disease-free survival.

**III-2.** Which of the following statements regarding polycythemia vera is correct?

A. An elevated plasma erythropoietin level excludes the diagnosis.

B. Transformation to acute leukemia is common.

C. Thrombocytosis correlates strongly with thrombotic risk.

D. Aspirin should be prescribed to all these patients to reduce thrombotic risk.

E. Phlebotomy is used only after hydroxyurea and interferon have been tried.

**III-3.** A 31-year-old female is referred to your clinic for an evaluation of anemia. She describes a 2-month history of fatigue. She denies abdominal pain but notes that her abdomen has become slightly more distended in recent weeks. Past medical history is otherwise unremarkable. The patient's parents are alive, and she has three healthy

**III-3.** *(Continued)*
siblings. Physical examination is significant for pale conjunctiva and a palpable spleen 4 cm below the left costal margin. Hematocrit is 31% and bilirubin is normal. The reticulocyte percentage is low. Haptoglobin and lactic dehydrogenase (LDH) are normal. A peripheral blood smear shows numerous teardrop-shaped red cells, nucleated red cells, and occasional myelocytes. A bone marrow aspirate is unsuccessful, but a biopsy shows a hypercellular marrow with trilineage hyperplasia and findings consistent with the presumed diagnosis of chronic idiopathic myelofibrosis. You transfuse her to a hematocrit of 40%. What is the most appropriate next management step?

A. Administer erythropoietin.

B. Follow up in 6 months.

C. Institute combined-modality chemotherapy.

D. Perform HLA matching of her siblings.

E. Perform a splenectomy.

**III-4.** A 51-year-old male presents to your clinic with "hip" pain for 3 months despite conservative treatment with exercise and analgesics. Plain films of the pelvis show a lytic lesion in the right ilium. He denies other sites of bony pain and also denies fevers, weight loss, bowel or bladder incontinence, or lower extremity weakness. An examination shows point tenderness over the right gluteal region. Sphincter tone is normal, as is the neurologic examination. Laboratories, including a complete blood count and renal function, are normal. You arrange for a computed tomography (CT)-guided biopsy of the lesion, which shows numerous plasma cells. Serum and urine protein electrophoreses are normal. A skeletal survey shows no other lytic lesions. Bone marrow biopsy does not show an increased number of plasma cells. What is the most appropriate treatment at this time?

A. Pain control, reassurance, and serial follow-up examinations

B. External-beam radiation therapy

C. Chemotherapy

D. Preparation for stem cell transplantation

E. Glucocorticoids

**III-5.** Which of the following statements is not a feature of monoclonal gammopathy of uncertain significance (MGUS)?

A. MGUS affects up to 10% of patients over age 75.
B. Anemia and bone lesions are usually absent.
C. About 1% of these patients per year go on to develop overt myeloma.
D. Median survival is similar to that of age-matched controls.
E. Periodic treatment with glucocorticoids has been shown to improve survival.

**III-6.** 65-year-old female presents with lethargy and confusion for the last 2 days. Her past medical history is significant for Waldenström's macroglobulinemia. On physical examination the patient is alert but disoriented. She is moving all extremities. The cranial nerves and reflexes are grossly normal. She has diffuse lymphadenopathy and hepatosplenomegaly. Complete blood count shows a hematocrit of 31% but is otherwise normal. A peripheral blood smear shows rouleaux formation. All the following are appropriate management steps *except*

A. zoledronic acid
B. checking a plasma viscosity level
C. plasmapheresis
D. cladribine
E. rituximab

**III-7.** A 32-year-old male presents complaining of a testicular mass. On examination you palpate a 1- by 2-cm painless mass on the surface of the left testicle. A chest x-ray shows no lesions, and a CT scan of the abdomen and pelvis shows no evidence of retroperitoneal adenopathy. The $\alpha$ fetoprotein (AFP) level is elevated at 400 ng/mL. Beta human chorionic gonadotropin ($\beta$-hCG) is normal, as is LDH. You send the patient for an orchiectomy. The pathology comes back as seminoma limited to the testis alone. The AFP level declines to normal at an appropriate interval. What is the appropriate management at this point?

A. Radiation to the retroperitoneal lymph nodes
B. Adjuvant chemotherapy
C. Hormonal therapy
D. Retroperitoneal lymph node dissection (RPLND)
E. Positron emission tomography (PET) scan

**III-8.** A 34-year-old female with a past medical history of sickle cell anemia presents with a 5-day history of fatigue, lethargy, and shortness of breath. She denies chest pain or bone pain. She has had no recent travel. Of note, the patient's 4-year-old daughter had a "cold" 2 weeks before the presentation. On examination she has pale conjunctiva, is anicteric, and is mildly tachycardic. Abdominal examination is unremarkable. Laboratories show a hemoglobin of 3 g/dL; her baseline is 8 g/dL. The white

**III-8.** *(Continued)*
blood cell count and platelets are normal. Reticulocyte count is undetectable. Total bilirubin is 1.4 mg/dL. Lactic dehydrogenase is at the upper limits of the normal range. Peripheral blood smear shows a few sickled cells but a total absence of reticulocytes. The patient is given a transfusion of 2 units of packed red blood cells and admitted to the hospital. A bone marrow biopsy shows a normal myeloid series but an absence of erythroid precursors. Cytogenetics are normal. What is the most appropriate next management step?

A. Make arrangements for exchange transfusion.
B. Tissue type her siblings for a possible bone marrow transplant.
C. Check parvovirus titers.
D. Start prednisone and cyclosporine.
E. Start broad-spectrum antibiotics.

**III-9.** All the following cause prolongation of the activated partial thromboplastin time (aPTT) that does not correct with a 1:1 mixture with pooled plasma *except*

A. lupus anticoagulant
B. factor VIII inhibitor
C. heparin
D. factor VII inhibitor
E. factor IX inhibitor

**III-10.** You are asked to consult on a 31-year-old male with prolonged bleeding after an oral surgery procedure. He has no prior history of bleeding diathesis or family history of bleeding disorders. The patient's past medical history is remarkable for infection with the human immunodeficiency virus, with a CD4 count of $51/mL^3$. The examination is remarkable only for spotty lymphadenopathy. The platelet count is 230,000 cells/mL. His international normalized ratio (INR) is 1.5. Activated partial thromboplastin time is 40 s. Peripheral blood smear shows no schistocytes and is otherwise unremarkable. A 1:1 mixing study corrects both conditions immediately and after a 2-h incubation. Fibrinogen level is normal. Thrombin time is prolonged. What is the diagnosis?

A. Disseminated intravascular coagulation (DIC)
B. Dysfibrinogenemia
C. Factor V deficiency
D. Liver disease
E. Factor XIII deficiency

**III-11.** All the following are vitamin K–dependent coagulation factors *except*

A. factor X
B. factor VII
C. protein C
D. protein S
E. factor VIII

**III-12.** All but which of the following statements about the lupus anticoagulant (LA) are true?

A. Lupus anticoagulants typically prolong the aPTT.
B. A 1:1 mixing study will not correct in the presence of lupus anticoagulants.
C. Bleeding episodes in patients with lupus anticoagulants may be severe and life-threatening.
D. Female patients may experience recurrent midtrimester abortions.
E. Lupus anticoagulants may occur in the absence of other signs of systemic lupus erythematosus (SLE).

**III-13.** The most common inherited prothrombotic disorder is

A. activated protein C resistance
B. prothrombin gene mutation
C. protein C deficiency
D. protein S deficiency
E. antithrombin deficiency

**III-14.** The risk of graft-versus-host disease (GVHD) is higher in hematopoietic stem cell transplantation (HSCT) from syngeneic donors than in that from allogeneic donors.

A. True
B. False

**III-15.** You are asked to consult for hyperbilirubinemia in a 32-year-old female on the bone marrow transplant service. Fifteen days ago she had an allogeneic bone marrow transplant for poor-risk acute myeloid leukemia. She received busulfan and high-dose cyclophosphamide as a preparative regimen. At 13 days after transplantation she started to develop icterus. Total bilirubin started to rise. She also developed abdominal swelling and peripheral edema. The patient's medications include valacyclovir, cefepime, and liposomal amphotericin. On examination she has scleral icterus. The abdomen is distended. There are bowel sounds. There is mild right upper quadrant tenderness. Ascites is present. She has 2+ pedal edema. She is neutropenic and transfusion-dependent for red blood cells and platelets. Direct bilirubin is 7 mg/dL. Aspartate aminotransferase (AST) is 98 U/L, and alanine aminotransferase (ALT) is 86 U/L. Alkaline phosphatase is 50 U/L. Right upper quadrant ultrasound shows hepatomegaly. Sonographic Murphy's sign is negative. What is the most likely diagnosis?

A. Leukemic infiltration of the liver
B. Graft-versus-host disease
C. Medication side effect
D. Venooclusive disease
E. Acalculous cholecystitis

**III-16.** All the following are late complications of bone marrow transplant preparative regimens *except*

**III-16.** *(Continued)*
A. growth retardation
B. azoospermia
C. hypothyroidism
D. cataracts
E. dementia

**III-17.** All but which of the following statements about graft-versus-host disease (GVHD) are true?

A. Up to 50% of patients surviving more than 6 months after allogeneic transplantation develop chronic GVHD.
B. T cell depletion is associated decreased GVHD and improvement in cure rates.
C. GVHD is more common in recipients from unrelated donors than in recipients from matched siblings.
D. Sicca syndrome is a common manifestation of chronic GVHD.
E. Acute GVHD typically manifests with an erythematous maculopapular rash, persistent diarrhea, or elevations in transaminases.

**III-18.** All but which of the following statements about cancer of unknown primary site (CUPS) are true?

A. Median survival is under 1 year.
B. Most patients with CUPS are over age 60.
C. Positron-emission tomography scan is recommended for identification of the primary site.
D. The majority of CUPS tumors will be adenocarcinomas on light microscopy.
E. Men with CUPS who have midline tumors and elevated $\alpha$ fetoprotein or $\beta$-hCG levels may be cured with combination chemotherapy.

**III-19.** All but which of the following statements about iron metabolism and erythropoiesis are true?

A. Hemolytic anemias result in increased red blood cell destruction and iron deficiency.
B. The average life span of a red blood cell is 120 days.
C. Iron is absorbed in the proximal intestine.
D. There is no physiologic excretory pathway for iron in humans.
E. Apoferritin acts as the intracellular storage protein for iron in red blood cells.

**III-20.** All the following are suggestive of iron deficiency anemia *except*

A. koilonychia
B. pica
C. decreased serum ferritin
D. decreased total iron-binding capacity (TIBC)
E. low reticulocyte response

**III-21.** You are asked to consult on a 45-year-old male with anemia whose hematocrit is 31%. A peripheral smear reveals hypochromic, microcytic red cells. All the following are appropriate initial laboratory tests *except*:

A. serum ferritin
B. total iron-binding capacity
C. hemoglobin electrophoresis
D. red cell protoporphyrin levels
E. serum iron

**III-22.** All but which of the following statements about aspirin (acetylsalicylic acid) are true?

A. Aspirin acts by irreversibly inhibiting cyclooxygenase (COX).
B. Aspirin reduces mortality in patients with unstable angina and myocardial infarction.
C. Aspirin reduces morbidity and mortality in patients who have had a stroke.
D. Aspirin is first-line therapy in elderly patients (over 65 years of age) with atrial fibrillation.
E. There is evidence for primary prevention of death and myocardial infarction in patients with risk factors for coronary artery disease.

**III-23.** All the following match the anticoagulant with its correct mechanism of action *except*

A. abciximab — GpIIb/IIIa receptor inhibition
B. clopidogrel — inhibition of thromboxane $A_2$ release
C. fondaparinux — inhibition of factor Xa
D. argatroban — thrombin inhibition
E. warfarin — vitamin K — dependent carboxylation of coagulation factors

**III-24.** You are asked to consult on a 34-year-old male with thrombocytopenia. He sustained a motor vehicle collision 10 days ago, resulting in shock, internal bleeding, and acute renal failure. An exploratory laparotomy was performed that showed a ruptured spleen requiring a splenectomy. He also underwent an open reduction and internal fixation of the left femur. The platelet count was 260,000 cells/$\mu$L on admission. Today it is 68,000 cells/$\mu$L. His medications are oxacillin, morphine, and subcutaneous heparin. On examination the vital signs are stable. The examination is significant for an abdominal scar that is clean and healing. The patient's left leg is in a large cast and is elevated. The right leg is swollen from the calf downward. Ultrasound of the right leg shows a deep venous thrombosis. Antiheparin antibodies are positive. Creatinine is 3.2 mg/dL. What is the most appropriate next management step?

A. Discontinue heparin.
B. Stop heparin and start enoxaparin.
C. Stop heparin and start argatroban.
D. Stop heparin and start lepirudin.
E. Observe the patient.

**III-25.** All but which of the following statements about chronic idiopathic myelofibrosis are true?

A. The median survival of patients with chronic idiopathic myelofibrosis is longer than the median survival of patients with polycythemia vera.
B. About 10% of patients with chronic idiopathic myelofibrosis will develop an aggressive form of acute leukemia.
C. Splenectomy worsens extramedullary hematopoiesis.
D. The only curative therapy is allogeneic bone marrow transplantation.
E. Abnormal cytogenetics portends a worse prognosis than does normal cytogenetics.

**III-26.** A 50-year-old female presents to your clinic for evaluation of an elevated platelet count. The latest complete blood count is white blood cells (WBC) 7,000/mm³, hematocrit 34%, and platelets 600,000/mm³. All the following are common causes of thrombocytosis *except*

A. iron-deficiency anemia
B. essential thrombocytosis
C. chronic myeloid leukemia
D. myelodysplasia
E. pernicious anemia

**III-27.** Which of the following statements about cardiac toxicity from cancer treatment is true?

A. Doxorubicin-based cardiac toxicity is idiosyncratic and dose-independent.
B. Anthracycline-induced congestive heart failure is reversible with time and control of risk factors.
C. Mediastinal irradiation often results in acute pericarditis during the first few weeks of treatment.
D. Chronic constrictive pericarditis often manifests symptomatically up to 10 years after treatment.
E. The incidence of coronary atherosclerosis in patients who have a history of mediastinal irradiation is the same as that in age-matched controls.

**III-28.** Which of the following pairs of chemotherapy and complication is incorrect?

A. Daunorubicin — CHF
B. Bleomycin — interstitial fibrosis
C. Cyclophosphamide — hematuria
D. Cisplatin — liver failure
E. Ifosfamide — Fanconi syndrome

**III-29.** A 30-year-old male is admitted for acute myeloid leukemia. His past medical history is significant for treatment of early-stage non-Hodgkin's lymphoma (cyclophosphamide, doxorubicin, vincristine, prednisone) and involved-field radiation 9 years earlier. He has a 12 pack-year history of tobacco and works as a welder. He has no

**III-29.** *(Continued)*

family history of cancer. The examination is notable only for pallor and some petechiae on the torso and lower extremities. Complete blood counts show that all three cell lineages are low. Cytogenetics shows a deletion in chromosome 5. What is the most likely cause of his acute myeloid leukemia?

A. Chemotherapy
B. Radiation
C. Combined modality therapy
D. Tobacco
E. Lynch syndrome

**III-30.** A 60-year-old male with a long history of tobacco use presents to the emergency room with headache, neck pain, and a swollen face. He has also noted a 10-lb weight loss over the last 2 months. He is tachypneic and tachycardic. Oxygen saturation is 92% on room air. The examination is notable for right supraclavicular lymphadenopathy. He has bilateral polyphonic end-expiratory wheezes. A chest x-ray shows a right upper lung mass. The patient is admitted to the intensive care unit for monitoring. All the following are appropriate management steps *except*

A. bronchoscopy
B. interventional radiology consultation
C. radiation oncology consultation
D. chemotherapy
E. glucocorticoids

**III-31.** A 40-year-old female complains of lower back pain for the last 2 weeks. She denies recent trauma or exertion. She also denies radiation down her legs, fevers, chills, or sweats. The past medical history is significant for treated stage II breast cancer. Her treatment chemotherapy and radiation ended 1 year ago. The patient is currently on tamoxifen. The physical examination is notable for a left lumpectomy scar. There is no point tenderness over the spine. The straight leg test is negative bilaterally. Sphincter tone and reflexes are normal. What is the most appropriate management?

A. Observation
B. Physical therapy
C. X-ray of the spine
D. Magnetic resonance imaging (MRI) of the spine
E. Bone scan

**III-32.** All the following types of cancer commonly metastasize to the central nervous system (CNS) *except*

A. ovarian
B. breast
C. hypernephroma
D. melanoma
E. acute lymphoblastic leukemia (ALL)

**III-33.** A 23-year-old male presents to the emergency room with headache and dizziness. He has also noted epistaxis and easy bruising for the last 3 days. The examination is notable for numerous petechiae. The spleen is not palpable. Initial laboratories show a white blood cell count of 150,000 cells/mL. Hematocrit is 15%. Platelets are 4000 cells/mL. A peripheral blood smear is consistent with acute myeloid leukemia. All the following are appropriate management steps *except*

A. bone marrow biopsy
B. cytotoxic chemotherapy
C. leukapheresis
D. red blood cell transfusion
E. human leukocyte antigen typing of his siblings

**III-34.** An 81-year-old male is admitted to the hospital for altered mental status. He was found at home, confused and lethargic, by his son. His past medical history is significant for metastatic prostate cancer. The patient's medications include periodic intramuscular goserelin injections. On examination he is afebrile. Blood pressure is 110/50 mmHg, and the pulse rate is 110 beats/min. He is lethargic and minimally responsive to sternal rub. He has bitemporal wasting, and his mucous membranes are dry. On neurologic examination he is obtunded. The patient has an intact gag reflex and withdraws to pain in all four extremities. Rectal tone is normal. Laboratory values are significant for a creatinine of 4.2 mg/dL, a calcium level of 12.4 meq/L, and an albumin of 2.6 g/dL. All the following are appropriate initial management steps *except*

A. normal saline
B. pamidronate
C. furosemide when the patient is euvolemic
D. calcitonin
E. dexamethasone

**III-35.** All the following are characteristic of tumor lysis syndrome *except*

A. hyperkalemia
B. hypercalcemia
C. lactic acidosis
D. hyperphosphatemia
E. hyperuricemia

**III-36.** You are about to begin chemotherapy for a 40-year-old male with abdominal Burkitt's lymphoma. All the following management steps to minimize the effects of tumor lysis syndrome are reasonable *except*

A. cardiac monitoring
B. sevelamer (Renagel) administration
C. normal saline infusion
D. allopurinol
E. acidification of urine

**III-37.** A 42-year-old male presents to the emergency room with fatigue, lethargy, and decreased urine output. His past medical history is notable for squamous cell cancer of the anus, which recently was treated with combination chemotherapy that included cisplatin and mitomycin. His only current medication is dolasetron. On physical examination the patient is pale. Vital signs are stable. $O_2$ saturation is 96% on room air. The examination is otherwise unremarkable. Laboratory values include a white blood cell count of 11,000 cells/$\mu$L. Hematocrit is 20%. Platelets are 40,000 cells/$\mu$L. Serum lactic dehydrogenase is 528 U/L. Creatinine is 5.1 mg/dL. INR is 1.1. The aPTT ratio is 1.0. You ask for a peripheral blood smear to be performed. What is the most likely diagnosis?

A. Hemolytic-uremic syndrome
B. Autoimmune hemolytic anemia
C. Evans syndrome
D. Disseminated intravascular coagulation
E. Sepsis

**III-38.** Which of the following statements is true?

A. Factor VIII deficiency is characterized clinically by bleeding into soft tissues, muscles, and weight-bearing joints.
B. Congenital factor VIII deficiency is inherited in an autosomal recessive fashion.
C. Factor VIII deficiency results in prolongation of the prothrombin time.
D. Factor VIII complexes with Hageman factor, allowing for a longer half-life.
E. Factor VIII has a half-life of nearly 24 h.

**III-39.** A 31-year-old male with hemophilia A is admitted with persistent gross hematuria. He denies recent trauma or any history of genitourinary pathology. The examination is unremarkable. Hematocrit is 28%. All the following are treatments for hemophilia A *except*

A. desmopressin (DDAVP)
B. fresh-frozen plasma (FFP)
C. cryoprecipitate
D. recombinant factor VIII
E. plasmapheresis

**III-40.** A 40-year-old male with hemophilia A presents with recurrent gum bleeding. He has had several transfusions in the last 4 months for epistaxis and hematuria. After multiple transfusions of fresh-frozen plasma (FFP) and recombinant human factor VIII, his bleeding persists and his factor VIII level is below 10%. Activated partial thromboplastin time (aPTT) is prolonged. Prothrombin time is normal. Platelets are 240,000 cells/$\mu$L. You perform a mixing study, which shows correction of the 1:1 aPTT immediately but fails to correct the 1:1 aPTT after a 2-h incubation. All the following are treatments for this condition *except*

**III-40.** *(Continued)*
A. recombinant factor VIIa
B. purified porcine factor VIII
C. prothrombinase complex
D. desmopressin
E. prednisone

**III-41.** You are called to the leukemia service to evaluate a 32-year-old female with right lower quadrant pain. She has noted fevers and sweats for 1 day and diarrhea that is streaked with blood. She has acute myeloid leukemia (AML) and completed induction chemotherapy with cytarabine and daunorubicin 10 days ago. The examination is notable for stable vital signs, petechiae throughout the skin, and right lower quadrant tenderness. There is no rebound. Bowel sounds are present, and her stool is heme-positive. Laboratory values are notable for a white blood cell count of 100 cells/m³. Lactate is normal. *Clostridium difficile* toxin of the stool is negative. A CT scan is performed, which shows a thickened cecal wall with some fat stranding. There is no abscess or free intraabdominal air. You draw blood cultures, start broad-spectrum antibiotics, and call for a surgical consult. What is the diagnosis?

A. Typhlitis
B. Bowel infarction
C. Diverticulitis
D. Leukemic infiltration of the colon
E. Cytarabine toxicity

**III-42.** A 40-year-old male with acute myeloid leukemia develops a fever of 39.4°C (103°F). He has just completed consolidation chemotherapy. The patient has no other focal complaints and otherwise feels well. The neutrophil count is 34 cells/$\mu$L. On examination he is in no apparent distress. Vital signs are stable. The rest of the examination is unremarkable. What is the most appropriate next management step?

A. Draw blood and urine cultures and observe the patient at home.
B. Do a panculture and admit for inpatient observation.
C. Do a panculture, admit to the hospital, and start intravenous cefepime.
D. Do a panculture, admit to the hospital, and start intravenous aztreonam.
E. Do a panculture, admit to the hospital, and start voriconazole.

**III-43.** All but which of the following statements about non-Hodgkin's lymphoma are true?

A. The incidence of non-Hodgkin's lymphoma increased from the 1950s to the 1990s.
B. Adult T cell lymphoma is associated with a viral infection.

**III-43.** *(Continued)*

   C.  Antibiotics are useful in the treatment of gastric MALT (mucosa-associated lymphoid tissue).

   D.  The majority of primary central nervous system lymphomas in HIV infected patients are associated with Epstein-Barr virus (EBV) infection.

   E.  The incidence of T cell lymphomas is highest in North America.

**III-44.** A 55-year-old male is referred to you for evaluation of an elevated white blood cell count. He has no specific complaints and denies fevers, chills, lymphadenopathy, or weight loss. His past medical history is unremarkable. The examination shows no evidence of lymphadenopathy. There is no hepatosplenomegaly. The white blood cell count is 15,000 cells/$\mu$L with 50% lymphocytes on the differential. Hematocrit and platelet count are normal. LDH is normal. Peripheral smear shows smudge cells and many circulating lymphocytes. Flow cytometry of the peripheral blood shows a clonal population of lymphoid cells that express CD20 and CD5 and are cyclin D1–negative. Which of the following statements about this condition is true?

   A.  Patients with unmutated immunoglobulins have a longer median survival than do patients with mutated immunoglobulins.

   B.  These patients are more prone to viral and fungal infections.

   C.  This is the least common lymphoid malignancy.

   D.  Combination chemotherapy has been shown to be curative in this disease.

   E.  The median survival for this patient is more than 10 years.

**III-45.** You are asked to consult on a 46-year-old patient with mucosa-associated lymphoid tissue (MALT) of the stomach. He is *Helicobacter pylori*–positive. Computed tomography does not show any other evidence of disease outside the stomach. The lesion is 3 to 4 cm and confined to the fundus. A bone marrow biopsy is negative. Which of the following statements about localized MALT lymphoma is not true?

   A.  *H. pylori* infection is associated in 95% of cases of gastric MALT.

   B.  Treatment of *H. pylori* may achieve remission of disease.

   C.  Gastric MALT may evolve into diffuse large B-cell lymphoma.

   D.  Some tumors bear t(11; 18).

   E.  Combination chemotherapy is used as the first curative approach.

**III-46.** A 41-year-old male presents with neck swelling. He notes subjective fevers, chills, and night sweats for the last 3 weeks. On physical examination you note a 3- by

**III-46.** *(Continued)*

4-cm left anterior cervical lymph node. It is nontender and mobile. The oropharynx is clear. He has no evidence of other lymphadenopathy or hepatosplenomegaly. In light of the size of the lymph node, you send him for surgical excision of the lymph node. The pathology comes back as diffuse large B cell lymphoma. All the following are predictors of his prognosis *except*

   A.  serum lactic dehydrogenase

   B.  tumor stage

   C.  tumor grade

   D.  extranodal involvement

   E.  age

**III-47.** A 22-year-old previously healthy college student presents with a 3-day history of fever, headache, malaise, and a hacking nonproductive cough. Physical examination is notable for a temperature of 38.5°C (101.3°F) and normal blood pressure and heart rate. Respiratory rate is 22/min, and Sa$_{O_2}$ is 93% on room air. The lungs have bilateral rare crackles. Chest x ray shows bilateral lower lobe lower lobe interstitial and alveolar infiltrates. Complete blood count revealed:

WBC: 11.5K
Hemoglobin: 8.9 g/dL
Hematocrit: 27%
Mean corpuscular volume: 104 fL
Platelets: 290,000/mm$^3$
Reticulocyte index: 8%

    Which of the following statements is not correct?

   A.  A detailed ear examination may suggest the causative agent.

   B.  The bone marrow probably will show erythroid hyperplasia.

   C.  The bilirubin will be elevated.

   D.  The haptoglobin level will be reduced.

   E.  The pneumonia probably will respond to cefuroxime.

**III-48.** All the following are associated with pure red cell aplasia *except*

   A.  anterior mediastinal masses

   B.  connective tissue disorders

   C.  giant pronormoblasts

   D.  low erythropoietin levels

   E.  parvovirus B19 infection

**III-49.** A 74-year-old male is referred to you for evaluation of newly diagnosed prostate cancer. He was noted by his primary care physician to have a slightly elevated prostate-specific antigen (PSA) level on routine evaluation. The examination is unremarkable. Digital rectal examination shows no palpable mass. Transrectal ultrasound

**III-49.** *(Continued)*
shows that the mass is confined to one lobe. The biopsy shows a Gleason score of 3. Which of the following statements regarding prostate cancer is not true?

A. This patient has a greater than a 50% risk of death from prostate cancer at 10 years.
B. Prostatectomy carries a risk of immediate impotence with possible improvement over time.
C. Watchful waiting is a reasonable option in this scenario.
D. PSA levels slowly decline after external-beam radiation.
E. Neoadjuvant hormonal therapy before prostatectomy has not been shown to improve disease-free survival.

**III-50.** Approximately what percentage of cases of breast cancer can be linked directly to a germ-line mutation?

A. 10%
B. 25%
C. 50%
D. 75%
E. 90%

**III-51.** All the following are associated with a reduced lifetime risk of developing breast cancer *except*

A. absence of a history of maternal nursing
B. first full-term pregnancy before age 18 years
C. menarche after age 15 years
D. natural menopause before age 42 years
E. surgical menopause before age 42 years

**III-52.** A 54-year-old male presents with 2 months of increasing dyspnea and a persistent cough. He has a 75 pack-year history of cigarette smoking. He denies any fevers or chills but has lost 20 lb over the last 6 months because of anorexia. The physical examination is normal except for cachexia and dullness to percussion with decreased breath sounds over the right chest. Chest radiography is shown in the following figure. Which of the following statements regarding this patient's diagnosis and treatment is not true?

**III-52.** *(Continued)*

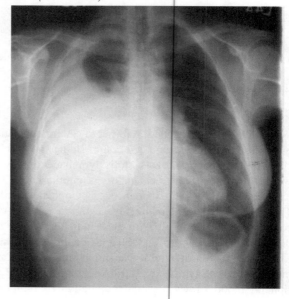

A. A pleural fluid cytology showing adenocarcinoma of the lung aids choice of therapy.
B. A pleural fluid cytology showing adenocarcinoma of the lung has diagnostic utility.
C. A pleural fluid pH above 7.2 is very likely.
D. A pleural fluid white cell count above 10,000/mm³ is likely.
E. An exudative pleural fluid is likely.

**III-53.** A 26-year-old female who is 4 months pregnant is seen for a standard evaluation. She reports feeling well with decreasing nausea over the last 1 month. The physical examination is normal except for the presence of a 1.5-cm hard nodule in the upper outer quadrant of the right breast. She does not recall the nodule being present previously and has not performed self-examination since becoming pregnant. Which of the following is the next most appropriate action?

A. Aspiration of the nodule
B. Mammogram after delivery
C. Prescription of oral progesterone therapy
D. Recommendation of genetic testing for *BRCA-1*
E. Repeat physical examination after delivery

**III-54.** Breast cancer screening with mammography has been shown to decrease mortality in which of the following groups of women?

A. Under 40 years old with a positive family history
B. Between 40 and 50 years old
C. Over 50 years old
D. Over 75 years old
E. On hormone replacement therapy

**III-55.** All the following conditions are associated with an increased incidence of cancer *except*

**III-55.** *(Continued)*

A. Down's syndrome
B. Fanconi's anemia
C. Von Hippel–Lindau syndrome
D. neurofibromatosis
E. fragile X syndrome

**III-56.** A 65-year-old postmenopausal female was found to have a 3.5-cm mass in the breast and axillary lymphadenopathy that was presumed to be malignant. For personal reasons she refused further evaluation. She returns 1 year later and agrees to undergo evaluation. The physical examination is notable for a palpable 6-cm mass and hard mobile axillary lymph nodes. Biopsy of the mass and the lymph nodes confirm the diagnosis of breast cancer. At this point what do you may inform her?

A. Her clinical stage is improved because of her post-menopausal status.
B. Her 5-year survival is approximately 50%.
C. Staging of postmenopausal breast cancer has little impact on the prognosis.
D. The presence of ipsilateral supraclavicular lymph nodes would not change the staging.
E. Waiting 1 year did not change her clinical stage.

**III-57.** A 68-year-old male with a history of coronary artery disease presents with symptoms of slurred speech and weakness and clumsiness of the left arm that lasted less than 2 h. At the time of presentation to the emergency department, his symptoms had resolved entirely and the neurologic examination was normal. Current medications include aspirin 325 mg daily, atenolol 50 mg daily, and enalapril 20 mg twice daily. The workup does not show any significant carotid stenosis or atrial fibrillation. You diagnose a transient ischemic attack. What treatment do you advise?

A. Increase the aspirin dose to twice daily.
B. Initiate therapy with clopidogrel.
C. Initiate therapy with warfarin.
D. Discontinue aspirin and initiate therapy with dipyridamole.
E. Make no changes in the patient's current regimen.

**III-58.** Which of the following anticoagulant therapies is incorrectly matched with its mechanism of action?

A. Heparin—inhibition of antithrombin
B. Dermatan sulfate—activation of heparin cofactor II
C. Fondaparinux—inhibition of factor Xa
D. Lepirudin—direct inhibition of thrombin
E. Ximelgatran—inhibition of antithrombin

**III-59.** A 29-year-old male is found on routine chest radiography for life insurance to have right hilar adenopa-

**III-59.** *(Continued)*

thy. He is otherwise healthy. Besides biopsy of the lymph nodes, which of the following is indicated?

A. Angiotension-converting enzyme (ACE) level
B. β-hCG
C. Thyroid stimulating hormone (TSH)
D. PSA
E. C-reactive protein

**III-60.** You are asked to consult on a 54-year-old female in the cardiac surgical intensive care unit. She is currently postoperative day 4 after mechanical aortic valve replacement for rheumatic heart disease. She underwent mitral valve replacement 6 years ago. Since surgery the patient's platelet count has fallen from 168,000/mm$^3$ to 56,000/mm$^3$. She has no known arterial or venous thromboses currently, although her heparin–platelet factor 4 antibody is positive. She remains on heparin by intravenous infusion at 1800 U/h. Which of the following drugs can be safely used without potential cross-reactivity with heparin in this patient?

A. Dermatan sulfate
B. Lepirudin
C. Argatroban
D. A and C
E. B and D

**III-61.** A 78-year-old African-American female presents to the emergency department with acute onset of dense left-sided hemiparesis and aphasia. A thrombotic cerebrovascular accident was confirmed by CT of the head. She has a prior history of left middle cerebral artery stroke. Blood pressure at presentation is 160/96. She receives 60 mg (0.9 mg/kg) of tissue-type plasminogen activator intravenously over 60 min. Approximately 2 h after administration the patient is noted to have worsening neurologic status and becomes obtunded. Follow-up CT of the head shows hemorrhagic conversion of the ischemic territory. All the following are risk factors for intracranial bleeding with thrombolysis *except*

A. female sex
B. systolic blood pressure >140 mmHg
C. diastolic blood pressure >90
D. African-American ethnicity
E. prior history of stroke

**III-62.** A 36-year-old female presents 1 week after a cholecystectomy, complaining of calf pain with walking. Physical examination reveals a positive Homan's sign with pain and redness of the right extremity below the knee. Doppler ultrasonography reveals evidence of deep venous thrombosis in the calf without proximal extension. What advice and/or treatment do you prescribe?

**III-62.** *(Continued)*

A. Repeat ultrasonography twice weekly for the next 2 weeks with initiation of anticoagulation if proximal extension is identified.

B. Initiate therapy with low-molecular-weight heparin and warfarin as proximal extension of the clot is inevitable.

C. No treatment is necessary unless the patient develops increasing symptoms.

D. If treatment is introduced, therapy should be continued for 12 months.

E. Catheter-directed thrombolysis is indicated to decrease the risk of postphlebitic syndrome.

**III-63.** A 63-year-old female is seen in clinic to follow up on test results for an unexplained anemia. As part of that testing the patient had a serum protein electrophoresis sent as well as a bone marrow biopsy. Laboratory studies were consistent with anemia of chronic disease, but incidental note was made of a monoclonal gammopathy measuring 0.5 g/dL and 5% plasma cells on bone marrow biopsy. What do you tell this patient about her disease?

A. There is no need for serial quantitative measurements of the monoclonal protein.

B. Her risk of developing multiple myeloma is approximately 10% per year.

C. The presence of Bence-Jones proteinuria predicts the likelihood of progression to multiple myeloma.

D. Her long-term survival is equal to that of age-matched controls.

E. She should initiate therapy with melphalan and prednisone.

**III-64.** A 64-year-old male presents to the emergency department with a chief complaint of blurred vision and headache. He has had a recent prolonged illness that has included symptoms of fatigue and recurrent upper respiratory infections. In addition, the patient has had a 30-lb weight loss and a feeling of abdominal fullness. On physical examination the patient is alert initially but becomes progressively obtunded over 12 h. The ophthalmologic examination reveals dilation of the retinal veins. He is noted to have hepatosplenomegaly and diffuse lymphadenopathy. The initial laboratory results include a hemoglobin of 7.2 mg/dL, white blood cell count of 8,300/$\mu$L, and platelets of 140,000/$\mu$L. He has normal renal function. The extended panel shows a total protein of 11.2 g/dL, an albumin of 3.3 g/dL, a total bilirubin of 3.2 mg/dL, and a direct bilirubin 0.4 mg/dL. A direct Coombs' test is positive. A peripheral blood smear shows rouleaux formation and spherocytosis. There is a plasma viscosity of 5.3 CP. Serum protein electrophoresis shows a monoclonal gammopathy measuring 6 g/dL. What is the most likely diagnosis?

**III-64.** *(Continued)*

A. Multiple myeloma

B. POEMS syndrome

C. Waldenström's macroglobulinemia

D. Angioimmunoblastic lymphoma

E. Multicentric Castleman's disease

**III-65.** What is the most appropriate treatment at this time?

A. Plasmapheresis

B. Rituximab

C. Fludarabine

D. Allogeneic bone marrow transplantation

E. Chemotherapy with cyclophosphamide, prednisone, doxorubicin, and vincristine

**III-66.** A 34-year-old female presents complaining of abdominal fullness in the right upper quadrant that has been present for 2 months. More recently she has noted a discrete mass in this area. She otherwise has no symptoms, including no fevers, chills, jaundice, or weight loss. The patient's only medication is oral contraceptive pills. She is originally from Alabama and has not traveled outside the United States. She does not use illicit drugs and drinks alcohol approximately once monthly. She received a blood transfusion at age 6 after a bicycle accident that resulted in a splenic rupture. On physical examination a 7-cm mass is palpated in the right upper quadrant. Hepatitis C antibody is negative, and the patient has a positive antibody for hepatitis B surface antigen. On contrast-enhanced CT, a mass measuring 7 cm by 7 cm is noted in the right lobe of the liver. What is the next step in the management of this patient?

A. Discontinuation of oral contraceptives and observation

B. Percutaneous needle biopsy of the lesion

C. Surgical removal of the lesion

D. Referral for liver transplantation

E. Treatment with oral metronidazole

**III-67.** A patient with hepatocellular carcinoma may be considered for liver transplantation if the patient meets which of the following criteria?

A. Single lesion less than 3 cm

B. Fewer than three lesions measuring less than 3 cm

C. Single lesion less than 5 cm

D. A and B

E. B and C

**III-68.** A 58-year-old female presents to the emergency department with symptoms of nausea, vomiting, and diarrhea after eating chicken salad at a picnic. The patient was diagnosed with a case of self-limited *Staphylococcus aureus* food poisoning. However, the patient has an abdominal radiogram showing diffuse calcification of the gallbladder wall. What is the next step in the treatment of this patient?

**III-68.** *(Continued)*

   A.  Watchful waiting
   B.  Referral for biopsy
   C.  Laparoscopic cholecystectomy
   D.  Open cholecystectomy
   E.  Radiation therapy

**III-69.** A 20-year-old female presents with anemia caused by menorrhagia. She has known type III von Willebrand's disease (vWD). Which of the following statements regarding this disease is not true?

   A.  This disorder is inherited in an autosomal dominant manner.
   B.  This patient has a marked reduction in factor VIII activity.
   C.  Type III von Willebrand's disease is the rarest type of vWD.
   D.  Ristocetin cofactor assay shows a marked reduction in platelet aggregation.
   E.  In addition to mucosal bleeding, these patients are at increased risk of hemarthroses.

**III-70.** A 68-year-old male presents with subacute onset of shortness of breath and is found to have a new anemia. The patient's hematologic studies and peripheral blood smear are shown below.

| | |
|---|---|
| Hemoglobin: | 6.3 g/dL |
| Hematocrit: | 19.7% |
| RDW: | 27.2% |
| Mean corpuscular volume | 107.7 fL |
| Total bilirubin: | 3.3 mg/dL |
| Direct bilirubin: | 0.8 mg/dL |
| Reticulocyte count: | 11.8% |
| Direct Coombs' test: | Positive for anti-IgG, negative for anti-C3 |

There is no evidence of cold agglutinins. The patient has a history of hypertension and coronary artery disease. His current medications include $\alpha$-methyldopa, atenolol, irbesartan, and aspirin. What is the most appropriate next step in the management of this patient?

   A.  Plasmapheresis
   B.  Discontinuation of irbesartan and initiation of prednisone
   C.  Discontinuation of $\alpha$-methyldopa and initiation of prednisone
   D.  Danazol
   E.  Treatment with antibiotics for *Mycoplasma pneumoniae*

**III-71.** A 42-year-old female presents for evaluation of a low platelet count found incidentally on a complete blood count drawn for an insurance evaluation. She denies easy bruising, gingival bleeding, or menorrhagia. She has not had any notable illnesses recently. She does not drink al-

**III-71.** *(Continued)*

cohol. The physical examination is unremarkable. There is no hepatosplenomegaly or lymphadenopathy. Laboratory studies reveal a platelet count of 19,000/$\mu$L, a hematocrit of 37%, and a white blood cell count of 7,660/$\mu$L. There are no abnormal cells on the differential. HIV antibody is positive. The CD4 count is 264/$\mu$L with a viral load of 250,000 copies. Bone marrow biopsy shows increased numbers of megakaryocytes without evidence of viral, fungal, or mycobacterial infection. What is the best way to treat the thrombocytopenia?

   A.  Prednisone 60 mg daily
   B.  Platelet transfusion
   C.  No treatment, as the patient has no symptoms of bleeding
   D.  Initiation of antiretroviral therapy with a regimen containing zidovudine
   E.  Intravenous immunoglobulin for 5 days

**III-72.** Which of the following statements regarding the primary treatment of breast cancer is not true?

   A.  Lumpectomy with radiation has equivalent survival to mastectomy with radiation.
   B.  Lumpectomy without radiation has equivalent survival to mastectomy without radiation.
   C.  Most women with primary breast cancer should receive a mastectomy.
   D.  Postlumpectomy nodal radiation improves 10-year survival.
   E.  Postlumpectomy radiation reduces the risk of local recurrence.

**III-73.** All the following patients with breast cancer should receive adjuvant chemotherapy *except*

   A.  a 28-year-old premenopausal female with a positive family history and an 8-mm tumor with negative axillary lymph nodes
   B.  a 35-year-old premenopausal female with a 2.2-cm tumor and negative axillary lymph nodes
   C.  a 40-year-old premenopausal female with a 1.8-cm tumor and one positive axillary lymph node
   D.  a 63-year-old postmenopausal female with a 2.2-cm tumor and one positive axillary lymph node
   E.  a 74-year-old postmenopausal female with a 3.5-cm tumor and negative axillary lymph nodes

**III-74.** Which of the following tumor characteristics confers a poor prognosis in patients with breast cancer?

   A.  Estrogen receptor-positive
   B.  Good nuclear grade
   C.  Low proportion of cells in S-phase
   D.  Overexpression of *erbB2 (HER-2/neu)*
   E.  Progesterone receptor-positive

**III-75.** A 44-year-old male seeks medical attention for recurrent headaches, particularly with exertion. The physical examination is notable for blood pressure of 150/95 mmHg, heart rate of 72/min, and a ruddy complexion. Hematocrit is 54%, and a chromium-labeled blood study shows increased red blood cell mass. The serum erythropoietin level is low. Based on this information, the most likely diagnosis is

A. high-affinity hemoglobinopathy
B. polycythemia vera
C. pulmonary arteriovenous (AV) malformation
D. smoker's polycythemia
E. spurious polycythemia

**III-76.** A 73-year-old male presents to the clinic with 3 months of increasing back pain. He localizes the pain to the lumbar spine and states that the pain is worst at night while he is lying in bed. It is improved during the day with mobilization. Past history is notable only for hypertension and remote cigarette smoking. Physical examination is normal. Laboratory studies are notable for an elevated alkaline phosphatase. A lumbar radiogram shows a lytic lesion in the L3 vertebra. Which of the following malignancies is most likely?

A. Gastric carcinoma
B. Non-small cell lung cancer
C. Osteosarcoma
D. Pancreatic carcinoma
E. Thyroid carcinoma

**III-77.** A 63-year-old male is brought to the physician by his wife because she is worried about his eyes. On questioning he reports right shoulder pain at rest and states that for approximately 2 months he has had some flushing and sweating on the right side of the face; however, that gradually decreased approximately 3 weeks ago. Now he notes that when he exercises on the treadmill, the right side of his face sweats less than the left side does. Past medical history is significant for hypertension and hypercholesterolemia. He smoked one pack of cigarettes a day until 3 years ago. His medications include hydrochlorothiazide, atenolol, and simvastatin. Physical examination is normal except for the findings shown below. Which of the following diagnostic tests is most likely to explain the history and physical findings?

A. CT scan of the chest
B. CT scan of the orbit/sinus
C. Electromyogram (EMG) of the right neck/shoulder
D. MRI of the brainstem
E. Myelogram of the cervical spine

**III-78.** A 52-year-old female is evaluated for abdominal swelling with a computed tomogram that shows ascites and likely peritoneal studding of tumor but no other ab-

**III-78.** *(Continued)*
normality. Paracentesis shows adenocarcinoma but cannot be further differentiated by the pathologist. A thorough physical examination, including breast and pelvic examination, shows no abnormality. CA-125 levels are elevated. Pelvic ultrasound and mammography are normal. Which of the following statements is true?

A. Compared with other women with known ovarian cancer at a similar stage, this patient can be expected to have a less than average survival.
B. Debulking surgery is indicated.
C. Surgical debulking plus cisplatin and paclitaxel is indicated.
D. Bilateral mastectomy and bilateral oophorectomy will improve survival.
E. Fewer than 1% of patients with this disorder will remain disease-free 2 years after treatment.

**III-79.** A 75-year-old male with a history of alcohol and tobacco abuse is seen for evaluation of a lump in the neck. Physical examination shows normal head, eyes, ears, nose, and throat. His neck has a 3- by 3-cm fixed, hard lymph node in the anterior cervical chain. Lungs are normal. Excisional biopsy of the lymph node shows squamous cell carcinoma. Which of the following is the most appropriate recommendation?

A. Hospice placement
B. Bilateral mammogram
C. Chest CT
D. Referral to otolaryngology
E. Empirical adriamycin and cyclophosphamide

**III-80.** A 48-year-old male is referred for evaluation by an acute care center because of a nodule on chest radiography. Three weeks ago he was diagnosed with pneumonia after reporting 3 days of fever, cough, and sputum production. The chest radiogram showed a small right lower lobe alveolar infiltrate and a left upper lobe 1.5-cm round nodule. He was treated with antibiotics and is now asymptomatic. A repeat chest radiogram shows that the right lower lobe pneumonia is resolved, but the nodule is still present. He is asymptomatic. He smoked one pack of cigarettes per day for 25 years and quit 3 years ago. He never had a prior chest radiogram. CT scan shows that the nodule is 1.5 by 1.7 cm and is located centrally in the left upper lobe, has no calcification, and has slightly scalloped edges. There is no mediastinal adenopathy or pleural effusion. Which of the following is the appropriate next step in his management?

A. Bronchoscopy
B. Mediastinoscopy
C. MRI scan
D. $^{18}$FDG PET scan
E. Repeat chest CT in 6 months

**III-81.** A 40-year-old male presents to the emergency room with headaches and nausea for 1 week. The patient's past medical history is unremarkable. He takes a multivitamin and atorvastatin. The examination is notable for pale conjunctiva and numerous petechiae on the skin and extremities. The spleen is not palpable. The neurologic examination is nonfocal. Laboratory examination shows a platelet count of 11,000/$\mu$L and a hematocrit of 23%. Other abnormalities include an elevated lactic dehydrogenase level and a low serum haptoglobin. Serum creatinine is normal. INR is 1.1, and the aPTT ratio is 1.0. A peripheral blood smear is shown in Figure III-81 (Color Atlas). What is the diagnosis?

A. Autoimmune hemolytic anemia
B. Disseminated intravascular coagulation (DIC)
C. Immune-mediated thrombocytopenia (ITP)
D. Paroxysmal nocturnal hemoglobinuria
E. Thrombotic thrombocytopenic purpura

**III-82.** A 22-year-old recent college graduate presents to her new primary care physician for an initial evaluation. She has been sexually active since age 19 with two to four partners per year and uses oral contraceptives. Her medical records from college show that 1 year ago she had her first Pap smear, which was normal. Her mother died at age 48 of cervical cancer. She is asymptomatic with normal menstrual periods and has a normal physical examination. Based on this information, you recommend which of the following?

A. Cervical smear for human papilloma virus (HPV) testing
B. Cervical smear for HSV testing
C. Colonoscopy
D. Pap smear now
E. Pap smear in 3 years

**III-83.** A 58-year-old male presents with fatigue. The physical examination is normal except for the presence of splenomegaly. A complete blood count (CBC) discloses hematocrit 29%, platelet count 90,000/$\mu$L, white blood cells (WBCs) 2700/$\mu$L, and an essentially normal red cell morphology (differential: 12% monocytes, 12% granulocytes, 76% lymphocytes). A bone marrow aspirate and a biopsy were performed. The aspirate was dry, and the biopsy results are pending. Based on the available information, the most likely diagnosis in this case is

A. chronic lymphocytic leukemia (CLL)
B. hairy cell leukemia
C. chronic myeloid leukemia (CML)
D. myelofibrosis
E. multiple myeloma

**III-84.** Coumarin-induced skin necrosis is occasionally associated with the institution of oral anticoagulants in patients with

**III-84.** *(Continued)*
A. antithrombin III deficiency
B. protein C deficiency
C. factor VIII deficiency
D. plasminogen deficiency
E. dysfibrinogenemias

**III-85.** An 18-year-old black male undergoing a physical examination before playing college sports is found to have a normal CBC except that the MCV is 72 fL. Subsequent testing reveals a normal metabisulfite test and a normal hemoglobin electrophoresis. Which of the following conditions most likely accounts for these findings?

A. Hemoglobin E trait
B. Sickle C disease
C. Sickle $\beta$ thalassemia
D. $\beta$-Thalassemia trait
E. $\alpha$-Thalassemia trait

**III-86.** Which of the following statements describes the relationship between testicular tumors and serum markers?

A. Pure seminomas produce $\alpha$ fetoprotein (AFP) or beta human chorionic gonadotropin ($\beta$-hCG) in more than 90% of cases.
B. More than 40% of nonseminomatous germ cell tumors produce no cell markers.
C. Both $\beta$-hCG and AFP should be measured in following the progress of a tumor.
D. Measurement of tumor markers the day after surgery for localized disease is useful in determining completeness of the resection.
E. $\beta$-hCG is limited in its usefulness as a marker because it is identical to human luteinizing hormone.

**III-87.** Two years ago a 68-year-old male was found to have a prostate nodule on routine examination. Biopsy revealed poorly differentiated prostatic adenocarcinoma; staging studies failed to reveal any evidence of extraprostatic spread. Because of a desire to maintain potency, the patient opted for radiation therapy as the primary treatment. Except for requiring lower extremity revascularization for intractable claudication, he did well until recently, when he developed pain in the right hip. Prostate-specific antigen was elevated. Bone scan revealed areas of positive uptake in the pelvis and ribs (not present on the original staging study). The patient expresses a desire not to have a bilateral orchiectomy "unless it would significantly improve my quality of life or survival compared with other therapies."

The most appropriate strategy at this point is to

A. biopsy one of the bony lesions
B. administer cisplatin and 5-fluorouracil
C. administer leuprolide and flutamide

**III-87.** *(Continued)*

  D.   administer diethylstilbestrol (DES) at a low dose

  E.   perform an orchiectomy

**III-88.** Which of the following statements regarding ovarian cancer is correct?

  A.   A surgical debulking procedure is unhelpful.

  B.   Nulliparity is a risk factor.

  C.   A history of cervical cancer is a risk factor.

  D.   Stromal cell and germ cell tumors of the ovary are the most common histologic subtypes.

  E.   Histologic grade is not an important prognostic factor.

**III-89.** Each condition listed below is associated with an increased risk of cancer of the esophagus. Which one is most closely linked to adenocarcinoma of the esophagus?

  A.   Achalasia

  B.   Smoking

  C.   Barrett's esophagus

  D.   Tylosis

  E.   Alcoholism

**III-90.** Which of the following is correct regarding small-cell lung cancer compared with non-small cell lung cancer?

  A.   Small-cell lung cancer is more radiosensitive.

  B.   Small-cell lung cancer is less chemosensitive.

  C.   Small-cell lung cancer is more likely to present peripherally in the lung.

  D.   Small-cell lung cancer is derived from an alveolar cell.

  E.   Bone marrow involvement is more common in non-small cell lung cancer.

**III-91.** A 28-year-old male with embryonal carcinoma of the testicle is undergoing chemotherapy with a regimen containing bleomycin, etoposide, and cisplatin. Toxicity to which one of the following organs bears close scrutiny in this situation?

  A.   Brain

  B.   Eye

  C.   Lungs

  D.   Liver

  E.   Heart

**III-92.** A 65-year-old male with a long history of smoking presents with progressive weakness of both legs. Specifically, he has had difficulty arising from a sitting position. The patient also complains of a cough. Physical examination is remarkable for a mildly chronically ill-appearing male with weakness of the proximal muscles of the arms and legs. Chest x-ray reveals a large right hilar mass. Which tumor-associated pathophysiologic abnormality

**III-92.** *(Continued)*

most likely accounts for the patient's neurologic symptoms?

  A.   Small-cell lung cancer and abnormalities in the presynaptic component of neuromuscular transmission

  B.   Non-small cell lung cancer and abnormalities in the presynaptic component of neuromuscular transmission

  C.   Small-cell lung cancer and abnormalities of axonal transmission

  D.   Non-small cell lung cancer and abnormalities of axonal transmission

  E.   Non-Hodgkin's lymphoma and abnormalities at the motor neuron

**III-93.** A 55-year-old female presents with progressive incoordination. Physical examination is remarkable for nystagmus, mild dysarthria, and past-pointing on finger-to-nose testing. She also has an unsteady gait. MRI reveals atrophy of both lobes of the cerebellum. Serologic evaluation reveals the presence of anti-Yo antibody. Which of the following is the most likely cause of this clinical syndrome?

  A.   Non-small cell cancer of the lung

  B.   Small-cell cancer of the lung

  C.   Breast cancer

  D.   Non-Hodgkin's lymphoma

  E.   Colon cancer

**III-94.** The most common cause of high serum calcium in a patient with a known cancer is

  A.   ectopic production of parathyroid hormone

  B.   direct destruction of bone by tumor cells

  C.   local production of tumor necrosis factor and IL-6 by bony metastasis

  D.   high levels of 1,25-hydroxyvitamin D

  E.   production of parathyroid hormone–like substance

**III-95.** A 43-year-old male presents with severe midthoracic back pain. His past medical history is remarkable for the removal of a malignant melanoma (depth 1.5 mm) approximately 3 years ago. The patient's back pain is severe and has been waking him up at night over the last week. Physical examination is unremarkable. Plain films of the spine reveal loss of the left pedicle in the fifth thoracic vertebra. Magnetic resonance images are obtained, and the patient is begun on glucocorticoids. Which of the following treatment modalities is most appropriate in this situation?

  A.   Surgery

  B.   Radiation therapy

  C.   Chemotherapy

  D.   Hormonal therapy

  E.   Immunotherapy

**III-96.** A 65-year-old male develops superficial thrombophlebitis in multiple sites, including the arms and chest. He has had several episodes in the last couple of months, each of which lasted a few days. Which of the following neoplasms is most closely associated with this patient's clinical problem?

A. Prostate carcinoma
B. Lung carcinoma
C. Pancreatic carcinoma
D. Acute promyelocytic leukemia
E. Paroxysmal nocturnal hemoglobinuria

**III-97.** Which of the following statements best characterizes the hemolysis associated with glucose-6-phosphate dehydrogenase (G6PD) deficiency?

A. It is more severe in affected blacks than in affected persons of Mediterranean ancestry.
B. It is more severe in females than in males.
C. It causes the appearance of Heinz bodies on Wright staining of a peripheral smear.
D. It most often is precipitated by infection.
E. The best time to perform the diagnostic test is during a hemolytic crisis.

**III-98.** A 65-year-old male with a benign past medical history presents to his internist for a routine medical checkup. The physical examination and laboratory studies are normal except for a serum prostate-specific antigen (PSA) value of 8 ng/mL (normal 0 to 3 ng/mL). Which of the following is a true statement about the man's condition?

A. His likelihood of prostate cancer is 75%.
B. If he does have prostate cancer, the disease is likely to be confined to the gland.
C. Assuming there is no evidence of metastatic spread, the patient should undergo a radical prostatectomy.
D. Assuming there is no evidence of spread, the patient should receive radiation therapy to the prostate.
E. The patient should receive therapy with leuprolide and flutamide.

**III-99.** A 28-year-old male presents with chest pain. Chest x-ray reveals a large mediastinal mass. Abdominal CT reveals periaortic lymphadenopathy. Physical examination, including examination of the testes, is negative. Mediastinoscopic biopsy reveals poorly differentiated carcinoma. Which of the following laboratory tests is most likely to be positive?

A. Prostate-specific antigen (PSA)
B. Beta human chorionic gonadotropin ($\beta$-hCG)
C. Carcinoembryonic antigen (CEA)
D. CA-125
E. CA19-9

**III-100.** Which of the following is likely to be a neoplasm of T-lymphocyte lineage?

A. Chronic lymphocytic leukemia (CLL)
B. Follicular lymphomas
C. Burkitt's lymphoma
D. Mycosis fungoides
E. Small lymphocytic (well-differentiated) lymphomas

**III-101.** A 55-year-old Japanese businessman visiting the United States was in excellent health until 6 months ago, when he first noted mild upper abdominal fullness after meals. On examination the man is noted to have hyperpigmented, heaped-up velvety lesions confined to the neck, axillae, and groin. Which of the following conditions is associated with the skin findings (see color Fig. III-101)?

A. Non-Hodgkin's lymphoma
B. Anorexia nervosa
C. Acute leukemia
D. Adenocarcinoma of the stomach
E. Addison's disease

# III. ONCOLOGY AND HEMATOLOGY

## ANSWERS

**III-1. The answer is B.** *(Chap. 70)* In 25% of selected patients with colon cancer, fewer than five hepatic metastases in one lobe, and no evidence of other metastatic disease, hepatic lobectomy may result in prolonged disease-free survival. 5-Fluorouracil, leucovorin, and irinotecan may prolong the median survival of patients with unresectable metastatic disease from approximately 14 to 18 months. BCG vaccine is used as intravesicle treatment for bladder cancer but has no role in the treatment of colon cancer.

**III-2. The answer is A.** *(Chap. 95)* Polycythemia vera (PV) is a clonal disorder that involves a multipotent hematopoietic progenitor cell. Clinically, it is characterized by a proliferation of red blood cells, granulocytes, and platelets. The precise etiology is unknown. Erythropoiesis is regulated by the hormone erythropoietin. Hypoxia is the physiologic stimulus that increases the number of cells that produce erythropoietin. Erythropoietin may be elevated in patients with hormone-secreting tumors. Levels are usually "normal" in patients with hypoxic erythrocytosis. In polycythemia vera, however, because erythrocytosis occurs independently of erythropoietin, levels of the hormone are usually low. Therefore, an elevated level is *not* consistent with the diagnosis. Polycythemia is a chronic, indolent disease with a low rate of transformation to acute leukemia, especially in the absence of treatment with radiation or hydroxyurea. Thrombotic complications are the main risk for PV and correlate with the erythrocytosis. Thrombocytosis, although sometimes prominent, does not correlate with the risk of thrombotic complications. Salicylates are useful in treating erythromelalgia but are not indicated in asymptomatic patients. There is no evidence that thrombotic risk is significantly lowered with their use in patients whose hematocrits are appropriately controlled with phlebotomy. Phlebotomy is the mainstay of treatment. Induction of a state of iron deficiency is critical to prevent a reexpansion of the red blood cell mass. Chemotherapeutics and other agents are useful in cases of symptomatic splenomegaly. Their use is limited by side effects, and there is a risk of leukemogenesis with hydroxyurea.

**III-3. The answer is D.** *(Chaps. 94 and 95)* Chronic idiopathic myelofibrosis is a clonal disorder of a multipotent hematopoietic progenitor cell of unknown etiology that is characterized by marrow fibrosis, myeloid metaplasia, extramedullary hematopoiesis, and splenomegaly. The peripheral blood smear reflects the features of extramedullary hematopoiesis, with teardrop-shaped red cells, immature myeloid cells, and abnormal platelets. Leukocytes and platelets may both be elevated. The median survival is poor at only 5 years. These patients eventually succumb to increasing organomegaly, infection, and possible transformation to acute leukemia. There is no specific therapy for chronic idiopathic myelofibrosis. Erythropoietin has not been shown to be consistently effective and may exacerbate splenomegaly. Supportive care with red blood cell transfusions is necessary as anemia worsens. Chemotherapy has no role in changing the natural history of the disease. Some newer agents, such as interferon and thalidomide, may play a role, but their place is not clear. Splenectomy may be necessary in symptomatic patients with massive splenomegaly. However, extramedullary hematopoiesis may worsen with rebound thrombocytosis and compensatory hepatomegaly. The only potential curative modality is allogeneic bone marrow transplantation. Morbidity and mortality are high, particularly in older patients. In light of this patient's young age and the presence of three healthy siblings, HLA matching of her siblings is the most reasonable step.

**III-4.** **The answer is B.** *(Chap. 98)* Plasma cell dyscrasias are monoclonal neoplasms within the B lymphocyte lineage. Multiple myeloma is characterized classically by marrow plasmacytosis (>10%), multiple lytic bone lesions, and a serum and/or urine monoclonal gammopathy. The prognosis varies with the extent of the disease and organ dysfunction, and treatment is often glucocorticoids together with thalidomide and/or alkylating agents. Bone pain is typically exacerbated with movement in myeloma patients and responds well to opiate analgesics, bisphosphonates, and control of tumor bulk. Stem cell transplantation may confer a survival benefit in selected patients. However, this patient has a variant of myeloma: solitary bone plasmacytoma. This is characterized by a local collection of plasma cells without a marrow plasmacytosis. M protein is often absent, and as a result, organ function is preserved. Solitary plasmacytoma, either of bone or in an extramedullary site, has an excellent long-term prognosis. It is highly responsive to radiotherapy. These patients have prolonged disease-free survival. Relapse at another site may be treated with another dose of local radiotherapy. Development of marrow plasmacytosis or frank myeloma requires systemic therapy. In this patient there is no evidence of any disease besides the one isolated spot in the pelvis; therefore, the treatment modality of choice is radiation therapy.

**III-5.** **The answer is E.** *(Chap. 98)* MGUS is characterized by the presence of an M component. By definition, there is no significant marrow plasmacytosis, anemia, renal dysfunction, bone lesions, or hypercalcemia. MGUS is extremely common, affecting about 1% of individuals over age 50 and 10% of individuals over age 75. Observational studies have indicated that about 1% of these patients per year will develop myeloma. However, for the remainder, the prognosis is excellent with median survival only 2 years shorter than that of age-matched controls. There is no proven benefit to treatment with any modality in patients with MGUS.

**III-6.** **The answer is A.** *(Chap. 98)* Waldenström's macroglobulinemia is characterized by a malignancy of lymphoplasmacytoid cells that secrete IgM. Clinical features include lymphadenopathy, hepatosplenomegaly, anemia, neuropathy, and symptoms related to hyperviscosity syndrome. These symptoms include weakness, fatigue, visual disturbances, mental status changes, headache, and transient paresis. Hyperviscosity syndrome is more common in patients with Waldenström's because of the size of the IgM. Peripheral blood smear often shows a normocytic, normochromic anemia. Rouleaux are a common feature. A positive Coombs' test and cryoglobulins may be present. Treatment includes therapy acutely for symptoms of hyperviscosity. A plasma viscosity level should be checked and therapeutic plasmapheresis should be initiated regardless of the viscosity level if the symptoms are significant. Therapy with purine nucleoside agents such as cladribine and fludarabine is effective. Monoclonal antibodies to CD20 (rituximab) may result in responses. Waldenström's macroglobulinemia does not produce bone lesions or hypercalcemia; therefore, therapy with a bisphosphonate such as zoledronic acid is unnecessary.

**III-7.** **The answer is D.** *(Chap. 82)* Testicular cancer occurs most commonly in the second and third decades of life. The treatment depends on the underlying pathology and the stage of the disease. Germ cell tumors are divided into seminomatous and nonseminomatous subtypes. Although the pathology of this patient's tumor was seminoma, the presence of AFP is suggestive of occult nonseminomatous components. If there are any nonseminomatous components, the treatment follows that of a nonseminomatous germ cell tumor. This patient therefore has a clinical stage I nonseminomatous germ cell tumor. As his AFP returned to normal after orchiectomy, there is no obvious occult disease. However, between 20 and 50% of these patients will have disease in the retroperitoneal lymph nodes. Because numerous trials have indicated no survival difference in this cohort between observation and RPLND and because of the potential side effects of RPLND, either approach is reasonable. Radiation therapy is the appropriate choice for stage I and stage II seminoma. It has no role in nonseminomatous lesions. Adjuvant chemotherapy is not indicated in early-stage testicular cancer. Hormonal therapy is effective for prostate cancer and receptor-positive breast cancer but has no role in testicular cancer. PET scan has no currently defined clinical role.

**III-8.   The answer is C.**   *(Chap. 94)*   Pure red cell aplasia (PRCA) is a condition characterized by the absence of reticulocytes and erythroid precursors. A variety of conditions may cause PRCA. It may be idiopathic. It may be associated with certain medications, such as trimethoprim-sulfamethoxazole (TMP-SMX) and phenytoin. It can be associated with a variety of neoplasms, either as a precursor to a hematologic malignancy such as leukemia or myelodysplasia or as part of an autoimmune phenomenon, as in the case of thymoma. Infections also may cause a pure red cell aplasia. Parvovirus B19 is a single-strand DNA virus that is associated with erythema infectiosum, or fifth disease in children. It is also associated with arthropathy and a flulike illness in adults. It is thought to attack the P antigen on proerythroblasts directly. Patients with a chronic hemolytic anemia, such as sickle cell disease, or with an immunodeficiency are less able to tolerate a transient drop in reticulocytes as their red blood cells do not survive in the peripheral blood for an adequate period. In this patient, her daughter had an illness before the appearance of her symptoms. It is reasonable to check her parvovirus IgM titers. If they are positive, a dose of intravenous immunoglobulin is indicated. Because her laboratories and smear are not suggestive of dramatic sickling, an exchange transfusion is not indicated. Immunosuppression with prednisone and/or cyclosporine may be indicated if another etiology of the PRCA is identified. However, that would not be the next step. Similarly, a bone marrow transplant might be a consideration in a young patient with myelodysplasia or leukemia, but there is no evidence of that at this time. Antibiotics have no role in light of her normal white blood cell count and the lack of evidence for a bacterial infection.

**III-9.   The answer is D.**   *(Chap. 102)*   The aPTT involves the factors of the intrinsic pathway of coagulation. Prolongation of the aPTT reflects either a deficiency of one of these factors (factor VIII, IX, XI, XII, etc.) or inhibition of the activity of one of the factors or components of the aPTT assay (i.e., phospholipids). This may be further characterized by the "mixing study," in which the patient's plasma is mixed with pooled plasma. Correction of the aPTT reflects a deficiency of factors that are replaced by the pooled sample. Failure to correct the aPTT reflects the presence of a factor inhibitor or phospholipid inhibitor. Common causes of a failure to correct include the presence of heparin in the sample, factor inhibitors (factor VIII inhibitor being the most common), and the presence of antiphospholipid antibodies. Factor VII is involved in the extrinsic pathway of coagulation. Inhibitors to factor VII would result in prolongation of the prothrombin time.

**III-10.   The answer is B.**   *(Chap. 102)*   Fibrinogen is a 340-kDa dimeric molecule made up of two sets of three covalently linked polypeptide chains. Thrombin cleaves multiple peptides to produce fibrin monomer that factor XIII stabilizes by cross-linking. Although fibrinogen is needed for platelet aggregation and fibrin formation, even severe fibrinogen deficiency such as afibrinogenemia produces mild, rare bleeding episodes, most often after surgery. Dysfibrinogenemia refers to a constellation of disorders that involve mutations that alter the release of fibrinopeptides, affect the rate of polymerization of fibrin monomers, or alter the sites of fibrin cross-linking. Dysfibrinogenemia is either inherited in an autosomal dominant fashion or acquired. Patients with liver disease, hepatomas, AIDS, and lymphoproliferative disorders may develop an acquired form of dysfibrinogenemia. The presence of altered partial thromboplastin time (PTT) and prothrombin time (PT)/INR reflects an abnormality in coagulation from the prothrombinase complex downstream to fibrin. Correction with a mixing study eliminates factor inhibition as a cause of the coagulation disorder. Other causes of prolongation of the PT and PTT include factor deficiencies in factor V or X, afibrinogenemia or dysfibrinogenemia, and consumption of coagulation factors from DIC. The absence of schistocytes from the blood smear makes DIC unlikely. The thrombin time tests the interaction with thrombin directly on fibrinogen. Its prolongation indicates an abnormality with that interaction and suggests a diagnosis of dysfibrinogenemia. Factor XIII deficiency is a bleeding disorder that manifests in childhood and is not consistent with this presentation.

**III-11.   The answer is E.**   *(Chap. 102)*    Vitamin K is a fat-soluble vitamin that plays an essential role in hemostasis. It is absorbed in the small intestine and stored in the liver. It serves as a cofactor in the enzymatic carboxylation of glutamic acid residues on prothrombin-complex proteins. The three major causes of vitamin K deficiency are poor dietary intake, intestinal malabsorption, and liver disease. The prothrombin complex proteins (factors II, VII, IX, and X and protein C and protein S) all decrease with vitamin K deficiency. Factor VII and protein C have the shortest half-lives of these factors and therefore decrease first. Therefore, vitamin K deficiency manifests with prolongation of the prothrombin time first. With severe deficiency, the aPTT will be prolonged as well. Factor VIII is not influenced by vitamin K.

**III-12.   The answer is C.**   *(Chap. 102)*    Lupus anticoagulants cause prolongation of coagulation tests by binding to phospholipids. Although most often encountered in patients with SLE, they may develop in normal individuals. The diagnosis is first suggested by prolongation of coagulation tests. Failure to correct with incubation with normal plasma confirms the presence of a circulating inhibitor. Contrary to the name, patients with LA activity have normal hemostasis and are not predisposed to bleeding. Instead, they are at risk for venous and arterial thromboembolisms. Patients with a history of recurrent unplanned abortions or thrombosis should undergo lifelong anticoagulation. The presence of lupus anticoagulants or anticardiolipin antibodies without a history of thrombosis may be observed as many of these patients will not go on to develop a thrombotic event.

**III-13.   The answer is A.**   *(Chap. 102)*    Factor V Leiden refers to a point mutation in the factor V gene (arginine to glutamine at position 506). This makes the molecule resistant to degradation by activated protein C. This disorder alone may account for up to 25% of inherited prothrombotic states, making it the most common of these disorders. Heterozygosity for this mutation increases an individual's lifetime risk of venous thromboembolism sevenfold. A homozygote has a 20-fold increased risk of thrombosis. Prothrombin gene mutation is probably the second most common condition that causes "hypercoagulability." Antithrombin, protein C, and protein S deficiencies are more rare. Antithrombin complexes with activated coagulation proteins and blocks their biologic activity. Deficiency in antithrombin therefore promotes prolonged activity of coagulation proteins, resulting in thrombosis. Similarly, protein C and protein S are involved in the proteolysis of factors Va and VIIIa, which shuts off fibrin formation. Because proteins C and S are dependent on vitamin K for carboxylation, administration of warfarin anticoagulants may lower the level of proteins C and S more quickly relative to factors II, VII, IX, and X, thereby promoting coagulation. Patients with protein C deficiency may develop warfarin-related skin necrosis.

**III-14.   The answer is B.**   *(Chap. 100)*    GVHD results when immune cells from the donor react against the patient. Syngeneic transplantation involves a donor and a recipient who are immunologically identical (i.e., identical twins). Allogeneic transplantation involves a donor and a recipient who are not immunologically identical. The risk of GVHD is related to the degree of immunologic mismatch. This may be minimized by matching major antigens from the human leukocyte antigen (HLA) molecules, particularly A, B, C, and D. These molecules are closely linked and therefore tend to be inherited as haplotypes, with only rare crossovers. Syngeneic transplantation, although not creating a risk of GVHD, paradoxically offers less chance of a cure for a number of hematologic malignancies. This is thought to relate to a "graft-versus-tumor" effect of the allogeneic transplant.

**III-15.   The answer is D.**   *(Chap. 100)*    Transplant preparative regimens cause a spectrum of acute toxicities. Nausea and vomiting are common. Regimens that include high-dose cyclophosphamide may result in hemorrhagic cystitis. Oral mucositis and alopecia are ubiquitous. Infectious complications are common in the early transplant period, and broad-spectrum antibiotics must be inititated at the first sign of fever regardless of the presence of positive cultures. Approximately 10% of these patients develop venoocculsive disease of the liver. This is related to direct cytotoxic injury to hepatic-venular and sinusoidal endothelium, with the subsequent development of a hypercoagulable state. These symptoms may occur at any time during the first month after transplantation, with a peak incidence around day 16. Clinical symptoms and signs include tender hepatomegaly, ascites, jaundice, and fluid retention. Mortality is high, with progressive hepatic failure culminating in a terminal hepatorenal syndrome. There are no proven therapies. The absence of leukocytes makes leukemic infiltration and graft-versus-host disease less likely. Medications may certainly produce liver disease, but the picture fits better with venoocclusive disease. The absence of gallbladder wall thickening or sonographic Murphy's sign does not support the diagnosis of acalculous cholecystitis.

**III-16.  The answer is E.**  *(Chap. 100)*   In addition to chronic GHVD, there are late complications of bone marrow transplantation that result from the chemotherapy and radiotherapy preparative regimen. Children may experience decreased growth velocity and delay in the development of secondary sex characteristics. Hormone replacement may be necessary. Gonadal dysfunction is common. Men frequently become azoospermic, and women develop ovarian failure. Patients who receive total body irradiation are at risk for cataract formation and thyroid dysfunction. Although cognitive dysfunction may occur in the peritransplant period for many reasons, there is no definitive evidence that dementia occurs at an increased frequency.

**III-17.  The answer is B.**  *(Chap. 100)*   GVHD results from allogeneic T cells that transferred with the donor's stem cells reacted with antigenic targets on host cells. Acute GVHD is defined as developing within the first 3 months after a transplant. Acute GVHD is manifested clinically by a rash, persistent anorexia or diarrhea, and liver disease with increased serum levels of bilirubin, transaminases, and alkaline phosphatase. Biopsy is required for confirmation. The grade of GVHD predicts the prognosis. Recipients from unrelated donors have a much higher rate of GVHD than do matched siblings. This accounts for the much higher mortality from unrelated donor transplants. Depletion of T cells from the donor results in a lower incidence of GVHD. However, it also results in a higher relapse rate, and there is no evidence that this approach improves cure rates in any specific setting. Chronic GVHD occurs in up to 50% of patients who survive more than 6 months after an allogeneic bone marrow transplantation. This disease resembles an autoimmune disorder, with malar rash, sicca syndrome, arthritis, obliterative bronchiolitis, and bile duct degeneration and cholestasis. In most patients chronic GVHD resolves, but it may require years of immunosuppressive treatment before these agents can be withdrawn without disease recurrence.

**III-18.  The answer is C.**  *(Chap. 85)*   Cancer of unknown primary site accounts for about 2% of all cancer diagnoses, with about 24,000 cases in the year 2000. The majority of these patients are older than 60 years of age. Survival is generally dismal, with a median survival between 4 and 11 months. Although there is no universally accepted definition of CUPS syndrome, some important criteria include (1) a biopsy-proven malignancy that is not consistent with a primary tumor at the biopsy site and (2) unrevealing history, physical examination, abdominal and pelvic CT, chest film, initial laboratory values, $\alpha$ fetoprotein, prostate-specific antigen (PSA), $\beta$-hCG levels, and mammography. The most common pathology is adenocarcinoma, followed by poorly differentiated carcinoma. Some groups may have a better prognosis. These groups include patients with an extragonadal germ cell tumor or lymphoma, women with peritoneal carcinomatosis, carcinoma in an axillary lymph node in a female, males with bone metastases and elevated PSA levels, and cervical lymph node metastases with squamous cell pathology. In patients whose pathology cannot yield a primary site and whose clinical scenario does not fit with one of these groups, extensive diagnostic studies do not prolong survival and therefore cannot be recommended. PET scans may identify the primary site but have not been shown to improve survival.

**III-19.**    **The answer is A.**    *(Chap. 90)*    Iron is a critical element in the function of all cells. The major role of iron in mammals is to carry $O_2$ as part of the heme protein. Iron is also critical in certain enzymes, including the cytochrome system in mitochondria. Iron is absorbed in the proximal small bowel. After absorption, it circulates in the plasma bound to transferrin, the iron transport protein. After binding to specific transferrin receptors on the surface of erythroid cells, this iron-transferrin complex is internalized and transported to an acidic endosome, where the iron is released. Within the erythroid cell, iron that is in excess binds to the storage protein apoferritin, forming ferritin. Red blood cell (RBC) life span is approximately 120 days. After that time red blood cells are recognized by the reticuloendothelial (RE) system and undergo phagocytosis. The hemoglobin is broken down, the globin portion of hemoglobin is returned to the amino acid pool, and the iron is presented back to circulating transferrin and recycled. This results in an efficient and highly conserved recycling of iron. Although hemolysis results in increased RBC destruction, this conservation process allows iron to be recovered from the red blood cells efficiently and prevents iron deficiency. In contrast, blood loss anemia results in a loss of total iron from the system. There is no excretory pathway for iron, and the only mechanisms by which iron is lost from the body are blood loss and the loss of epidermal cells from the skin and gut.

**III-20.**    **The answer is D.**    *(Chap. 90)*    Iron deficiency anemia is a condition in which there is anemia and clear evidence of iron deficiency. Initially, a state of negative iron balance occurs during which iron stores become slowly depleted. Serum ferritin may decrease, and the presence of stainable iron on bone marrow preparation decreases. When iron stores are depleted, serum iron begins to fall. TIBC starts to increase, reflecting the presence of circulating unbound transferrin. Once the transferrin saturation falls to 15 to 20%, hemoglobin synthesis is impaired. The peripheral blood smear reveals the presence of microcytic and hypochromic red cells. Reticulocytes may also become hypochromic. Reticulocyte numbers are reduced relative to the level of anemia, reflecting a hypoproduction anemia secondary to iron deficiency. Clinically, these patients exhibit the usual signs of anemia: fatigue, pallor, and reduced exercise capacity. Cheilosis and koilonychia are signs of advanced tissue iron deficiency. Some patients may experience pica, a desire to ingest certain materials, such as ice (pagophagia) and clay (geophagia).

**III-21.**    **The answer is D.**    *(Chap. 90)*    The differential diagnosis of a hypochromic, microcytic anemia is limited. The workup starts with measurement of the serum iron level, total iron-binding capacity, and serum ferritin level. Iron deficiency is distinguished by a low ferritin level, a low serum iron, and an elevated TIBC. Other than iron deficiency, only three other conditions must be considered. The first consists of inherited defects in globin chain synthesis, the thalassemias. In this case iron levels are typically normal. Hemoglobin electrophoresis will often detect an abnormal pattern. The second condition consists of chronic inflammatory states. In this case, the ferritin level is normal or increased and the TIBC is typically lower than normal. Third, sideroblastic anemia, resulting from impaired protoporphyrin synthesis, may result in microcytosis. In this case iron values are normal. Peripheral smear or bone marrow biopsy may yield the diagnosis. Protoporphyrin levels are not useful in this setting. They will be elevated in a number of conditions that impair heme formation, including iron deficiency and lead poisoning.

**III-22.**    **The answer is D.**    *(Chap. 103)*    Aspirin acts by irreversibly inhibiting cyclooxygenase activity in platelets. This prevents thromboxane synthesis and impairs platelet secretion and aggregation. The effects peak at 1 h and last for the duration of the platelets' life span: approximately 1 week. Toxicities include gastrointestinal discomfort, blood loss, and systemic bleeding. Aspirin has a number of convincing indications. It has been shown to reduce morbidity and mortality in patients with acute myocardial infarction (MI), unstable angina, transient ischemic attacks, and stroke. It prevents recurrent cardiovascular events (secondary prevention) in patients with a history of MI or stroke. In patients older than 50 years who have risk factors for coronary heart disease, there is evidence for a primary prevention benefit with aspirin. The risk of thrombosis in patients with atrial fibrillation increases with age, prior events, risk factors for coronary heart disease, and LEFT ventricular dysfunction. Aspirin is indicated in patients with atrial fibrillation who are younger than 65 years of age and have no structural heart disease. In these patients the yearly stroke risk is less than 1%. However, in elderly patients warfarin provides significant risk reduction and should be considered the first-line treatment.

**III-23. The answer is B.** *(Chap. 103)* Antiplatelet and anticoagulant agents act by a variety of mechanisms. Platelet aggregation is dependent initially on the binding of von Willebrand factor and platelet glycoprotein IB. This initiates the release of a variety of molecules, including thromboxane $A_2$ and adenosine diphosphate (ADP), resulting in platelet aggregation. Glycoprotein IIB/IIIa receptors recognize the amino acid sequence that is present in adhesive proteins such as fibrinogen. Coagulation occurs by a convergence of different pathways on the prothrombinase complex, which mediates the conversion of fibrinogen to fibrin, thus forming the clot. Factor Xa and factor Va are two of the essential components of the prothrombinase complex. Abciximab is a monoclonal antibody of human and murine protein that binds to GpIIb/IIIa. It and other inhibitors have been studied extensively in patients with unstable angina, patients with MI, and those undergoing percutaneous coronary intervention. Clopidigrel acts by inhibiting ADP-induced platelet aggregation. It has been evaluated in many of the same settings either in place of or in conjunction with aspirin. Heparin acts to bind factor Xa and activate antithrombin. Low-molecular-weight heparins primarily act through anti–factor Xa activity. Fondaparinux is a synthetic pentasaccharide that causes selective indirect inhibition of factor Xa. Lepirudin and argatroban are direct thrombin inhibitors. They are indicated in patients with heparin-induced thrombocytopenia. Warfarin acts by inhibiting vitamin K–dependent carboxylation of factors II, VII, IX, and X.

**III-24. The answer is C.** *(Chap. 103)* Heparin-induced thrombocytopenia (HIT) is common in patients who receive heparin products. Because the risk of death is significantly increased in patients with HIT type II and thrombosis if no anticoagulation is given, observation or simply discontinuation of heparin is not an option. Although enoxaparin and other low-molecular-weight heparins have less of a propensity to cause HIT, they are cross-reactive in patients who already have HIT and thus are contraindicated. Direct thrombin inhibitors are the treatment of choice. Lepirudin is a recombinant direct thrombin inhibitor. It may be given intravenously or subcutaneously. It is excreted throught the kidney and lacks an antidote. Therefore, it is relatively contraindicated in patients with renal insufficiency. Argatroban is another direct thrombin inhibitor. Because it is hepatically metabolized, it is a reasonable option in patients with HIT and renal insufficiency.

**III-25. The answer is A.** *(Chaps. 94 and 95)* Chronic idiopathic myelofibrosis (MF) follows a natural history of progressive marrow failure with worsening organomegaly and transfusion-dependent anemia. The median survival is only 5 years, far worse than that of polycythemia vera and essential thrombocytosis. Like chronic myeloid leukemia (CML), MF may progress to acute leukemia. This is generally incurable. Complications resulting from organomegaly and extramedullary hematopoiesis dominate the progression of disease. Splenectomy may be required for symptomatic splenomegaly. This will worsen extramedullary hematopoieis, particularly in the liver. Extramedullary hematopoiesis may occur anywhere in the body and cause symptoms related to local growth (e.g., ureteral obstruction from sites near the bladder or kidney). Although hydroxyurea may control organomegaly, the only potentially curative option is allogeneic bone marrow transplantation. This is an option for younger patients (age less than 40 years). However, transplant-related morbidity and mortality are significant, particularly in older patients. Investigational agents such as thalidomide are being studied.

**III-26.   The answer is E.** *(Chap. 95)*   Thrombocytosis may be "primary" or "secondary." Essential thrombocytosis is a myeloproliferative disorder that involves a multipotent hematopoietic progenitor cell. Unfortunately, there is no clonal marker that can reliably distinguish it from more common nonclonal, reactive forms of thrombocytosis. Therefore, the diagnosis is one of exclusion. Common causes of secondary thrombocytosis include infection, inflammatory conditions, malignancy, iron deficiency, hemorrhage, and postsurgical states. Other myeloproliferative disorders, such as CML and myelofibrosis, may result in thrombocytosis. Similarly, myelodysplastic syndromes, particularly the 5q- syndrome, may cause thrombocytosis. Pernicious anemia caused by vitamin $B_{12}$ deficiency does not typically cause thrombocytosis. However, correction of $B_{12}$ deficiency or folate deficiency may cause a "rebound" thrombocytosis. Similarly, cessation of chronic ethanol use may also cause a rebound thrombocytosis.

**III-27.   The answer is D.** *(Chap. 89)*   Cancer is the second leading cause of mortality in the United States. Millions of Americans who are alive today have cancer in their past history. Cardiac toxicity is typically related to prior treatment with anthracycline-based chemotherapy or mediastinal irradiation. This is seen most commonly in patients who have survived Hodgkin's or non-Hodgkin's lymphoma. Anthracycline-related cardiotoxicity is dose-dependent. About 5% of patients who receive more than 550 mg/m² of doxorubicin will develop congestive heart failure (CHF). Rates are higher in those with other cardiac risk factors and those who have received mediastinal irradiation. Unfortunately, anthracycline-related CHF is typically not reversible. Intracellular chelators or liposomal formulations of the chemotherapy may prevent cardiotoxicity, but their impact on cure rates is unclear. Radiation has both acute and chronic effects on the heart. It may result in acute and chronic pericarditis, myocardial fibrosis, and accelerated atherosclerosis. The mean time to onset of "acute" pericarditis is 9 months after treatment, and so caretakers must be vigilant. Similarly, chronic pericarditis may manifest years later.

**III-28.   The answer is D.** *(Chap. 89)*   The focus of cancer care is cure. Many individuals who are fortunate enough to survive the malignancy will nevertheless bear chronic stigmata, both psychological and medical, of the treatment. Anthracyclines, which are used frequently in the treatment of breast cancer, Hodgkin's disease, lymphoma, and leukemia, are toxic to the myocardium and, at high doses, can lead to heart failure. Bleomycin results in pulmonary toxicity. Pulmonary fibrosis and pulmonary venoocclusive disease may result. Liver dysfunction is common with a number of chemotherapy agents. However, cisplatin primarily causes renal toxicity and acute renal failure. It may also cause neuropathy and hearing loss, but liver dysfunction is not a common complication. Ifosfamide may cause significant neurologic toxicity and renal failure. Also, it may cause a proximal tubular defect resembling Fanconi syndrome. Cyclophosphamide may result in cystitis and increases the long-term risk of bladder cancer. Administration of mesna ameliorates but does not completely eliminate this risk.

**III-29.   The answer is C.** *(Chap. 89)*   Long-term complications of cancer treatment are common. Because the care of cured oncology patients often is the responsibility of primary care specialists, awareness of potential long-term complications is crucial. Patients treated with radiation therapy have a significantly increased risk of developing second solid tumors, usually in or adjacent to the radiation field. Some populations followed for 25 years or more have more than a 25% chance of developing a second treatment-related tumor. The risk of hematologic malignancy is much lower. Tobacco poses a risk of malignancy, particularly lung, bladder, esophageal, and head and neck cancer. It does not pose a significant risk for leukemia. Lynch syndrome refers to genetic defects in mismatch repair that predispose to a variety of malignancies. It encompasses the hereditary nonpolyposis colon cancer syndrome. Establishment of the familial nature of the disorder often requires identification of multiple individuals with cancer in different generations. Certain chemotherapeutics pose risks for myelodysplasia and acute leukemia. Patients treated with alkylating agents in combination with radiation therapy may develop malignant leukemic cells that typically carry deletions in chromosome 5 or 7. The peak incidence is 4 to 6 years after treatment. Topoisomerase II inhibitors used at high doses may result in leukemias showing defects in particular chromosomes (e.g., 11q23). The incidence of leukemia in this situation peaks 1 to 3 years after treatment.

**III-30.    The answer is D.**    *(Chap. 88)*    This patient has superior vena cava syndrome (SVCS). The diagnosis of SVCS is a clinical one. It involves obstruction of the SVC, most commonly by malignant tumors. Rarer causes include benign tumors, aortic aneurysm, thyroid enlargement, and fibrosing mediastinitis. The most common malignancy is lung cancer, particularly squamous cell and small-cell lung cancer. In younger patients lymphoma is the most common cause. Symptoms include neck and facial swelling, dyspnea, and cough. Other symptoms include hoarseness, headaches, nasal congestion, hemoptysis, dysphagia, dizziness, and syncope. Cardiorespiratory symptoms at rest suggest significant airway and vascular obstruction. Upper airway obstruction poses an immediate risk. Bronchoscopy is mandatory if upper airway obstruction is suspected. Interventional radiology may involve intravascular stenting in selected cases. Early consultation is reasonable. Radiation is the mainstay of non-small cell lung cancer treatment. Early consultation is critical as significant palliation may occur if it is begun early. Glucocorticoids are useful in the treatment of lymphoma and are often begun before tissue diagnosis. Although chemotherapy is potentially curative in limited-stage small-cell lung cancer and lymphoma, pathologic diagnosis is mandatory before the administration of chemotherapy as it is less effective in non-small cell lung cancer and other solid tumors.

**III-31.    The answer is D.**    *(Chap. 88)*    Back pain is an extremely common occurrence. Normally, the presence of back pain in a young woman would not prompt further evaluation. However, concerning features here are the lack of trauma or exertion to explain the onset of pain and the prior history of malignancy. Patients with cancer who develop back pain must be evaluated for spinal cord compression as quickly as possible. Symptoms may precede neurologic changes by many weeks to months. Treatment is far more successful in ambulatory patients with minimal symptoms than it is in patients with significant neurologic compromise. Indeed, only 10% of patients with paraplegia recover the ability to walk. Conservative measures such as observations, serial examinations, and physical therapy are therefore not options. Imaging of the spine should be done. Plain films may show obvious erosion of the bony architecture. Bone scans may show metabolic changes throughout the spine. However, their sensitivity in evaluating the spinal cord is limited. For proper visualization of the spinal cord and nerve roots, an MRI of the spine is mandatory. If evidence of neurologic compromise develops or metastatic disease is definitively identified, glucocorticoids are required and consultation with the radiation oncology department is necessary. In tumors that are less radiosensitive or in selected patients, surgical laminectomy may be considered.

**III-32.    The answer is A.**    *(Chap. 88)*    About 25% of patients with cancer die with intracranial metastases. Symptoms may relate to parenchymal or leptomeningeal involvement. The signs and symptoms of metastatic brain tumor are similar to those of other intracranial expanding lesions: headache, nausea, vomiting, behavioral changes, seizures, and focal neurologic deficits. Three percent to 8% of patients with cancer develop a tumor involving the leptomeninges. These patients typically present with multifocal neurologic signs and symptoms. Signs include cranial nerve palsies, extremity weakness, paresthesias, and loss of deep tendon reflexes. CT and MRI are useful in establishing the diagnosis of intraparenchymal lesions. The treatment of choice is radiotherapy. Solitary lesions in selected patients may be resected to achieve improved disease-free survival. The diagnosis of leptomeningeal disease is made by demonstrating tumor cells in the cerebrospinal fluid (CSF).

Each attempt has limited sensitivity, and so patients with clinical features suggestive of leptomeningeal disease should undergo three serial CSF samplings. Neoplastic meningitis usually occurs in the setting of uncontrolled cancer outside the CNS. Therefore, the prognosis is typically dismal, with a median survival between 10 and 12 weeks.

**III-33.**    **The answer is D.**    *(Chap. 88)*    Hyperleukocytosis and the leukostasis syndrome are potentially fatal complications of acute leukemia, particulary acute myeloid leukemia (AML). It typically occurs with an elevated blast cell count. The frequency of hyperleukocytosis is 3 to 13% in AML patients and 10 to 30% in ALL patients. High blast cell counts may result in elevated blood viscosity. Symptoms of hyperviscosity include stupor, headache, dizziness, tinnitus, visual disturbances, confusion, and frank coma. Pulmonary leukostasis may present as respiratory distress, hypoxemia, and progressive respiratory failure. The presence of hyperleukocytosis constitutes an oncologic emergency. These patients must be admitted to an intensive care unit setting. Bone marrow aspiration and biopsy will aid in the ultimate diagnosis of the type of leukemia and in prognostication. HLA typing of siblings is useful but not emergent. AML with poor-risk cytogenetics is rarely curable with chemotherapy alone, and allogeneic bone marrow transplantation is often the preferred option. In the acute setting, patients are given cytotoxic chemotherapy (and differentiating agents in the case of acute promyelocytic leukemia) to bring the blast count down. Leukapheresis may be helpful in decreasing the number of circulating blasts. Transfusion of blood products, however, will raise blood viscosity, may worsen symptoms, and should be avoided if possible until the blast cell count is reduced.

**III-34.**    **The answer is E.**    *(Chaps. 86 and 332)*    Hypercalcemia is a common oncologic complication of metastatic cancer. Symptoms include confusion, lethargy, change in mental status, fatigue, polyuria, and constipation. Regardless of the underlying disease, the treatment is similar. These patients are often dehydrated, as hypercalcemia may cause a nephrogenic diabetes insipidus, and are often unable to take fluids orally. Therefore, the primary management entails reestablishment of euvolemia. Often hypercalcemia will resolve with hydration alone. Bisphosphonates are another mainstay of therapy as they stabilize osteoclast resorption of calcium from the bone. However, their effects may take 1 to 2 days to manifest. Care must be taken in cases of renal insufficiency as rapid administration of pamidronate may exacerbate renal failure. Once euvolemia is achieved, furosemide may be given to increase calciuriesis. Nasal or subcutaneous calcitonin further aids the shift of calcium out of the intravascular space. Glucocorticoids may be useful in patients with lymphoid malignancies as the mechanism of hypercalcemia in those conditions is often related to excess hydroxylation of vitamin D. However, in this patient with prostate cancer, dexamethasone will have little effect on the calcium level and may exacerbate the altered mental status.

**III-35.**    **The answer is B.**    *(Chap. 88)*    Tumor lysis syndrome is a well recognized clinical entity that is characterized by metabolic derangements secondary to the destruction of tumor cells. Lysis of cells causes the release of intracellular pools of phosphate, potassium, and nucleic acids, leading to hyperphosphatemia and hyperuricemia. Lactic acidosis frequently develops for similar reasons. The increased urine acidity may promote the formation of uric acid nephropathy and subsequent renal failure. Hyperphosphatemia promotes a reciprocal depression in serum calcium. This hypocalcemia may result in severe neuromuscular irritability and tetany.

**III-36.**    **The answer is E.**    *(Chap. 88)*    Tumor lysis syndrome is a complication related to the rapid destruction of tumor cells and the subsequent metabolic derangements that result. Hyperkalemia, hyperphosphatemia, hyperuricemia, lactic acidosis, and hypocalemia are the typical manifestations. Nephropathy may result from both urate deposition and precipitation of calcium phosphate stones in the kidney. Treatment centers on prevention. Patients with rapidly growing tumors (e.g., Burkitt's lymphoma, aggressive non-Hodgkin's lymphomas, acute leukmias) are typically given allopurinol and phosphate binders (e.g., aluminum hydroxide, calcium acetate, sevelamer) before the institution of chemotherapy. Cardiac monitoring is often performed, as disturbances in potassium and calcium may result in arrhythmia. Patients are aggressively hydrated, and the urine is alkalinized with intravenous sodium bicarbonate. Alkalinization decreases the formation of uric acid stones. However, paradoxically, alkalosis may precipitate calcium phosphate stone formation and worsen hypocalcemia.

**III-37.** **The answer is A.** *(Chap. 88)* The presence of anemia, thrombocytopenia, and renal failure should always evoke the possibility of hemolytic-uremic syndrome (HUS) or thrombotic thrombocytopenic purpura (TTP). Their occurrence in a patient with cancer raises the question of treatment-related side effects. Mitomycin is by far the most common agent implicated in HUS. Other implicated antineoplastic agents include cisplatin, bleomycin, and gemcitabine. Autoimmune hemolytic anemia would not explain renal failure or thrombocytopenia. Evans syndrome (autoimmune hemolytic anemia and autoimmune thrombocytopenia) is seen more commonly in children. It may be idiopathic or may be related to hematologic malignancies. The normal coagulation studies eliminate DIC as a potential diagnosis. Sepsis may be seen commonly in patients undergoing chemotherapy. In this case the clinical scenario does not support that diagnosis.

**III-38.** **The answer is A.** *(Chap. 102)* Hemophilia A results from an inherited deficiency of factor VIII. The gene for factor VIII is on the X chromosome. Therefore, its X-linked inheritance pattern results in approximately 1 in 10,000 male patients being born with some level of dysfunction. Clinically, it is characterized by bleeding into soft tissues, muscles, and weight-bearing joints. Symptomatic patients usually have levels below 5%. Bleeding occurs hours or days after an injury and can involve any organ. Factor VIII is involved in the intrinsic pathway of coagulation. Therefore, deficiency usually results in abnormalities of the activated partial thromboplastin time. Factor VIII has a very short half-life of 8 to 12 h. Therefore, repeated transfusions of plasma, cryoprecipitate, or purified factor VIII must be given at least twice daily. Factor VIII complexes to von Willebrand factor, not Hageman factor.

**III-39.** **The answer is E.** *(Chap. 102)* Hemophilia A results from a deficiency of factor VIII. Replacement of factor VIII is the centerpiece of treatment. Cessation of aspirin or nonsteroidal anti-inflammatory drugs (NSAIDs) is highly recommended. FFP contains pooled plasma from human sources. Cryoprecipitate refers to FFP that is cooled, resulting in the precipitation of material at the bottom of the plasma. This product contains about half the factor VIII activity of FFP in a tenth of the volume. Both agents are therefore reasonable treatment options. DDAVP causes the release of a number of factors and von Willebrand factor from the liver and endothelial cells. This may be useful for patients with mild hemophilia. Recombinant or purified factor VIII (i.e., Humate P) is indicated in patients with more severe bleeding. Therapy may be required for weeks, with levels of factor VIII kept at 50%, for postsurgical or severe bleeding. Plasmapheresis has no role in the treatment of hemophilia A.

**III-40.** **The answer is D.** *(Chap. 102)* The correction of the mixing study immediately, only to have prolongation of the aPTT at a 2-h incubation, is suggestive of a factor VIII inhibitor. This occurs in patients who have received multiple transfusions. It may occur in older individuals idiopathically or in relation to autoimmune disorders. The inhibitors are typically IgG antibodies that rapidly neutralize factor VIII activity. Treatments are aimed at bypassing the role of factor VIII in coagulation and, in severe cases, suppression of the immune system. Prothrombinase complexes are highly effective as they activate fibrinogen conversion to fibrin independent of the intrinsic pathway. Similarly, porcine factor VIII may not be affected by inhibitors. Factor VIIa directly activates factor X and bypasses the inhibitor-induced block. In severe cases immunosuppression with glucocorticoids, chemotherapy, and rituximab may play a role. Desmopressin, which results in increased factor VIII levels, confers no added benefit over FFP or human factor VIII concentrates.

**III-41.** **The answer is A.** *(Chap. 72)* Infections in patients who are undergoing chemotherapy are extremely common, particularly in neutropenic patients (neutrophils <500/mL$^3$). Typhlitis, also referred to as necrotizing enterocolitis, is a poorly understood phenomenon that occurs primarily in immunocompromised patients. It probably involves a combination of mucosal injury to the bowel wall from cytotoxic chemotherapy, neutropenia, and impaired host defense against microorganisms. The cecum is almost always involved, but other parts of the ascending colon and terminal ileum also may be involved. Blood, stool, and *C. difficile* cultures should always be performed. A surgical consult is mandatory, and patients with evidence of bowel perforation or infarction should receive an exploratory laparotomy. Others may be treated conservatively with broad-spectrum antibiotics, serial examinations, and periodic CT scans.

**III-42.** **The answer is C.** *(Chap. 72)* Oncologic patients with neutropenic fever pose a clinical dilemma. Many of these patients do not grow positive blood cultures. However, observation alone has been shown to result in increased morbidity and mortality. Therefore, the presence of neutropenic fever in a cancer patient demands a thorough workup for potential sources of infection, with particular attention paid to catheter sites, the oral cavity, and pulmonary processes. Empirical antibiotics are the rule, with coverage of both gram-negative and gram-positive bacteria necessary in the initial regimen. Single agents without activity against gram-positive organisms are inadequate and should be avoided. After 48 to 72 h, if a fever persists, empirical antibiotics with activity against fungal infections (e.g., amphotericin, voriconazole) should be initiated. Although some trials have indicated that it may be safe to treat "low-risk" patients with neutropenic fever, data from large randomized trials have not demonstrated the superiority of this approach.

**III-43.** **The answer is E.** *(Chap. 97)* For unknown reasons, non-Hodgkin's lymphomas increased in frequency in the United States at a rate of 4% per year between 1950 and the late 1990s. This led investigators to speculate that environmental causes, including infectious agents, chemical exposures, and medical treatments, played a role in that epidemiologic phenomenon. Indeed, further evidence for an environmental influence has come from the variation in the pattern of expression of the various subtypes based on geography. T cell lymphomas are more common in Asia than in Western countries, whereas B cell lymphomas are more common in Western countries. Angiocentric nasal T/natural killer (NK) cell lymphoma has a particular geographic occurrence, being most common in southern Asia and parts of Latin America. Adult T cell lymphoma is seen particularly in southern Japan and the Caribbean, in association with infection with human T cell lymphotropic virus (HTLV) I. Patients with HIV infection are predisposed to the development of an aggressive B cell non-Hodgkin's lymphoma. Primary CNS lymphomas are associated with EBV infection. Infection with *Helicobacter pylori* induces the development of gastric MALT lymphomas. Treatment with antibiotics to eradicate *H. pylori* has led to regression of MALT lymphomas.

**III-44.** **The answer is E.** *(Chap. 97)* Chronic lymphocytic leukemia (CLL) is the most common lymphoid malignancy, accounting for about 7% of non-Hodgkin's lymphomas. It is characterized by increased numbers of circulating B lymphocytes that are monoclonal and display the CD5 antigen. Mantle cell lymphoma may have this phenotype but also expresses a translocation between chromosomes 11 and 14 with the expression of cyclin D1. Clinically, patients may range from being asymptomatic to having fatigue, weight loss, fevers, lymphadenopathy, autoimmune hemolytic anemia, or autoimmune thrombocytopenia. B cell CLL has also been associated with pure red cell aplasia. Patients may be hypogammaglobulinemic and prone to bacterial infections. The prognosis historically has been determined by the stage of disease (i.e., the extent of lymphadenopathy and the presence of anemia and/or thrombocytopenia). However, in recent years, it has been noted that patients with mutated immunoglobulins have a much better median survival than do patients with unmutated immunoglobulins. Unfortunately, analysis of somatic mutation is difficult, and investigators have tried to identify markers that reflect mutational status.

CD38, ZAP-70, and activation-induced cytidinedeaminase are under investigation as prognostic tools. Patients with no evidence of cytopenia and no lymphadenopathy or organomegaly have median survivals greater than 10 years. Some of these patients, particularly if their cells have a mutated status, do not require treatment and may not become symptomatic with their disease. For patients who develop progression of CLL, treatment with purine nucleosides, monoclonal antibodies, or combination chemotherapy is an option. These agents are not curative, however. Allogeneic bone marrow transplantation may be curative, but transplant-associated mortality limits this option to selected younger patients.

**III-45. The answer is E.** *(Chap. 97)*   Marginal zone B cell lymphoma is another type of clonal malignancy of B cells. It is characterized immunophenotypically by CD20 positivity. Morphologically, the cells are small lymphocytes that are CD5-negative. Clinically, the disease is indolent. Extranodal marginal zone B cell lymphoma may occur in mucosa-associated lymphoid tissue, hence the name MALT lymphoma. This may occur in the stomach, orbit, intestine, lung, thyroid, salivary gland, skin, soft tissues, bladder, kidney, and CNS. The stomach is the most common site. Among the MALT lymphomas of the gastric type, *H. pylori* infection is associated in 95% of cases. The significance of *H. pylori* infection is demonstrated by the remission of disease seen in some patients treated for this infection. If the disease is localized to the stomach, antibiotic treatment is the first option. This alone may result in remission. In patients who do not respond to antibiotics, tumors often contain cytogenetic abnormalities, e.g., t(11; 18). Combination chemotherapy is reserved for patients in whom antibiotic treatment fails or those with disease that shows evidence of transformation into more aggressive lymphoma.

**III-46. The answer is C.** *(Chap. 97)*   The International Prognostic Index (IPI) was formulated to evaluate prognosis in patients with diffuse large B cell lymphoma (DLBCL). Other infections that may lead to MALT lymphoma in other sites include *Campylobacter jejuni* (small intestines), *Chlamydia psittaci* (ocular adrenal), and *Borrelia* sp. (skin). Patients with high scores respond poorly to chemotherapy, have shorter median survivals, and may have better outcomes with stem cell transplantation. The five clinical risk factors in the IPI are age over 60 years, elevated serum lactic dehydrogenase, ECOG performance status greater than or equal to 2 or Karnofsky score below 70, Ann Arbor stage III or IV, and more than one site of extranodal involvement. Patients with no risk factors or one risk factor have a 5-year survival of 73% with combination chemotherapy. Patients with four to five risk factors have a median survival of 26%. Tumor grade is not considered in the IPI. All patients who are diagnosed with DLBCL should have a CT scan of the chest, abdomen, and pelvis; a serum lactate dehydrogenase level; and a bone marrow biopsy. The role of autologous bone marrow transplantation in patients with high IPI scores is being defined. Allogeneic transplantation is potentially curative but is limited by transplant-related toxicity, and its role is debated.

**III-47. The answer is E.** *(Chap. 93)*   This patient has an autoimmune hemolytic anemia with cold agglutinins secondary to *Mycoplasma pneumoniae*. Approximately 50 to 70% of patients with mycoplasma pneumonia will develop cold agglutinins as a result of the development of IgM antibodies to the I-antigen on red blood cells. The hemolysis may cause a significant fall in the hematocrit. The reticulocytosis, increase in the mean corpuscular volume (MCV), increase in indirect bilirubin, and decreased (or absent) haptoglobin are characteristic. The bone marrow will show erythroid hyperplasia, which can be seen in any cause of acute hemolysis. White blood cells and platelets are not involved. The clinical diagnosis of mycoplasma pneumonia may be supported by finding myringitis bullosa on the tympanic membrane. *Mycoplasma* will not respond to any cephalosporins. Effective antibiotics include macrolides, quinolones, and tetracyclines.

**III-48. The answer is D.** *(Chap. 94)*   Pure red cell aplasia is a normochromic, normocytic anemia with absent erythoblasts on the bone marrow, hence the diminished number or lack of reticulocytes. The bone marrow shows red cell aplasia and the presence of giant pronormoblasts. Several conditions have been associated with pure red cell aplasia, including viral infections such as B19 parvovirus (which can have cytopathic bone marrow changes), HIV, EBV, HTLV, and hepatitis B virus; malignancies such as thymomas and lymphoma (which often present with an anterior mediastinal mass); connective tissue disorders such as SLE and rheumatoid arthritis (RA); pregnancy; drugs; and hereditary disorders. Erythropoietin levels are elevated because of the anemia.

**III-49.  The answer is A.** *(Chap. 81)*   Approximately 200,000 prostate cancer diagnoses occurred in the United States in 2003. The prognosis is dependent on the stage and grade of the tumor. Grade is assigned by the Gleason score, in which the dominant and secondary glandular histologic patterns are scored from 1 (well differentiated) to 5 (undifferentiated) and summed to give a total score of 2 to 10 for each tumor. Stage reflects the degree of extension out of the prostatic capsule. Early-stage tumors are confined to one lobe of the prostate and are often not palpable. Later-stage lesions are palpable and may invade locally into the seminal vesicles or metastasize to the pelvis or skeleton. Early-stage lesions with a low tumor grade, as in this case, have a low risk of death, with 10-year median survivals up to 80%. This compares favorably with either surgical or radiation therapy for early-stage tumors. Watchful waiting is appropriate in patients with life expectancies less than 10 years who have early-stage and/or low-grade tumors. Radical retropubic prostatectomy may be curative in patients with early-stage disease. Impotence and incontinence are the primary side effects. Impotence often occurs immediately, but in patients <70 years old undergoing nerve-sparing procedures at experienced institutions, a significant proportion of patients recover function within 4 to 6 months. Radiation therapy is also an effective procedure, and the choice is dependent on the institution and personal preference. PSA levels typically decline slowly over time after radiation therapy. Side effects also develop more slowly. Neoadjuvant hormonal therapy is unproven in the treatment of prostate cancer.

**III-50.  The answer is A.** *(Chap. 76)*   At this point only approximately 10% of cases of human breast cancer can be linked directly to a germ-line mutation. Inherited mutations of the tumor suppressor genes p53, *PTEN*, *BRCA-1*, and *BRCA-2* increase the risk of breast cancer. Women who inherit a mutation in the *BRCA-1* gene have a 60 to 80% lifetime risk of developing breast cancer and a 33% risk of developing ovarian cancer. Men with this mutation have an increased risk of developing breast and prostate cancer. Men and women with a mutation in *BRCA-2* have an increased risk of developing breast cancer. Mutations in *BRCA-1* and *BRCA-2* can be detected diagnostically. Men and women (particularly women of Ashkenazi Jewish descent) with a strong history of breast cancer should receive genetic testing and counseling. Whether these genes and their proteins are important in the pathogenesis of sporadic cases of breast cancer is undetermined.

**III-51.  The answer is A.** *(Chap. 76; Lancet 360:187–195, 2002.)*   Approximately 80 to 90% of the variation in breast cancer frequency in different countries can be attributed to differences in menarche, first pregnancy, and menopause. Women who experience menarche at age 16 have 40 to 50% the risk of breast cancer of women who experience menarche at age 12 years. Menopause, surgical or natural, occurring 10 years before the median age of 52 years reduces the risk of breast cancer by 35%. Women who have the first full-term pregnancy by age 18 have a 30 to 40% reduced risk of breast cancer compared with nulliparous women. These data taken together suggest that a substantial portion of the risk of developing breast cancer is related directly to the length of menstrual life, particularly the fraction occurring before the first full-term pregnancy. Independently of these factors, the duration of maternal nursing is associated with a reduction in breast cancer risk.

**III-52.  The answer is D.** *(Chap. 75)*   The chest radiogram shows a large right pleural effusion with a contralateral mediastinal shift. Combined with the history, this most likely represents a malignant pleural effusion resulting from non-small cell carcinoma of the lung. A single diagnostic thoracentesis has more than a 60% yield in non-small cell lung cancer. The yield increases with the volume of fluid and with repeated sampling. A positive fluid cytology for non-small cell carcinoma stages the patient as IIIB (positive fluid cytology is T4), and the patient therefore is not a candidate for curative surgical therapy. The 5-year survival of patients with stage IIIb non-small cell lung cancer is less than 10%. Most malignant pleural effusions are exudative with a pH over 7.3; however, a pH below 7.2 identifies a group of patients with an even poorer prognosis. Effusions with a pH below 7.2 generally also have a low glucose concentration. The number of white blood cells in malignant pleural effusions is generally <4000/mm³ with a lymphocyte predominance and less than 25% neutrophils. A higher white blood cell count or percentage of neutrophils suggests active inflammation or superimposed infection.

**III-53.  The answer is A.**  *(Chap. 76)*   During pregnancy the breast grows under the influence of estrogen, progesterone, prolactin, and human placental lactogen. However, the presence of a dominant breast nodule/mass during pregnancy should never be attributed to hormonal changes. Breast cancer develops in 1:3000 to 4000 pregnancies. The prognosis for breast cancer by stage is no different in pregnant compared with pregnant women. Nevertheless, pregnant women are often diagnosed with more advanced disease because of delay in the diagnosis. Pregnant patients with persistent lumps in the breast should be receive prompt diagnostic evaluation.

**III-54.  The answer is C.**  *(Chap. 76; CA Cancer J Clin 54:41–52, 2004.)*   Multiple studies have demonstrated a benefit of mammography on mortality in women over 50 years old. The magnitude of the survival benefit ranges from 25 to 30%. However, there are insufficient data to demonstrate a benefit in women older than age 70 years. The effect of screening mammography on survival for women 40 to 50 years old is less conclusive and more controversial. Increasing breast density (less fat) decreases the sensitivity of mammography as a screening tool. Increased breast density is associated with younger age, hormone replacement therapy, and the luteal (versus follicular) phase of the menstrual cycle.

**III-55.  The answer is E.**  *(Chap. 68)*   A small proportion of cancers occur in patients with a genetic predisposition. Roughly 100 syndromes of familial cancer have been reported. Recognition allows for genetic counseling and increased cancer surveillance. Down's syndrome, or trisomy 21, is characterized clinically by a variety of features, including moderate to severe learning disability, facial and musculoskeletal deformities, duodenal atresia, congenital heart defects, and an increased risk of acute leukemia. Fanconi's anemia is a condition that is associated with defects in DNA repair. There is a higher incidence of cancer, with leukemia and myelodysplasia being the most common cancers. Von Hippel—Lindau syndrome is associated with hemangioblastomas, renal cysts, pancreatic cysts and carcinomas, and renal cell cancer. Neurofibramotosis (NF) type I and type II are both associated with increased tumor formation. NF II is more associated with a schwannoma. Both carry a risk of malignant peripheral nerve sheath tumors. Fragile X is a condition associated with chromosomal instability of the X chromosome. These patients have mental retardation, typical morphologic features including macroorchidism and prognathia, behavioral problems, and occasionally seizures. Increased cancer incidence has not been described.

**III-56.  The answer is B.**  *(Chap. 76)*   The staging of breast cancer is vital to determining a patient's prognosis and, often, therapy. Staging of breast cancer has changed over the last two decades. The current staging system depends not on menopausal state but solely on characteristics of the tumor, nodes and the presence of metastases. In this case the tumor growing from 3.5 cm to 6 cm changed the tumor classification from T2 to T3, and so waiting a year may have worsened the prognosis. Pathologic ipsilateral supraclavicular lymph nodes qualify as metastases (M1) and therefore would place a patient in stage IV. Note also that the quality of the axillary lymph nodes distinguishes between N1 and N2.

which is also important for staging. With the information provided, this patient has T3N1M0 disease. This places her in stage IIIA disease, with a 47% 5-year survival.

**Staging of Breast Cancer**

**Primary Tumor (T)**

| T0 | No evidence of primary tumor | T2 | Tumor >2 cm but ≤5 cm |
|---|---|---|---|
| TIS | Carcinoma in situ | T3 | Tumor >5 cm |
| T1 | Tumor ≤2 cm | T4 | Extension to chest wall, inflammation, satellite lesions, ulcerations |

**Regional Lymph Nodes (N)**

| N0 | No regional lymph nodes | N2 | Metastasis to matted or fixed ipsilateral nodes |
|---|---|---|---|
| N1 | Metastasis to movable ipsilateral nodes | N3 | Metastasis to ipsilateral internal mammary nodes |

**Distant Metastasis (M)**

| M0 | No distant metastasis | M1 | Distant metastasis (includes spread to ipsilateral supraclavicular nodes) |
|---|---|---|---|

**Stage Grouping**

| Stage 0 | TIS | N0 | M0 | Stage IIIA | T0 | N2 | M0 |
|---|---|---|---|---|---|---|---|
| Stage I | T1 | N0 | M0 | | T1 | N2 | M0 |
| Stage IIA | T0 | N1 | M0 | | T2 | N2 | M0 |
| | T1 | N1 | M0 | | T3 | N1, N2 | M0 |
| | T2 | N0 | M0 | Stage IIIB | T4 | Any N | M0 |
| Stage IIB | T2 | N1 | M0 | | Any T | N3 | M0 |
| | T3 | N0 | M0 | Stage IV | Any T | Any N | M1 |

*Source*: Modified from the American Joint Committee on Cancer, 1992.

**III-57.   The answer is B.**   *(Chap. 103; Lancet 348:1329, 1996.)*   Therapy with the antiplatelet agents ticlopidine and clopidogrel has been demonstrated to have superior effects compared with aspirin in preventing thromboembolic cerebrovascular disease. Ticlopidine and clopidogrel are structurally similar compounds that selectively inhibit ADP-induced platelet aggregation. The CAPRIE trial showed a small absolute risk reduction from 8% to 7% in cerebrovascular events in patients taking clopidogrel compared with aspirin. Ticlopidine is rarely used currently because of the risk of hematologic toxicities, including thrombotic thrombocytopenic purpura. Clopidogrel is associated with occasional thrombocytopenia but only rarely causes severe hematologic toxicity.

There is no proven benefit in increasing aspirin doses to more than 325 mg daily, and increased gastrointestinal intolerance is likely at this dose. Dipyridamole inhibits platelet activation by inhibiting phosphodiesterase. The use of dipyridamole alone has increased the risk of recurrent events although there may additional benefit in terms of decreasing cerebrovascular events when it is used in combination with aspirin. Warfarin would be appropriate if the patient had atrial fibrillation.

**III-58.   The answer is E.**   *(Chap. 103)*   Traditionally, anticoagulant therapy was done primarily with the broad-spectrum anticoagulants heparin and warfarin. Recent advances in anticoagulation have seen the introduction of a range of specific anticoagulants. Unfractionated heparin (UFH) is a heterogeneous mixture of highly sulfated glycosaminoglycans that bind to antithrombin. Once it is bound, the anticoagulant effect of antithrombin is potentiated. Antithrombin and anti–factor Xa activities are approximately equal when heparin is used. In contrast, low-molecular-weight heparins (LMWHs) have limited antithrombin activity compared with their activity against anti–factor Xa. LMWHs are derived from UFH by enzymatic or chemical cleavage of the glycosaminoglycans into smaller molecules. Dermatan sulfate is a heparanoid compound that activates heparin cofactor II and has a anti–

factor Xa activity greater than 22 times that of its antithrombin activity. More recently, fondaparinux has been developed as a synthetic polysaccharide that indirectly inhibits factor Xa. It has recently been approved for the prevention of deep venous thrombosis, and trials are under way to discover its efficacy in other areas of venous thromboembolism.

Multiple direct thrombin inhibitors also have been developed recently. Lepirudin is a recombinant hirudin (the anticoagulant produced by the medicinal leech) that irreversibly binds to thrombin but has a short half-life. It is contraindicated in renal failure, and there is no effective antidote. Additionally, 40% of patients treated with lepirudin develop anti-IgG antibodies to it, and this decreases renal elimination of the drug. Other direct thrombin inhibitors include argatroban, bivalirudin, and ximelagatran, a new oral direct thrombin inhibitor that does not require laboratory monitoring of its efficacy.

**III-59. The answer is B.** *(Chap. 85)* The patient is a young man with asymmetric hilar adenopathy. The differential diagnosis would include lymphoma, testicular cancer, and, less likely, tuberculosis or histoplasmosis. Because of his young age, testicular examination and ultrasonography would be indicated, as would measurement of $\beta$-hCG and AFP, which are generally markedly elevated. In men with carcinoma of unknown primary source, AFP and $\beta$-hCG should be checked as the presence of testicular cancer portends an improved prognosis compared with possible primary sources. Biopsy would show lymphoma. The ACE level may be elevated but is not diagnostic of sarcoidosis. Thyroid disorders are not likely to present with unilateral hilar adenopathy. Finally, PSA is not indicated in this age category, and C-reactive protein would not differentiate any of the disorders mentioned above. Biopsy is the most important diagnostic procedure.

**III-60. The answer is E.** *(Chap. 103)* This patient has developed heparin-induced thrombocytopenia (HIT). Type I HIT is self-limited and not immune-mediated, whereas type II HIT is frequently associated with the adverse consequences of both arterial and venous thromboses. It is caused by the development of antibody to heparin–platelet factor 4 complexes and results in activation of platelet aggregation. This immune-mediated disease is seen after prolonged treatment with heparin or after the reintroduction of heparin after a prior exposure, such as prior cardiac surgery requiring cardiopulmonary bypass. Treatment consists of discontinuation of heparin and anticoagulation with another type of anticoagulant. Of note, these patients can have a prolonged hypercoagulable state after discontinuation of heparin and should remain anticoagulated. Options for treatment of HIT include the direct thrombin inhibitors: argatroban, lepirudin, bivalirudin, and ximelagatran. Argatroban is hepatically metabolized but can be safely used in those with renal dysfunction, whereas lepirudin is contraindicated with creatinine clearance <60 mL/min. Low-molecular-weight heparin has a lower incidence of associated HIT, but once HIT has developed, there is significant cross-reactivity. Dermatan sulfate is a heparinoid compound that is occasionally used in HIT, but it does exhibit cross-reactivity with heparin. Thus, it is not the drug of choice for this disease.

**III-61. The answer is C.** *(Chap. 103)* Thrombolytic therapy has been approved for use in thrombotic cerebrovascular accidents when it is given within 3 h of the onset of symptoms at a dose no higher than 0.9 mg/kg over 60 min. Risk factors for intracranial bleeding after thrombolytic infusion include older age, female sex, African-American or black ethnicity, history of stroke, systolic blood pressure >140 mmHg, and diastolic blood pressure >100 mmHg.

**III-62. The answer is A.** *(Chap. 103)* The management of deep venous thrombosis (DVT) in the calf is controversial. Approximately 15 to 25% of these thromboses will propagate proximally with an increased incidence of pulmonary emboli. Proximal conversion will occur during the first 2 weeks in the majority of these patients and should be treated with anticoagulant therapy. Careful surveillance with serial Doppler ultrasonography twice weekly for 2 weeks is the recommended treatment. As this is a situational DVT occurring after a surgical intervention, 6 weeks of therapy will be appropriate if proximal extension occurs. There is no indication for catheter-directed thrombolysis in this patient, although it should be considered in patients with large proximal clot burden and severe symptoms, including phlegmasia cerulea dolens (venous limb gangrene).

**III-63.   The answer is C.**   *(Chap. 98)*   The patient demonstrates a monoclonal gammopathy of unknown significance (MGUS) with monoclonal protein and a limited expansion of plasma cells in the bone marrow. Approximately 1% of the population over age 50 and 10% over age 75 will demonstrate MGUS. Multiple myeloma develops in approximately 1% of these patients per year. Factors that suggest progression to multiple myeloma include more than 10% plasma cells in the bone marrow, an M protein spike >3 g/dL, presence of Bence-Jones proteinuria, and development of renal failure, anemia, lytic bone lesions, or hypercalcemia. Once a patient has been identified as having MGUS, serial serum and urine electrophoresis should be performed every 6 to 12 months to quantify the monoclonal protein. Patients with MGUS have a decrease in survival of about 2 years compared with age-matched controls. No treatment is necessary with MGUS. Treatment approaches to multiple myeloma include bisphosphonates and therapy directed at the tumor, either dexamethasone plus thalidomide or melphalan plus prednisone.

**III-64 and III-65.   The answers are C and A.**   *(Chap. 98)*   This patient presents with a history and physical and laboratory examinations consistent with the diagnosis of Waldenström's macroglobulinemia. This is a malignancy of lymphoplasmacytoid cells in which there is secretion of large IgM proteins. Clinically, the disease is associated with symptoms of the hyperviscosity syndrome, lymphadenopathy, and hepatosplenomegaly. Often the patient complains of prolonged fatigue and weight loss. Large multimers of IgM proteins result in the hyperviscosity syndrome. Clinically, symptoms are usually seen when the serum viscosity exceeds 4 CP. Symptoms include headache, visual changes, dizziness, epistaxis, and neuropathy. Laboratory examination shows normal renal function, a large globulin fraction, and often anemia. A positive direct Coombs' test and autoimmune hemolytic anemia are often present. Peripheral blood smear shows rouleaux formation resulting from the hyperviscosity and spherocytosis related to extravascular hemolytic anemia.

    Treatment for this patient should initially consist of plasmapheresis to relieve symptoms related to the hyperviscosity. Once the symptoms of hyperviscosity have been addressed, therapy directed toward the Waldenström's macroglobulinemia can be undertaken. Fludarabine and cladribine are effective as single agents. Rituximab, a monoclonal antibody directed against CD20-positive cells, is also effective alone or in combination with other therapy. About 80% of patients will respond to chemotherapy, with a median survival longer than 3 years.

**III-66.   The answer is A.**   *(Chap. 78)*   The patient's clinical presentation is consistent with the diagnosis of hepatocellular adenoma. These benign tumors of the liver are more common in women, and an association with oral contraceptive use has been demonstrated. The risk of hepatocellular adenomas is also increased with the use of androgens and anabolic steroids. Hepatic adenomas occur most commonly in the right lobe of the liver and present clinically as a mass in the right upper quadrant. Pain is occasionally present. The diagnosis is usually made by diagnostic imaging. Angiographically, these tumors are usually hypervascular. The risk of malignant change is low. Treatment consists of discontinuation of oral contraceptives and watchful waiting. Patients are advised not to become pregnant as the risk of hemorrhage is increased with pregnancy. Surgical resection should be considered for lesions that do not regress with discontinuation of oral contraceptives or lesions larger than 10 cm.

**III-67.  The answer is E.**  *(Chap. 78)*  Hepatocellular carcinoma most commonly occurs in patients with chronic hepatitis B or C or alcoholic cirrhosis. The development of hepatocellular carcinoma in these patients should not preclude them from liver transplantation if the size or number of tumors identified is not prohibitive. In fact, liver transplantation is considered a therapeutic option in these patients if there is a single lesion less than 5 cm or three or fewer lesions less than 3 cm. After liver transplantation survival in patients meeting these criteria is identical to that in patients transplanted for nonmalignant disease.

**III-68.  The answer is D.**  *(Chap. 78)*  This patient's abdominal radiogram demonstrates a porcelain gallbladder, which is associated with an approximately 25% risk of gallbladder cancer. The finding of a porcelain gallbladder is thus an indication for open cholecystectomy because of this risk. Biopsy and laparascopic cholecystectomy are not options because of the risk of rupture of the calcified gallbladder. Gallbladder cancer is often found at an advanced stage. If the tumor is found incidentally and is resected, the 5-year survival rate is 50%. However, most gallbladder cancers present with unresectable disease with a 1-year mortality of over 95%.

**III-69.  The answer is A.**  *(Chaps. 101 and 102)*  Von Willebrand's disease is the most common inherited bleeding disorder. Multiple genetic mutations have been identified as causative of the clinical phenotype of vWD. Based on inheritance pattern, pathophysiology, and risk of bleeding, three broad types of vWD have been identified. Type III vWD is the rarest, occurring in 1 per million population, and is the only type of vWD that is inherited in an autosomal recessive fashion. Most patients with type I vWD have reductions in their Von Willebrand factor to just below normal, and their risk of bleeding is greatest after surgery or trauma. Spontaneous bleeding is rare. In contrast, patients with type III vWD often have no detectable von Willebrand factor (vWF) or activity. These patients often present with severe mucosal bleeding, especially with menorrhagia in women. In addition, as vWF is the plasma carrier for factor VIII, these patients may also present with hemarthroses in a fashion similar to that of patients with hemophilia A. Plasma levels of factor VIII are severely reduced, as is the ristocetin cofactor assay of platelet aggregation. Treatment of patients with type III vWD requires infusion of cryoprecipitate or, preferably, factor VIII concentrates, which retain high-molecular-weight multimers of vWF. Desmopressin is frequently used for the treatment of type I vWD as it stimulates the release of vWF from endothelial cells, raising the plasma level of vWF in these patients. However, type III vWD does not respond to this therapy.

**III-70.  The answer is C.**  *(Chap. 93)*  This patient has evidence of autoimmune hemolytic anemia with warm agglutinins. Multiple causes of warm agglutinins have been described, including drug-related causes, viral infections, autoimmune diseases, and malignancies, particularly hematologic malignancies. Methyldopa is among the more common causes of drug-induced autoimmune hemolytic anemia. In fact, 10 to 20% of patients treated with methyldopa develop a positive direct Coombs' test with IgG antibody directed against the Rh complex. Antibody does not develop to complement that is seen in IgM-mediated cold agglutinin disease, such as that seen with *M. pneumoniae* infection. Clinically, however, only 1 to 5% of patients on methyldopa develop significant hemolysis. Treatment should include discontinuation of suspected agents such as methyldopa and initiation of glucocorticoids. With methyldopa, this usually produces remission of the disease, but it may take weeks to months for the response to be seen. The appropriate dose and duration of treatment with glucocorticoids are not well established. Most hematologists recommend initial doses of the equivalent of 60 mg of prednisone with tapering over 1 month if a response is seen. Glucocorticoids should be decreased to the minimum dose that induces a response. If hemolysis persists despite these measures, other therapies to consider include cytotoxic therapy with cyclophosphamide or azathioprine, danazol, and intravenous immunoglobulin. Refractory cases should be considered for possible therapy with rituximab or splenectomy.

**III-71.** **The answer is D.** *(Chap. 101; N Engl J Med 327:1779–1784, 1992.)* The patient has HIV-associated thrombocytopenia without current symptoms of bleeding. These patients often have very low platelet counts ($<20,000/\mu$L) with infrequent bleeding complications. However, the risk of spontaneous bleeding increases with platelet counts below 20,000/$\mu$L, and treatment for this patient should be considered. HIV-associated thrombocytopenia that is not associated with acute bleeding may be managed with antiretroviral therapy. Zidovudine (AZT) as monotherapy has been shown to increase platelet counts, although current treatment guidelines do not support monotherapy because of the development of resistance. AZT acts at the bone marrow to increase platelet production and should be included in the combination of drugs used as an initial highly active antiretroviral combination. Treatment with highly active antiretroviral therapy (HAART) containing AZT causes platelets to rise over several weeks to months. For patients who are acutely bleeding and require a more rapid increase in platelets, multiple therapies in addition to platelet transfusion have been used with success, including glucocorticoids, intravenous immunoglobulin, and anti-RhD immunoglobulin. In refractory cases splenectomy may be considered.

**III-72.** **The answer is C.** *(Chap. 76)* Multiple randomized clinical trials have demonstrated the equivalency of breast-conserving surgical therapy (lumpectomy) with or without postoperative radiation to mastectomy. Lumpectomy does incur a risk of local recurrence of tumor, but this does not translate into a decrease in 10-year survival, probably because the local recurrence is not the cause of distant metastases. Postoperative radiation therapy does reduce the rate of local recurrence, and nodal radiation therapy improves survival. Lumpectomy is not suitable for women with tumors larger than 5 cm, tumors involving the nipple/areola, extensive intraductal disease, collagen vascular disease, or lack of access to postoperative radiation therapy. These patients should be considered for mastectomy. Currently, approximately a third of patients with breast cancer who are receiving surgical therapy undergo lumpectomy. Many patients currently receiving mastectomy are candidates for lumpectomy and breast conservation.

**III-73.** **The answer is A.** *(Chap. 76)* Adjuvant chemotherapy after local therapy for breast cancer improves survival by decreasing the incidence of metastatic disease. The need for adjuvant therapy is generally determined by staging. Currently, this therapy is not routinely recommended for females with tumors smaller than 1 cm and negative axillary lymph nodes. New techniques for assessing tumor biology and genetics may allow refinement in the indications for adjuvant chemotherapy. Any patient with a tumor larger than 2 cm or positive lymph nodes should receive adjuvant therapy. The choice of therapy depends on the endocrine receptor (ER) status. Premenopausal women and patients with tumors that are ER-negative should receive multidrug chemotherapy. Postmenopausal women with ER-positive tumors should receive tamoxifen.

**III-74.** **The answer is D.** *(Chap. 76)* Pathologic staging remains the most important determinant of overall prognosis. Other prognostic factors have an impact on survival and the choice of therapy. Tumors that lack estrogen and/or progesterone receptors are more likely to recur. The presence of estrogen receptors, particularly in postmenopausal women, is also an important factor in determining adjuvant chemotherapy. Tumors with a high growth rate are associated with early relapse. Measurement of the proportion of cells in S-phase is a measure of the growth rate. Tumors with more than the median number of cells in S-phase have a higher risk of relapse and an improved response rate to chemotherapy. Histologically, tumors with a poor nuclear grade have a higher risk of recurrence than do tumors with a good nuclear grade. At the molecular level, tumors that overexpress *erbB2* (*HER-2/neu*) or that have a mutated p53 gene portend a poorer prognosis for patients. The overexpression of *erbB2* is also useful in designing optimal treatment regimens, and a human monoclonal antibody to *erbB2* (Herceptin) has been developed.

**III-75.** **The answer is B.** *(Chaps. 52 and 95)* The demonstration of an elevated hemoglobin/hematocrit with an elevated red blood cell mass rules out spurious or relative erythrocytosis. Erythropoietin levels distinguish primary (polycythemia vera) from secondary causes of polycythemia (erythrocytosis). Polycythemia vera is a myeloproliferative disorder characterized by clonal expansion of myeloid precursor cells. Secondary causes of polycythemia are an elevation of erythropoietin caused by reduced arterial oxygen saturation (lung disease, hypoventilation, pulmonary AV malformation, intracardiac right-to-LEFT shunting, altitude), an elevated carboxyhemoglobin level (smoker's, accidental CO poisoning), a high-affinity hemoglobinopathy, and tumors (renal cell carcinoma, hepatocellular carcinoma, uterine leiomyoma).

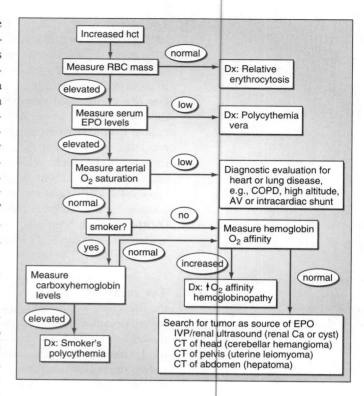

**III-76.** **The answer is B.** *(Chap. 84)* Bone pain resulting from metastatic lesions may be difficult to distinguish from degenerative disease, osteoporosis, or disk disease in the elderly. Generally, these patients present with insidious worsening localized pain without fevers or signs of infection. In contrast to pain related to disk disease, the pain of metastatic disease is worse when the patient is lying down or at night. Neurologic symptoms related to metastatic disease constitute an emergency. Lung, breast, and prostate cancers account for approximately 80% of bone metastases. Thyroid carcinoma, renal cell carcinoma, lymphoma, and bladder carcinoma may also metastasize to bone. Metastatic lesions may be lytic or blastic. Most cancers cause a combination of both, although prostate cancer is predominantly blastic. Either lesion may cause hypercalcemia, although lytic lesions more commonly do this. Lytic lesions are best detected with plain radiography. Blastic lesions are prominent on radionuclide bone scans. Treatment and prognosis depend on the underlying malignancy. Bisphosphanates may reduce hypercalcemia, relieve pain, and limit bone resorption.

**III-77.** **The answer is A.** *(Chaps. 15 and 75)* This patient presents with Horner's syndrome (miosis, ptosis, anhydrosis, and narrowing of the palpedral fissure), which is often the presenting finding for a superior sulcus (Pancoast) tumor resulting from non-small cell carcinoma of the lung. Up to two-thirds of patients with superior sulcus tumors will present with Horner's syndrome. Horner's syndrome is caused by the tumor compressing or invading the paravertebral sympathetic chain or the stellate ganglion. With early involvement, the irritation may cause flushing and increased sweating. Chest radiograms may show only capping of the apical pleura, but a CT scan shows the mass and the extent of invasion better. The staging of the disease depends mostly on the extent of the tumor invasion. T3N0M0 disease is considered stage IIB and may be amenable to combined-modality therapy, including surgery. Preoperative radiation therapy in these cases may improve survival. The differential diagnosis of Horner's syndrome includes brainstem or posterior circulation stroke, carotid artery dissection, cavernous sinus thrombosis, trauma, and metastatic disease.

**III-78.** **The answer is C.** *(Chap. 85)* The patient presents with symptoms suggestive of ovarian cancer. Although her peritoneal fluid is positive for adenocarcinoma, further speciation cannot be done. Surprisingly, the physical examination and imaging do not show a primary source. Although the differential diagnosis of this patient's disorder includes gastric cancer or another gastrointestinal malignancy and breast cancer, peritoneal carcinomatosis most commonly is due to ovarian cancer in women, even when the ovaries are normal at surgery. Elevated CA-125 levels or the presence of psamomma bodies is further suggestive of an ovarian origin, and such patients should receive surgical debulking and carboplatin or cisplatin plus paclitaxel. Patients with this presentation have a similar stage-specific survival compared with other patients with known ovarian cancer. Ten percent of patients with this disorder, also known as primary peritoneal papillary serous carcinoma, will remain disease-free 2 years after treatment.

**III-79. The answer is D.** *(Chap. 85)* This patient with risk factors for head and neck cancer is found to have an enlarged cervical lymph node, and a biopsy shows squamous cell carcinoma. Physical examination is not revealing of a source. In this case it is important to evaluate for thyroid carcinoma, which can have improved survival compared with carcinoma of an unknown primary. In addition, otolaryngology evaluation, including laryngoscopy, nasopharyngoscopy, and random punch biopsies, is indicated as definitive therapy, including radical neck dissection and/or radiation therapy. This may lead to prolonged survival in this patient population. Male breast cancer is most likely to be adenocarcinoma, not squamous carcinoma. Therefore, bilateral mammography is not indicated. Chest CT is less likely to be helpful with normal lung examination and a high cervical node, as this cancer is more likely to have a head or neck origin.

**III-80. The answer is D.** *(Chap. 75; N Engl J Med 348:2535–2542, 2003.)* The evaluation of a solitary pulmonary nodule (SPN) remains a combination of art and science. Approximately 50% of SPNs (less than 3.0 cm) turn out to be malignant, but studies have found a range between 10 and 70%, depending on patient selection. If the SPN is malignant, surgical therapy can result in 80% 5-year survival. Most benign lesions are infectious granulomas. Spiculated or scalloped lesions are more likely to be malignant, whereas lesions with central or popcorn calcification are more likely to be benign. Masses (larger than 3.0 cm) are usually malignant. $^{18}$FDG PET scanning has added a new test to the options for evaluating a SPN. PET has over 95% sensitivity and 75% specificity for identifying a malignant SPN. False negatives occur with small (less than 1 cm) tumors, bronchoalveolar carcinomas, and carcinoid tumors. False positives are usually due to inflammation. In this patient with a moderate risk of malignancy (age over 45, lesion larger than 1 cm, positive smoking history, suspicious lesion, no prior radiogram demonstrating the lesion) a PET scan would be the most reasonable choice. PET is also useful for staging disease. The diagnostic accuracy of PET for malignant mediastinal lymph nodes approaches 90%. Another option would be a transthoracic needle biopsy, with a sensitivity of 80 to 95% and a specificity of 50 to 85%. Transthoracic needle aspiration has the best results and the fewest complications (pneumothorax) with peripheral lesions versus central lesions. Bronchoscopy has a very poor yield for lesions smaller than 2 cm. Mediastinoscopy would be of little value unless PET or CT raised a suspicion of nodal disease. MRI scan will not add any information and is less able than CT to visualize lesions in the lung parenchyma. A repeat chest CT is a reasonable option for a patient with a low clinical suspicion.

**III-81. The answer is E.** *(Chap. 101)* The peripheral blood smear showing schistocytes (fragmented red blood cells) and the clinical picture, including the evidence of hemolysis and the absence of coagulopathy, are typical for thrombotic thrombocytopenic purpura (TTP). TTP and hemolytic-uremic syndrome (HUS) are often considered distinct syndromes. However, in adult patients their overlapping symptoms and signs, as well as their common treatment with plasma exchange, make the clinical distinction imprecise and sometimes challenging. TTP is classically defined by a pentad of abnormalities: microangiopathic hemolytic anemia, thrombocytopenia, renal failure, neurologic abnormalities, and fever. However, this fulminant classic presentation is rare. Indeed, the only two criteria required now are thrombocytopenia and microangiopathic hemolytic anemia without another clinically apparent etiology. HUS was initially described in children with acute renal failure who also had thrombocytopenia. This was recognized to have an association with enteric infection with a Shiga toxin–producing bacteria. TTP has been recognized to be a congenital or acquired deficiency in a von Willebrand factor protease, resulting in increased platelet activation. Acquired TTP may be idiopathic (after a viral infection?) or secondary to diseases (e.g., HIV infection, rheumatologic conditions) or drugs (clopidogrel, cyclosporine). Because it is often clinically difficult to distinguish the two entities at first presentation, the term TTP-HUS is often used. Plasma exchange has dramatically changed the natural history of these diseases from one of 85% mortality to one of 85% recovery. In the congenital form of TTP plasma replacement may be sufficient as opposed to exchange. Additional treatments, such as prednisone, splenectomy, and immunosuppression, are unproven but often are used in refractory cases. The blood smear showing microangiopathy with schistocytes excludes ITP, autoimmune hemolytic anemia, and paroxysmal nocturnal hemoglobinuria as the sole diagnosis. The presence of normal coagulation factors makes DIC unlikely.

**III-82.   The answer is D.**   *(Chap. 83; N Engl J Med 347:1645–1651, 2002.)*   The incidence of cervical carcinoma has fallen by at least 50% over the last 30 years, largely as a result of the use of Pap smear screening. However, it remains a significant health problem, particularly in underdeveloped countries and in patients with poor access to medical care in the United States. Sexually transmitted infection with many serotypes of human papilloma virus is associated with cervical intraepithelial neoplasia (CIN) that may progress to invasive cervical carcinoma. Pap smears are over 90% accurate in detecting early lesions of cervical carcinoma. Women after the onset of sexual activity or over 20 years old should have two consecutive yearly negative Pap smears. Afterward, Pap smears may be repeated every 3 years. Women with low-grade CIN should be tested for human papilloma virus (HPV). Women with high-grade CIN or worse should receive colposcopy. Recently, a vaccine to HPV-16 was shown to decrease the incidence of infection and CIN in women. In the absence of symptoms or physical findings, testing for HPV is not recommended.

**III-83.   The answer is B.**   *(Chap. 97; Pettitt et al, Br J Haematol 106:2–8, 1999.)*   Pancytopenia with a dry marrow aspirate argues against CLL and myeloma. Normal red blood cell (RBC) morphology argues against myelofibrosis. The WBC count and differential count argue against CML. Hairy cell leukemia is a neoplasm of mature B lymphocytes that typically presents with pancytopenia, splenomegaly, and a dry bone marrow aspirate. Patients with hairy cell leukemia are prone to infections with unusual microorganisms, such as atypical mycobacteria; they tend to be granulocytopenic and have a preponderance of mature-appearing lymphocytes in the peripheral blood that have, on close inspection or on ultrastructural analysis, multiple hairlike projections. Bone marrow biopsies typically yield a "fried egg" appearance in that the cells appear to be separated from one another as a result of these projections and fixation artifacts generated from them. Immunophenotypically, hairy cells are characterized by the presence of mature B cell markers as well as the CD25 antigen, which is the low-affinity IL-2 receptor. Fortunately, there are many treatment modalities available for patients with hairy cell leukemia. The current treatment of choice is a 7-day intravenous infusion of 2-chlorodeoxyadenosine. This single course of treatment results in complete remissions in approximately 80% of these patients. Other effective modalities include splenectomy, interferon $\alpha$, and pentostatin (deoxycoformycin).

**III-84.   The answer is B.**   *(Chap. 103)*   Several reports have described the association of coumarin-induced skin necrosis in patients with congenital protein C deficiency. The skin lesions occur on the breasts, buttocks, legs, and penis. They appear to result from diffuse thrombosis of the venules with interstitial bleeding. This condition is assumed to result from an imbalance in hemostatic mechanism activity favoring thrombosis during the early phases of coumarin administration. Protein C has a relatively short half-life within the circulation (about 14 h) compared with that of some of the vitamin K–dependent clotting factors (factor X and prothrombin), and a rapid drop in its effective concentration could produce such a situation. However, only about one-third of cases of coumarin-induced skin necrosis are related to protein C deficiency.

**III-85.   The answer is E.**   *(Chap. 91)*   Hemoglobinopathies are a diverse group of congenital disorders characterized by one or more mutations in one of the genes coding for hemoglobin chains. The clinical consequences can range from no effect to incompatibility with life. Microcytosis occurs in these conditions except for the silent $\alpha$-thalassemia carrier state, in which only one of the four $\alpha$-globin genes is deleted. Such persons have no hematologic abnormalities. Persons with deletion of two of the four $\alpha$-chain genes ($\alpha$-thalassemia trait) tend to have microcytic and slightly hypochromic red cells without significant hemolysis or anemia. Hemoglobin electrophoresis may be normal or may reveal a decreased amount of hemoglobin A2. Deletion of three of the four $\alpha$-chain genes, so-called hemoglobin H disease, is associated with significant anemia and with the production of hemoglobin H ($\beta$-chain tetramers) on hemoglobin electrophoresis. There are only two genes coding for the $\beta$-globin chain. Patients with abnormalities in one such chain have $\beta$-thalassemia trait characterized by microcytosis, abnormal-appearing red cells, and an elevated level of hemoglobin A2 or F or both on hemoglobin electrophoresis. Any patient who inherits at least one allele with a hemoglobin S mutation (sickle hemoglobin, valine to glutamic acid substitution at the sixth amino acid of the $\beta$-globin chain) will demonstrate red blood cell sickling under reduced oxygen tension, as is artificially produced by the addition of an oxygen-consuming agent such as metabisulfite to the blood. Therefore, any patient with sickle cell trait, sickle cell anemia, or a compound heterozygote such as sickle $\beta$-thalassemia or sickle C will have a positive metabisulfite test (and would also have a positive hemoglobin electrophoresis). Hemoglobin E is a very common hemoglobin variant that is highly prevalent in southeastern Asia. Patients with this disorder have an abnormal hemoglobin electrophoresis, slightly macrocytic red cells, and target cells but no anemia or other clinical manifestations unless they also inherit $\beta$ thalassemia.

**III-86.   The answer is C.**   *(Chap. 82)*   Ninety percent of persons with nonseminomatous germ cell tumors produce either AFP or $\beta$-hCG; in contrast, persons with pure seminomas usually produce neither. These tumor markers are present for some time after surgery; if the presurgical levels are high, 30 days or more may be required before meaningful postsurgical levels can be obtained. The half-lives of AFP and $\beta$-hCG are 6 days and 1 day, respectively. After treatment, unequal reduction of $\beta$-hCG and AFP may occur, suggesting that the two markers are synthesized by heterogeneous clones of cells within the tumor; thus, both markers should be followed. $\beta$-hCG is similar to luteinizing hormone except for its distinctive beta subunit.

**III-87.   The answer is C.**   *(Chap. 81; Morris, Scher, Cancer 89:1329–1348, 2000.)*   In light of the poorly differentiated histology at presentation with the associated high risk of recurrence and the characteristic indicators of metastatic prostate cancer, biopsy is unnecessary. Because the patient has symptomatic disease, he should be started on androgen deprivation therapy, which is likely to cause a decrease in his pain. An equivalent response rate has been demonstrated with bilateral orchiectomy, DES, and luteinizing hormone–releasing hormone (LHRH) analogues such as leuprolide. In light of his desire not to have an orchiectomy and his vascular disease, LHRH analogues would be the best approach. Although providing "total androgen blockade" may be beneficial, whether flutamide should be routinely combined with an LHRH agonist such as leuprolide is unclear. Chemotherapy, perhaps with taxanes, may have a role in treating hormone-refractory disease.

**III-88.   The answer is B.**   *(Chap. 83)*   Alhough the incidence of ovarian carcinoma is low, the propensity to present at an advanced stage (only 25% of patients have disease limited to one or both ovaries) helps explain why this disease is the most common cause of death among all gynecologic malignancies. As a result of the advanced stage at presentation, surgical debulking is the initial therapy for most of these patients. Only about 15% of ovarian cancers arise from nonepithelial elements. Epithelial tumors are most common in peri- or postmenopausal women, especially nulliparous women and those with few children. Prior breast cancer increases the risk of developing ovarian cancer by twofold to fourfold. An advanced stage and a larger size of residual tumor after initial surgery carry an adverse prognosis, as do poorly differentiated ovarian carcinomas, which are associated with a 5-year survival well under 20%.

**III-89. The answer is C.** *(Chap. 77)* Squamous cell cancer of the esophagus accounts for approximately 10,000 deaths annually in the United States. Worldwide, incidence rates vary greatly, but it is particularly common in a belt from the Caspian Sea to northern China. In the United States, epidemiologic studies have linked smoking and alcohol to squamous cell cancer of the esophagus and may explain the association of this tumor with head and neck carcinoma. Exposure to agents that damage the mucosa (e.g., very hot tea, lye, radiation) or ingestion of carcinogens such as nitrites, smoked opiates, and fungal toxins is associated with an increased risk of esophageal carcinoma. The long-term stasis associated with achalasia leads to chronic irritation of the esophagus, which is thought to predispose to cancer formation. Tylosis is a genetic disease characterized by thickening of the skin on the hands and feet and is associated with squamous cell cancer of the esophagus. Chronic gastric reflux (Barrett's esophagus) is associated with adenocarcinoma but not with squamous cell carcinoma of the esophagus.

**III-90. The answer is A.** *(Chap. 75)* Approximately 20% of all lung cancers are small-cell cancers. These tumors tend to present centrally, be derived from neuroendocrine tissues, and be much more chemo- and radiosensitive than non-small cell cancer. Histologic subtypes of non-small cell cancer include adenocarcinoma (which has a more often peripheral presentation), large cell cancer, bronchoalveolar cell cancer, and squamous cell (or bronchogenic) lung cancer. All histologic types of lung cancer are associated with smoking. In the relatively uncommon patient who presents with a small non-small cell primary lesion and no lymph node involvement, surgery alone may be curative. Patients with small-cell lung cancer are divided into two staging groups: those with limited disease who have tumors generally confined to one hemithorax encompassable by a single radiation port and all others who are said to have extensive disease. About 20 percent of patients who present with limited-stage small-cell lung cancer are curable with a combination of radiation therapy and chemotherapy, with cisplatin and etoposide being the two most active agents.

**III-91. The answer is C.** *(Chaps. 70 and 82)* It is important to be familiar with the unique side effects of chemotherapeutic agents. Most drugs used to treat cancer inhibit cell division in one form or another. Tissues that undergo rapid turnover, such as the hair, gastrointestinal tract, and bone marrow, are most typically affected. Therefore, hair loss, mouth sores, diarrhea, and cytopenias are very commonly observed side effects after the administration of chemotherapy. However, certain commonly used drugs have a more specific side-effect spectrum. Bleomycin, an antitumor antibiotic that is used to treat patients with Hodgkin's disease and testicular cancer, can produce interstitial lung disease and pulmonary fibrosis. Patients who receive bleomycin-containing chemotherapy regimens are typically followed with serial lung examinations and pulmonary function studies, with a decrement in the diffusion capacity for carbon monoxide being a cause for concern. Because oxygen can potentiate the pulmonary damage mediated by bleomycin, patients receiving such chemotherapy must be supported with very low inspired concentrations of oxygen, if, for example, they need a surgical procedure.

**III-92. The answer is A.** *(Chap. 87)* The Lambert-Eaton neuromuscular syndrome—weakness of muscles caused by inability to release acetylcholine from the presynaptic fiber of the neuromuscular junction—is one of the most common paraneoplastic neurologic syndromes. However, patients with clinical Lambert-Eaton syndrome harbor a malignancy only about 50% of the time. Small-cell lung cancer accounts for the vast majority of those with malignancy-associated Lambert-Eaton syndrome; 3% of all patients with small-cell cancer of the lung have this type of paraneoplastic syndrome. Most of these patients have abnormalities of the peripheral nervous system, but occular (ptosis, diplopia) and bulbar (dysphasia, dysarthria) symptoms may also occur. The pathophysiology is believed to represent a neoplasm-induced IgG antibody against the voltage-gated calcium channels in the terminus of the motor neuron. The best therapy is control of the primary neoplasm; however, immunosuppression to reduce antibody formation and acetylcholine-enhancing drugs such as pyridostigmine have also been tried, with variable success.

**III-93. The answer is C.** *(Chap. 87; Sillevis Smith et al, N Engl J Med 342:21–27, 2000.)* One of the better characterized paraneoplastic neurologic syndromes is cerebellar ataxia caused by Purkinje cell drop-out in the cerebellum; it is manifested by dysarthria, limb and gait ataxia, and nystagmus. Radiologic imaging reveals cerebellar atrophy. Many antibodies have been associated with this syndrome, including anti-Yo, anti-Tr, and antibodies to the glutamate receptor. Although lung cancer, particularly small-cell cancer, accounts for a large number of patients with neoplasm-associated cerebellar ataxia, those with the syndrome who display anti-Yo antibodies in the serum typically have breast or ovarian cancer.

**III-94. The answer is E.** *(Chaps. 86 and 88)* Although it once was thought that most cases of hypercalcemia of malignancy are due to a direct resorption of bone by the tumor, it is now recognized that 80% of such instances occur because of the production of a protein called parathyroid hormone reactive protein (PTHrP) by the tumor. PTHrP shares 80% homology in the first 13 terminal amino acids with native parathyroid hormone. The aberrantly produced molecule is essentially functionally identical to native parathyroid hormone in that it causes renal calcium conservation, osteoclast activation and bone resorption, renal phosphate wasting, and increased levels of urinary cyclic adenine monophosphate (cAMP). Only about 20% of cases of the hypercalcemia malignancy are due to local production of substances, such as transforming growth factor and IL-1 or IL-6, which cause bone resorption at the local level and release of calcium from bony stores. Although aggressive hydration with saline and administration of a loop diuretic are helpful in the short-term management of patients with the hypercalcemia of malignancy, the most important therapy is the administration of a bisphosphonate, such as pamidronate, that will control the laboratory abnormalities and the associated symptoms in the vast majority of these patients. Symptoms of hypercalcemia are nonspecific and include fatigue, lethargy, polyuria, nausea, vomiting, and decreased mental acuity.

**III-95. The answer is A.** *(Chaps. 73 and 88)* Metastases to the spine are extremely common in patients with solid tumors, particularly those with breast cancer, renal cell carcinoma, multiple myeloma, melanoma, prostate cancer, and lung cancer. Back pain in a patient with cancer should always be taken seriously. Any finding suggesting cord compression on physical examination (extensor plantar response or loss of pinprick sensation in a sensory-level distribution) or an abnormal routine radiographic examination (particularly loss of pedicles on plain radiography of the spine) should prompt a definitive anatomic study. The most appropriate definitive study is an MRI of the entire spine to define the locus of disease, which most commonly would be metastases to a vertebral body growing into the canal. In this patient's case, there is a high likelihood of disseminated malignant melanoma in light of the fact that he had a deep lesion resected several years ago. However, other histologies are also theoretically possible. The uncertainty of the diagnosis coupled with the radioresistance and chemoresistance of this tumor should prompt primary consideration for surgery to resect the tumor, prevent cord compromise, and define the histology. A prolonged disease-free interval with subsequent development of aggressive metastatic disease is not unusual for patients with malignant melanoma.

**III-96. The answer is C.** *(Chap. 102; Bick, Hematol Oncol Clin North Am 10:875, 1996.)* A unifying pathophysiologic explanation for the association between malignancy and thrombosis has not been developed; however, many factors may play a role in increasing the likelihood of abnormal clotting in cancer patients. Those factors include immobilization and bed rest, dysproteinemias producing hyperviscosity, abnormal platelet function in myeloproliferative disorders, tumor-associated low-grade DIC, production of procoagulants by the tumor, and cancer-mediated thrombocytosis. Unlike the case for patients with coagulopathies, there is no useful laboratory test that will identify the hypercoagulable state. Different types of malignancies may be associated with specific thrombotic syndromes. For example, migratory superficial thrombophlebitis (Trousseau's syndrome) in the absence of apparent predisposing factors is most frequently associated with gastrointestinal malignancies, particularly pancreatic carcinoma. Hepatic vein thrombosis (Budd-Chiari syndrome) and portal vein thrombosis are associated with myeloproliferative disorders such as paroxysmal nocturnal hemoglobinuria, essential thrombocythemia, and polycythemia vera.

**III-97.   The answer is D.**   *(Chap. 93)*   The gene for G6PD is on the X chromosome; thus, G6PD deficiency is a sex-linked trait. Hemolytic anemia occurs much more commonly in males than in heterozygote female carriers, who are usually asymptomatic. Among the more than 100 variants of G6PD, the most commonly encountered variant of clinical significance in the United States is the A-type, which is found in about 15% of black males. It generally causes less severe hemolysis than does the Mediterranean variant. Hemolysis is usually precipitated by an environmental oxidant stress, most commonly viral or bacterial infection. Certain drugs, such as antimalarial agents, sulfonamides, phenacetin, and vitamin K, can also trigger hemolysis. These oxidant stresses cause precipitation of hemoglobin because affected persons are unable to maintain adequate intracellular levels of reduced glutathione. Precipitated hemoglobin forms Heinz bodies that are visualized only with supravital stains; these inclusions cause premature destruction of red blood cells. The diagnosis should be considered in any person experiencing a hemolytic episode. However, since decreased G6PD levels are found mainly in older cells, a false-negative test may be obtained during a hemolytic crisis, and the test should be repeated upon recovery.

**III-98.   The answer is B.**   *(Chap. 81; Carter et al, J Natl Cancer Inst 91:1733–1737, 1999.)* PSA determinations are assuming an increasingly important role in the diagnosis, screening, and staging of men with prostate cancer. Patients with urinary symptoms who are found to have an elevated level of serum PSA have a 60% percent likelihood of having prostate cancer. About 16% of patients with prostate cancer have an elevated level of serum PSA as the sole diagnostic abnormality. However, additional studies need to be done to delineate precisely the role of PSA evaluation in screening. Fewer than 10% of ambulatory volunteers older than age 50 years have elevated serum PSA values. A serum PSA between 4 and 10 ng/mL indicates that cancer is 25% likely, whereas values >10 ng/mL increase the likelihood of cancer to about 60%. About 20% of those with an elevated PSA (alone) compared with 10% of those with a suspicious digital rectal examination (alone) will have prostate cancer. The vast majority of cancers that are detected by screening for PSA are localized clinically and therefore have an excellent chance of being cured with either radiation or surgery. Moreover, few tumors detected by PSA screening are incidental as most have a high volume or a worrisome Gleason score (indicating a poor prognosis based on histologic grade). However, additional studies demonstrating a screening-induced decrease in cancer-related mortality are necessary to convince all that screening for prostate cancer with PSA determinations is beneficial. A clear use for serum PSA determination is in postoperative evaluation. If the postoperative serum PSA value is detectable, the presence of residual tumor is likely. A rising PSA value after definitive radiation therapy indicates a high likelihood of eventual metastatic spread. The use of systemic hormonal therapy for metastatic prostate cancer should be reserved for patients with certain evidence of locally advanced or metastatic disease.

**III-99.   The answer is B.**   *(Chap. 85; Lenzi et al, J Clin Oncol 15:2056–2066, 1997.)*   Approximately 10% of all cancer patients present in such a manner that assignment of the organ of origin of the tumor is unclear. Most patients who present in this fashion will have neoplasms that are poorly responsive to systemic therapy. However, it is important to recognize certain subgroups in which a specific approach to treatment might be beneficial or even associated with long-term disease-free survival. One such group has what has been termed the unrecognized extragonadal germ cell cancer syndrome. This includes patients displaying one or more of the following features: age less than 50 years; tumor involving midline structures, lung, or parenchymal lymph nodes; an elevated serum $\alpha$ fetoprotein or $\beta$-hCG level; or evidence of rapid tumor growth. If patients with these features do not have any histologic or immunohistochemical features suggesting a primary site, strong consideration should be given to treatment with a cisplatin-based chemotherapy regimen (as would be used for germ cell cancer). Approximately 20% of patients presenting in this fashion may be cured with the use of cisplatin, bleomycin, and etoposide chemotherapy.

**III-100. The answer is D.** *(Chap. 97)* Lymphoid neoplasms may be classified in regard to their cell of origin by the use of antisera and monoclonal antibodies against certain cell surface phenotypic markers and, more recently, by the use of DNA probes for immuno-globulin genes and genes for the beta chain of the T cell receptor. The malignant cell in CLL is a morphologically normal but functionally abnormal B lymphocyte. Follicular lymphomas arise from the lymphoid follicle, whereas the diffuse, small lymphocytic lymphomas (identical to CLL) are derived from the secretory compartment of the medullary cords. The Burkitt's lymphoma cell is a malignant cell of B lymphocyte lineage; in many cases it bears a characteristic chromosomal translocation: t(8;14). In contrast to these B cell neoplasms, mycosis fungoides is a peripheral T cell lymphoma in which helper cell function and phenotype have been identified in some cases.

**III-101. The answer is D.** *(Chap. 48)* Acanthosis nigricans is a skin disease that is associated with a number of disorders. The skin, which is thrown up into folds, appears velvety and hyperpigmented (brown to black) grossly and papillomatous microscopically. The lesions appear on the flexural areas of the neck, axillae, groin, and antecubital fossae; occasionally around the areolae, periumbilical and perianal areas, lips, and buccal mucosa; and over the surfaces of the palms, elbows, knees, and interphalangeal joints. The disorder may be hereditary or appear in association with obesity or an endocrinopathy (acromegaly, polycystic ovary syndrome, diabetes mellitus, and Cushing's syndrome but not adrenal insufficiency). Drugs such as nicotinic acid also can produce the condition. When acanthosis nigricans develops in a nonobese adult, neoplasia, particularly gastric adenocarcinoma, must be suspected.

# IV. INFECTIOUS DISEASES

## QUESTIONS

**DIRECTIONS:** Each question below contains four or five suggested responses. Choose the **one best** response to each question.

**IV-1.** A 19-year-old female from Guatemala presents to your office for a routine screening physical examination. At age 4 years she was diagnosed with acute rheumatic fever. She does not recall the specifics of her illness and remembers only that she was required to be on bed rest for 6 months. She has remained on penicillin V orally at a dose of 250 mg bid since that time. She asks if she can safely discontinue this medication. She has had only one other flare of her disease, at age 8, when she stopped taking penicillin at the time of her emigration to the United States. She is currently working as a day care provider. Her physical examination is notable for normal point of maximal impulse (PMI) with a grade III/VI holosystolic murmur that is heard best at the apex of the heart and radiates to the axilla. What do you advise the patient to do?

A. Penicillin prophylaxis can be discontinued because she has had no flares in 5 years.
B. An echocardiogram should be performed to determine the extent of valvular damage before deciding if penicillin can be discontinued.
C. She should change her dosing regimen to intramuscular benzathine penicillin every 8 weeks.
D. She should continue on penicillin indefinitely as she had a previous recurrence, has presumed rheumatic heart disease, and is working in a field with high occupational exposure to Group A streptococcus.
E. She should replace penicillin prophylaxis with polyvalent pneumococcal vaccine every 5 years.

**IV-2.** A 32-year-old female with AIDS and a CD4 count of $32/\mu L$ presents with a 3-week history of progressive dyspnea on exertion. The patient is homeless and currently takes no medication. On physical examination, she is tachypneic with a respiratory rate of 42/min, and her initial oxygen saturation is 84% on room air. A chest x-ray shows bilateral reticulonodular infiltrates. Arterial blood gases on room air are performed with the following results: pH 7.54, $Pa_{O_2}$ 48 mmHg, and $Pa_{CO_2}$ 28 mmHg. *Pneumoncystis carinii* (PCP) infection is strongly sus-

**IV-2.** *(Continued)*
pected. She is initiated on therapy with clindamycin and primaquine as she previously had an allergic reaction to sulfa drugs. Twenty-four hours later the patient develops hypoxemic respiratory failure and is intubated and mechanically ventilated. Which of the following statements regarding her care is true?

A. Her decline could have been prevented if treatment with trimethoprim-sulfamethoxazole had been used.
B. Her worsened oxygenation status probably is related to failure to prescribe steroids as part of the initial therapy.
C. Her 1-year mortality after recovery from an episode of *Pneumocystis carinii* pneumonia is 40%.
D. An elevated serum lactate dehydrogenase level would be diagnostic of PCP.
E. Highly active antiretroviral therapy should be started to improve her chances of survival.

**IV-3.** A 32-year-old female with AIDS and a CD4 count of $32/\mu L$ presents with a 3-week history of progressive dyspnea on exertion. The patient is homeless and currently takes no medication. On physical examination she is tachypneic with a respiratory rate of 42/min, and her initial oxygen saturation is 84% on room air. A chest x-ray shows bilateral reticulonodular infiltrates. Arterial blood gases on room air are performed, with the following results: pH 7.54, $Pa_{O_2}$ 48 mmHg, and $Pa_{CO_2}$ 28 mmHg. *Pneumoncystis carinii* infection is strongly suspected. She is started on therapy with clindamycin and primaquine as she previously had an allergic reaction to sulfa drugs. Twenty-four hours later the patient develops hypoxemic respiratory failure and is intubated and mechanically ventilated. Which of the following tests is mostly likely to provide a definitive diagnosis?

A. Bronchoalveolar lavage
B. Serum lactate dehydrogenase (LDH)
C. Induced sputum
D. High-resolution CT scan of the lung
E. PET scan of the lung

**IV-4.** A 44-year-old male with HIV presents to your office and asks whether he can discontinue prophylaxis against *Pneumocystis carinii*. His current CD4 T cell count is 330/μL, and his nadir count was 97/μl. He had an episode of PCP pneumonia 3 years previously, requiring prolonged hospitalization because of bilateral pneumothoraces. He has been on highly active antiretroviral therapy with lamivudine, efavirenz, and zidovudine for 18 months. His CD4 count has been >200/μL with an undetectable viral load for 9 months. What advice should you give this patient?

A. He can safely stop PCP prophylaxis as his CD4 count has been >200 for 3 months.
B. He will be able to stop PCP prophylaxis safely when his CD4 count has been >200 for 1 year.
C. He can safely stop PCP prophylaxis because his viral load has been undetectable for 6 months.
D. Because he had a complicated pneumonia with PCP, he can never safely discontinue prophylaxis.
E. He will be able to stop PCP prophylaxis safely when his viral load has been undetectable for 1 year.

**IV-5.** A 53-year-old male with a history of alcoholism presents with an enlarging mass at the angle of the jaw. The patient describes the mass slowly enlarging over a period of 6 weeks with occasional associated pain. He also has noted intermittent fevers throughout this period. Recently, he has developed yellowish drainage from the inferior portion of the mass. He takes no medications and has no other past history. He drinks six beers daily. On physical examination, the patient has a temperature of 37.9°C (100.2°F). His dentition is poor. There is diffuse soft tissue swelling and induration at the angle of the mandible on the left. It is mildly tender, and no discrete mass is palpable. The area of swelling is approximately 8 by 8 cm. An aspirate is sent for Gram stain and culture. The culture initially grows *Eikenella corrodens*. After 7 days you receive a call reporting growth of a gram-positive bacillus branching at acute angles on anaerobic media. What organism is causing this man's clinical presentation?

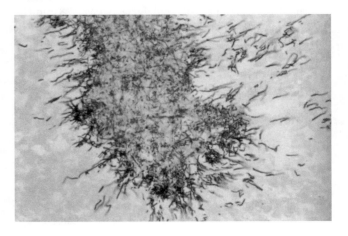

**IV-5.** *(Continued)*
A. *Nocardia*
B. *Actinomyces*
C. *Eikenella corrodens*
D. *Mucormycosis*
E. *Peptostreptococcus*

**IV-6.** What is the most appropriate therapy for this patient?

A. Surgical debridement
B. Amphotericin B
C. Itrakonazole
D. Penicillin
E. Tobramycin

**IV-7.** A 68-year-old female with end-stage renal disease and diabetes mellitus presents with an alteration in consciousness. She had been well until the day before admission, when she developed a mild gastrointestinal illness with several episodes of diarrhea and decreased oral intake. She receives hemodialysis three times weekly through a left upper extremity arteriovenous fistula. She takes multiple medications, including insulin, calcitriol, erythropoietin, and calcium acetate. On physical examination the patient is obtunded, moaning only to sternal rub. She is febrile to 39.6°C (103.3°F). Her blood pressure is 92/45. She has evidence of meningismus, with a positive Kernig sign. Her cerebrospinal fluid (CSF) is notable for 110 white blood cells in tubes 1 and 4 with a polymorphonuclear predominance at 93%. No red blood cells are present. The CSF glucose was 58 mg/dL, and protein was 93 mg/dL. Gram stain of the CSF reveals gram-positive rods. Which of the following antibiotic regimens along with an aminoglycoside is most effective against the organism that most likely is causing meningitis?

A. Ampicillin
B. Ceftriaxone
C. Rifampin
D. Trimethoprim-sulfamethoxazole
E. Vancomycin

**IV-8.** The primary means of transmission of donovanosis is

A. Fecal-oral
B. Sexual
C. Reduviid bug
D. Contaminated food source
E. Sandfly vector

**IV-9.** The bacterial organism responsible for donovanosis is

A. *Chlamydia trachomatis*
B. *Haemophilus ducreyi*
C. *Leishmania donovani*
D. *Calymmatobacterium granulomatis*
E. *Rickettsia prowazekii*

**IV-10.** You are a physician working on a cruise ship traveling from Miami to the Yucatán Peninsula. In the course of 24 h, 32 people are seen with acute gastrointestinal illness that is marked by vomiting and watery diarrhea. The most likely causative agent of the illness is

A. Enterohemorrhagic *Escherichia coli*
B. Norovirus
C. Rotavirus
D. Shigella
E. Salmonella

**IV-11.** What is the best method for diagnosis?

A. Acute and convalescent antibody titers
B. Demonstration of Norwalk toxin in the stool
C. Isolation in cell culture
D. Polymerase chain reaction to identify the Norwalk-associated calcivirus
E. Electron microscopy

**IV-12.** Which of the following has been shown to decrease the incidence of ventilator-acquired pneumonia?

A. Replacement of the ventilator circuit equipment every 24 h
B. Elevation of the head of the bed to more than 45 degrees
C. Selective gut decontamination with norfloxacin
D. Stress ulcer prophylaxis with sucralfate
E. Stress ulcer prophylaxis with a proton pump inhibitor

**IV-13.** You are an intensive care unit (ICU) physician caring for a 54-year-old female with chronic obstructive pulmonary disease who has had a prolonged intubation for hypercarbic respiratory failure. A recent urinalysis revealed the presence of many yeast with 3 to 5 WBC/hpf. She has been afebrile and is clinically stable. A Foley catheter is in place, draining dark yellow urine. A urine culture grows more than 10,000 colonies of *Candida albicans*. What is the best approach to treating this patient?

A. Treat only if a repeat urine culture reveals more than 100,000 colonies of *C. albicans*.
B. Initiate therapy with fluconazole through a nasogastric tube.
C. Initiate therapy with amphotericin B intravesicularly.
D. Remove the Foley catheter.
E. Treat only if a repeat urinalysis reveals more than 25 WBC/hpf.

**IV-14.** A 45-year-old male is admitted to the surgical ICU after a motor vehicle accident with multiple long bone fractures and lung contusions. He is placed on a mechanical ventilator and has bilateral chest tubes, a Foley catheter, and a triple-lumen central venous catheter infusing total parenteral nutrition. Four days after admission, he

**IV-14.** (*Continued*)
develops fever and blood cultures grow gram-positive cocci. What is the most likely source of his bacteremia?

A. Contamination of the parenteral nutrition
B. Contamination of the hubs of vascular devices
C. Hematogenous spread from an empyema
D. Migration of cutaneous microflora from the venous catheter insertion site
E. Urinary tract infection

**IV-15.** In assessing for infection related to a vascular access device, what is the most appropriate mode of culture?

A. Obtain cultures from each access port of the suspected line.
B. Obtain cultures peripherally from two separate sites with semiquantitative cultures of the catheter tip.
C. Obtain one culture from the central venous catheter and one peripherally.
D. Obtain semiquantitative cultures of the catheter tip.
E. Obtain a culture of skin from the exit site of the central venous catheter.

**IV-16.** Which of the following is true about the insertion and maintenance of central venous catheters?

A. Guidewire exchange is appropriate in replacing a malfunctioning catheter.
B. When one is sterilizing a site for insertion, povidine iodine 10% is most effective when the needle is introduced while the solution remains wet on the skin.
C. Scheduled guidewire exchange decreases the rate of catheter-related bacteremia.
D. Maximal barrier technique is not required in performing a guidewire exchange.
E. Application of bacitracin ointment to the catheter exit site has been proved to decrease subsequent infection rates.

**IV-17.** You are the on-call physician practicing in a suburban community. You receive a call from a 28-year-old female with a past medical history significant for sarcoidosis who is currently on no medications. She is complaining of the acute onset of crampy diffuse abdominal pain and multiple episodes of emesis that are nonbloody. She has not had any light-headedness with standing or loss of consciousness. When questioned further, the patient states that her last meal was 5 hours previously, when she joined her friends for lunch at a local Chinese restaurant. She ate from the buffet, which included multiple poultry dishes and fried rice. What should you do for this patient?

A. Initiate antibiotic therapy with clindamycin.
B. Reassure the patient that her illness is self-limited and no further treatment is necessary if she can maintain adequate hydration.

**IV-17.** *(Continued)*

C. Ask the patient to go to the nearest emergency department for resuscitation with intravenous fluids.

D. Refer the patient for CT to assess for appendicitis.

E. Refer the patient for admission for intravenous vancomycin because of her immunocompromised state resulting from sarcoidosis.

**IV-18.** The most common cause of traveler's diarrhea in Mexico is

A. *Campylobacter jejuni*
B. *Vibrio cholerae*
C. *Giardia lamblia*
D. Enterotoxigenic *Escherichia coli*
E. *Entamoeba histolytica*

**IV-19.** A 25-year-old male presents to your outpatient clinic with "swollen glands." He has noted subjective fevers at home, night sweats, and malaise for 10 days. He noted a mild sore throat 7 days ago that has resolved. He denies cough, chest pain, shortness of breath, or a rash. He has had four female sexual partners in the last year and denies illicit drug use. On exam, he has multiple 1-cm soft, nontender movable lymph nodes in the cervical chain. He has palpable, soft, movable, nontender 1-cm inguinal lymph nodes but no other adenopathy. His oropharynx has no lesions. His spleen is not palpable. The rest of the physical exam is unremarkable. All the following are reasonable initial management steps *except*

A. Observation
B. Monospot
C. HIV RNA polymerase chain reaction (PCR)
D. Complete blood count
E. Fine needle aspiration

**IV-20.** A 61-year-old male with a history of emphysema presents to the emergency room with a 3-day history of productive cough, diarrhea, and fever. A chest x-ray shows a patchy infiltrate in the right middle lobe. After 12 h, a urine sample comes back positive for *Legionella* antigen. The patient reports severe GI symptoms when taking macrolide antibiotics. The most appropriate antibiotic choice would be

A. Vancomycin
B. Clindamycin
C. Trimethoprim-sulfamethoxazole
D. Doxycycline
E. Levofloxacin

**IV-21.** A 30-year-old female complains of a week of bloody diarrhea, nausea, vomiting, and fever. She rapidly develops weakness in her lower extremities, beginning in the lower legs and ascending to the thighs. A diagnosis of Guillain-Barré syndrome is made. Which infectious agent is most strongly associated with the development of Guillain-Barré syndrome?

**IV-21.** *(Continued)*

A. *Campylobacter jejuni*
B. *E. coli* O:157:H7
C. Norwalk virus
D. *Shigella* species
E. *Yersinia enterocolitica*

**IV-22.** A 40-year-old male smoker with a history of asthma is admitted to the inpatient medical service with fever, cough, brownish-green sputum, and malaise. Physical exam shows a respiratory rate of 15, no use of accessory muscles of breathing, and bilateral polyphonic wheezes throughout the lung fields. There is no clubbing or skin lesions. You consider a diagnosis of allergic bronchopulmonary aspergillosis. All the following clinical features are consistent with allergic bronchopulmonary aspergillosis *except*

A. Bilateral, peripheral cavitary lung infiltrates
B. Elevated serum IgE
C. Peripheral eosinophilia
D. Positive serum antibodies to *Aspergillus* species
E. Positive skin testing for *Aspergillus* species

**IV-23.** A 35-year-old male presents to the emergency department in late summer with acute onset of fevers and severe pleuritic chest pain. He reports he felt well until the day before presentation, when he initially developed paroxysms of knifelike pleuritic chest pain. This was followed by a fever to 39.4°C (103.0°F). On physical examination the patient appears in marked distress, writhing in pain with rapid shallow breathing. His temperature currently is 38.8°C (101.8°F). The respiratory rate is 32 breaths per minute, and heart rate is 120 beats per minutes. Blood pressure is 112/68. Head, ears, eyes, nose, and throat (HEENT) exam is unremarkable. The patient is tachycardic with a regular rhythm and without murmurs or rubs. Chest examination reveals no accessory muscle use with shallow respirations. A focal pleural friction rub is heard posteriorly at the right lung base. There are no crackles. The remainder of the examination is unremarkable, including a normal abdominal exam and no evidence of joint inflammation or rashes. Laboratory examination shows a hemoglobin of 13.1 mg/dL and a white blood cell count of 9100 (62% polymorphonucleocytes, 28% lymphocytes, 7% monocytes, and 3% eosinophils). A chest radiograph shows no pulmonary infiltrates. What is the most likely cause of the patient's symptoms?

A. Systemic lupus erythematosis
B. *Pneumocystis* pneumonia
C. Coxsackie B virus infection
D. Echovirus infection
E. Familial Mediterranean fever

**IV-24.** A 19-year-old female is brought to the emergency department in September with fevers, headache, and change in mental status. The patient is a college freshman

**IV-24.** *(Continued)*

living in a dormitory. A week earlier the patient had a febrile gastrointestinal illness that subsequently resolved. The fevers returned on the morning of presentation and were followed by progressive headache. By the early evening the patient was lethargic with vomiting such that she was unable to tolerate liquids. On physical examination she is arousable but lethargic. She complains of pain with eye movement, but there are no focal neurologic deficits. She has a temperature of 39.1°C (102.3°F). Neck stiffness is present with positive Kernig and Brudzinski signs. A lumbar puncture is performed with an opening pressure of 27 cmH$_2$O. There are 130 white blood cells (97% lymphocytes) in the first tube and 110 white blood cells (95% lymphocytes) in the fourth tube. The protein is 76 mg/dL, and glucose is 56 mg/dL. A Gram stain shows many lymphocytes without any organisms. You admit the patient to the hospital for observation and further management. What do you tell the patient and her family about the prognosis and further therapy?

A. She should expect to recover with appropriate antibiotic therapy, but neurologic sequelae such as hearing loss are common.

B. Her illness could have been prevented by a vaccination that is recommended before moving into a college dormitory.

C. The mumps virus is most likely causing the patient's illness.

D. The patient's prognosis is excellent with appropriate supportive care, and she should expect to recover fully.

E. All the patient's contacts in the dormitory and classroom should be notified of the patient's illness and receive prophylactic antibiotic administration.

**IV-25.** A 32-year-old male presents to your clinic complaining of fevers, sore throat, and rash. He reports feelings of malaise for the last week. On the day before presentation the patient developed a vesicular rash on his palms and in his oropharynx (see Color Atlas, Fig. IV-25). His trunk and extremities are otherwise spared. He reports that the rash is tender, and some vesicles have ulcerated. What is the most likely diagnosis?

A. Disseminated gonococcal infection

B. Hand-foot-and-mouth disease

C. *Varicella zoster* infection

D. Secondary syphilis

E. Behçet's disease

**IV-26.** Oral polio vaccination is recommended in all the following instances *except*

A. An unvaccinated 20-year-old female who is traveling with the Red Cross to Pakistan, where there has been an epidemic polio outbreak

B. A 12-year-old child who is traveling with his parents to east Africa within the next 2 weeks

**IV-26.** *(Continued)*

C. A 6-month-old child whose father previously received a bone marrow transplant for treatment of acute myelogenous leukemia

D. An unvaccinated 32-year-old female who is traveling to an endemic area and is breast-feeding a 12-month-old infant.

**IV-27.** All the following infections are caused by *Bartonella* species *except*

A. Cat-scratch disease

B. Oroya fever

C. Peliosis hepatis

D. Q fever

E. Veruga peruana

**IV-28.** A 27-year-old male presents with painful lymphadenopathy and fevers for 1 week. On questioning, the patient reports that he has a 6-month-old kitten at home. Physical examination reveals a temperature of 37.9°C (100.3°F). There are multiple 3- to 5-cm enlarged tender lymph nodes in the right anterior cervical chain. Multiple scratches are noted on the patient's forearms in various stages of healing. You suspect cat-scratch disease. What is the best way to make the diagnosis?

A. Blood cultures for *Bartonella henselae*

B. Blood cultures for *Afipia felis*

C. Serologic tests for *B. henselae*

D. Demonstration of small gram-negative rods on Giemsa stain of lymph node biopsy

E. Polymerase chain reaction performed on tissue from lymph node biopsy.

**IV-29.** In the case in Question IV-28 the diagnosis of cat-scratch disease is confirmed. What treatment do you recommend?

A. No treatment is necessary as the disease is self-limited.

B. Oral azithromycin for 5 days.

C. Intravenous azithromycin plus gentamicin.

D. Oral cephalexin for 14 days.

E. A single dose of intramuscular penicillin.

**IV-30.** A 35-year-old male with acquired immune deficiency syndrome and a CD4 count of 32/mm$^3$ presents with a complaint of purple lesions on the lower extremities. In addition, the patient complains of daily fevers, right upper quadrant abdominal pain, and a 25-pound weight loss. The patient has a history of cryptococcal meningitis. He is not on highly active antiretroviral therapy. His medications include fluconazole and dapsone. The patient is allergic to sulfa drugs. He acquired HIV through homosexual contact. On physical examination the patient appears chronically ill with temporal wasting. He weighs 52 kg. His temperature is 38.2°C (100.8°F). Ab-

**IV-30.** *(Continued)*

dominal examination shows enlargement of the liver to 10 cm below the right costal margin with tenderness to palpation. There is also mild splenomegaly. No ascites is present. There are numerous purple papular lesions measuring 1 to 2 cm on the lower extremities. A biopsy of the skin lesion shows lobular proliferation of blood vessels with many bacilli seen on Warthin-Starry stain. What is the diagnosis?

A. Disseminated Kaposi's sarcoma
B. Epstein-Barr virus–associated B cell lymphoma
C. Disseminated cryptococcal disease
D. Bacillary angiomatosis and peliosis hepatis
E. Pyogenic granuloma

**IV-31.** A 24-year-old male is brought to the emergency department with shortness of breath and confusion. He recently returned from a retreat in New Mexico, where he stayed in rodent-infested cabins. For the past 3 or 4 days he has complained of fever, muscle aches, nausea, and vomiting. Today he became more short of breath and confused. His physical examination is notable for a temperature of 39°C (102.2°F), blood pressure of 90/60 mmHg, heart rate of 135/min, and respiratory rate of 28/min. Oxygen saturation on room air is 84%. His chest has minimal crackles. There are no petechiae or echymoses. Chest radiography shows bilateral pulmonary edema and pleural effusions. Laboratory studies demonstrate a low platelet count and atypical lympocytes on blood smear. Which of the following will be most useful in making a diagnosis?

A. Culture of blood
B. Culture of pleural fluid
C. Flow cytometry of the atypical lymphocytes
D. Measurement of IgM antibodies
E. Silver stain of bronchoalveolar lavage

**IV-32.** A 56-year-old male originally from St. Croix, Virgin Islands, presents to your hospital complaining of fatigue, fevers, and weight loss for 6 months. He has HIV that he acquired through heterosexual contact, with a CD4 count most recently of 156. He is not on any highly active antiretroviral therapy as he has been unable to tolerate many of these medications because of a variety of side effects. He currently is not taking any medications. On physical examination the patient is tachypneic and febrile to 39.1°C (102.3°F). He appears chronically ill. His liver is palpable 12 cm below the right costal margin. His spleen is also enlarged and is palpable 8 cm below the left costal margin. Scattered on his extremities and trunk are multiple purple papules measuring no more than 2 cm, as shown in Figure IV-32 (Color Atlas). The patient has diffuse lymphadenopathy. He undergoes a lymph node biopsy, which reveals the hyaline vascular variant of Castleman's disease. What is the cause of the patient's disease?

**IV-32.** *(Continued)*

A. Disseminated CMV infection
B. Bacillary angiomatosis
C. Disseminated Epstein-Barr virus infection
D. HTLV-1-associated lymphoma
E. Human herpesvirus 8 infection

**IV-33.** What is the causative organism of Lemierre's disease (septic thrombophlebitis of the internal jugular vein)?

A. *Peptostreptococcus*
B. *Fusobacterium necrophorum*
C. *Actinobacillus*
D. *Bacteroides fragilis*
E. *Enterococcus faecium*

**IV-34.** A 64-year-old female with an indwelling hemodialysis catheter develops fevers and chills. She subsequently grows *Enterococcus faecalis* and is found to have a mitral valve vegetation with preserved valvular function. The minimum inhibitory concentration for penicillin is <16 μg/mL, and the minimum inhibitory concentration of gentamicin is <2000 μg/mL. The patient has no allergies. The catheter is replaced and put in a new site. What is the treatment of choice for this patient?

A. Intravenous ampicillin plus gentamicin
B. Intravenous ampicillin
C. Valve replacement surgery followed by intravenous ampicillin
D. Intravenous vancomycin plus gentamicin
E. Intravenous ampicillin plus linezolid

**IV-35.** Which of the following drugs for HIV is incorrectly matched with its side effect?

A. Indinavir—kidney stones
B. Nelfinavir—lipodystrophy
C. Didanosine—pancreatitis
D. Efavirenz—lactic acidosis
E. Abacavir—hypersensitivity rash

**IV-36.** A 34-year-old male complains of a left frontal headache for 2 weeks that is not relieved by analgesics. One month ago he had extensive dental work for necrotic teeth and gingivitis. He has no other significant past medical history. His vital signs are normal except a temperature of 38°C (100.4°F). Physical examination is otherwise unremarkable. CT scan of the head demonstrates an abscess in the left frontal lobe. Which of the following organisms is most likely to be the predominant organism on sterile culture of the abscess?

A. *Bacteroides*
B. *Neisseria*
C. *Peptostreptococcus*
D. *Staphylococcus*
E. *Zygomyces*

**IV-37.** A 32-year-old female comes to the emergency department reporting 5 days of worsening left lower abdominal pain, nausea, and low-grade fever. Her past medical history is notable for prior episodes of gonorrhea and chlamydial sexually transmitted diseases (STDs). The only medication she is taking is an oral contraceptive. Physical examination is notable for a temperature of 38.9°C (102.2°F) and tenderness to palpation in the left lower quadrant without rebound. A pelvic examination reveals cervical motion tenderness and a possible mass in the left Fallopian area. A serum $\beta$-HCG is negative. Pelvic ultrasound reveals a 3- by 3-cm mass with an air-fluid level adjacent to the left ovary. Which of the following is most likely to be the predominant microbe on sterile culture of the mass?

A. *Bacteroides fragilis*
B. *Chlamydia trachomatis*
C. *Clostridium septicum*
D. *Gardnerella vaginalis*
E. *Neisseria gonorrhoeae*

**IV-38.** A previously healthy 19-year-old male college student presents to his physician's office with 3 weeks of progressive nonproductive cough, mild headache, and fevers. He has had no sick contacts and takes no medications. On further questioning, he mentions a painful rash over his hands and feet for the last 2 days, but he has had no other associated symptoms. His temperature is 38.9°C (102°F), pulse 110, respiratory rate 20, and blood pressure 120/70 with a finger pulse oximetry reading of 95% on room air. He is coughing frequently but has normal breath sounds bilaterally. A picture of his rash is shown in Figure IV-38 (Color Atlas). A chest radiograph shows bilateral diffuse interstitial infiltrates. The most likely etiology of this patient's illness is

A. Herpes simplex virus
B. *Chlamydia psittacosis*
C. *Mycoplasma pneumoniae*
D. Influenza
E. *Haemophilus influenzae*

**IV-39.** The most appropriate therapy for this patient is

A. Cefepime
B. Penicillin
C. Acyclovir
D. Gatifloxacin
E. Amantadine

**IV-40.** A 25-year-old male is seen in the emergency department for symptoms of fevers and abdominal swelling, early satiety, and weight loss. His symptoms began abruptly 2 weeks ago. He was previously healthy and is taking no medications. He denies illicit drug use and recently immigrated to the United States from Bangladesh.

**IV-40.** *(Continued)*
On physical exam, temperature is 39.0°C (102.2°F) and pulse is 120 with normal blood pressure and respiratory rate. The remainder of the exam is notable for cachexia and a distended abdomen with a massively enlarged spleen. The spleen is tender and soft. The liver is not palpable. Mild peripheral adenopathy is present. Which of the following statements is correct regarding this patient with presumed kala azar leishmaniasis?

A. He probably has normal cell counts on peripheral blood smear.
B. Splenic aspiration offers the highest diagnostic yield.
C. Leishmania-specific cell-mediated immunity probably is present.
D. Treatment can be delayed until the diagnosis is confirmed.
E. A thick and a thin smear are unlikely to be helpful in light of the duration of symptoms.

**IV-41.** A migrant worker is seen in the clinic for progressive weight loss and occasional diarrhea. A helminthic infection is strongly suspected. The patient collects a stool sample, and it is submitted for laboratory analysis. Cultures are negative, and stool ova and parasites are not seen. A computed tomogram with oral and IV contrast is unremarkable. Which of the following statements is most correct?

A. A minimum of three stools should be obtained to examine for ova and parasites to rule out helminthic infection.
B. The patient can be reassured that his symptoms are not due to helminthic infection.
C. All submitted samples would be from sequential bowel movements.
D. Stool analysis will not be affected by ingestion of oral contrast.
E. Empirical albendazole is indicated.

**IV-42.** A 21-year-old female is seen in the general medicine clinic for changes she has noted on her nipples after initiating breast-feeding with her now 3-month-old daughter. She recently immigrated to the United States from Senegal. She had a healthy childhood but noted that for several years she had patches within her mouth on the buccal mucosa that several other family members also had. On physical exam she has numerous patches over both nipples. A biopsy is obtained of one of the lesions, and it shows gummae. Endemic syphilis is suspected. Which of the following statements is true?

A. The etiologic agent is *Treponema pallidum* subspecies *pallidum*.
B. The patient probably has primary infection with this spirochete.

**IV-42.**  *(Continued)*

C.   The child probably has mucosal lesions similar to the patient's previous lesions.

D.   Rapid plasma reagin (RPR) is likely to be negative in the patient's serum.

E.   No therapy is indicated at this time.

**IV-43.**   A 57-year-old female with chronic renal insufficiency requiring hemodialysis complains of 2 months of increasing low back pain, malaise, and fatigue. She attends dialysis regularly three times a week and has a history of mild degenerative joint disease. Her physical examination is notable for normal vital signs and tenderness to palpation over the L4–L5 lumbar area. The neurologic examination is normal. Radiographs of the lumbar spine demonstrate irregular erosions in the end plates of the L4 and L5 disks with narrowing of the disk space. Which of the following most likely explains her back pain?

A.   Ankylosing spondylitis

B.   Bacterial osteomyelitis

C.   Multiple myeloma

D.   Rheumatoid arthritis

E.   Secondary hyperparathyroidism

**IV-44.**   A 43-year-old male with diabetes sees his physician, complaining of 4 weeks of lumbar back pain. He was discharged from the hospital 6 weeks ago after a motor vehicle accident. During his hospitalization he spent 2 weeks in the ICU receiving mechanical ventilation and parenteral nutrition. Bone scans of the lumbar spine reveal increased uptake in L3–L4, and a needle biopsy grows *Staphylococcus aureus*. He is treated with 4 weeks of intravenous oxacillin. Which of the following studies will be most helpful in deciding whether to continue antibiotics for another 2 to 4 weeks?

A.   Alkaline phosphatase

B.   Bone scan

C.   C-reactive protein

D.   Plain radiographs of the lumbar spine

E.   White blood cell count

**IV-45.**   A 50-year-old male is 4 months past a lung transplant for pulmonary fibrosis. His medications include tacrolimus, mycophenalate mofitil, and predinisone. He lives with his son and daughter-in-law. They are expecting their first child in the next 2 or 3 months. You advise your patient that it is safe for the child to receive all the routine vaccinations *except*

A.   Live oral polio

B.   Nonviable hepatitis A

C.   Polyvalent pneumococcal

D.   Recombinant hepatitis B

E.   Tetanus toxoid

**IV-46.**   A 28-year-old female is about to start a new job teaching at a preschool. Her past medical history is notable for a heart transplant 4 years ago. Her maintenance medications include tacrolimus, azathioprine, and prednisone. She does not recall anything about her immunization history. She is concerned about the development of disease and would like to repeat the recommended childhood vaccinations. You advise her that it will be safe to receive all the following vaccinations *except*

A.   *Haemophilus influenzae* B

B.   Hepatitis B

C.   Inactivated polio virus

D.   MMR (measles/mumps/rubella)

E.   Tetanus

**IV-47.**   A 53-year-old male is seen by his primary care physician for a routine visit. He has a history of chronic renal insufficiency, and his nephrologist recently told him that he probably will require dialysis within the next 1 or 2 years. The patient reports that he has not received any vaccinations since childhood. In light of his age and medical condition you recommend all the following vaccinations *except*

A.   Annual influenza vaccine

B.   Hepatitis A vaccine

C.   Hepatitis B vaccine

D.   Polyvalent pneumococcal polysaccharide vaccine

E.   Varicella vaccine

**IV-48.**   A 24-year-old college student is brought to the emergency department by friends from his dormitory for altered mental status. They state that he recently returned from a trip to South America and that many colleagues have upper respiratory tract infections. His physical examination is notable for confusion, fever, and a rigid neck. CSF examination reveals a white blood cell count of 1800 cells/$\mu$L with 98% neutrophils, glucose of 35 mg/dL, and protein of 100 mg/dL. He is placed on empirical treatment for meningitis. Which of the following statements about the CSF examination is true?

A.   A negative latex agglutination test for *Staphylococcus pneumoniae* rules out this organism as a cause of the meningitis.

B.   A negative latex agglutination test for *Neisseria meningitidis* rules out this organism as a cause of the meningitis.

C.   Meningeal enhancement on MRI is diagnostic of meningitis.

D.   A positive limulus amebocyte lysate assay is diagnostic of protozoal meningitis.

E.   A positive latex agglutination test for *S. pneumoniae* is diagnostic of *S. pneumoniae* meningitis.

**IV-49.**   A 19-year-old college student is brought to the emergency department by friends from his dormitory for

**IV-49.** *(Continued)*

confusion and altered mental status. They state that many colleagues have upper respiratory tract infections. He does not use alcohol or illicit drugs. His physical examination is notable for confusion, fever, and a rigid neck. CSF examination reveals a white blood cell count of 1800 cells/$\mu$L with 98% neutrophils, glucose of 35 mg/dL, and protein of 100 mg/dL. Which of the following antibiotic regimens is most appropriate as initial therapy?

A. Ampicillin plus vancomycin
B. Ampicillin plus gentamicin
C. Cefazolin plus doxycycline
D. Cefotaxime plus doxycycline
E. Cefotaxime plus vancomycin

**IV-50.** In addition to antibiotics, which of the following adjunctive therapies should be administered to improve the chance of a favorable neurologic outcome?

A. Dexamethasone
B. Dilantin
C. Gabapentin
D. L-Dopa
E. Parenteral nutrition

**IV-51.** A 24-year-old previously healthy office worker comes to the emergency department complaining of a severe bilateral headache, malaise, and photophobia for 1 day. Her physical examination is notable for a temperature of 38.8°C (101.8°F) and neck pain on extreme flexion. She is lethargic but fully oriented. CSF is clear with a white blood cell count of 50 cells/$\mu$L with 80% lymphocytes. CSF glucose is 80 mg/dL, and protein is 40 mg/dL. Which of the following tests is most likely to be diagnostic?

A. Cerebral angiogram
B. Cerebral MRI with gadolinium
C. CSF acid-fast stain
D. CSF india ink stain
E. CSF latex agglutination for *S. pneumoniae*

**IV-52.** A 64-year-old female is admitted to the hospital with altered mental status. She recently returned from a summer white-water rafting trip in Colorado. Her husband reports increasing confusion, alternating lethargy and agitation, and visual hallucinations over the last 3 days. There is no history of drug abuse or psychiatric illness. She takes no medications. Her physical examination is notable for a temperature of 39°C (102.2°F), myoclonic jerks, and hyperreflexia. She is delirious and oriented to person only when aroused. There is no nuchal rigidity. CSF examination reveals clear fluid with a white blood cell count of 15 cells/$\mu$L with 100% lymphocytes, protein of 100 mg/dL, and glucose of 80 mg/dL. Gram stain of the CSF shows no organisms. You suspect infection with West Nile virus. Which of the following studies will be most useful in making that diagnosis?

**IV-52.** *(Continued)*

A. CSF culture
B. CSF IgM antibodies
C. CSF PCR
D. CNS MRI
E. Stool culture

**IV-53.** A 44-year-old male is undergoing evaluation for altered mental status. His wife reports increasing confusion, forgetfulness, and decreased vision over the last month. She also notes that his mood has become very labile with frequent outbursts of anger. He has a history of intravenous drug abuse but quit 4 years ago. He is on no medications. Physical examination is notable for a normal temperature and vital signs, cachexia, and a left homonymous hemianopia. He is oriented only to person, cannot follow complex commands, and has marked short-term memory loss. A brain MRI shows bilateral periventricular white matter lesions on T2 imaging. There are no masses, and the ventricles are of normal size. CSF testing is notable for the presence of JC viral DNA on PCR testing. Additional testing most likely will be positive for

A. Anti-Hu antibody
B. Antinuclear antibodies
C. c-ANCA
D. Hepatitis B antibody
E. HIV antibody

**IV-54.** A 29-year-old female with a history of allergic rhinitis seeks medical attention, complaining of 3 days of purulent nasal drainage and headache. Vital signs are normal, and there is some tenderness to percussion over the left frontal sinus and bilateral nasal congestion. The remainder of the physical examination is normal. Which of the following is most appropriate at this time?

A. Nasal decongestants alone
B. Nasal decongestants plus amoxicillin
C. Nasal decongestants plus doxycycline
D. Nasal decongestants plus a sinus CT scan
E. Nasal decongestants plus sinus radiographs

**IV-55.** A 27-year-old male is brought to the emergency department with fever, confusion, and difficulty breathing. Five days ago he was evaluated for a sore throat and was found to have an exudate on the right tonsil. No antibiotics were prescribed. He works in an office, is sexually active in a monogamous relationship, does not smoke cigarettes, does not use illicit drugs, and is on no medications. On the day of admission he complained of worsening sore throat, right neck pain, dysphagia, and rigors. Physical examination is notable for a temperature of 39.2°C (102.6°F), blood pressure of 85/55 mmHg, heart rate of 125 /min, and swelling, redness, and pain over the right lateral neck. A chest radiograph shows multiple round opacities, some with an air-fluid level. Which of the

**IV-55.** *(Continued)*
following organisms is most likely to grow on blood culture?

A.  *Bacteroides fragilis*
B.  *Fusobacterium necrophorum*
C.  *Rhizopus oryzae*
D.  *Staphylococcus aureus*
E.  *Neisseria gonorrhoeae*

**IV-56.** A 45-year-old male reports to his internist because of fatigue. He gives a history of being treated successfully for testicular cancer 10 years earlier. The physical examination is unremarkable. Routine blood tests reveal a normal complete blood count, normal creatinine, normal $\alpha$-fetoprotein, and normal $\beta$-human chorionic gonadotropin, but his hepatic transaminases are each three times the upper limit of normal. Knowing that the patient had received blood transfusional therapy while receiving cancer chemotherapy, the physician orders serologic studies for hepatitis viruses, which reveal evidence of his having had a prior infection with hepatitis C virus (HCV). The next most appropriate diagnostic or therapeutic strategy would be to

A.  Send serum to detect HCV RNA by polymerase chain reaction (PCR) analysis
B.  Refer for liver biopsy
C.  Begin interferon (IFN) therapy
D.  Repeat the serologic test for hepatitis C virus
E.  Order tomographic scanning of the abdomen and pelvis

**IV-57.** A 55-year-old female from Oregon presents with diplopia 24 hours after eating home-canned fruit. Within a few hours of presentation she is also noted to have dysphonia and arm weakness. Other symptoms include nausea, vomiting, dizziness, blurred vision, and dry mouth. The patient is afebrile, alert, and oriented. Which of the following is *least* important in managing this patient's illness?

A.  Intravenous penicillin
B.  Spirometric monitoring
C.  Antitoxin therapy
D.  Laxatives
E.  Enema

**IV-58.** Several weeks after eating a meal in rural France that included meat from locally bred horses and pigs, a 35-year-old woman presents with muscle aches and swelling, particularly in both biceps and the neck. Physical examination reveals periorbital edema. Laboratory evaluation reveals eosinophilia, elevated serum IgE, and elevated creatinine phosphokinase levels. The most likely diagnosis is

**IV-58.** *(Continued)*
A.  Ocular larva migrans (*Toxocara canis* infection)
B.  Trichinosis
C.  Viral myositis
D.  Polymyositis (autoimmune)
E.  Typhoid fever

**IV-59.** Which of the following syndromes is least likely to be associated with parvovirus infection?

A.  A 5-year-old child with a 3-day history of low-grade fevers who presents with ruby-red cheeks
B.  A 35-year-old female with painful wrist and knees for 3 weeks
C.  A 20-year-old patient with sickle cell disease who presents with a marked drop in hematocrit
D.  A 55-year-old with hemolytic anemia and a normal white count and platelet count
E.  A 7-year-old boy with nausea, vomiting, and watery diarrhea for 3 days

**IV-60.** A 25-year-old intravenous drug abuser with fever has blood cultures obtained, and 24 hours later a report from the microbiology laboratory indicates the presence of gram-positive cocci in clusters. The identification of the organism and sensitivities are pending. The most appropriate antibiotic choice would be

A.  Penicillin
B.  Nafcillin
C.  Vancomycin
D.  Trimethoprim-sulfamethoxazole (TMP/SMZ)
E.  Ciprofloxacin

**IV-61.** What are the clinical consequences of *Bacillus anthracis* endospores coming in contact with an abrasion on the arm of a rancher?

A.  The endospores germinate in the skin, gain access to the blood, and cause death from massive sepsis.
B.  The endospores germinate in the skin, gain access to the lymphatic system, and cause significant axillary lymphadenopathy.
C.  The endospores germinate in the skin, gain access to the blood, and cause fatal pneumonia.
D.  The endospores are engulfed by dermal macrophages and are transported by them to the blood, at which point they germinate; the ensuing bacterial proliferation causes death from massive sepsis.
E.  The lesion that forms undergoes central necrosis and surrounding edema.

**IV-62.** A 23-year-old previously healthy female letter carrier works in a suburb in which the presence of rabid foxes and skunks has been documented. She is bitten by a bat, which then flies away. Initial examination reveals a clean

**IV-62.** *(Continued)*

break in the skin in the right upper forearm. She has no history of receiving treatment for rabies and is unsure about vaccination against tetanus. The physician should

A. Clean the wound with a 20% soap solution
B. Clean the wound with a 20% soap solution and administer tetanus toxoid
C. Clean the wound with a 20% soap solution, administer tetanus toxoid, and administer human rabies immune globulin intramuscularly
D. Clean the wound with a 20% soap solution, administer tetanus toxoid, administer human rabies immune globulin intramuscularly, and administer human diploid cell vaccine
E. Clean the wound with a 20% soap solution and administer human diploid cell vaccine

**IV-63.** A 73-year-old previously healthy male is hospitalized because of the acute onset of dysuria, urinary frequency, fever, and shaking chills. His temperature is 39.5°C (103.1°F), blood pressure is 100/60 mmHg, pulse is 140 beats per minute, and respiratory rate is 30 breaths per minute. Which of the following interventions would be the most important in the treatment of this acute illness?

A. Catheterization of the urinary bladder
B. Initiation of antibiotic therapy
C. Infusion of Ringer's lactate solution
D. Infusion of dopamine hydrochloride
E. Intravenous injection of methylprednisolone

**IV-64.** Which of the following organisms is most likely to cause infection of a shunt implanted for the treatment of hydrocephalus?

A. *Staphylococcus epidermidis*
B. *Staphylococcus aureus*
C. *Corynebacterium diphtheriae*
D. *Escherichia coli*
E. *Bacteroides fragilis*

**IV-65.** Exposure to which of the following mandates passive immunization with standard immune serum globulin?

A. Rabies
B. Hepatitis A
C. Hepatitis B
D. Tetanus
E. Cytomegalovirus

**IV-66.** Imipenem is coadministered with cilastatin because

A. The combination of these antibiotics is synergistic against *Pseudomonas* spp.
B. Cilastatin aids the gastrointestinal absorption of the active moiety, imipenem.

**IV-66.** *(Continued)*

C. Cilastatin inhibits a β-lactamase that destroys imipenem.
D. Cilastatin inhibits an enzyme in the kidney that destroys imipenem.
E. Cilastatin prevents the hypoprothrombinemic effect of imipenem.

**IV-67.** A 35-year-old male is seen 6 months after a cadaveric renal allograft. The patient has been on azathioprine and prednisone since that procedure. He has felt poorly for the past week with fever to 38.6°C (101.5°F), anorexia, and a cough productive of thick sputum. Chest x-ray reveals a left lower lobe (5 cm) nodule with central cavitation. Examination of the sputum reveals long, crooked, branching, beaded gram-positive filaments. The most appropriate initial therapy would include the administration of which of the following antibiotics?

A. Penicillin
B. Erythromycin
C. Sulfisoxazole
D. Ceftazidime
E. Tobramycin

**IV-68.** A previously healthy 28-year-old male describes several episodes of fever, myalgia, and headache that have been followed by abdominal pain and diarrhea. He has experienced up to 10 bowel movements per day. Physical examination is unremarkable. Laboratory findings are notable only for a slightly elevated leukocyte count and an elevated erythrocyte sedimentation rate. Wright's stain of a fecal sample reveals the presence of neutrophils. Colonoscopy reveals inflamed mucosa. Biopsy of an affected area discloses mucosal infiltration with neutrophils, monocytes, and eosinophils; epithelial damage, including loss of mucus; glandular degeneration; and crypt abscesses. The patient notes that several months ago he was at a church barbecue where several people contracted a diarrheal illness. Although this patient could have inflammatory bowel disease, which of the following pathogens is most likely to be responsible for his illness?

A. *Campylobacter*
B. *S. aureus*
C. *E. coli*
D. *Salmonella*
E. Norwalk agent

**IV-69.** A 19-year-old female visits the emergency room because of a swollen left knee. She has no past medical problems. She gives a history of several days of feeling feverish and having muscle and joint aches. Specifically, her hands and wrists were painful for a few days, but at this point she is bothered only by her knee. Physical examination is remarkable only for vesiculopustular skin le-

**IV-69.** *(Continued)*

sions and a mildly swollen left knee. The procedure most likely to yield a diagnosis at this point would be

A. Cervical culture
B. Blood culture
C. Sinovial culture
D. Serum complement assay
E. Skin biopsy

**IV-70.** A 65-year-old retired banker who spends the summer on Nantucket Island off the Massachusetts coast returned to his home in Boston early in September. He noted the gradual onset of a febrile illness with chills, sweats, myalgias, and yellow eyes. His doctor palpated the spleen and noted a macrocytic anemia, hyperbilirubinemia, and a high serum level of lactic dehydrogenase on laboratory examination. Which of the following would be the most helpful diagnostic procedure at this point?

A. Blood culture
B. Examination of leukocytes on blood film
C. Examination of erythrocytes on blood film
D. Splenic biopsy
E. Liver biopsy

**IV-71.** A 35-year-old intravenous drug abuser with HIV infection is being managed with combination antiretroviral therapy. The patient was doing well on his current medical regimen, which consists of lamivudine and saquinavir as well as methadone, trimethoprim-sulfamethoxazole (TMP/SMZ), and fluconazole. Although he has been stable clinically of late, efavirenz recently was added to his medical regimen in an attempt to decrease a rising viral load. After approximately 1 week of therapy with efavirenz, the patient develops abdominal cramps, malaise, sweats, and anxiety. The most likely reason for the patient's symptoms is

A. Primary efavirenz toxicity
B. Increased fluconazole levels
C. Infection with *Pneumocystis* as a result of decreased TMP/SMZ levels
D. Lamivudine toxicity secondary to decreased albumin binding
E. Reduced plasma methadone concentration

**IV-72.** A 19-year-old male comes to his physician complaining of 4 days of dysuria. He has no difficulty initiating his stream but has pain with urination. He denies fevers, chills, or testicular pain. He is heterosexually active with multiple partners. On examination, he is afebrile and there is no testicular pain, redness, or swelling. Milking the patient's urethra yields a small amount of purulent material. Gram stain reveals >5 white blood cells per high-power field with no gram-negative intracellular dip-

**IV-72.** *(Continued)*

lococci. Which of the following organisms is most likely to be causing his symptoms?

A. *Chlamydia trachomatis*
B. *Escherichia coli*
C. *Mycoplasma genitalium*
D. *Trichomonas vaginalis*
E. *Ureaplasma urealyticum*

**IV-73.** A 26-year-old male from Cape Cod sees his physician because of a 3-week history of an expanding, slightly burning ring of redness (as shown in Fig. IV-73, Color Atlas) that first surrounded a red papule on the posterior neck. He complains of headaches, generalized muscle aches, anorexia, and malaise. On examination he is noted to be febrile [38.3°C (101°F)]; his rash is slightly raised and slightly tender and displays central clearing but no scaling even after vigorous scraping. Which of the following vectors has been strongly associated with this type of rash?

A. Kissing bug
B. Spider
C. Flea
D. Tick
E. Housefly

**IV-74.** A 67-year-old male presents with a history of headache for 5 days and 2 days of swelling of the right part of the forehead and right eye (see Fig. IV-74, Color Atlas). A Tzanck preparation of the lesion reveals multinucleate giant cells on Giemsa stain. The patient is admitted to the hospital and put on intravenous acyclovir. The most important next step is

A. Ophthalmologic consultation
B. Administration of systemic glucocorticoids to prevent postherpetic neuralgia
C. Administration of antistaphylococcal antibiotics to prevent secondary bacterial infection
D. Application of an iodine-containing solution to prevent secondary bacterial infections
E. CT scan of the brain

**IV-75.** A person with liver disease caused by *Schistosoma mansoni* would be most likely to have

A. Gynecomastia
B. Jaundice
C. Esophageal varices
D. Ascites
E. Spider nevi

**IV-76.** A 25-year-old homosexual male presents with a diffuse maculopapular rash over the trunk, head, neck, palms, and soles. Generalized lymphadenopathy is also present. He has a history of 4 weeks of anal pain. Which

**IV-76.** *(Continued)*

of the following tests is likely to identify the etiologic agent?

A. Antinuclear antibody
B. Blood culture
C. Serum rapid plasma reagin (RPR)
D. Skin biopsy
E. Serum HIV antibody

**IV-77.** A 53-year-old female with breast cancer is receiving chemotherapy through an indwelling central venous catheter. She is not neutropenic but develops a fever. Evaluation reveals a bloodstream infection with *Candida krusei*. The catheter is removed, and therapy is initiated with amphotericin B. Physical exam shows no evidence of joint effusions, cellulitis, thrombophlebitis, or other skin abnormalities. Evaluation for thoracic or abdominal abcess is negative, lumbar puncture is negative, endoscopic evaluation is negative for esophagitis, and transesophageal echocardiogram is negative for vegetation. Despite premedications the patient developed bronchospasm and hypotension with the administration of the amphotericin B. How will you modify her therapy?

A. Discontinue amphotericin B and give amphotericin B lipid complex 5 mg/kg per day.
B. Discontinue amphotericin B and give fluconazole 800 mg per day.
C. Discontinue amphotericin B and give ketoconazole 400 mg/d.
D. Discontinue amphotericin B and give caspofungin 50 mg/kg per day.
E. Discontinue amphotericin B and give flucytosine 25 mg/kg qd.

**IV-78.** A 28-year-old female presents to her primary care physician with a complaint of painful fissures at the corner of the mouth that have been present for 2 weeks. She does not complain of odynophagia. Her past medical history is unremarkable without a history of diabetes. The patient is on no medications and has no allergies. She has smoked one pack per day of cigarettes for 5 years but denies alcohol or illicit drug use. She is monogamous with a new sexual partner for the last 3 months. Exam is significant for oral lesions (Fig. IV-78, Color Atlas). Complete blood count and Chem-7 are within normal limits, urine human chorionic gonadotropin (hCG) is negative, and HIV antibody is negative. What is the best recommendation?

A. Check glucose tolerance test.
B. Check HIV RNA PCR viral load.
C. Do not check further lab tests. Reevaluate in 2 weeks.
D. Check serum HCG.

**IV-79.** A 72-year-old male is admitted to the hospital with bacteremia and pyelonephritis. He is HIV-negative and

**IV-79.** *(Continued)*

has no other significant past medical history. Two weeks into his treatment with antibiotics a fever evaluation reveals a blood culture positive for *Candida albicans*. Exam is unremarkable. White blood cell count is normal. The central venous catheter is removed, and systemic antifungal agents are initiated. What further evaluation is recommended?

A. Repeat blood cultures
B. Abdominal CT scan to evaluate for abscess
C. Transthoracic echocardiogram
D. Chest x-ray
E. Funduscopic examination

**IV-80.** A 33-year-old, 60-kg male with HIV has a diagnosis of esophageal candidiasis by endoscopic evaluation and biopsy. Herpes virus evaluation was negative. He has been treated successfully with fluconazole. Five months later he is diagnosed again with esophageal candidiasis and treated successfully with fluconazole. He did not have any complications of candidemia, esophageal perforation, or significant malnutrition. He continues on HAART therapy and is currently without complaints. What is your next recommendation?

A. Initiate oral fluconazole 200 mg once a day
B. Initiate oral fluconazole 400 mg once a day
C. Intitiate oral itraconazole 300 mg once a day
D. Initiate oral voriconazole 200 mg twice a day
E. No added therapy at this time

**IV-81.** A 62-year-old female with a history of diabetes mellitus presents to the emergency room with a 3-day history of fever, complaints of aching pain across her sinuses, and a nasal discharge occasionally streaked with blood. Her family reports that the patient has been demonstrating signs of mild confusion over the last few days. Her past medical history is significant for allergic rhinitis. Her medications include insulin and an antihistamine. She has no allergies. Physical exam reveals a temperature of 37.8°C (100.1°F), heart rate of 110, and normal blood pressure. Extraocular movements are intact and visual fields are full without deficit, ear examination is normal, and nasal turbinate on the right is a dusky red color and is very painful. The oropharynx shows numerous necrotic eschars on the right soft and hard palate. Laboratories are significant for serum glucose of 400 mg/dL and serum bicarbonate of 10 meq/dL. Blood cultures are negative. What is the most likely diagnosis?

A. Diabetic ketoacidosis
B. *Aspergillus* sinusitis
C. Mucormycosis sinusitis
D. *Staphylococcus pneumonia* sinusitis
E. *S. aureus* sinusitis

**IV-82.** How is the diagnosis made?

A. Checking of arterial blood gas and serum ketones titer
B. Serial blood cultures
C. Sinus CT scan
D. Biopsy of the oropharynx
E. Lumbar puncture with culture of the cerebrospinal fluid

**IV-83.** A 38-year-old female pigeon keeper who has no significant past medical history, is taking no medications, has no allergies, and is HIV-negative presents to the emergency room with a fever, headache, and mild nuchal rigidity. Neurologic exam is normal. Head CT exam is normal. Lumbar puncture is significant for an opening pressure of 20 cmH$_2$O, white blood cell count 15 (90% monocytes), protein 50 mg/mL, glucose 50 mg/dL, and positive india ink stain. What is the appropriate therapy for this patient?

A. Intravenous ceftriaxone and vancomycin for 2 weeks
B. Amphotericin B for 10 weeks followed by oral fluconazole 400 mg daily for 6 to 12 months
C. Amphotericin B for 2 weeks
D. Amphotericin B with flucytosine for 2 weeks
E. Amphotericin B for 2 weeks followed by oral fluconazole 400 mg daily

**IV-84.** An HIV-positive patient with a CD4 count of 110/$\mu$L who is not taking any medications presents to an urgent care center with complaints of a headache for the past week. He also notes nausea and intermittently blurred vision. Exam is notable for normal vital signs without fever but mild papilledema. Head CT does not show dilated ventricles. The definitive diagnostic test for this patient is

A. Ophthalmologic examination including visual field testing
B. MRI with gadolinium imaging
C. Serum cryptococcal antigen testing
D. Urine culture
E. CSF culture

**IV-85.** A 63-year-old male complains of 10 years of intermittent purulent cough associated with shortness of breath since he had a severe case of influenza pneumonia. These episodes typically respond to oral antibiotics. Over the last 10 years he has averaged two to three courses of antibiotics a year. Pulmonary function tests show moderate obstruction. He now presents with purulent cough for 3 days with fever and shortness of breath. A chest radiograph demonstrates focal bronchial dilation and a nodular infiltrate in the right lower lobe. Sputum culture grows an acid-fast organism. For which of the following organisms would therapy be indicated at this point?

**IV-85.** *(Continued)*
A. *Mycobacterium avium*
B. *M. gordonae*
C. *M. intracellulare*
D. *M. kansasii*
E. *M. marinum*

**IV-86.** A 64-year-old female complains of 3 weeks of progressive shortness of breath and a productive cough. She has a history of mild chronic obstructive pulmonary disease (COPD) treated with long-acting beta agonists. She has no prior hospitalizations and is on no other medications. She is a schoolteacher and reports that her yearly purified protein derivatives (PPDs) have always been negative. Physical examination is notable for a temperature of 38.0°C (100.4°F) and a focal area of crackles and wheezes in the right lateral chest. A chest CT shows small nodules and cylindrical bronchiectasis in the middle lobe. Bronchoalveolar lavage and transbronchial lung biopsy show acid-fast organisms. While awaiting culture identification of the acid-fast organisms she should receive

A. No antibiotic therapy
B. Isoniazid and rifampin
C. Clarithromycin, ethambutol, and rifabutin
D. Isoniazid, rifampin, and ethambutol
E. Amikacin, cefoxitin, and clarithromycin

**IV-87.** You are a physician for an undergraduate university health clinic in Arizona. You have evaluated three students with similar complaints of fever, malaise, diffuse arthralgias, cough without hemoptysis, and chest discomfort, and one of the patients has a skin rash on her extremities consistent with erythema multiforme. Chest radiography is similar in all three, with hilar adenopathy and small pleural effusions. Upon further questioning you learn that all three students are in the same archaeology class and participated in an excavation 1 week ago. Your leading diagnosis is

A. Mononucleosis
B. Primary pulmonary coccidioidomycosis
C. Primary pulmonary aspergillosis
D. Streptococcal pneumonia
E. Primary pulmonary histoplasmosis

**IV-88.** A 40-year-old male with HIV who recently arrived in United States from Panama presents to the emergency room with a 3-day history of fever to 38.9°C (102°F), cough, shortness of breath, and malaise. He is emaciated, and examination is significant for an oxygen saturation of 88% while breathing room air, hepatomegaly, and diffuse lymphadenopathy. Examination of his skin shows small erythematous papules on the upper extremities. His previous form of employment was as a farm hand responsible for chicken coops. Laboratory assessment shows a hematocrit of 31%, white blood cell count of 3200/mm$^3$,

**IV-88.** *(Continued)*

platelet count of 75,000/mm³, and lactate dehydrogenase of 4250 U/dL. Chest radiography shows bilateral diffuse reticulonodular infiltrates. Microscopic evaluation of bronchiolar lavage reveals multiple organisms in the cytoplasm of alveolar macrophages as shown below. What is the recommended treatment for this patient?

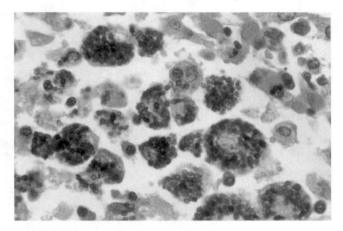

A.  IV amphotericin B
B.  IV vancomycin
C.  IV trimethoprim-sulfamethoxazole
D.  IV acyclovir
E.  Observation

**IV-89.** A 55-year-old male is admitted to the hospital with aspiration pneumonia. Over the last 8 months he has had a relentless neurologic decline characterized by dementia with severe memory loss and decline in intellectual function. These symptoms were preceded by 2 to 3 months of labile mood, weight loss, and headache. Currently he is awake but unable to answer questions. Neurologic examination is notable for normal cranial nerves and sensation. He has marked myoclonus provoked by startle or bright lights, but it also occurs spontaneously during sleep. Prior evaluation revealed normal serum chemistries, negative serologic tests for syphilis, and normal CSF studies. Head CT scan in normal. The infectious agent that caused his neurologic syndrome is most likely a

A.  DNA virus
B.  Fungus
C.  Protein lacking nucleic acid
D.  Protozoan
E.  RNA virus

**IV-90.** A 55-year-old male is admitted to the intensive care unit for severe community-acquired pnemonia. He is treated with ceftriaxone and azithromycin. His fever resolves after 3 days of therapy. On hospital day 5 he develops fever, abdominal pain, and nonbloody diarrhea. Which of the following statements regarding *Clostridium difficile*–associated diarrhea is true?

**IV-90.** *(Continued)*

A.  A negative toxin assay for *C. difficile* toxin A rules out the diagnosis.
B.  A positive stool culture for *C. difficile* confirms the diagnosis.
C.  Endoscopy will demonstrate pseudomembranes in the colon and distal ileum.
D.  Oral therapy is as effective as intravenous therapy.
E.  The patient's stool probably was colonized with *C. difficile* before admission.

**IV-91.** A 33-year-old male with altered mental status is brought to the emergency department by his wife. She tells you that he has a history of sickle cell disease that has been well controlled with hydroxyurea. Two days ago he developed upper respiratory symptoms and fever that was treated with over-the-counter medications. Today he became confused and lethargic. His physical examination is notable for a blood pressure of 75/45 with a heart rate of 130/min and a temperature of 40°C (104°F). His extremities are warm. Blood cultures are most likely to grow which of the following organisms?

A.  *Candida albicans*
B.  *Pseudomonas aeruginosa*
C.  *Staphylococcus aureus*
D.  *Streptococcus pneumoniae*
E.  *Salmonella typhii*

**IV-92.** All the following patient characteristics are included in the calculation of the Pneumonia Patient Outcomes Research Team (PORT) score that is used in the evaluation of patients with community acquired pneumonia *except*

A.  Age
B.  Coexisting illness
C.  Laboratory findings
D.  Radiographic findings
E.  Smoking history

**IV-93.** A 23-year-old previously healthy maintenance worker is admitted to the hospital with fever, cough, and a right lower lobe infiltrate on chest radiography. He has no past medical history other than a 10-pack-year history of cigarette smoking. All the following organisms, if isolated from sputum, should be considered pathogens *except*

A.  *Blastomycosis dermatidis*
B.  *Coccidioidomycosis immitis*
C.  *Histoplasma capsilatum*
D.  *Legionella pneumophila*
E.  *Moraxella catarrhalis*

**IV-94.** A 40-year-old female with a history of mitral valve replacement undergoes dental cleaning and extraction of two teeth. Several weeks later she notes intermittent fevers

**IV-94.** *(Continued)*
and chills, with weight loss. She presents to her primary care doctor, who suspects bacterial endocarditis. Her previously noted murmur is louder on physical exam, and Janeway lesions (Fig. IV-94, Color Atlas) are seen on her hands. Blood cultures are negative at 4 days. Which of the following statements is correct?

A.   HACEK organisms are unlikely to cause her endocarditis as this illness was acquired during a dental procedure.
B.   HACEK endocarditis on a prosthetic valve is unlikely to be cured by antibiotics alone.
C.   HACEK organisms generally grow within 1 week of culture.
D.   Valvular vegetations are unlikely to be found on an echocardiogram in HACEK endocarditis.
E.   *Actinobacillus* spp. are the most common source of HACEK endocarditis.

**IV-95.** Cultures later turn positive for *Haemophilus parainfluenza*, and a 1-cm vegetation is seen on the prosthetic valve. Therapy at this point should include

A.   Ceftriaxone for 6 weeks
B.   Surgical debridement
C.   Penicillin for 6 weeks
D.   A and B
E.   B and C

**IV-96.** A 45-year-old patient with severe fistulizing Crohn's disease has undergone numerous bowel surgeries, leaving him with chronic malabsorption and short gut syndrome. There is an outbreak of a viral illness in the local preschool in which he works. The patient develops cough, coryza, fever, conjunctivitis, and Kopkick's spots. Which of the following statements is correct?

A.   The patient probably contracted this illness through fecal-oral contact.
B.   A rash can be expected to follow the oral findings by 1 or 2 days, beginning at the periphery and marching centrally.
C.   The causative organism can be diagnosed at this stage by checking IgM titers to the virus.
D.   Therapy with vitamin A should be instituted.
E.   The patient is at high risk for subacute sclerosing panencephalitis.

**IV-97.** A 24-year-old female comes to her physician complaining of a 3-day history of malodorous vaginal discharge. She recently had unprotected intercourse with a new male partner. Her only medication is oral contraceptives. She denies any fever, dysuria, joint pain, or neurologic findings. Physical examination is normal except for a malodorous white vaginal discharge. Placing 10% KOH on the vaginal secretions yields a fishy odor. A wet mount

**IV-97.** *(Continued)*
of vaginal secretions is shown below. This patient should be treated with which of the following antibiotics?

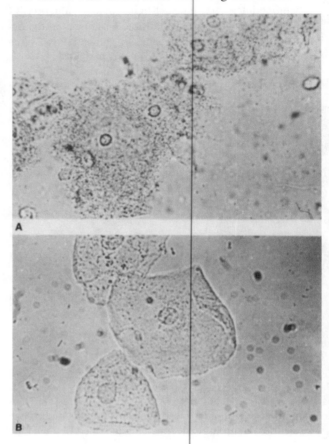

A.   Acyclovir
B.   Ceftriaxone
C.   Doxycycline
D.   Fluconazole
E.   Metronidazole

**IV-98.** A 25-year-old medical student living in Maryland comes to the emergency department with sudden-onset fever, headache, retroorbital pain, epistaxis, and severe myalgias. He has been working on the clinical wards for 3 months, although 1 week ago he returned from a vacation in the Caribbean. On weekends he has been hiking and camping in the nearby forests. Physical examination is notable for a temperature of 39.2°C (102.6°F), a macular rash on the trunk and extremities, axillary adenopathy, small vesicles on the palate, severe muscle tenderness, and scattered petechiae on the arms. Laboratory examination reveals thrombocytopenia and leukopenia. A rapid HIV PCR is negative. This patient's illness most likely was transmitted by

A.   A mosquito bite
B.   A tick bite
C.   Aerosol inhalation of a nosocomial infection

**IV-98.** *(Continued)*

D. Exposure to infected blood

E. Exposure to rodent urine

**IV-99.** A 48-year-old female presents to her physician with a 2-day history of fever, arthralgias, diarrhea, and headache. She recently returned from an ecotour in tropical sub-Saharan Africa, where she went swimming in inland rivers. Notable findings on physical examination include a temperature of 38.7°C (101.7°F); 2-cm tender mobile lymph nodes in the axilla, cervical, and femoral regions; and a palpable spleen. Her white blood cell count is 15,000/mm$^3$ with 50% eosinophils. She should receive treatments with which of the following medications?

A. Chloroquine

B. Mebendazole

C. Metronidazole

D. Praziquantel

E. Thiabendazole

**IV-100.** A sputum culture from a patient with cystic fibrosis showing which of the following organisms has been associated with a rapid decline in pulmonary function and a poor clinical prognosis?

A. *Burkholderia cepacia*

B. *Pseudomonas aeruginosa*

C. *Staphylococcus aureus*

D. *Staphylococcus epidermidis*

E. *Stenotrophomonas maltophilia*

**IV-101.** An 18-year-old sexually active male presents to your clinic complaining of a penile lesion for 2 weeks. Examination reveals an indurated ulcer, and the edge has a cartilaginous consistency upon palpation. There is also associated painless inguinal lymphadenopathy. Rapid plasma reagin and FTA-ABS testing is positive. A single dose of penicillin G 2.4 mU IM is given. Upon arrival home the patient calls your office to report new symptoms

**IV-101.** *(Continued)*
of fever, chills, headache, and diffuse myalgias. He denies rash or respiratory complaints. You recommend which of the following?

A. Acetominophen for symptom-based therapy

B. Return to the clinic for another dose of penicillin G

C. Return to the clinic for lumbar puncture

D. HIV viral load testing and CD4 count

**IV-102.** A 48-year-old male Boy Scout troop leader who has led numerous camping trips in Maine presents to the urgent care clinic with complaints of right knee pain for the last 3 weeks. He denies any trauma to the knee. His past history is significant only for mild hypertension treated with a beta blocker. He does not drink alcohol. Exam shows a warm erythematous knee with an effusion. He is afebrile. Radiology does not show a fracture or destructive lesions. Arthrocentesis show a white blood cell count of 25,000/$\mu$L with 90% polymorphonuclear leukocytes. No crystals are seen, and there are no organisms on Gram stain. Antinucleolar antibody and rheumatoid factor are negative. The most likely diagnosis is

A. Gout

B. Pseudogout

C. Lyme disease

D. Osteoarthritis

E. Septic arthritis

**IV-103.** A 20-year-old female is 36 weeks pregnant and presents for her first evaluation. She is diagnosed with *Chlamydia trachomatis* infection of the cervix. Upon delivery, what complication is her infant most at risk for?

A. Jaundice

B. Hydrocephalus

C. Hutchinson triad

D. Conjunctivitis

E. Sensorineural deafness

# IV. INFECTIOUS DISEASES

## ANSWERS

**IV-1.  The answer is D.**  *(Chap. 302)*   Recurrent episodes of rheumatic fever are most common in the first 5 years after the initial diagnosis. Penicillin prophylaxis is recommended for at least this period. After the first 5 years secondary prophylaxis is determined on an individual basis. Ongoing prophylaxis is currently recommended for patients who have had recurrent disease, have rheumatic heart disease, or work in occupations that have a high risk for reexposure to Group A streptococcal infection. Prophylactic regimens are penicillin V PO 250 mg bid, benzathine penicillin 1.2 million units IM every 4 weeks, and sulfadiazine 1 g PO daily. Polyvalent pneumococcal vaccine has no cross-reactivity with Group A streptococcus.

**IV-2 and IV-3.  The answers are B and A.**  *(Chap. 191)*   PCP pneumonia is among the most common opportunistic infections in HIV patients. *Pneumocystis carinii* is ubiquitous throughout the world, and most children have been exposed by age 4 years. In the era of HIV, PCP has emerged as a frequent cause of morbidity and death. Before the 1980s PCP was seen primarily in chronically immunosuppressed cancer and transplant patients who were receiving chronic steroids. Mortality in AIDS patients after a bout of PCP pneumonia is 50% at 1 year and is over 60% in patients requiring mechanical ventilation. This patient's clinical course is typical for PCP pneumonia, developing over weeks, with a chest radiograph showing bilateral interstitial infiltrates. The best diagnostic test to determine if PCP is present is demonstration of the organism on Giemsa-Wright or another cytopathologic stain. Induced sputum has a sensitivity of 30 to 75%, whereas bronchoalveolar lavage (BAL) has a sensitivity over 90% in patients who are not receiving prophylaxis. BAL remains useful diagnostically even a week after therapy has been initiated. In patients who have not been on prophylaxis, transbronchial biopsy adds little to lavage for diagnosis. Although LDH levels are often elevated in patients with PCP, this is not a specific finding as many other pulmonary infections or inflammatory diseases may cause similar elevations of LDH. CT scans will show bilateral infiltrates but are not specific. Positron emission tomography (PET) scans have not been studied in PCP but are unlikely to be helpful diagnostically. Although the treatment of choice for PCP is clearly trimethoprim-sulfamethoxazole, the combination of clindamycin and primaquine is an option for those with sulfa allergy. Other options include intravenous pentamidine. Patients receiving appropriate therapy for PCP often undergo clinical deterioration soon after the onset of therapy if steroids are not also given. Prednisone at an initial dose of 40 mg bid is recommended when $Pa_{O_2}$ is less than 70 mmHg on room air at presentation. This is thought to be due to rapid death of the organisms and the resultant inflammatory response. Therefore, the most likely reason for this patient's clinical decline is failure to receive steroid therapy concurrent with antibiotic drugs.

**IV-4.  The answer is A.**  *(Chap. 191; N Engl J Med 340:1301, 1999; Lancet 353:1293, 1999.)*  PCP prophylaxis is recommended for anyone with a CD4 count $<200/\mu L$. The incidence of PCP in patients with prior PCP is 40 to 60% per year and is 40 to 50% in patients with a CD4 count $<100/\mu L$. If a patient requires hospitalization, the mortality for a given episode of PCP is 15 to 20%. In an era of highly active antiretroviral therapy, many patients have undergone immune reconstitution. Discontinuation of PCP prophylaxis has been evaluated in several trials and shown to be safe when a patient has achieved a CD4 count higher than 200 for 3 months. These studies have included patients receiving secondary prophylaxis as well, showing that there is no difference in rates of PCP among patients who have discontinued prophylaxis. The severity of prior PCP does not make a difference in the discontinuation of PCP prophylaxis, and viral load should not be taken into account other than to suggest that there may be resistance to the chosen highly active antiviral therapy (HAART) regimen. If the CD4 count again drops $<200/\mu L$, PCP prophylaxis should be resumed.

**IV-5 and IV-6. The answers are B and D.** *(Chap. 147)* The most common site of actinomycosis infection is the craniofacial area. Often the infection is associated with poor dentition, facial trauma, or tooth extraction. Clinically this presents as a chronic cellulitis of the face, often with drainage through sinus tracts. The infection may spread without regard for tissue planes, and adjacent bony structures may be involved. Diagnosis requires a high degree of suspicion. The drainage is frequently contaminated with other organisms, especially gram-negative rods. The characteristic sulfur granules may not be seen unless deep tissue is sampled. On Gram stain, the characteristic appearance is shown in Figure V-5, with an intense gram-positive center and branching rods at the periphery. As opposed to the strictly aerobic *Nocardia* species, *Actinomyces* grows slowly in anaerobic and microaerobic conditions. Therapy requires a long course of antibiotics even though the organism is very sensitive to penicillin therapy. This is presumed to be due to the difficulty of using antibiotics to penetrate the thick-walled masses and sulfur granules. Current recommendations are for penicillin intravenously for 2 to 6 weeks followed by oral therapy for a total of 6 to 12 months. Surgery should be reserved for patients who are not responsive to medical therapy.

**IV-7. The answer is A.** *(Chap. 123)* The patient is elderly with relative immunocompromise associated with diabetes mellitus and renal disease. Gram stain reveals the presence of gram-positive rods that are most likely to be *Listeria monocytogenes*. The therapy of choice for this organism is ampicillin or penicillin G intravenously, often in combination with an aminoglycoside for synergy. Rifampin should not be used as it may antagonize the effects of ampicillin. Trimethoprim-sulfamethoxazole is a second-line agent that may be used in patients with penicillin allergy. *Listeria* is resistant to cephalosporin therapy, and single-agent therapy with ceftriaxone is contraindicated in elderly or immunocompromised patients.

**IV-8 and IV-9. The answers are B and D.** *(Chap. 145)* Donovanosis is primarily a sexually transmitted disease that also is called granuloma inguinale or granuloma venereum. It is caused by the gram-negative intracellular organism *Calymmatobacterium granulomatis*. Although infection rates have fallen dramatically in the United States, with fewer than 20 cases reported yearly, it remains endemic in many parts of the Caribbean and Africa and among the Aboriginal population of Australia. Clinically, it presents with one or more subcutaneous nodules that erode to form clean painless ulcers. Genital swelling resembling lymphedema may occur, leading to the term *pseudoelephantiasis*. The finding of intracellular Donovan bodies within mononuclear cells on smear confirms the diagnosis. However, *C. granulomatis* has never been grown on solid media. Treatment includes a range of antibiotics that are effective against intracellular pathogens, including azithromycin, doxycycline, trimethoprim-sulfamethoxazole, and chloramphenicol.

**IV-10 and IV-11. The answers are B and D.** *[Chap. 113; Sherris' Medical Microbiology, Chap. 39, p. 581; MMWR 50(RR09)1–18, June 1, 2001.]* Norovirus, or the so-called Norwalk-like agent, was initially described as a cause of food-borne illness in Norwalk, Ohio, in 1968. Since that time the virus responsible has been identified as a small RNA virus of the Calciviridae family. The initial detection of the Norwalk agent was poor, relying on electron microscopy or immune electron microscopy. Using these techniques, the Norwalk agent was identified as the causative agent in 19 to 42% of nonbacterial diarrheal outbreaks. With the development of more sensitive molecular assays (RT-PCR, ELISA), Norwalk-like viruses are being found as increasingly frequent causes of diarrheal outbreaks. Treatment is supportive as symptoms improve within 10 to 51 hours. Rotavirus is the most common cause of viral diarrhea in infants but is uncommon in adults. Salmonella, shigella, and *E. coli* present with more colonic and systemic manifestations.

**IV-12.   The answer is B.**   *[Chap. 116; Ann Intern Med 138(6):494–501, 2003.]*   Hospital-acquired pneumonia accounts for approximately 20% of nosocomial infections. In patients in intensive care units an attributable mortality rate of 6 to 14% has been associated with ventilator-associated pneumonia (VAP). Aspiration is felt to be a common contributor to the development of VAP. Three trials have demonstrated a decreased incidence of VAP with a semirecumbent position more than 45-degrees. Stress ulcer prophylaxis does not prevent VAP; instead, it may increase the incidence because of its effect in changing the microbial gastric flora to gram-negative organisms. This is especially true in the case of $H_2$ blockers and proton pump inhibitors. Sucralfate has been demonstrated to have less associated VAP compared with $H_2$ blockers but offers less protection against gastrointestinal (GI) bleed and is no better than placebo for the prevention of VAP. Increasing the frequency of ventilator circuitry changes has also been associated with an increased frequency of VAP. Finally, there are insufficient data to support selective gut decontamination, and in light of worries about the selection of resistant organisms, it is not recommended.

**IV-13.   The answer is D.**   *[Chap. 116; Clin Infect Dis 38(2):161–189, 2004.]*   *Candida albicans* is the organism most commonly recovered from the urinary tract in patients hospitalized in ICUs. In most instances of asymptomatic candiduria treatment is not warranted. Removal of the catheter alone results in clearance of candiduria in 40% of cases. If it is imprudent to remove the Foley catheter, changing devices may be beneficial. Treatment is recommended in instances of immunosuppression, neutropenia, obstruction, and invasion into the upper pole. The antimicrobial treatment of choice is fluconazole or intravenous amphotericin. Bladder irrigation with amphotericin B may transiently eliminate candiduria, but the effect is not persistent. If candiduria persists in an immunocompromised host, further bladder imaging is warranted.

**IV-14.   The answer is D.**   *(Chap. 116)*   Migration of cutaneous flora is the most common cause of catheter-related bloodstream infection. The most common bacteria causing line-associated bacteremia is *Staphylococcus epidermidis*. Contamination of the hubs of a central venous catheter does occur in long-term vascular access devices, particularly in surgically placed or cuffed catheters. Ventilator-associated pneumonia provides a clear explanation of fever but less commonly causes bacteremia. Urinary tract infection is common in ICU patients but usually does not cause bacteremia. Multiple chest tubes are a potential cause of empyema, but this is usually clinically apparent and usually does not cause bacteremia.

**IV-15.   The answer is B.**   *(Chap. 116)*   The best way to determine if a catheter-related bloodstream infection is present is to demonstrate the same species of microorganisms from two separate peripheral blood cultures and from a semiquantitative culture from the culture tip. Culturing only the catheter may demonstrate contamination of the line but is unacceptable for diagnosing catheter-related bloodstream infection. Other methods that can be used less commonly include differential time to positivity and differential increase in quantitative cultures between central and peripheral cultures.

**IV-16.   The answer is A.**   *[Chap. 116; Clin Infect Dis 38(2):161–189, 2004.]*   Scheduled guidewire exchange of central venous catheters has not been shown to decrease infection rates. Guidewire exchange may be used when a catheter is malfunctioning; however, if the catheter exit site appears to be infected, a new venous puncture must be attempted. Maximal barrier technique should be used for the placement of all central venous catheters, including guidewire exchanges. Antisepsis preferably should be with chlorhexidine solution, but if povidone iodine is used, it must be allowed to dry before the introduction of the needle. Application of antibacterial ointments to the skin is not recommended as no study has shown that it decreases the rates of bacterial colonization, and it may increase the risk of contamination with *Candida* species.

**IV-17.   The answer is B.**   *(Chap. 113)*   The patient most likely has food poisoning because of contamination of the fried rice with *Bacillus cereus*. This toxin-mediated disease occurs when heat-resistant spores germinate after boiling. Frying before serving may not destroy the preformed toxin. The emetic form of illness occurs within 6 hours of eating and is self-limited. No therapy is necessary unless the patient develops severe dehydration. This patient currently has no symptoms consistent with volume depletion; therefore, she does not need intravenous fluids at present. Sarcoidosis does not predispose patients to infectious diseases.

**IV-18.   The answer is D.**   *(Chap. 113)*   Enterotoxigenic *E. coli* is responsible for 50% of traveler's diarrhea in Latin America and 15% in Asia. *E. histolytica* and *V. cholerae* account for smaller percentages in Mexico. *Campylobacter* is more common in Asia and during the winter in subtropical areas. *Giardia* is associated with a contaminated water supply in Russia and the northern United States, especially in campers who drink from freshwater streams.

**IV-19.   The answer is E.**   *(Chap. 54)*   Lymphadenopathy is a component of numerous medical conditions, particularly infectious, autoimmune, and malignant disorders. The critical features of lymphadenopathy are the distribution (local versus generalized), location (e.g., supraclavicular versus occipital), size, texture, and tenderness. Constitutional symptoms of fever, sweats, and weight loss may indicate a more systemic process. Age and tobacco use heighten the risk of malignancy. This patient's age, constitutional symptoms, and diffuse distribution of lymphadenopathy make one suspect an infectious process. Mononucleosis from Epstein-Barr virus or cytomegalovirus is possible. Acute HIV infection and acute toxoplasmosis are also considerations. The lack of adenopathy greater than a centimeter and the soft movable texture make one less concerned about an oncologic process. In light of these features, observation with a follow-up physical exam in 2 to 4 weeks is reasonable. Monospot or HIV testing is not unreasonable in this patient. A complete blood count (CBC) may indicate atypical lymphocytes that would point toward an acute viral illness. Evidence for lymphoma or leukemia may be seen in the CBC as well. If this patient's lymphadenopathy persisted or worsened, a tissue diagnosis would be warranted. However, most diagnoses, especially lymphoma, require nodal architecture, and so the diagnostic procedure of choice would be an excisional biopsy, not a fine-needle aspiration.

**IV-20.   The answer is E.**   *(Chap. 132)*   Legionnaire's disease (pneumonia) is included in the differential diagnosis of atypical pneumonia. The species associated with the vast majority of human infections is the aerobic gram-negative bacillus *Legionella pneumophila*. Clinical features include cough, malaise, myalgias, fatigue, and fever. Gastrointestinal features may be pronounced, including abdominal pain, nausea, vomiting, and diarrhea. The chest x-ray often shows patchy infiltrates. Since members of the Legionellaceae do not grow on routine microbiologic media, the diagnosis requires special microbiologic tests. Sputum may be assayed by using direct fluorescent antibody (DFA) staining, which is specific but not sensitive. Culture requires buffered charcoal yeast extract (BCYE) agar. The urinary antigen test is available for *L. pneumophila* serogroup 1, which is responsible for up to 80% of *Legionella* infections. The antibiotics of choice for these infections include the macrolides and the respiratory tract quinolones, which display a superior ability to reach intracellular concentrations as well as good penetration of lung tissue. Intitial therapy should be through the intravenous route. Oral therapy may be substituted when the patient's clinical status is stable.

**IV-21. The answer is A.** *(Chap. 139)* *Campylobacter* species are motile, non-spore-forming, curved gram-negative rods. They are found in the gastrointestinal tracts of many animals. In most cases they are transmitted to humans in undercooked meats. Clinical manifestations include diarrhea, abdominal pain, and fever. The diarrhea may range from loose stools to grossly bloody stools. Enteritis is usually self-limited and rarely may be complicated by bacteremia, local suppurative complications such as peritonitis, cystitis, and endocarditis. In 1 in 1000 cases *Campylobacter* infection may be complicated by the ascending polyneuropathy Guillain-Barré syndrome (GBS). It is estimated that 20 to 40% of all GBS cases are triggered by *Campylobacter* infection. Although *E. coli, Shigella*, and *Yersinia* species are in the differential diagnosis of bloody diarrhea, none of them are associated with GBS to the degree that *Campylobacter* infection is. *E. coli* O:157 species are associated with bloody diarrhea and an increased propensity to hemolytic-uremic syndrome. Norwalk virus typically does not cause bloody diarrhea.

**IV-22. The answer is A.** *(Chap. 188)* *Aspergillus* has many clinical manifestations. Invasive aspergillosis typically occurs in immunocompromised patients and presents as rapidly progressive pulmonary infiltrates. Infection progresses by direct extension across tissue planes. Cavitation may occur. Allergic bronchopulmonary aspergillosis is a different clinical entity. It often occurs in patients with preexisting asthma or cystic fibrosis. It is characterized by an allergic reaction to *Aspergillus* species. Clinically, it is characterized by intermittent wheezing, bilateral pulmonary infiltrates, brownish sputum, and peripheral eosinophilia. IgE may be elevated, suggesting an allergic process, and a specific reaction to *Aspergillus* species that is manifested by serum antibodies or skin testing is common. Although central bronchiectasis is common in allergic bronchopulmonary aspergellosis (ABPA), the presence of peripheral cavitary lung lesions is *not* a common feature.

**IV-23. The answer is C.** *(Chap. 175)* The patient is suffering from pleurodynia, which is also known by the eponym Bornholm disease. Pleurodynia is most commonly caused by coxsackie B viral infection. An RNA virus, coxsackie B virus is a member of the enterovirus family. In temperate areas these viruses most commonly cause symptoms in late summer and early fall. In tropical areas they cause disease year-round. Paroxysms of knifelike pleuritic chest pain in adults or abdominal pain in children lasting 15 to 30 minutes are followed by fevers with diaphoresis and tachycardia. The white blood cell count and chest radiographs are most frequently normal, and the disease is self-limited. Treatment is symptomatic with high-dose nonsteroidal anti-inflammatory drugs to control pain.

**IV-24. The answer is D.** *(Chap. 175)* This patient most likely has aseptic meningitis related to an enteroviral infection. Enteroviruses cause up to 90% of cases of aseptic meningitis and are most common in late summer and early fall. A preceding febrile illness may be reported before the development of headaches, meningismus, and lethargy. Cerebrospinal fluid shows normal glucose and a mild elevation in protein, most often less than 100 mg/dL. CSF pleocytosis is notable for a lymphocytic predominance, although very early in the illness polymorphonucleocytes may be the predominant cell. Symptoms usually resolve within 1 week with an excellent neurologic prognosis. Mumps may cause aseptic meningitis, but this is much less likely than enterovirus and usually occurs only in the winter months.

Meningococcal meningitis is a feared bacterial meningitis that often occurs in epidemics, especially among patients living in close quarters. The case fatality rate is approximately 13%, but permanent neurologic sequelae occur in one-third to one-half of these patients. When meningococcal meningitis is diagnosed, all contacts are instructed to receive a single dose of rifampin to prevent disease. In addition, a meningococcal vaccine is available and is recommended for people planning to live in dormitories in the military or at college.

**IV-25. The answer is B.** *(Chap. 175)* The patient is suffering from hand-foot-and-mouth disease, which is characterized by a tender vesicular rash primarily involving the oropharynx and the dorsum of the hands. An additional one-third of patients also have a rash on the feet. Unlike varicella infection, these vesicular lesions do not extend to the trunk. The vesicles form bullae and rapidly ulcerate. Within the oropharynx they may be seen on the hard palate, tongue, buccal mucosa, or uvula. The causative agents are found in the Enterovirus family, most frequently coxsackie virus A16 and enterovirus 71.

**IV-26.** **The answer is D.** *(Chap. 175)* Inactivated injectable polio vaccination is currently recommended for all children in the United States, given in four doses at ages 2, 4, and 6 to 18 months and at 4 to 6 years. Oral polio vaccination (OPV) contains three strains of live attenuated polio viruses. Approximately 50% of recipients develop protective antibodies after a single dose; thus, OPV is the vaccination of choice for controlling polio outbreaks. In addition, OPV promotes better intestinal immunity as well as increasing immunity within the community by secondary spread with gastrointestinal shedding. In the United States OPV vaccination is also recommended for unvaccinated persons traveling to endemic or epidemic areas in less than 4 weeks. Breast-feeding was once felt to be a contraindication but has been shown to be safe. Oral polio vaccination should not be administered to individuals with immunodeficiency or their household contacts.

**IV-27.** **The answer is D.** *(Chap. 144)* Q fever is caused by *Coxiella burnetti*. All other infections are the result of infection with either *Bartonella henselae* (cat-scratch disease and peliosis hepatis) or *B. bacilliformis* (Oroya fever and veruga peruana).

**IV-28.** **The answer is C.** *(Chap. 144)* *Bartonella henselae* is the causative organism of cat-scratch disease. Serologic tests are currently the diagnostic test of choice for the diagnosis of *B. henselae* infection. Growth in blood cultures requires cocultivation with endothelial cell monolayers and requires prolonged incubation for 1 to 4 weeks. Demonstration on pathologic biopsy specimens may also be diagnostic but requires Warthin-Starry silver stains. Currently, polymerase chain reaction testing is not commercially available. *Afipia felis* is a gram-negative organism that once was thought to be the causative organism of cat-scratch disease.

**IV-29.** **The answer is B.** *(Chap. 144)* In most cases cat-scratch disease is self-limited, but the systemic symptoms and tender regional lymphadenopathy may be debilitating. A randomized, placebo-controlled trial has shown that a 5-day course of oral azithromycin provides significant clinical improvement in typical cases. Aminoglycosides may be added for more significant infection, as in the case of endocarditis or encephalitis. The β-lactam antibiotics are not useful for treatment of cat-scratch disease.

**IV-30.** **The answer is D.** *(Chap. 144)* The patient has bacillary angiomatosis with concurrent peliosis hepatis caused by *Bartonella henselae* as demonstrated by the finding of bacillus organisms on Warthin-Starry stain. *B. quintana* also may cause bacillary angiomatosis but does not cause liver disease. Instead, *B. quintana* frequently causes bony invasion and destruction. Presenting symptoms of bacillary angiomatosis include a purple vascular-appearing lesion on the extremities. If peliosis hepatis is also present, focal right upper quadrant abdominal pain is a common complaint. Nonspecific systemic symptoms such as fevers, malaise, and weight loss are also frequent complaints. This disease is rare in patients without immunocompromise. The major confounding diagnosis is Kaposi's sarcoma (KS) because the lesions look very similar and may coexist in the same patient. Pathologically, bacillary angiomatosis also appears similar to KS lesions with prominent angiogenesis. However, bacillary angiomatosis may be differentiated from KS by the finding of bacilli on Warthin-Starry silver stain. Treatment with oral azithromycin or doxycycline alone may be used if there is only skin involvement. However, intravenous antibiotics are recommended for systemic involvement.

**IV-31.** **The answer is D.** *(Chap. 180)* Hantavirus pulmonary syndrome is a rodent-borne hemorrhagic fever caused by a member of the Bunyaviridae. Other hemorrhagic fevers include Lassa fever, Rift Valley fever, yellow fever, *Ebola*, and dengue. Hantavirus may also present with a renal syndrome that is more prevalent outside the United States. Hantavirus pulmonary syndrome was first recognized in the United States in 1993; however, serologic studies demonstrate prior episodes. The disease is strongly linked to rodent exposure in dwellings or during occupational activities, particularly in rural areas. The disease begins with a viral prodrome and then usually progresses to respiratory failure within a week. Mortality in those with respiratory failure is 30 to 40%; patients who survive the first 48 hours of the fulminant illness generally recover without serious sequelae. The differential diagnosis of a patient in respiratory failure includes rickettsial disease, meningococcemia, plague, tularemia, and sepsis. IgM testing of acute-phase serum, which may be positive during the prodrome, is best for making a specific diagnosis. Cultures of blood or pleural fluid will not be positive. Flow cytometry is useful for the diagnosis of malignancy but in this case will not be helpful. Silver stain of bronchoalveolar lavage is useful in the diagnosis of *Pneumocystis carazii* pneumonia (PCP). Bronchoalveolar lavage in patients with hantavirus pulmonary syndrome may be consistent with alveolar hemorrhage, but this is a nonspecific finding.

**IV-32.    The answer is E.**    *(Chap. 166)*    Kaposi's sarcoma was originally described in 1872 as a rare vascular neoplasm seen primarily in people of Eastern European and Mediterranean descent. There was a rapid increase in the number of cases reported during the AIDS epidemic in the 1980s. In 1994, KS was shown to be related to a unique herpesvirus infection that subsequently was named human herpesvirus-8 or Kaposi's sarcoma–associated herpesvirus. HHV-8 has been shown to be sexually transmitted and is more common among homosexual men. The incidence of new cases of KS has decreased dramatically since the institution of highly active antiretroviral therapy. KS presents clinically with the finding of red- to purple-appearing raised skin lesions on the extremities and oropharynx. It may become disseminated and progress, in which case immunocompromise worsens. Lesions may occur anywhere and can cause hemoptysis with lung lesions or gastrointestinal bleeding with lesions in the GI tract. Treatment of KS alone should be focused on improving immune function and local therapy. KS is rarely fatal except in cases of diffuse pulmonary parenchymal involvement.

Since the initial description of HHV-8 as the causative agent in KS, two other disease entities have been found to also be associated with HHV-8 infection: multicentric Castleman's disease and primary effusion lymphoma. Multicentric Castleman's disease, also known as angiofollicular lymphoid hyperplasia, usually presents with fevers, diffuse lymphadenopathy, and hepatosplenomegaly. Pathology shows distortion of lymphoid architecture of either hyaline vascular or plasma cell variants. Primary effusion lymphoma is a body cavity–based lymphoma of B cell origin. Clinical manifestations include fevers, malaise, and the presence of pleural effusions, although it may present with pericardial effusion or ascites as well. These findings also are seen almost exclusively in immunocompromised patients, especially those with HIV. Compared with patients with KS alone, the prognosis is very poor, with most patients dying within 1 year.

**IV-33.    The answer is B.**    *(Chap. 148)*    Lemierre's disease was first described by an English physician in 1936, with septic internal jugular vein thrombophlebitis occurring in the setting of an oropharyngeal infection. The causative organism has been shown to be *Fusobacterium necrophorum*, an anaerobic gram-negative rod. In the era before antibiotics this infection was frequently fatal, with multiple septic abscesses. With improved oral hygiene the disease is much less frequently reported today, and prolonged intravenous antibiotics directed toward anaerobes are usually curative. Occasionally surgical intervention is necessary.

**IV-34.    The answer is A.**    *(Chaps. 109 and 121; JAMA 274:1706, 1995.)*    *Enterococcus* species account for 5 to15% of cases of endocarditis. Treatment requires prolonged antibiotic therapy with two antibiotics for 4 to 6 weeks. In patients who do not have a penicillin allergy ampicillin or penicillin intravenously in combination with gentamicin or streptomycin is the preferred regimen. Four weeks of therapy is indicated for patients with less than 3 months of symptoms, and 6 weeks of therapy is recommended for patients with symptoms for more than 3 months, those with prosthetic valve endocarditis, and those with relapsed infection. Patients with penicillin allergy should receive vancomycin in combination with gentamicin or streptomycin for 4 to 6 weeks. Valve replacement surgery is reserved for patients with poor valvular function or heart failure, recurrent emboli, or perivalvular abscess. Linezolid is not recommended for patients with enterococcal endocarditis that is penicillin-sensitive as it is a bacteriostatic agent.

IV-35.   **The answer is D.**   *(Chap. 173)*   Lactic acidosis is a class effect of the nucleoside analogue reverse transcriptase inhibitors, which include didanosine, zidovudine, and lamivudine, among others. Abacavir is another nucleoside analogue reverse transcriptase inhibitor that has a significant association with a hypersensitivity rash in 2 to 5% of the patients who receive it. Patients should be told to be evaluated if a rash develops on abacavir as the rash is indicative of a systemic hypersensitivity reaction that may be life-threatening. Efavirenz is a nonnucleoside analogue reverse transcriptase inhibitor that does not cause lactic acidosis. The major side effect with efavirenz is vivid dreams and nightmares that usually subside over time. Nelfinavir and indinavir are protease inhibitors. Lipodystrophy has been described as a class effect of these drugs and causes fat accumulation centrally and in the upper back (buffalo hump). Gynecomastia is also seen. Indinavir also causes nephrolithiasis in 10 to 20% of patients, and patients are advised to increase their fluid intake to more than 1.5 L daily.

IV-36.   **The answer is C.**   *(Chaps. 148 and 360)*   Brain abscess is a serious complication of extensive dental work with damage to the oral mucosal barrier. Symptoms are usually vague, with headache the most likely symptom. Fever is variable. Proper culture of brain abcesses usually reveals anaerobic bacteria, with peptostreptococci being most common, followed by fusobacterium and *Bacteroides* species. Facultative and microaerophilic streptococci and coliforms constitute the balance of microbes. In the absence of bacteremia or underlying immunosuppression, staphylococcal bacteria and zygomyces are less likely.

IV-37.   **The answer is A.**   *(Chap. 148)*   Tuboovarian abscess (TOA) is a common complication of pelvic inflammatory disease (PID) and is usually due to anaerobic infection. *Neisseria* and chlamydial infections are the most common cause of PID. TOA is likely to result from mucosal disruption and ascending colonization of anerobes. The most common anaerobes isolated from TOA are *Bacteroides* species. *Gardnerella* is commonly associated with bacterial vaginosis. *Clostridium septicum* is the thought to be the primary pathogen of neutropenic enterocolitis (see Chaps. 72, 88).

IV-38.   **The answer is C.**   *(Chap. 159)*   This is a classic presentation of *Mycoplasma pneumoniae* in a young male. *M. pneumoniae*, which lacks a cell wall, can cause pneumonia in any age group but most commonly affects people age 5 to 20. The organism has an incubation period of 2 to 3 weeks and is associated with severe nonproductive cough and headache. Although chest wall tenderness after coughing is common, myalgias, shaking chills, and gastrointestinal symptoms are rare. *M. pneumoniae* has a number of extrapulmonary manifestations, including erythema multiforme (shown in the question), maculopapular exanthems, myocarditis and pericarditis, encephalitis, and hemolytic anemia. When these conditions occur, it is rare to isolate *M. pneumoniae* from the extrapulmonary site. Thus, their etiology remains controversial but generally is believed to be immunologic.

IV-39.   **The answer is D.**   *(Chap. 159)*   This patient presented with a syndrome of atypical community-acquired pneumonia caused by *Mycoplasma pneumoniae*. Appropriate empirical therapy for outpatient community-acquired pneumonia must include coverage for typical and atypical organisms, including *Legionella pneumophila*. Antibiotics with activity against *L. pneumophila* are doxycycline, macrolides, and fluoroquinolones. Although second- and third-generation fluoroquinolones and macrolides generally cover the pneumococcus and constitute acceptable therapy in the outpatient setting, in a hospitalized severely ill patient it is recommended to use either a later-generation fluoroquinolone or a macrolide plus a second- or third-generation cephalosporin. Doxycycline is generally not recommended for empirical therapy in a hospitalized patient, but it can be used in the outpatient setting.

**IV-40.   The answer is B.**   *(Chap. 196)*   This patient comes from an area endemic for visceral leishmaniasis that includes Bangladesh, India, Nepal, Sudan, and Brazil. Although many species can cause cutaneous or mucosal disease, the *L. donovani* complex generally is associated with visceral leishmaniasis. The organism is transmitted by the bite of the sandfly in the majority of cases. Although many patients remain asymptomatic, malnourished persons are at particular risk for progression to symptomatic disease or kala azar, the life-threatening form. The presentation of this disease generally includes fever, cachexia, and splenomegaly. Hepatomegaly is rare compared with other tropical diseases associated with organomegaly, such as malaria, miliary tuberculosis, and schistosomiasis. Pancytopenia is associated with severe disease, as are hypergammaglobulinemia and hypoalbuminemia. Although active investigation is under way to determine a means of diagnosing leishmaniasis by molecular techniques, the current standard remains demonstration of the organism on a stained slide or in tissue culture of a biopsy specimen. Splenic aspiration has the highest yield, with reported sensitivity of 98% (Chap. 196). In light of the high mortality associated with this disease, treatment should not be delayed. The mainstay of therapy is a pentavalent antimonial, but newer therapies including amphotericin and pentamidine can be indicated in certain situations. In this case it would be prudent to rule out malaria with a thick and a thin smear. Rarely, the intracellular amastigote forms of *Leishmania* spp. can be seen on a peripheral smear.

**IV-41.   The answer is A.**   *(Chap. 192)*   In the evaluation of helminthic infection, stool analysis is the mainstay of diagnosis. Stool should be collected in clean cardboard containers on alternate days for a minimum of three samples because of the cyclic nature of parasitic shedding. Oral contrast and antidiarrheal agents can change the consistency of feces, making laboratory diagnosis more challenging. At this point there is no urgent indication for empirical therapy, which should be avoided until a diagnosis is made. Helminthic infection cannot be ruled out by the information provided.

**IV-42.   The answer is C.**   *(Chap. 154)*   The patient comes from an area where endemic syphilis caused by *Treponema pallidum* subspecies *endemicum* is prevalent in more than 10% of the population. Other affected countries include Mali, Niger, and Burkina Faso. Yaws is most commonly seen in Asia but has occasionally been seen in the Caribbean and South America; pinta is limited to Central and South America. In endemic syphilis primary infection occurs in childhood as a result of contact with mucosal surfaces and is manifest by an oral papule, which may be painless and asymptomatic. Secondary disease presents with extensive mucous patches on the oral mucosa that last for months to years. Other findings include periostitis and lymphadenopathy. Late disease is characterized by cutaneous and osseous gummae. Nipple gummae are common among breast-feeding women when their infants have oral lesions. The RPR is positive generally in all patients with endemic treponematoses, and the titer will decrease with therapy. Penicillin is indicated in all stages of the disease to prevent transmission in early disease and progression and destruction by gummae in late disease.

**IV-43.   The answer is B.**   *(Chap. 111)*   Bacterial osteomyelitis from a hematogenous source most commonly affects the lumbar spine in adults. Hemodialysis and degenerative joint disease are risk factors. The disease is often indolent over 2 or 3 months, and fever may not be present. Markers of inflammation such as the erythrocyte sedimentation rate (ESR) and C-reachtive protein (CRP) will be elevated. White blood cell count is normal or elevated slightly. Blood cultures will be positive less than half the time. *Staphylococcus aureus* is most common in adults, followed by gram-negative bacilli. End plate bony erosions crossing adjacent disk spaces with narrowing of the disk space are virtually diagnostic of bacterial osteomyelitis. Tumors and other spinal diseases usually do not cross the disk space. Radiographically, hyperparathyroidism causes subperiosteal resorption, myeloma causes osteopenia and lytic lesions, rheumatoid arthritis (RA) causes erosions of bone cortex and cartilage at joint spaces, and anklyosing spondylitis causes squaring of the vertebral bodies.

**IV-44.  The answer is C.**  *(Chap. 111)*  This patient has vertebral osteomyelitis caused by *S. aureus*. A 4- to 6-week course of appropriate antibiotics should be adequate to cure the infection. Surgical therapy is seldom necessary. Failure of the C-reactive protein to normalize is an indication for reevaluation for a longer treatment course.

**IV-45.  The answer is A.**  *(Chap. 107)*  Live oral polio virus vaccine is contraindicated in immunosuppressed children or children with immunosuppressed household contacts because of the potential for the development of vaccine-associated polio via fecal shedding. Killed, partial component, and nonviable vaccines are safe.

**IV-46.  The answer is D.**  *(Chap. 107)*  MMR is composed of live viruses and therefore is contraindicated in immunosuppressed invidiuals. All the other vaccines mentioned are noninfectious and safe. Inactivated polio virus is composed of three different strains of inactivated viruses to enhance immunogenicity. *Haemophilus influenzae* B vaccine is a bacterial polysaccharide–protein complex. Hepatitis B vaccine is an inactivated serum-derived antigen. Tetanus is a toxoid.

**IV-47.  The answer is E.**  *(Chap. 107)*  Annual influenza vaccine is recommended for patients with chronic illness, close contacts with patients with chronic illness, and anyone over 50 years old. Hepatitis B vaccine is recommended for any patient with risk factors for clinical, occupational, behavioral, or travel acquisition. In this case the patient has impending hemodialysis. Hepatitis A vaccine is recommended for the same patients as hepatitis B vaccine plus those with chronic liver disease or coagulopathy. Pneumococcal vaccine is recommended for patients over 65 years old and those with chronic illness. Varicella virus is not indicated in this patient and, because it is a live virus, may impose risks because of the immune suppression of hemodialysis.

**IV-48.  The answer is E.**  *(Chap. 360)*  The sensitivity of the latex agglutination (LA) test for *S. pneumoniae* is 70 to 100%. The LA test for *N. meningitides* is substantially lower at 33 to 70%. Thus, a negative test does not rule out disease. The specificity of these tests is 95 to 100%, and so a positive test is virtually diagnostic. MRI will be abnormal in most patients with bacterial meningitis, but the findings of cerebral edema, ischemia, and diffuse meningeal enhancement are not diagnostic. Meningeal enhancement occurs in any disease process that increases permeability of the blood-brain barrier. The limulus amebocyte lysate assay tests for endotoxin, and a positive test suggests gram-negative meningitis.

**IV-49 and IV-50.  The answers are E and A.**  *(Chap. 360)*  In a previously healthy student, particularly one living in a dormitory, *Staphylococcus pneumoniae* and *Neisseria meningitides* are the pathogens most likely to be causing community-acquired bacterial meningitis. As a result of the increasing prevalence of penicillin- and cephalosporin-resistant streptococci, initial empirical therapy should include a third- or fourth-generation cephalosporin plus vancomycin. Dexamethasone has been shown in children and adults to decrease meningeal inflammation and unfavorable outcomes in acute bacterial meningitis. In a recent study of adults the effect on outcome was most notable in patients with *S. pneumoniae* infection. The first dose (10 mg intravenous) should be administered 15 to 20 min before or with the first dose of antibiotics and is unlikely to be of benefit unless it is begun 6 h after the initiation of antibiotics. Dexamethasone may decrease the penetration of vancomycin into the CSF.

**IV-51. The answer is F.** *(Chap. 360)*  This patient has viral (aseptic) meningitis. The CSF showing mild pleocytosis with predominant lymphocytes and normal CSF glucose and protein is typical. Enteroviruses cause over 75% of cases of viral meningitis when a specific etiology is found. Enteroviral (coxsackievirus, echovirus, poliovirus, and human enterovirus 68-71) meningitis typically occurs in the summer and early fall but may occur year-round. PCR of CSF is useful for the identification of enteroviruses, herpes simplex virus (HSV), Epstein-Barr virus, varicella virus, and cytomegalovirus infection. MRI and cerebral angiography are useful for the diagnosis of subarachnoid hemorrhage; however, the CSF findings make this unlikely. The CSF findings in this case are less likely to be due to bacterial, fungal, or tuberculosis meningitis.

**IV-52. The answer is B.** *(Chap. 360)*  In 2002 West Nile virus (WNV) caused over 4000 cases of encephalitis with approximately 300 deaths. Cases typically occur in the summer, often in community outbreaks, associated with dead crows. WNV cannot be cultured, and there is not yet a PCR test. IgM antibodies normally do not cross the blood-brain barrier, and so their presence in the CSF is due to intrathecal production during acute infection with WNV. MRI is abnormal in only 30% of cases of WNV, significantly less often than is the case in HSV encephalitis. Stool culture may be useful in the diagnostic evaluation of enteroviral meningitis or encephalitis but not in cases of WNV.

**IV-53. The answer is D.** *(Chap. 360)*  This patient has progessive multifocal leukoencephalopathy (PML). The combination of MRI findings and the presence of JC virus in the CSF is diagnostic. The CSF may have a mild pleocytosis (25%) and a slightly elevated protein. PML almost always is seen in patients with advanced immunosuppression. Over 60% of cases are seen in patients with HIV, but PML can also be seen in patients with other conditions, such as lymphoproliferative and myeloproliferative disorders. There is no effective specific therapy. Patients with HIV may be treated with antiretroviral therapy to reduce the degree of immunosuppression.

**IV-54. The answer is A.** *(Chap. 27)*  Acute bacterial sinusitis is uncommon in patients with symptoms for less than 7 days and in the absence of severe symptoms (facial or tooth pain, soft tissue swelling). Even among patients with nasal discharge and symptoms for more than 7 days, fewer than half have true bacterial sinusitis. The initial management of patients with mild to moderate symptoms for less than a week is targeted toward facilitating sinus drainage with decongestants, saline lavage, and nasal steroids. Antibiotics are recommended in patients whose symptoms do not improve after 7 days of drainage-targeted therapy. Empirical therapy should target *S. pneumoniae* and *H. influenzae*. There is no current evidence to support broader therapy than amoxicillin or trimethoprim-sulfamethoxazole (TMP/SMX) in uncomplicated patients. Sinus CT or radiography is not recommended in early routine cases. In complicated, recurrent, or refractory cases sinus CT is superior to plain radiographs.

**IV-55. The answer is B.** *(Chap. 148; Lancet, March 28, 1936.)*  This patient has Lemierre's disease, jugular vein suppurative thrombophlebitis, or postanginal septicemia. First described by Lemierre in 1936 , in this disease young adults develop septic thrombophlebitis 3 to 10 days after a sore throat, exudative tonsillitis, or peritonsillar abscess. Infection of the deep pharyngeal tissues extends to the lateral pharyngeal space that includes the jugular vein and carotid artery. Bacteremia may lead to septic pulmonary and systemic emboli. The infection classically is due to *Fusobacterium necrophorum*. In the presence of poor dentition or malnutrition, Bacteroides would be a consideration. Intravenous drug abuse would make staphylococcus more likely. Rhizopus (zygomycosis) is usually seen in diabetic patients with poor control or immunosuppressed patients. Gonococcal pharyngitis may disseminate to the joints but rarely causes sepsis.

**IV-56. The answer is A.** *(Chaps. 282 and 287; Catalina, Navarro, Hosp Pract 35:97–108, 2000.)*  Risk factors for the acquisition of HCV include receiving a blood transfusion before 1992, intravenous drug use, hemodialysis, sexual relations with an infected individual, and a history of a sexually transmitted disease. Most patients with HCV infection remain asymptomatic for a long time after the initial infection. The biggest concern in chronically infected patients is the development of cirrhosis, along with the complications of portal hypertension and an increased risk of hepatocellular carcinoma. It is best to confirm a positive serology result with the PCR-based test for HCV mRNA. Moreover, quantitative tests for the level of HCV RNA may be useful in measuring response to therapy. Liver biopsy would not be indicated until the PCR test confirmed the presence of disease, although such a procedure would be very helpful in assessing the magnitude of histologic change. In addition to counseling a patient with a confirmed infection to eliminate behaviors that could result in transmission to others, treatment with recombinant IFN-$\alpha$-2b may result in some degree of benefit. Patients most likely to respond to interferon therapy are those with cirrhosis, a low but present serum HCV mRNA level, and an HCV genotype other than type 1. Interferon in combination with ribavirin may be more effective than therapy with either agent alone.

**IV-57.** **The correct answer is A.** *(Chap. 125)* Botulism is caused by protein neurotoxins elaborated by the *Clostridium botulinum* anaerobic gram-positive organism. These organisms form spores that are found in soils and marine environments throughout the world. Eight toxin types have been described; each can be inactivated by cooking at high temperatures. In the United States toxin types A, B, and E are usually associated with food-borne botulism, often from home-canned food, particularly vegetables, fruit, and occasionally meat and fish.

The incubation period after the ingestion of food containing the toxin is usually 18 to 36 hours but can vary. The disease is usually heralded by cranial neuropathies and then generally progresses to symmetric descending paralysis that is sometimes associated with nausea, vomiting, abdominal pain, dizziness, blurred vision, dry mouth, and dry sore throat. Although potentially anxious, patients are generally alert and oriented.

The diagnosis must be suspected clinically and should be distinguished from Guillain-Barré syndrome, Lambert-Eaton syndrome, polymyositis, tick paralysis, diphtheria, and chemical intoxication.

Treatment should include hospitalization and close monitoring for a potential decline in respiratory function, which should be treated with intubation and mechanical ventilation. Trivalent (including types A, B, and E) equine antitoxin should be administered immediately. Anaphylaxis and serum sickness may occur. In the absence of ileus, cathartics and enemas should be given to purge the toxin; gastric lavage will help only in cases in which the time after ingestion is brief. Antimicrobial therapy plays no role in this situation, since the disease is not caused by a proliferation of bacteria but instead by previously elaborated toxins.

**IV-58.** **The answer is B.** *(Chap. 200)* *Trichinella* spp. are members of the nematode phylum (roundworms). Trichinosis occurs after a person eats meat containing *Trichinella* nematode oocytes. After the consumption of affected meat, the encysted larvae are released by the action of gastric acid and pepsin. The larvae penetrate the small interstitial mucosa and rapidly mature into adult worms. In 1 week female worms release newborn larvae that travel via the circulation to striated muscle and then encyst. Clinical symptoms follow each of these phases. Initially gut invasion may be marked by abdominal pain, nausea, and constipation or diarrhea. Larval migration, which occurs during the second week after infection, produces a local and systemic hypersensitivity reaction manifested by fever, hypereosinophilia, and periorbital and facial edema. Myocarditis, encephalitis, and pneumonitis are rare but potentially life-threatening complications that may occur during this phase. After larval encystment in muscle for 2 to 3 weeks, edema and symptoms of myositis, including muscle edema and weakness, develop. The symptoms subside gradually during what may be a prolonged convalescence. Antihelminthic drugs are ineffective against the encysted larvae. Trichinosis, which typically is associated with eosinophilia and an elevated IgE level, may be prevented by cooking pork until it is no longer pink or freezing it at −15°C for 3 weeks. Ocular larva migrans, another nematode infection, is caused by the invasion of *Toxocara* larvae into the eye, typically producing a granulomatous mass, usually in the posterior pole of the retina.

**IV-59.    The answer is E.**    *(Chap. 168; Takahashi et al, Proc Natl Acad Sci USA 95:8227–8232, 1998.)*    Parvovirus subtype B19 is a nonenveloped single-stranded DNA virus. Several clinical syndromes have been found to be associated with parvovirus B19 infection. These syndromes generally occur on the basis of intranasal respiratory infection with the virus. Normal immunocompetent hosts generally clear the parvoviral infection but may experience a clinical syndrome of aching joints, fever, and chills. Patients may develop an exanthem more common in children, termed *fifth disease*, which is characterized by a facial rash with a "slapped cheek" appearance. Anemia may result from parvovirus infection even in normal hosts. In those with chronic hemolysis, such as patients with spherocytosis or sickle cell disease, parvoviral infection can result in a very serious aplastic crisis, which can produce life-threatening anemia. Immunodeficient patients may also experience profound anemias after infection with this virus. Moreover, B19 infection in adults may present as a rash or an acute, peripheral, symmetric, nondestructive polyarthritis. Studies have suggested a link between parvovirus B19 infection and rheumatic disease, including rheumatoid arthritis, vasculitis, lupus, and dermatomyositis. Parvovirus is not known to cause primary gastrointestinal infection, which is more likely to be caused by infection with a rotavirus or Norwalk agent.

**IV-60.    The answer is C.**    *(Chap. 120; Lowy, N Engl J Med 339:520–532, 1998.)*    This patient must be considered to have a life-threatening infection with *S. aureus* with possible valvular involvement. Only 5% of isolates are sensitive to penicillin; methicillin resistance is extremely common. Vancomycin with or without an aminoglycoside is recommended for such suspected community- or hospital-acquired *S. aureus* infections. Although drugs such as TMP/SMZ and clindamycin and fluoroquinolones such as ciprofloxacin are effective, they are not as efficacious as vancomycin and are more likely to induce resistance during therapy. There have been isolated case reports of vancomycin-resistant *S. aureus* strains; however, the mechanism of resistance is not due to the same genes that cause vancomycin resistance in enterococci, which is a major clinical problem at this time.

**IV-61.    The answer is E.**    *(Chap. 205; Dixon et al, N Engl J Med 341:815–826, 1999.)*    The endospores of *B. anthracis*, a gram-positive organism, are generally hearty and difficult to eradicate. The endospores are introduced into the body via the skin (abrasion or cut), inhalation, or ingestion or are phagocytosed by macrophages and carried to regional lymph nodes. Germination occurs in the lymph node; bacteria released into the bloodstream cause massive septicemia, which is almost always fatal. When anthrax endospores are ingested or inhaled or if bacteria reach the meninges, fatality is common. However, 80 to 90% of cutaneous anthrax is self-limited. The primary skin lesion is a pruritic papule that appears 3 to 5 days after the introduction of endospores. One to two days later the lesion forms a vesicle that eventually undergoes central necrosis, giving a typical black eschar. The eschar is surrounded by edema and purplish vesicles. This so-called malignant edema can, if present in the neck and thoracic region, lead to a tracheal compromise. Antibiotic treatment for cutaneous anthrax is recommended but probably not required.

**IV-62.    The answer is D.**    *(Chap. 179; Fishbein, Robinson, N Engl J Med 329:1632–1638, 1993.)*    The patient has been bitten by a member of a species known to carry rabies in an area in which rabies is endemic. Based on the animal vector and the facts that the skin was broken and that saliva possibly containing the rabies virus was present, postexposure rabies prophylaxis should be administered. If an animal involved in an unprovoked bite can be captured, it should be killed humanely and the head should be sent immediately to an appropriate laboratory for rabies examination by the technique of fluorescent antibody staining for viral antigen. If a healthy dog or cat bites a person in an endemic area, the animal should be captured, confined, and observed for 10 days. If the animal remains healthy for this period, the bite is highly unlikely to have transmitted rabies. Postexposure prophylactic therapy includes vigorous cleaning of the wound with a 20% soap solution to remove any virus particles that may be present. Tetanus toxoid and antibiotics should also be administered. Passive immunization with antirabies antiserum in the form of human rabies immune globulin (rather than the corresponding equine antiserum because of the risk of serum sickness) is indicated at a dose of 10 units/kg into the wound and 10 units/kg intramuscularly into the gluteal region. Second, one should actively immunize with an antirabies vaccine [either human diploid cell vaccine or rabies vaccine absorbed (RVA)] in five 1-mL doses given intramuscularly, preferably in the deltoid or anterior lateral thigh area. The five doses are given over a 28-day period. The administration of either passive or active immunization without the other modality results in a higher failure rate than does the combination therapy.

**IV-63.** **The answer is B.** *(Chaps. 116 and 134; Wheeler, Bernard, N Engl J Med 240:207–214, 1999.)* In this case the history and physical examination strongly suggest gram-negative sepsis stemming from a urinary tract infection. In older men obstruction resulting from prostatic hypertrophy is usually the cause. Prompt initiation of appropriate antibiotic therapy is most important. The choice of antibiotics can be guided by the history and microscopic examination of a Gram-stained urine specimen. In the absence of definitive laboratory information, initial treatment with maximal doses of broad-spectrum antibiotics such as gentamicin or tobramycin plus ampicillin or a cephalosporin is indicated. Bladder catheterization may be necessary to relieve the obstruction or monitor urine flow. Intravenous infusion of bicarbonate solutions and Ringer's lactate or dextrose-in-saline solutions is needed acutely to correct acidosis, restore vascular volume, and maintain renal perfusion. Glucocorticoids may protect against the lethal effects of endotoxin in experimental animals, but recent placebo-controlled trials have not supported their use in most clinical situations. Antiendotoxin antibodies and agents that interfere with the action of cytokines (e.g., tumor necrosis factor $\alpha$ and interleukin 1$\beta$) that mediate the manifestations of septic shock are under investigation.

**IV-64.** **The answer is A.** *(Chaps. 120 and 122)* Probably because of its ubiquity and ability to stick to foreign surfaces, *S. epidermidis* is the most common cause of infections of central nervous system shunts as well as an important cause of infections on artificial heart valves and orthopedic prostheses. *Corynebacterium* spp. (diphtheroids), just like *S. epidermidis*, colonize the skin. When these organisms are isolated from cultures of shunts, it is often difficult to be sure if they are the cause of disease or simply contaminants. Leukocytosis in cerebrospinal fluid, consistent isolation of the same organism, and the character of a patient's symptoms are all helpful in deciding whether treatment for infection is indicated.

**IV-65.** **The answer is B.** *(Chap. 107)* Passive immunization can be used to provide temporary immunity in a person who is exposed to an infectious disease and previously was not actively immunized. Standard human immune serum globulin does not contain known antibody content for a specific agent, unlike special immune serum globulins that exist for the treatment of susceptible patients exposed to hepatitis B, varicella (which is indicated for postexposure prophylaxis of susceptible immunocompromised persons, susceptible pregnant women, and exposed newborn infants), rabies, tetanus, and cytomegalovirus (used in bone marrow and kidney transplant recipients). Intramuscular immune globulin can be used for hepatitis A pre- and postexposure prophylaxis as well as hepatitis C postexposure prophylaxis; it is of questionable efficacy as postexposure prophylaxis for hepatitis B and rubella but may play a role in postexposure prophylaxis for immunocompromised persons exposed to measles.

**IV-66.** **The answer is D.** *(Chap. 118)* Imipenem is a $\beta$-lactam antibiotic in the carbapenem class with activity against most gram-positive organisms, including those which produce $\beta$-lactamase. Imipenem's antibacterial spectrum is quite broad and extends to all pathogens except xanthomonas, resistant *Pseudomonas* spp., methicillin-resistant staphylococci, and *E. faecium*. This drug must be given intravenously because of its instability in gastric acid. Since imipenem is hydrolyzed in the renal tubule by dihydropeptidase I, the coadministration of cilastatin, an inhibitor of this enzyme, markedly boosts levels of this broad-spectrum antibiotic. Clavulanate is a β-lactamase inhibitor that has been used with partial success when combined with amoxicillin (Augmentin) for the treatment of resistant otitis and urinary tract infections.

**IV-67.**   **The answer is C.**   *(Chap. 117)*   This patient is chronically immunosuppressed from his antirejection prophylactic regimen, which includes both glucocorticoids and azathioprine. However, the finding of a cavitary lesion on chest x-ray considerably narrows the possibilities and increases the likelihood of nocardial infection. The other clinical findings, including production of profuse thick sputum, fever, and constitutional symptoms, are also quite common in patients who have pulmonary nocardiosis. The Gram stain, which demonstrates filamentous branching gram-positive organisms, is characteristic. Most species of *Nocardia* are acid-fast if a weak acid is used for decolorization (e.g., modified Kinyoun method). These organisms also can be visualized by silver staining. They grow slowly in culture, and the laboratory must be alerted to the possibility of their presence on submitted specimens. Once the diagnosis, which may require an invasive approach, is made, sulfonamides are the drugs of choice. Sulfadiazine or sulfisoxazole from 6 to 8 g/d in four divided doses generally is administered, but doses up to 12 g/d have been given. The combination of sulfamethoxazole and trimethoprim has also been used, as have the oral alternatives minocycline and ampicillin and intravenous amikacin. There is little experience with the newer β-lactam antibiotics, including the third-generation cephalosporins and imipenem. Erythromycin alone is not effective, although it has been given successfully along with ampicillin. In addition to appropriate antibiotic therapy, the possibility of disseminated nocardiosis must be considered; sites include brain, skin, kidneys, bone, and muscle.

**IV-68.**   **The answer is A.**   *(Chap. 139)*   Campylobacters are motile, curved gram-negative rods. The principal diarrheal pathogen is *C. jejuni*. This organism is found in the gastrointestinal tract of many animals used for food production and is usually transmitted to humans in raw or undercooked food products or through direct contact with infected animals. Over half the cases are due to insufficiently cooked contaminated poultry. *Campylobacter* is a common cause of diarrheal disease in the United States. The illness usually occurs within 2 to 4 days after exposure to the organism in food or water. Biopsy of an affected patient's jejunum, ileum, or colon reveals findings indistinguishable from those of Crohn's disease and ulcerative colitis. Although the diarrheal illness is usually self-limited, it may be associated with constitutional symptoms, lasts more than 1 week, and recurs in 5 to 10% of untreated patients. Complications include pancreatitis, cystitis, arthritis, meningitis, and Guillain-Barré syndrome. The symptoms of *Campylobacter* enteritis are similar to those resulting from infection with *Salmonella*, *Shigella*, and *Yersinia*; all these agents cause fever and the presence of fecal leukocytes. The diagnosis is made by isolating *Campylobacter* from the stool, which requires selective media. *E. coli* (enterotoxogenic) generally is not associated with the finding of fecal leukocytes; nor is the Norwalk agent. *Campylobacter* is a far more common cause of a recurrent relapsing diarrheal illness that could be pathologically confused with inflammatory bowel disease than are *Yersinia, Salmonella, Shigella*, and enteropathogenic *E. coli*.

**IV-69.**   **The answer is A.**   *(Chap. 128)*   One of the most common causes of infectious arthritis in young adults, particularly in urban medical centers, is gonococcal infection. Entry occurs via sites of sexual contact: the genitourinary tract, oropharynx, and rectum. Infection at one of these sites, particularly in menstruating females, pregnant women, and those with complement deficiencies, may lead to dissemination. Such an occurrence produces a biphasic illness that is first manifested by constitutional symptoms, migratory arthritis (particularly in the knee, shoulder, wrists, and interphalangeal joints of the hand), tenosynovitis, and vesiculopustular skin lesions. Although these symptoms may abate, joint involvement may progress to a purulent mono- or polyarticular arthritis. Synovial culture and Gram stain are usually negative early in the course of the illness but may be positive at later stages. Blood cultures may be positive, but only in the early stage of the illness. Complement deficiencies are present only in patients who have congenital hypocomplementemia. Gonococci are demonstrable by Gram stain in the skin lesions in about two-thirds of cases. However, diagnosis is best made by observing the intracellular gram-negative diplococci in leukocytes from Gram-stained smears of urethral or endocervical exudates. Because of the presence of other gram-negative diplococci in normal oral flora, Gram stains of pharyngeal smears are not specific. Selective media, such as Thayer-Martin, should be used to culture gonococcus from the urethra, endocervix, pharynx, or rectum. The endocervical culture is positive in 80 to 90% of women with gonorrhea. Treatment for disseminated gonococcal infection includes hospitalization and the administration of ceftriaxone, ceftizoxime, or cefotaxime. If the patient is proved to have gonorrhea, a serologic test for syphilis and confidential testing for HIV infection should also be undertaken.

**IV-70.** **The answer is C.** *(Chap. 195)* This patient was in the right location and has the typical clinical features of a patient infected with *Babesia*, a tick-borne protozoa that multiplies in red blood cells. The clinical manifestations can be more severe in splenectomized persons. The best way to make the diagnosis is to demonstrate the parasite's presence in erythrocytes in Giemsa-stained peripheral blood smears. Serologic confirmation can also be helpful. The combination of quinine and clindamycin constitutes the most effective treatment.

**IV-71.** **The answer is E.** *(Chap. 173; Piscitelli, Gallicano, N Engl J Med 344:984–996, 2001.)* The mainstay of treatment of patients with HIV infection is combination antiretroviral therapy, or HAART. When to initiate such therapy is controversial, but it is reasonable to treat patients with the acute HIV syndrome, those with symptomatic disease, those with CD4+ T cell counts $<500/\mu L$, and those with $>20,000$ copies of HIV RNA/mL. Combination therapy usually consists of two nucleoside analogues, one of which is usually lamivudine, and a protease inhibitor. Another regimen uses two nucleoside analogues plus a nonnucleoside reverse transcriptase inhibitor. The increase in the plasma HIV RNA load is often considered an indication to change therapy, as is a failure to achieve an improvement in the CD4 counts. It is very important to consider drug-drug interactions in patients taking complicated medical regimens that include antiretroviral drugs in addition to prophylactic antibiotics and/or other medicines. There are numerous such interactions among the antiretroviral drugs. For example, efavirenz, a nonnucleoside reverse transcriptase inhibitor, can decrease serum levels of the HIV protease inhibitor indinavir, requiring an increase in the indinavir dose. Second, both efavirenz and another nonnucleoside reverse transcriptase inhibitor, nevirapine, can reduce plasma methadone concentrations by approximately 50% in those receiving methadone maintenance therapy. Such a decrease in the methadone concentration could precipitate methadone withdrawal, which would yield the symptoms evidenced by this patient. It is therefore very important to consider the effect of any new drugs in HIV patients with a stable regimen by consulting the appropriate sources in the literature or on an Internet-based site.

**IV-72.** **The answer is A.** *(Chap. 115)* Since the 1990s chlamydia has been the most common cause of nongonococcal urethritis (NGU) in men. Gram-negative intracellular diplococci in the presence of polymorphonuclear leukocytes are seen in 70% of cases of gonocccoccal urethritis. Despite common belief, men can be infected with trichomonas and develop urethritis. Recently, mycoplasma and ureaplasma have been implicated in a some cases of NGU. Herpes simplex virus may also cause similar symptoms. Coliforms may cause urethritis in men who engage in anal intercourse. In the absence of any other symptoms or systemic findings, Reiter's syndrome is unlikely. In the absence of gonococci on culture or DNA testing, NGU is treated with single-dose azithromycin or doxycycline for 7 days. Sexual partners should be treated with the same regimen.

**IV-73.   The answer is D.**   *(Chap. 157)*   An expanding erythematous rash not associated with scaling is characteristic of erythema chronicum migrans. The disease first appears weeks to months after a tick bite. The lesion begins as a red macule at the site of the bite; the borders of the lesion then expand to form a red ring, with central clearing, as wide as 20 to 30 cm or more in diameter. Occasionally, secondary rings may occur within the original one. The lesion may itch or burn and may be accompanied by fever, headache, vomiting, fatigue, and regional adenopathy.

**IV-74.   The answer is A.**   *(Chap. 164)*   Herpes zoster, caused by the varicella zoster virus, which resides in ganglia after primary infection, usually produces a vesicular eruption limited to the dermatome innervated by the corresponding sensory ganglia. Frequently the characteristic rash, grouped vesicles on an erythematous base, is preceded by several days of pain and paresthesia in the involved area. The most common site of involvement is thoracic dermatomes, but trigeminal, lumbar, and cervical regions may also be affected. Immunosuppressed persons may display dissemination of zoster, which certainly mandates systemic therapy. Nasociliary branch involvement is not uncommon in patients with ophthalmic zoster and may be heralded by vesicular lesions on the side or tip of the nose. In light of the possibility of associated conjunctivitis, keratitis, scleritis, or iritis, an ophthalmologist should always be consulted. Although the risk of postherpetic neuralgia is significant in patients over age 60, it is unclear if early use of steroids prevents this complication. Although it is reasonable to undertake measures to contain bacterial superinfection, including the use of antibacterial compresses, administration of prophylactic systemic antibiotics is not indicated.

**IV-75.   The answer is C.**   *(Chap. 203)*   *Schistosoma mansoni* infection of the liver causes cirrhosis from vascular obstruction resulting from periportal fibrosis but relatively little hepatocellular injury. Hepatosplenomegaly, hypersplenism, and esophageal varices develop quite commonly, and schistosomiasis is usually associated with eosinophilia. Spider nevi, gynecomastia, jaundice, and ascites are observed less commonly than they are in alcoholic and postnecrotic fibrosis.

**IV-76.   The answer is C.**   *(Chap. 153)*   The rash of secondary syphilis is a maculopapular squamous eruption characterized by scattered reddish-brown lesions with a thin scale. The eruption often involves the palms and the soles; this is an important clue in the differential diagnosis. This rash can resemble atypical pityriasis rosea or erythema multiforme. The nontreponemal serologic tests such as the Venereal Disease Research Laboratory (VDRL) and RPR tests are positive. Patients usually give a history of a chancre at the site of the primary infection—in a heterosexual male usually the penis but possibly the anus or pharynx. Treatment for both HIV-positive and HIV-negative adults is 2.4 million units of benzathine penicillin by intramuscular injection. If this treatment is successful, the nontreponemal serologic tests should become negative.

**IV-77.   The answer is D.**   *[Chaps. 182 and 187; Clin Infect Dis 3(12):772–785, 2003.]*   A common risk factor for fungemia is indwelling central venous catheters, and the most commonly identified species is *Candida albicans*. However, other species, such as *C. glabrata, C. tropicalis, C. parapsilosis,* and *C. krusei,* are also identified. This is one of the rare patients (1%) with evidence of an anaphylactic response to amphotericin. Although the prevalence of anaphylaxis in the use of lipid formulations of amphotericin is also rare, it has been described. Thus, these formulations should be avoided in this patient. *C. krusei* is most often azole-resistant. Therefore, high-dose fluconazole is unlikely to be effective. Also, because of the many toxic side effects ketoconazole is rarely used and has been replaced by itraconazole. Itraconzaole has a broader spectrum of clinical efficacy with less described hepatotoxicity and arrhythmias. Flucytosine is an antimetabolite agent that is converted to 5-fluorouracil within the fungal cell. It is often effective against candidiasis but would never be given as monotherapy because of the rapid development of drug resistance. Therefore, in this patient an effective and optimal treatment choice would be caspofungin. This is an echinocandin drug that acts by inhibiting synthesis of the $(1,3)\beta$-D-glucan in the fungal cell wall. This drug shows activity against all *Candida* species independent of azole resistance except for *C. parapsilosis*. Toxicity is low except for possible hepatotoxicity.

**IV-78.  The answer is B.**  *(Chap. 187)*   Oral thrush, or mucocutaneous candidiasis, presents with discrete and confluent adherent white plaques on the oral and pharyngeal mucosa. Unexplained oral thrush must raise the possibility of HIV infection and is common in patients with acute HIV infection. Thus, the HIV antibody test may be negative in acute seroconversion and it is important to check the HIV viral load to make the diagnosis. With no history of diabetes and a normal serum glucose there is no need to proceed with a glucose tolerance test. Urine hCG testing is a highly sensitive test, and oral thrush is uncommon during pregnancy; vulvovaginal candidiasis is much more common, especially in the third trimester. The diagnosis may be confirmed with a scraping for a smear from the oral plaque. Therapy for oral candidiasis includes clotrimazole troches five times per day; this is as effective as oral fluconazole 100 mg/d. Oral nystatin suspension is less effective.

**IV-79.  The answer is E.**  *(Chap. 187)*   *Candidemia* may lead to seeding of other organs. Among nonneutropenic patients up to 10% develop retinal lesions; therefore, it is very important to perform thorough funduscopy. Focal seeding can occur within 2 weeks of the onset of candidemia and may occur even if the patient is afebrile or the infection clears. The lesions may be unilateral or bilateral and are typically small white retinal exudates. However, retinal infection may progress to retinal detachment, vitreous abscess, or extension into the anterior chamber of the eye. Patients may be asymptomatic initially but also may report blurring, ocular pain, or scotoma. Abdominal abscess are possible but usually occur in patients recovering from profound neutropenia. Fungal endocarditis is also possible but is more common in patients who use intravenous drugs and may have a murmur on cardiac examination. Fungal pneumonia and pulmonary abscesses are very rare and are not likely in this patient.

**IV-80.  The answer is E.**  *[Chap. 187. Clin Ther 25(5):1321–1381, 2003.]*   Although this patient has had a recurrence of esophageal candidiasis, neither episode was severe and the frequency of episodes is not considered high at this time. Therefore, prophylaxis therapy is not indicated. In HIV-positive patients, if recurrent esophageal candidiasis is considered very frequent or severe, the recommended therapy is fluconazole (3 to 6 mg/kg) or itraconazole (5 mg/kg). Voriconazole is reserved for severe fungal infections and may be considered in patients who are unresponsive to fluconazole treatment.

**IV-81 and IV-82.  The answers are C and D.**  *(Chap. 189)*   Mucormycosis is an opportunistic fungal infection commonly caused by species of *Rhizopus, Rhizomucor*, and *Cunninghamella*. Patients at risk for developing mucormycosis infection are those with diabetes mellitus, organ transplant recipients, those with a hematologic malignancy, and those who have received long-term deferoxamine therapy. Other sites of infection include pulmonary, gastrointestinal, and cutaneous. Although the infection is rare, its prognosis is poor, with a mortality rate up to 50% for localized disease even with appropriate therapy. Diagnosis is most often made by biopsy and histologic evaluation. Cultures of affected sites should be attempted, but they are often negative. Imaging by CT or MRI/MRA is important to assess the extent of invasive disease, including vascular invasion, but this is not the standard for diagnosis. Diabetic ketoacidosis increases the risk of the development of this infection, and an important part of therapy is good regulation of diabetes. Intravenous amphotericin B should be initiated and a surgical consult should be obtained for evaluation for the need for debridement, including possible orbital exenteration. Therapy is continued for 10 to 12 weeks.

**IV-83.  The answer is B.**  *(Chap. 186)*   The goal of therapy for cryptococcal meningoenceph-alitis in an HIV-negative patient is cure of the fungal infection, not simply control of symptoms. Thus, the course of intravenous amphotericin is recommended to be 10 weeks with negative CSF cultures, a decreasing CSF cryptococcal antigen titer, and a normalized CSF glucose value. Once this is completed and clinical response has been achieved, therapy is followed by fluconazole to complete a 6- to 12-month course. The 2-week amphotericin can be used in clinically responding HIV-positive patients, who then will require 8 weeks of fluconazole 400 mg daily followed by lifelong suppressive therapy with fluconazole 200 mg daily. Flucytosine has been used to accelerate a negative culture response, but its use exposes the patient to potentially severe toxicities. Ceftriaxone and vancomycin are the recommended treatments for bacterial meningitis in an immunocompetent patient less than 50 years of age.

**IV-84.  The answer is E.**  *(Chap. 186)*   Cryptococcal meningoencephalitis presents with early manifestations of headache, nausea, gait disturbance, confusion, and visual changes. Fever and nuchal rigidity are often mild or absent. Papilledema is present in approximately 30% of cases. Asymmetric cranial nerve palsies occur in 25% of cases. Neuroimaging is often normal. If there are focal neurologic findings, an MRI with T2 or FLARE and gadolinium may be used to diagnose cryptococcomas in the basal ganglia or caudate nucleus, although they are more common in immunocompetent patients with *C. neoformans* var. *gattii.* Imaging does not make the diagnosis. The definitive diagnosis remains CSF culture. How-ever, capsular antigen testing in both the serum and the CSF is very sensitive. Approxi-mately 90% of patients, including all with a positive CSF smear, and the majority of AIDS patients have detectable cryptococcal antigen. However, because of a very small false-positive rate in antigen testing, CSF culture remains the definitive diagnostic test. In this condition *C. neoformans* often can also be cultured from the urine; however, other testing methods are more rapid and useful.

**IV-85.  The answer is D.**  *(Chap. 152)*   Patients with bronchiectasis characterized by repeated episodes of purulent bronchitis and dilated bronchi on radiographs may develop nontu-berculous mycobacterium (NTM). However, NTM may also cause progressive destructive lung infection in patients with normal or abnormal lungs. The diagnosis of invasive disease requires a compatible clinical syndrome, radiographic abnormalities, and either repeated positive sputum cultures despite courses of bronchodilators or evidence of tissue invasion on biopsy. In this case a single positive culture with all the above organisms except *M. kansasii* could represent colonization. *M. kansasii* is usually pathogenic, and a single iso-late in a clinically and radiographically compatible patient warrents therapy. *M. kansasii* is treated with rifampin, isoniazid, and ethambutol for at least 18 months. If isolates are resistant to rifampin, clarithromycin or azithromycin is substituted.

**IV-86.  The answer is C.**  *(Chap. 152)*   This patient most likely has infection with a nontuber-culous mycobacterium. *M. avium* complex organisms, especially *M. intracellulare*, are the most common cause of nontuberculous mycobacterium infections in otherwise normal hosts. Typical patients are elderly women with indolent respiratory deterioration, fever, and purulent cough. Radiographs typically demonstrate small nodular infiltrates and cy-lindrical bronchiectasis. These infections often involve the middle lobe. Indications for treatment include a compatible clinical and radiographic presentation plus either repeated positive sputum cultures or demonstration of organisms on tissue biopsy. Isoniazid/rif-ampin and isoniazid/rifampin/ethambutol are effective regimens for *M. tuberculosis.* Ami-kacin/cefoxitin/clarithromycin is effective for treatment of *M. fortuitum.*

**IV-87.  The answer is B.**  *(Chap. 184)*   *Coccidioides immitis* is a mold that is found in the soil in the southwestern United States and Mexico. Case clusters of primary disease may appear 10 to 14 days after exposure, and the activities with the highest risk include archaeologic excavation, rock hunting, military maneuvers, and construction work. Only 40% of primary pulmonary infections are symptomatic. Symptoms may include those of a hypersensitivity reaction such as erythema nodosum, erythema multiforme, arthritis, or conjunctivitis. Diagnosis can be made by culture of sputum; however, when this organism is suspected, the laboratory needs to be notified as it is a biohazard level 3 fungus. Serologic tests of blood may also be helpful; however, seroconversion of primary disease may take up to 8 weeks. Skin testing is useful only for epidemiologic studies and is not done in clinical practice.

**IV-88. The answer is A.** *(Chap. 183)* Given the high-risk endemic area and employment behavior in an HIV-positive patient with classic symptomatology, the most likely diagnosis is disseminated *histoplasmosis*. Although the differential diagnosis includes *Pneumocystis* pneumonia or disseminated *M. tuberculosis*, the pancytopenia, very elevated lactic dehydrogenase, skin findings, and high exposure risk are more typical for histoplasmosis. The small budding yeast may be seen in alveolar macrophages from bronchoalveolar lavage. Diagnosis can be made from culture of the skin lesions, although this is often difficult. Blood cultures require 15 mL of blood at a minimum and may take over 2 weeks to grow. Cultures of sputum, bone marrow, mucosal lesions, bronchoalveolar lavage, or liver biopsy may be helpful. Antigen detection in serum or blood is an available and rapid test used for diagnosis; however, this still requires confirmation by culture and histopathology. For disseminated disease in an immunocompromised host the recommended treatment is amphotericin B for 10 to 12 weeks, followed by conversion to lifelong itraconazole suppression therapy. For an immunocompetent patient with acute pulmonary histoplasmosis, if the clinical evaluation is stable, the recommended treatment is observation.

**IV-89. The answer is C.** *(Chap. 362)* Prions are infectious proteins that lack nucleic acids and cause neurodegenerative diseases. The most common prion disease in humans is sporadic Creutzfeld-Jakob disease (s-CJD). Others include familial CJD, fatal familial insomnia, kuru, and iatrogenic CJD. Prions result when an abnormal prion protein binds to a normal isoform of the prion protein, stimulating its conversion into the abnormal isoform. Abnormal prion isoforms have a greater proportion of beta structure and less alpha helix than do normal isoforms. The alpha-to-beta structural transition underlies the etiology of the CNS degeneration. The patient described has a typical presentation of s-CJD with sleep disturbance, fatigue, and defects in higher cortical functions. CJD progresses quickly to dementia. Over 90% of patients with CJD exhibit myoclonus during the illness. Typically the myoclonus is provoked by startle, loud noises, or bright lights and will occur even during sleep. The diagnosis requires an appropriate clinical presentation and no other etiologies on CSF examination. There is no widely available laboratory test for diagnosis. Brain biopsy may demonstrate spongiform degeneration and the presence of prion proteins.

**IV-90. The answer is D.** *(Chap. 114)* The diagnosis of *C. difficile*–associated diarrhea (CDAD) requires a combination of the appropriate clinical circumstances and demonstration of either toxin A or toxin B in the stool, toxin producing *C. difficile* on stool culture, or pseudomembranes in the colon. Not all strains of *C. difficile* produce toxin, and so the diagnosis requires the demonstration of a toxin-producing strain. The sensitivity of assays for *C. difficile* toxins A and B is not high, and so repeated testing is necessary to rule out the disease in symptomatic patients. Pseudomembranes are seen in approximately 50% of patients with CDAD. Pseudomembranous colitis usually involves the entire colon but may spare the rectum in approximately 10% of cases. The small bowel is not involved. Prospective studies have demonstrated that patients colonized with *C. difficile* have a decreased risk of developing CDAD. Oral therapy with vancomycin or metronidazole for 10 to 14 days is the suggested initial therapy, with response rates of approximately 95%. The diarrhea generally responds in 2 to 4 days.

**IV-91. The answer is C.** *(Chaps. 119, 239)* Patients with SS sickle cell disease are considered functionally asplenic by middle childhood. Thus, they are at risk for serious infections from encapsulated bacteria. Eighty percent of cases of overwhelming infections in this patient population are due to *S. pneumoniae*, usually from a pulmonary source. Pneumonia in this population may have a mortality as high as 45%.

**IV-92.  The answer is E.**  *(Chap. 239)*   The PORT score is a system used to classify community-acquired pneumonia (CAP) from mild to severe. The score assigns points to 20 items associated with mortality, including age, nursing home residence, coexisting illness (neoplastic disease, liver disease, congestive heart failure, cerebrovascular disease, renal disease), physical examination findings (mental status, respiratory rate, blood pressure, temperature, pulse rate), and laboratory/radiographic findings (pH, blood urea nitrogen, sodium, glucose, hematocrit, PaO$_2$, pleural effusion). The resulting scores are used to define five classes with progressively increasing mortality. These classes correlate with mortality and have been used to derive suggested management and site of treatment (home versus hospital) criteria. Cigarette smoking is a risk factor for the development of pneumonia but is not used in the prognostic scoring system.

**IV-93.  The answer is E.**  *(Chap. 239)*   *Moraxella* can colonize the upper airways of cigarette smokers. The diagnosis of pneumonia in these cases requires an appropriate clinical condition and a suitable Gram stain. Sputum samples with more than 25 white blood cells and fewer than 10 squamous epithelial cells per low-power field are suitable for culture. Growth of *B. dermatidis, C. immitis, H. capsilatum, Legionella* spp., or *M. tuberculosis* on culture is considered to reflect pathogens, not colonizers.

**IV-94 and IV-95.  The answers are C and A.**  *(Chap. 131)*   HACEK organisms (*Haemophilus* spp., *Actinobacillus actinomycetemcomitans, Cardiobacterium hominus, Eikenella corrodens*, and *Kingella kingae*) are most commonly acquired from the oral cavity, and in this case the dental cleaning led to the introduction of bacteria that probably caused bacterial endocarditis. *Haemophilus* spp. account for over 50% of cases of HACEK endocarditis. Cultures for the organisms are generally positive after 1 week, but in rare cases it may take up to 1 month to grow these fastidious organisms. Of note, the presentation can be relatively acute, with over 60% of patients with *Haemophilus* endocarditis coming to medical attention after less than 2 months of illness. Echocardiography is helpful in making the diagnosis, with over 85% of patients having vegetations present. Antibiotic therapy is highly successful; indeed, prosthetic valve endocarditis with HACEK organisms is often cured with antibiotic therapy alone. *Haemophilus* spp. are treated with ceftriaxone.

**IV-96.  The answer is D.**  *(Chap. 176)*   The patient has a classic presentation for measles, which despite an effective vaccination program still has sporadic miniepidemics in the United States. Most outbreaks occur among preschool children. The virus is contracted by exposure to respiratory secretions. The first 2 days of the illness are characterized by cough, coryza, and fevers that can be as high at *40.6°(105°*F) and are followed closely by the development of Kopkick's spots, which are depicted in the question. The spots are found in the buccal mucosa and are blue-white on a red background. As the rash appears, marching from the head to the trunk and finally the periphery, Kopkick's spots fade. The rash is classically confluent. Diagnosis can be made by finding characteristic multinucleated giant cells with inclusion bodies from the respiratory epithelium. However, IgM against measles is unlikely to be positive until at least 1 to 2 days after development of the rash. Subacute sclerosing panencephalitis (SSPE) is a very rare complication of measles encephalitis and is generally found only in children who have acquired the illness before 2 years of age. Therapy with vitamin A has been shown to decrease mortality among infected children, and it is now recommended for this population, but also for patients with immunodeficiency, vitamin A deficiency, impaired intestinal absorption, or moderate to severe malnutrition *and for* recent immigrants from areas with high measles mortality.

**IV-97.  The answer is D.**  *(Chap. 115)*   This patient has bacterial vaginosis (BV). BV is usually diagnosed clinically by the presence of three of the four following findings: increased white vaginal discharge, pH of the discharge >4.5, liberation of a fishy odor when the discharge is mixed with 10% KOH, and microscopic demonstration of clue cells (the figure above demonstrates vaginal epithelial cells coated with coccobacillary organisms) on a wet mount. BV is treated with oral metronidazole or vaginal metronidazole or clindamycin. BV recently was demonstrated to increase the risk of preterm delivery. Vulvovaginal candidiasis will have more symptoms of itching or irritation, a lower vaginal discharge pH, and fungal elements on KOH stain. *Trichomonas* vaginitis is characterized by a profuse purulent discharge, vaginal itching, and motile organisms on wet mount microscopy. Trichomonas is also treated with metronidazole.

**IV-98. The answer is A.** *(Chap. 180)* This patient has acute dengue fever acquired from a mosquito bite while he was in the Caribbean. The 1-week incubation and symptoms including severe myalgias, petechiae, and epistaxis are typical. Diagnosis is best made by IgM ELISA or paired serology. The disease may progress into a case of hemorrhagic fever with severe shock and gastrointestinal hemorrhage. The differential would include rickettsial illness transmitted by a tick. Acute HIV seroconversion can present with fever, adenopathy, and myalgias; however, the HIV PCR would be postitive with symptoms (although the HIV antibody test would be negative). Exposure to rodent urine could cause leptospirosis.

**IV-99. The answer is E.** *(Chaps. 193 and 203)* This patient has Katayama fever caused by infection with *Schistosoma mansoni*. Approximately 4 to 8 weeks after exposure the parasite migrates through the portal and pulmonary circulations. This phase of the illness may be asymptomatic but in some cases evokes a hypersensitivity response and a serum-sickness-type illness. Eosinophilia is usual. Since there is not a large enteric burden of parasites during this phase of the illness, stool studies may not be positive and serology may be helpful, particularly in patients from nonendemic areas. Praziquantel is the treatment of choice because Katayama fever may progress to include neurologic complications. Chloroquine is used for treatment of malaria; mebendazole for ascariasis, hookworm, trichinosis, and visceral larval migrans; metronidazole for amebiasis, giardiasis, and trichomoniasis; and thiabendazole for strongyloides.

**IV-100. The answer is A.** *(Chaps. 116 and 241)* *B. cepacia* is an opportunistic pathogen that has been responsible for nosocomial outbreaks. It also colonizes and infects the lower respiratory tract of patients with cystic fibrosis, chronic granulomatous disease, and sickle cell disease. In patients with cystic fibrosis it portends a rapid decline in pulmonary function and a poor clinical prognosis. It also may cause a resistant necrotizing pneumonia. *B. cepacia* is often intrinsically resistant to a variety of antimicrobials, including many β-lactams and aminoglycosides. Trimethoprim-sulfamethoxazole (TMP/SMX) is usually the first-line treatment. *P. aeruginosa* and *S. aureus* are common colonizers and pathogens in patients with cystic fibrosis. *Stenotrophomonas maltophilia* is the pathogen, particularly in patients with cancer, transplants, and critical illness. *S. maltophilia* is a cause of pneumonia, urinary tract infection, wound infection, and bacteremia. TMP/SMX is usually the treatment of choice for *Stenotrophomonas* infections.

**IV-101. The answer is A.** *(Chap. 153)* This patient presents with classic manifestations of primary syphilis caused by *Treponema pallidum*. Recommended treatment is one dose of penicillin G IM, which is curative in 95% of cases. This patient then develops symptoms consistent with the Jarisch-Herxheimer reaction, which usually begins within 1 to 2 hours after treatment and resolves within 24 to 48 hours. These symptoms are hypothesized to be due to release of treponemal lipopolysaccharide from dying spirochetes. Symptoms can be controlled with acetaminophen or nonsteroidal anti-inflammatory drugs, but there is no indication for additional antibiotic therapy or steroids. Although neurosyphilis can present in any phase of the infection, because of the timing of the development of these symptoms without other specific neurologic signs, there is no indication for lumbar puncture at this time. In light of the fact that syphilis is a sexually transmitted disease, this patient should indeed undergo HIV screening with HIV antibody testing.

**IV-102.   The answer is C.**   *(Chap. 157)*   Lyme borreliosis is caused by a spirochete, *Borrelia burgdorferi*, that is transmitted by the tick *Ixodes ricinus* complex. The principal vector is the northeastern United States from Maine to Maryland and the Midwestern states of Wisconsin and Minnesota. Lyme disease can also be seen in northern California and Oregon. Characteristic of early infection is the expanding annular lesion erythema migrans (EM). Most patients do not remember the tick bite, and up to 20% do not exhibit EM. Stage 2, or disseminated, infection may present as diffuse symptomatology or even meningitis with neurologic deficits. Eight percent of patients develop cardiac involvement, usually in the form of an atrioventricular block. This patient has a classic description of arthritis secondary to Lyme disease. It typically affects the knees and may last for weeks to months. Gout is not the diagnosis because there is no evidence of crystals on the arthrocentesis. Pseudogout, or calcium pyrophosphate dihydrate disease, is possible because the rhomboid crystals in this disease are often difficult to find; however, the definitive diagnosis can be made only if the crystals are identified or there are classic findings of chondrocalcinosis on radiography. Inflammatory effusions are not typical of osteoarthritis, and although septic arthritis must always be considered in the differential diagnosis of a monoarthritis, the Gram stain did not support this diagnosis. The diagnosis of Lyme arthritis can be made by serologic testing of the synovial fluid by ELISA and Western blot for anti–*B. burgdorferi* antibody. Synovial fluid for PCR of the *Borellia* genome can be performed, but there is concern about laboratory standards and the significance of a positive finding. Recommended treatment is either penicillin or ceftriaxone.

**IV-103.   The answer is D.**   *(Chap. 160)*   Congenital infection from maternal transmission can lead to severe consequences for the neonate; thus, prenatal care and screening for infection are very important. *C. trachomatis* is associated with up to 25% of exposed neonates who develop inclusion conjunctivitis. It can also be associated with pneumonia and otitis media in the newborn. Hydrocephalus can be associated with toxoplasmosis. Hutchinson triad, which is Hutchinson teeth (blunted upper incisors), interstitial keratitis, and eighth nerve deafness, is due to congenital syphilis. Sensorineural deafness can be associated with congenital rubella exposure. Treatment of *C. trachomatis* in this patient consists of oral erythromycin.

# V. DISORDERS OF THE CARDIOVASCULAR SYSTEM

## QUESTIONS

**DIRECTIONS:** Each question below contains five suggested responses. Choose the **one best** response to each question.

**V-1.** All the following are included in the revised cardiac risk index to predict patients at high risk of sustaining perioperative cardiovascular complications *except*

A. chronic kidney disease with a preoperative creatinine greater than 2.0 mg/dL
B. current tobacco use
C. history of congestive heart failure
D. history of ischemic heart disease
E. insulin therapy for diabetes mellitus

**V-2.** You are asked to evaluate a 66-year-old male for preoperative cardiovascular risk before the surgical removal of a 2-cm sigmoid colon cancer. The patient has an 80-pack-year history of cigarette use but quit 6 months before this presentation. His past medical history is also significant for hypertension and hypercholesterolemia. He has no past cardiac history and has never received cardiac imaging or stress testing. He currently is taking lisinopril 20 mg/d, hydrochlorothiazide 25 mg/d, and pravastatin 20 mg/d. He has not tolerated atenolol in the past because of fatigue and decreased libido. Functionally, the patient is quite healthy and continues to play golf weekly while carrying his own golf bag. He lives on the fourth floor of an apartment complex and prefers climbing the stairs to using the elevator. He has no limiting dyspnea or chest pain. On physical examination the patient appears his stated age and has a blood pressure of 136/88. Heart rate is 90. Cardiovascular and pulmonary examinations are normal. The patient has good peripheral pulses and no carotid bruits. His electrocardiogram reveals no evidence of prior ischemia or left ventricular hypertrophy, but he does have a right bundle branch block. What do you advise the patient and his surgeon about his operative risk?

A. He should undergo cardiac stress testing with imaging before surgery to rule out silent ischemia in the setting of a right bundle branch block.
B. His hypertension, hypercholesterolemia, and tobacco use place him in a high-risk surgical category, and he should undergo immediate cardiac catheterization before abdominal surgery.

**V-2.** *(Continued)*

C. Functional status is such that the patient can perform to greater than four metabolic equivalents, and the patient has only one risk factor for predicting cardiovascular events. Thus, he can proceed to surgery without further investigation.
D. The patient should not receive preoperative metoprolol because he had a bad reaction to it in the past.
E. Because of his smoking history, the patient's pulmonary risk outweighs his cardiovascular risk.

**V-3.** A 35-year-old female undergoes a physical examination while obtaining new insurance coverage. She reports 1 year of slowly progressive dyspnea on exertion and a change in skin color. Her physical examination is notable for the presence of cyanosis, an elevated jugular venous pulse, a fixed split loud second heart sound, and peripheral edema. Arterial oxygen saturation is 84%. Chest radiography shows an enlarged heart and normal lung parenchyma. Ten years ago, at her last insurance physical examination, her physical examination, oxygen saturation, and chest radiogram were normal. Echocardiography most likely will reveal

A. atrial septal defect
B. Ebstein's anomaly
C. tetralogy of Fallot
D. truncus arteriosis
E. ventricular septal defect

**V-4.** A 24-year-old male seeks medical attention for the recent onset of headaches. The headaches are described as "pounding" and occur during the day and night. He has had minimal relief with acetaminophen. Physical examination is notable for a blood pressure of 185/115 mmHg in the right arm, a heart rate of 70/min, arterioventricular (AV) nicking on funduscopic examination, normal jugular veins and carotid arteries, a pressure-loaded PMI with an apical $S_4$, no abdominal bruits, and reduced pulses in both lower extremities. Review of symptoms is positive only for leg fatigue with exertion. Additional measurement of blood pressure reveals the following:

**V-4.** *(Continued)*

    Right arm    185/115
    Left arm     188/113
    Right thigh  100/60
    Left thigh   102/58

Which of the following diagnostic studies is most likely to demonstrate the cause of the headaches?

A.    MRI of the head
B.    MRI of the kidney
C.    MRI of the thorax
D.    24-h urinary 5-HIAA
E.    24-h urinary free cortisol

**V-5.** The patient described in Question VII-4 is most likely to have which of the following associated cardiac abnormalities?

A.    Bicuspid aortic valve
B.    Mitral stenosis
C.    Preexcitation syndrome
D.    Right bundle branch block
E.    Tricuspid atresia

**V-6.** A 52-year-old male with a history of injection drug use presents to the emergency department with several days of dyspnea, occasional fevers, and new-onset syncope. He has no other medical problems and takes no medications. On physical exam his temperature is 38.1°C (100.5°F), pulse (P) 30, respiratory rate (R) 26, and blood pressure 70/40 mmHg. He is ill-appearing and diaphoretic. Lungs are clear, and cardiac exam is notable for a nondisplaced PMI, bradycardia, normal $S_1$ and $S_2$, and a II/VI systolic murmur at the apex, radiating to the axilla. Electrocardiography shows third-degree heart block. Chest plain film is normal. Management at this point should include all the following *except*

A.    intensive care unit admission
B.    transthoracic echocardiogram
C.    serial cardiac marker measurement
D.    placement of a permanent pacemaker
E.    empirical antibiotics to cover gram-positive organisms

**V-7.** A transthoracic echocardiogram is obtained and shows no evidence of vegetation. Blood cultures grow *Staphylococcus aureus* on multiple occasions. The next most appropriate diagnostic step after clinical stabilization is

A.    transesophageal echocardiogram
B.    cardiac catheterization
C.    brain natriuretic peptide measurement
D.    cardiac surgical consultation
E.    dobutamine stress echocardiogram

**V-8.** A 79-year-old male undergoes elective aortic valve replacement with a porcine valve. One month after the operation he develops daily low-grade temperatures. A thorough history and physical exam do not localize the symptoms. A CT is obtained of the thorax, abdomen, and pelvis and shows no abnormality. Blood cultures are likely to grow which of the following?

A.    *Streptococcus faecium*
B.    *Staphylococcus epidermidis*
C.    *Haemophilus* species
D.    *Pseudomonas aeruginosa*
E.    *Streptococcus pneumoniae*

**V-9.** Appropriate empirical therapy for the most likely organism in Question VII-8 is

A.    oxacillin
B.    ceftriaxone
C.    vancomycin
D.    ampicillin and gentamicin
E.    oxacillin and gentamicin

**V-10.** A 30-year-old female is seen in the clinic before undergoing an esophageal dilation for a stricture. Her past medical history is notable for mitral valve prolapse with mild regurgitation. She takes no medications and is allergic to penicillin. Her physician should recommend which of the following?

A.    Clarithromycin 500 mg PO 1 h before the procedure.
B.    Clindamycin 450 mg PO 1 h before the procedure.
C.    Vancomycin 1 g intravenously before the procedure.
D.    The procedure is low-risk, and therefore no prophylaxis is indicated.
E.    Her valvular lesion is low-risk, and therefore no prophylaxis is indicated.

**V-11.** You are working in the cardiac intensive care unit and are called to deal with a cardiac arrest. The patient is a 36-year-old female who was admitted with dehydration in the setting of a gastrointestinal illness. She has had profound vomiting and diarrhea for the last 4 days with 10 recorded stools. In addition, the patient is known to be an alcoholic who drinks a pint of vodka daily. On arrival,

**V-11.** *(Continued)*
the patient is in full cardiac arrest without a pulse, and the nursing staff has initiated basic cardiopulmonary life support. The patient has been intubated. The patient's rhythm is shown below. Which of the following drugs would be most helpful in correcting this rhythm?

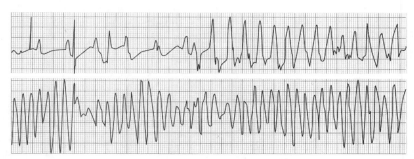

A. Magnesium sulfate
B. Amiodarone
C. Sodium bicarbonate
D. Calcium chloride
E. Lidocaine

**V-12.** A 66-year-old male is admitted to the cardiac care unit for treatment of an inferior wall myocardial infarction and undergoes successful percutaneous intervention with stent placement to the midright coronary artery. His clinical course was complicated by prolonged symptoms for 24 h before the intervention. It is noted at the time of cardiac catheterization that he has right-dominant circulation with blood supply to the posterior descending artery from the right coronary artery. Five days after the original presentation you are called emergently to his bedside when he develops acute shortness of breath and hypotension. The patient appears to be in marked respiratory distress, sitting upright at the edge of the bed with diaphoresis. His vital signs include a heart rate of 120 beats per minute, blood pressure of 86/42, respiratory rate of 40, and oxygen saturation by pulse oximetry of 80% on room air. Jugular venous pressure is elevated at 8 cm above the sternal notch. The respiratory exam shows diffuse bilateral crackles in both lung fields. The cardiovascular exam reveals a regular tachycardia without muffled heart sounds. There is no palpable thrill or heave. There has been interval development of a loud III/VI blowing, holosystolic murmur heard throughout the precordium. The extremities are cool to palpation. A typical pulmonary capillary wedge tracing is shown in the following figure. The right atrial oxygen saturation is 72%, and the pulmonary artery oxygen saturation is 69%. What is the most likely diagnosis?

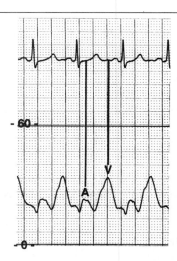

A. Acute mitral regurgitation
B. Acute ventricular septal defect
C. Left ventricular wall rupture
D. Recurrent myocardial ischemia
E. Acute aortic regurgitation

**V-13.** In the patient described in Question VII-12 what is the most appropriate next step in management?

A. Placement of an intra-aortic balloon pump
B. Emergent surgical intervention
C. Repeat cardiac catheterization with angioplasty

**V-13.** *(Continued)*
D.   Intravenous dobutamine
E.   Intravenous nitroprusside

**V-14.** All the following ECG findings are suggestive of left ventricular hypertrophy *except*

A.   (S in $V_1$ + R in $V_5$ or $V_6$) >35 mm
B.   R in aVL >11 mm
C.   R in aVF >20 mm
D.   (R in I + S in III) >25 mm
E.   R in aVR >8 mm

**V-15.** A 35-year-old Hispanic female is admitted to the hospital for hemoptysis and a 1-month history of progressive shortness of breath. The cardiac exam shows a loud opening snap at $S_1$ and a low-pitched diastolic murmur that is loudest at the apex. Chest x-ray shows Kerley B lines and evidence of pulmonary edema. A diagnosis of mitral stenosis is made. Echocardiography shows a dilated left atrium and a mitral orifice size of 1.1 cm². The mitral valve leaflets have minimal calcification. There is no mitral regurgitation. What is the appropriate management?

A.   Antibiotic prophylaxis for dental procedures, adequate diuresis, and a repeat echocardiogram in 6 months
B.   Coronary angiogram
C.   Balloon valvotomy
D.   Surgical valvotomy
E.   Mitral valve replacement

**V-16.** All the following statements regarding aortic stenosis (AS) are true *except*

A.   Rheumatic heart disease is the most common cause of AS in North America and Western Europe.
B.   The majority of adult patients with symptomatic valvular AS are male.
C.   A large transvalvular pressure gradient may exist for years without a reduction in cardiac output or left ventricular dilatation.
D.   AS is rarely of clinical importance until the valve orifice has narrowed to approximately 0.5 cm²/m².
E.   Symptoms of congestive heart failure are associated with a shorter mean survival time than are symptoms of syncope.

**V-17.** An 80-year-old male presents to your clinic with a 5-month history of progressive shortness of breath, dyspnea on exertion, orthopnea, and lower extremity edema. He notes "chest pressure" while walking up a flight of stairs that is relieved with rest. He denies any episodes of syncope but has felt "dizzy" at various times over the last 2 months. On exam, jugular venous pressure is elevated. There is an audible grade IV systolic ejection murmur

**V-17.** *(Continued)*
heard at the base with radiation to the carotid arteries. There are bibasilar crackles and pitting edema. An electrocardiogram shows evidence of left ventricular hypertrophy. You order an echocardiogram, which shows a stenotic, calcified aortic valve with an estimated valve area of 0.7 cm² with an elevated transvalvular gradient. Ejection fraction is estimated at 40%. What management step should you recommend to improve his long-term survival?

A.   Furosemide
B.   Atorvastatin
C.   Nitroglycerin
D.   Aortic valve replacement
E.   Balloon valvuloplasty

**V-18.** All the following patients should undergo operative repair or replacement of the mitral valve *except*

A.   a 64-year-old male with mitral regurgitation, congestive heart failure, and an ejection fraction of 20%
B.   a 70-year-old asymptomatic female with mitral regurgitation and an ejection fraction of 45%
C.   a 45-year-old male with dyspnea on exertion, fatigue, mitral regurgitation, and an ejection fraction of 55%
D.   a 60-year-old female with symptomatic mitral stenosis and mitral regurgitation
E.   a 55-year-old asymptomatic female with an end-systolic cavity dimension of 55 mm

**V-19.** All the following disorders may be associated with thoracic aortic aneurysm *except*

A.   osteogenesis imperfecta
B.   Takayasu's arteritis
C.   Ehlers-Danlos syndrome
D.   ankylosing spondylitis
E.   Klinefelter's syndrome

**V-20.** All the following are true about cardiac valve replacement *except*

A.   Bioprosthetic valve replacement is preferred to mechanical valve replacement in younger patients because of the superior durability of the valve.
B.   Bioprosthetic valves have a low incidence of thromboembolic complications.
C.   The risk of thrombosis with mechanical valve replacement is higher in the mitral position than in the aortic position.
D.   Mechanical valves are relatively contraindicated in patients who wish to become pregnant.
E.   Double-disk tilting mechanical prosthetic valves offer superior hemodynamic characteristics over single-disk tilting valves.

**V-21.** A 50-year-old male comes into your clinic for a new patient visit. His past medical history is notable for an anterior myocardial infarction 2 years ago. At that time he underwent a coronary angiogram that showed a ruptured atheromatous plaque in the left anterior descending artery but no other evidence of coronary artery disease. He underwent an angioplasty and stent placement with excellent results. He currently denies chest pain, dyspnea, or orthopnea. He walks 1 mile a day. His medications include aspirin, metoprolol, furosemide, lisinopril, atorvastatin, and clopidigrel. His exam is notable for a normal jugular venous pulsation, a normal $S_1$ and $S_2$, and an $S_3$ gallop. His lungs are clear, and he has no edema. An echocardiogram shows an ejection fraction of 25% with an akinetic anterior wall. There is no evidence of thrombus. What is the most appropriate next management step?

A. Addition of digoxin
B. Addition of amiodarone
C. Repeat cardiac catheterization
D. Referral for coronary artery bypass graft (CABG)
E. Referral for implantable cardioverter defibrillator (ICD) placement

**V-22.** A 56-year-old male is brought to the emergency department after collapsing at home. Initial cardiopulmonary resuscitation (CPR) was performed in the field, and he was intubated. A peripheral intravenous line was placed. On arrival at your station the patient has no spontaneous pulse or respiration. A rhythm strip shows monomorphic ventricular tachycardia (VT). You order additional defibrillatory shocks: first 200 J, then 300 J, and finally 360 J. A dose of vasopressin is administered. CPR is continued. What is the most appropriate drug to administer at this time?

A. Sodium bicarbonate
B. Amiodarone
C. Procainamide
D. Bretylium
E. Lidocaine

**V-23.** All the following patients should be evaluated for secondary causes of hypertension *except*

A. a 37-year-old male with strong family history of hypertension and renal failure who presents to your office with a blood pressure of 152/98
B. a 26-year-old female with hematuria and a family history of early renal failure who has a blood pressure of 160/88
C. a 63-year-old male with no past history with a blood pressure of 162/90
D. a 58-year-old male with a history of hypertension since age 45 whose blood pressure has become increasingly difficult to control on four antihypertensive agents

**V-23.** *(Continued)*
E. a 31-year-old female with complaints of severe headaches, weight gain, and new-onset diabetes mellitus with a blood pressure of 142/89

**V-24.** A 46-year-old white female presents to your office with concerns about her diagnosis of hypertension 1 month previously. She asks you about her likelihood of developing complications of hypertension, including renal failure and stroke. She denies any past medical history other than hypertension and has no symptoms that suggest secondary causes. She currently is taking hydrochlorothiazide 25 mg/d. She smokes half a pack of cigarettes daily and drinks alcohol no more than once per week. Her family history is significant for hypertension in both parents. Her mother died of a cerebrovascular accident. Her father is alive but has coronary artery disease and is on hemodialysis. Her blood pressure is 138/90. Body mass index is 23. She has no retinal exudates or other signs of hypertensive retinopathy. Her point of maximal cardiac impulse is not displaced but is sustained. Her rate and rhythm are regular and without gallops. She has good peripheral pulses. An electrocardiogram reveals an axis of $-30$ degrees with borderline voltage criteria for left ventricular hypertrophy. Creatinine is 1.0 mg/dL. Which of the following items in her history and physical examination is a risk factor for a poor prognosis in a patient with hypertension?

A. Family history of renal failure and cerebrovascular disease
B. Persistent elevation in blood pressure after the initiation of therapy
C. Ongoing tobacco use
D. Ongoing use of alcohol
E. Presence of left ventricular hypertrophy on ECG

**V-25.** Which of the following conditions is not associated with sinus bradycardia?

A. Brucellosis
B. Leptospirosis
C. Hypothyroidism
D. Advanced liver disease
E. Typhoid fever

**V-26.** A 55-year-old male presents with severe substernal chest pain for the last hour. It began at rest and is associated with dyspnea and nausea. The electrocardiogram shows bradycardia with a Mobitz type II second-degree block. Chest plain film is normal. Which of the following is likely to be found in addition on the electrocardiogram?

A. ST elevation $V_1-V_3$
B. Wellen's T waves
C. ST elevation II, III, and aVF
D. ST depression in I and aVL
E. No other abnormality

**V-27.** Which of the following patients has an indication for permanent pacemaker placement?

A. A 25-year-old female with a history of recurrent idiopathic syncope is noted to have a heart rate of 65 on physical exam. An electrocardiogram shows sinus rhythm at 65. Carotid sinus massage results in 4-s ventricular asystole with presyncope.

B. A 54-year-old male has an inferior myocardial infarction complicated by a Mobitz type II second-degree block with a narrow QRS complex. After emergent percutaneous intervention the patient feels well. The electrocardiogram shows sinus bradycardia with a heart rate of 50 while the patient is taking low-dose metoprolol.

C. An 85-year-old female with no symptoms. Electrocardiography shows first-degree atrioventricular block and right bundle branch block.

D. A 65-year-old asymptomatic male referred for Holter monitoring before obtaining a life insurance policy. He is found to have intermittent third-degree atrioventricular block.

E. A 25-year-old male with acute Lyme disease is noted to have syncope with third-degree heart block. After treatment, electrocardiography shows sinus rhythm at 55.

**V-28.** A 30-year-old female with a history of irritable bowel syndrome presents with complaints of palpitations. On further questioning, the symptoms occur randomly throughout the day, perhaps more frequently after caffeine. The primary sensation is of her heart "flip-flopping" in her chest. The patient has never had syncope. Her vital signs and exam are normal. An electrocardiogram is obtained, and it shows normal sinus rhythm with no other abnormality. A Holter monitor is obtained and shows premature ventricular contractions occurring approximately six times per minute. The next most appropriate step in her management is

A. referral to a cardiologist for electrophysiologic study
B. beta blocker administration
C. amiodarone administration
D. reassurance that this is not pathologic
E. verapamil administration

**V-29.** All the following are associated with a high risk of stroke in patients with atrial fibrillation *except*

A. diabetes mellitus
B. hypercholesterolemia
C. congestive heart failure
D. hypertension
E. age over 65

**V-30.** A 29-year-old male presents to the emergency department feeling light-headed and dizzy and with new-

**V-30.** *(Continued)*
onset palpitations. His symptoms began suddenly 30 minutes before presentation. His past medical history is notable only for a laproscopic cholecystectomy 1 year ago. He takes no medications, does not take alcohol, and does not use tobacco or illicit drugs. On physical exam, he is ill-appearing, diaphoretic, but oriented and conversant with a temperature of 36.9°C (98.4°F), pulse of 220, respiratory rate of 25, and blood pressure of 110/50. His cardiac exam, besides being tachycardic, is irregular. His electrocardiogram shows an irregular wide complex tachycardia. The preoperative electrocardiogram is shown here. The most appropriate therapy at this point is

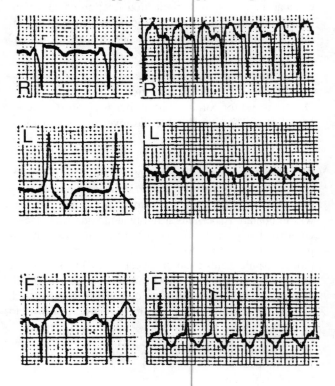

A. direct-current cardioversion
B. IV metoprolol
C. IV diltiazem
D. IV procainamide
E. IV adenosine

**V-31.** After stabilization and restoration of normal sinus rhythm, which of the following statements should be made about the patient?

A. The patient is at very low risk of this happening again and should need no further specific therapy.
B. The patient should be anticoagulated to prevent cardioembolic stroke.
C. The patient should be chronically maintained on digoxin to prevent a future recurrence.
D. The patient should be referred to an electrophysiologist for bypass tract ablation.

**V-31.** *(Continued)*
E.  The patient should be referred for pacemaker placement.

**V-32.**  A 65-year-old male is seen in the emergency department with palpitations. His symptoms began 30 min before arrival. He has not had any dizziness, light-headedness, or chest pain. His past medical history is notable for a myocardial infarct 2 years ago, chronic atrial fibrillation, and a three-vessel coronary artery bypass graft surgery 1 year ago. Medications include aspirin, metoprolol,

**V-32.** *(Continued)*
warfarin, and lisinopril. An electrocardiogram shows wide complex tachycardia at a rate of 170. Which of the following will prove definitively that his rhythm is ventricular tachycardia?

A.  Hypotension
B.  Cannon *a* waves
C.  An odd electrocardiogram with similar QRS morphology
D.  Irregular rhythm
E.  Syncope

**V-33.**  A 40-year-old male with diabetes and schizophrenia is started on antibiotic therapy for chronic osteomyelitis in the hospital. His osteomyelitis has developed just underlying an ulcer where he has been injecting heroin. He is found unresponsive by the nursing staff suddenly. His electrocardiogram is shown here. The most likely cause of this rhythm is which of the following substances?

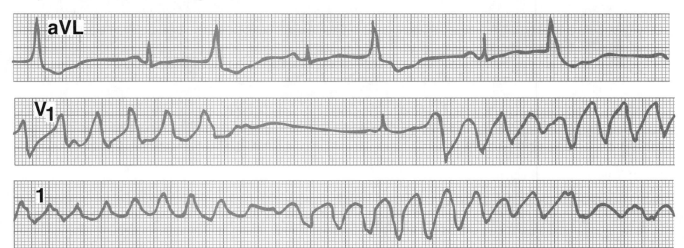

A.  Furosemide
B.  Metronidazole
C.  Droperidol

D.  Metformin
E.  Heroin

**V-34.**  Normal sinus rhythm is restored with electrical cardioversion. A 12-lead electrocardiogram is notable for a prolonged QT interval. Besides stopping the offending drug, the most appropriate management for this rhythm disturbance should include intravenous administration of which of the following?

A.  Amiodarone
B.  Lidocaine
C.  Magnesium
D.  Metoprolol
E.  Potassium

**V-35.** A 44-year-old female is brought to the emergency department by her husband with 6 h of chest pain and shortness of breath. The chest pain began about 2 h after she finished dinner, while she was cleaning up. The pain is sharp and constricting, predominantly around the left sternum and radiating to the back. She has a history of hypertension treated with a diuretic and smokes a pack of cigarettes a day. Physical examination is notable for a blood pressure of 160/100 and a heart rate of 105/min. The lungs are clear to auscultation. A chest radiogram is normal. The electrocardiogram is shown below. What is the most appropriate next intervention?

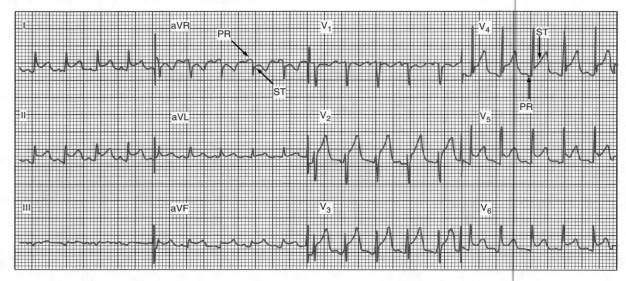

A. Coronary artery catheterization
B. CT aortogram
C. CT pulmonary angiogram
D. Ibuprofen 600 mg PO qd
E. Omeprazole 20 mg/d

**V-36.** Which of the following physical findings is most likely to be found in a patient with the following recordings from simultaneous measurement of left ventricular and right ventricular pressure?

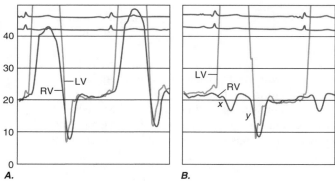

A. Holodiastolic low-pitched murmur at the cardiac apex
B. Kussmaul's sign
C. Pansystolic murmur at the lower sternal border
D. Pericardial friction rub
E. Pulsus paradoxus

**V-37.** A 78-year-old female with a past medical history remarkable for ischemic cardiomyopathy, chronic atrial fibrillation, and diabetes is admitted to the hospital with *Escherichia coli* urosepsis. She is started on intravenous antibiotics. The course is unremarkable except for the development of delirium. The day of discharge she develops syncope, and she is found to be in polymorphic ventricular tachycardia. Which drug is the *least* likely to have caused this arrhythmia?

**V-37.** *(Continued)*
A. Clarithromycin
B. Haloperidol
C. Levofloxacin
D. Olanzapine
E. Sotalol

**V-38.** 42-year-old male from El Salvador complains of several months of dyspnea on exertion. Physical examination reveals an elevated jugular venous pressure, clear lungs, a third heart sound, a pulsatile liver, ascites, and dependent edema. Chest radiography reveals no cardiomegaly and clear lung fields. An echocardiogram demonstrates normal to mildly decreased left ventricular systolic function. The initial diagnostic workup should include all the following *except*

A. computed tomography of the chest
B. coronary angiogram
C. fat pad biopsy
D. iron studies
E. tuberculin skin test

**V-39.** Each of the following patients should have a goal low-density lipoprotein cholesterol (LDL-C) <100 mg/dL to reduce the risk of coronary heart disease *except*

A. a 49-year-old male smoker with a history of exertional angina
B. a 49-year-old female who is asymptomatic with diabetes mellitus type 1
C. a 62-year-old male with long-standing hypertension and a family history of coronary heart disease
D. a 68-year-old asymptomatic male with a 60% right carotid obstruction
E. a 68-year-old female with a history of a femoral popliteal bypass

**V-40.** A 23-year-old female is brought to the emergency department after witnessed syncope. The patient reports having been at church, where she was standing for approximately 45 min. She noted feeling sweaty and lightheaded and "seeing spots." She was aware of the sensation of her heart beating and then fell to the ground with loss of consciousness. After the fall, according to witnesses, she had a thready pulse and a few clonic jerks of the legs. She regained consciousness in about 3 min. Which of the following aspects of this history is not consistent with neurocardiogenic syncope?

A. Clonic jerks of the legs
B. Prodrome of seeing spots, diaphoresis, and lightheadedness
C. Palpitations
D. Thready pulse
E. None of the above

**V-41.** A 78-year-old male presents to the clinic complaining that every time he shaves with a straight razor, he passes out. His symptoms have been occurring for the last 2 months. Occasionally, when he puts on a tight collar, he passes out as well. The loss of consciousness is brief, he has no associated prodrome, and he feels well afterward. His past medical history is notable for hypertension and hypercholesterolemia. His only medication is hydrochlorothiazide. On physical exam his vital signs are normal, and his cardiac exam is normal with the exception of a fourth heart sound. Which of the following is the most appropriate next diagnostic test?

A. Stress echocardiography
B. Adenosine thallium scan
C. Computed tomogram of the neck
D. Carotid sinus massage
E. Tilt table test

**V-42.** An 88-year-old female is admitted to the hospital with syncope that occurred after she stood up to use the bathroom in the middle of the night. This has happened to her several times over the last month, according to her family, each time in the context of transitioning from a lying to a sitting position. Her past medical history is notable for hypertension, diabetes mellitus, remote myocardial infarction, polymyalgia rheumatica, and depression. Her medications include hydrochlorothiazide 25 mg PO qd, atenolol 25 mg PO qd, metformin 500 mg PO bid, aspirin 81 mg PO qd, a multivitamin, prednisone 15 mg PO qd, sertraline 100 mg PO qd, and simvastatin 40 mg PO qd. Physical exam is notable for orthostatic hypotension but no other abnormalities. Despite adequate volume resuscitation in the hospital, she remains orthostatic. Which of the following is the most appropriate next step in her management?

A. Increased prednisone to 40 mg PO qd
B. Tilt table testing
C. Echocardiogram
D. Discontinuation of metformin and hydrochlorothiazide
E. Discontinuation of atenolol and sertraline

**V-43.** Which of the following disorders is not associated with ventricular tachycardia as a cause of syncope?

A. Hypertrophic obstructive cardiomyopathy
B. Prior myocardial infarction
C. Atrial myxoma
D. Aortic valvular stenosis
E. Congenital long QT syndrome

**V-44.** A 48-year-old male is admitted to the hospital after an episode of syncope. The patient reports approximately

**V-44.** *(Continued)*

1 week of viral upper respiratory tract infection with nasal congestion, sore throat, and dry cough. The cough has progressed to the point where after one bout of severe tussis, he transiently lost consciousness. The pathophysiologic cause of this syncope is most likely

A. increased sympathetic tone with tachycardia and decreased left ventricular filling time
B. peripheral vasodilation from cytokines and subsequent arterial hypotension
C. increased intrathoracic pressure with subsequent decreased right ventricular venous return
D. intracranial hypertension during coughing as a result of venous congestion
E. decreased vagal tone with tachycardia and decreased left ventricular filling time

**V-45.** A patient presents with unstable angina and is admitted to the intensive care unit. A cardiac catheterization is planned with likely stent placement. The patient can be counseled to expect which of the following outcomes with this management technique compared with a more conservative plan that includes medical therapy but no catheterization during this admission?

**V-45.** *(Continued)*

A. Decreased incidence of malignant arrhythmias
B. More rapid return to work
C. Fewer readmissions
D. A and B
E. B and C

**V-46.** Which of the following patients undergoing diagnostic catheterization for chronic stable angina does not have an indication for coronary bypass graft surgery?

A. A 60-year-old male with 90% stenosis of the left anterior descending, left circumflex, and right coronary arteries.
B. A 75-year-old male with hypertension and hypercholesterolemia and 80% left main stenosis
C. A 50-year-old male with diabetes mellitus and 70% stenosis of the left anterior descending and right coronary arteries
D. A 68-year-old male with tobacco abuse and a 70% stenosis of the left circumflex artery and mild mitral regurgitation and normal left ventricular function
E. An 80-year-old female with symptomatic critical aortic stenosis and 90% left anterior descending stenosis

**V-47.** This echocardiographic image most likely was obtained from which of the following patients?

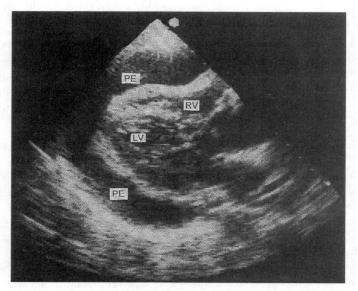

A. A 17-year-old athlete with atypical chest pain who has a midsystolic click and murmur on auscultation
B. A 22-year-old female who grew up in Central America who presents with 2 years of dyspnea and newly diagnosed atrial fibrillation
C. A 33-year-old postpartum female with hypotension, tachycardia, elevated jugular venous pressure, and diffuse lung crackles on auscultation

D. A 63-year-old male with a history of lung cancer who presents with hypotension, tachycardia, jugular venous distention, clear lungs, and an enlarged heart on chest radiography
E. A 77-year-old male with a history of a systolic heart murmur who presents with syncope

**V-48.** A 54-year-old male is brought to the emergency department with 1 hour of substernal crushing chest pain, nausea, and vomiting. He developed the pain while playing squash. The pain was improved with the administration of sublingual nitroglycerine in the field. His ECG is shown below. Emergent cardiac catheterization is most likely to show acute thrombus in which of the following vessels?

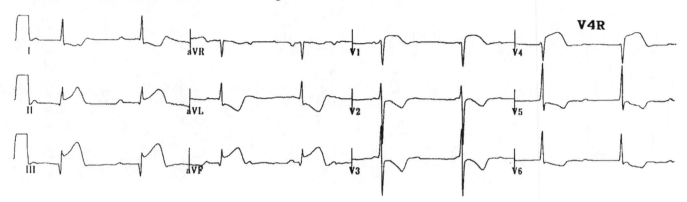

A. Left anterior descending coronary artery
B. Left circumflex coronary artery
C. Left main coronary artery

D. Obtuse marginal coronary artery
E. Right main coronary artery

---

**V-49.** The patients described below present to a rural emergency room with 2 hours of substernal chest pain, acute ST-segment elevations in leads $V_2$–$V_4$ on ECG, and elevated serum troponin. Cardiac catheterization is not available. All the following patients should receive intravenous thrombolytics *except*

A. A 44-year-old male lost consciousness in a casino. He received cardiopulmonary resuscitation (CPR) by trained personnel for 1 to 2 min and was revived with one shock from an on-site defibrillator that showed he was in ventricular fibrillation.
B. A 55-year-old female with five admissions in the last year for hypertensive urgency resulting from medical noncompliance. Her blood pressure in the emergency department is 140/90.
C. A 59-year-old female former smoker who is receiving coumadin for a deep venous thrombosis. Her international normalized ratio (INR) is 1.7.
D. A 62-year-old male who had a thrombotic cerebrovascular accident (CVA) 6 weeks ago. He did not receive thrombolytics at that time.
E. A 72-year-old female who underwent an abdominal hysterectomy 3 weeks ago.

**V-50.** A 73-year-old male with a long history of diabetes, cigarette smoking, and hypertension is admitted to the hospital with shortness of breath, near syncope, and hy-

potension. A Swan-Ganz catheter is placed and reveals a cardiac index of 1.3 L/min per m², pulmonary artery (PA) pressure of 44/22 mmHg, renal artery (RA) pressure of 18 mmHg, and pulmonary capillary wedge (PCW) pressure of 5 mmHg. The patient most likely has

A. aortic stenosis
B. cor pulmonale
C. mitral stenosis
D. occlusion of the left anterior descending coronary artery
E. pericardial tamponade

**V-51.** A 73-year-old female develops substernal chest pain, severe nausea, and vomiting while mowing the lawn. In the emergency department she has cool extremities, right arm and left arm blood pressure of 85/70 mmHg, heart rate of 65/min, clear lungs, and no murmurs. She has no urine output. A Swan-Ganz catheter is placed and reveals cardiac index of 1.1 L/min per m², PA pressure of 20/14 mmHg, PCW pressure of 6 mmHg, and RA pressure of 24 mmHg. The patient most likely has

A. gram-negative sepsis
B. occlusion of the left main coronary artery
C. occlusion of the right coronary artery
D. perforated duodenal ulcer
E. ruptured aortic aneurysm

**V-52.** The ECG shown below, most likely was obtained from which of the following patients?

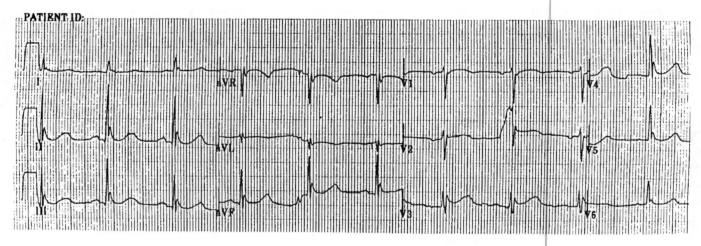

A. A 24-year-old female with fever, anterior chest pain, and a pericardial friction rub

B. A 33-year-old female 1 day after thyroid resection with a serum calcium of 6.4 mEq/dL

C. A 44-year-old alcoholic found unconscious with a core temperature of 31°C (87.8°F)

D. A 54-year-old male on diuretics with a serum potassium of 3.1 mEq/dL

E. A 63-year-old male with a history of coronary artery disease complaining of 3 h of substernal chest pain

---

**V-53.** The ECG most likely was obtained from which of the following patients?

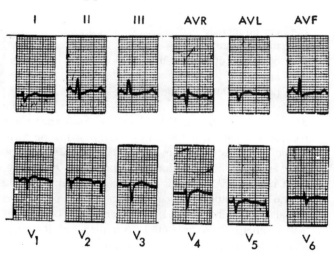

A. A 33-year-old female with acute-onset severe headache, disorientation, and intraventricular blood on head CT scan

B. A 42-year-old male with sudden-onset chest pain while playing tennis

C. A 54-year-old female with a long history of smoking and 2 days of increasing shortness of breath and wheezing

D. A 64-year-old female with end-stage renal insufficiency who missed dialysis for the last 4 days

E. A 78-year-old male with syncope, delayed carotid upstrokes, and a harsh systolic murmur in the right second intercostal space

**V-54.** All the following are complications of cardiac catheterization and stent placement *except*

A. coronary dissection
B. hematoma at the insertion site
C. in-stent restenosis
D. jugular venous thrombosis
E. pseudoaneurysm at insertion site

**V-55.** A 58-year-old female undergoes successful cardiac catheterization after a non-ST-elevation myocardial infarction. Two stents are placed in the left anterior descending and left circumflex arteries. She should be discharged on all the following medications *except*

A. aspirin
B. atenolol
C. clopidogrel
D. lisinopril
E. warfarin

**V-56.** All the following may cause elevation of serum troponin *except*

A. congestive heart failure
B. myocarditis
C. myocardial infarction
D. pneumonia
E. pulmonary embolism

**V-57.** A 55-year-old male with a past medical history of tobacco abuse, hypertension, and diabetes mellitus is ad-

**V-57.** *(Continued)*

mitted to the hospital with a 3-h history of severe retrosternal chest pain radiating to the arm and neck with associated diaphoresis. His initial serum troponin is normal, as is CK-MB. The electrocardiogram shows deep symmetric T-wave inversions in the precordial leads. The patient undergoes cardiac catheterization. Which of the following findings can be expected based on his electrocardiogram?

A.  90% stenosis in the right coronary artery
B.  90% left main stenosis
C.  80% stenosis of the right coronary artery, left circumflex artery, and left anterior descending artery after the branch for the first septal perforator
D.  90% left circumflex artery stenosis
E.  No predictions because T-wave inversions do not localize coronary lesions

**V-58.** A 49-year-old male is found to have persistently elevated total cholesterol and low-density lipoprotein (LDL) despite lifestyle modification. You prescribe an HMG-CoA reductase inhibitor to reduce the risk of coronary events. This medication will exert all the following beneficial effects *except*

A.  direct action on atheroma progression
B.  improvement in endothelial-dependent vasomotion
C.  long-term reduction of serum LDL
D.  regression of existing coronary stenosis
E.  stabilization of exisiting atherosclerotic lesions

**V-59.** A 54-year-old male with type 2 diabetes mellitus reports 3 months of exertional chest pain. His physical examination is notable for obesity with a body mass index (BMI) of 32 kg/m², blood pressure of 150/90, an $S_4$, no cardiac murmurs, and no peripheral edema. Fasting glucose is 130 mg/dL, and serum triglycerides are 200 mg/dL. Which of the following is most likely in this patient?

A.  Elevated high-density lipoprotein (HDL) cholesterol
B.  Insulin resistance
C.  Larger than normal LDL particles
D.  Reduced serum endothelin level
E.  Reduced serum homocysteine level

**V-60.** All the following interventions have demonstrated a decrease in macrovascular complications (coronary artery disease, stroke) in patients with diabetes and dyslipidemia *except*

A.  ACE inhibitors
B.  gemfibrazil therapy
C.  goal blood pressure below 130/85
D.  HMG-CoA reductase therapy
E.  tight glycemic control

**V-61.** A 51-year-old female seeks advice regarding medical therapy for menopause. Initiation of oral estrogen/progesterone replacement therapy will result in a reduction in all the following effects *except*

A.  cardiovascular events
B.  hip fractures
C.  LDL cholesterol
D.  vaginal dryness
E.  vasomotor symptoms

**V-62.** Which of the following parameters adds predictive information regarding cardiovascular risk stratification and the measurement of serum cholesterol?

A.  Anti–*Chlamydia pneumoniae* antibodies
B.  C-reactive protein
C.  Homocysteine
D.  Lipoprotein A
E.  Plasminogen activator inhibitor 1

**V-63.** A 62-year-old female with a history of chronic left bundle branch block is admitted to the coronary care unit with 4 hours of substernal chest pain and shortness of breath. She has elevation of serum troponin-T. She receives urgent catheterization with angioplasty and stent placement of a left anterior descending (LAD) artery lesion. Three days after admission she develops recurrent chest pain. Which of the following studies is most useful for detecting new myocardial damage since the initial infarction?

A.  Echocardiogram
B.  Electrocardiogram
C.  Serum myoglobin
D.  Serum troponin-I
E.  Serum troponin-T

**V-64.** A 28-year-old female has hypertension that is difficult to control. She was diagnosed at age 26. Since that time she has been on increasing amounts of medication. Her current regimen consists of labetalol 1000 mg bid, lisinopril 40 mg qd, clonidine 0.1 mg bid, and amlodipine 5 mg qd. On physical examination she appears to be without distress. Blood pressure is 168/100, and heart rate is 84 beats per minute. Cardiac examination is unremarkable, without rubs, gallops, or murmurs. She has good peripheral pulses and has no edema. Her physical appearance does not reveal any hirsutism, fat maldistribution, or abnormalities of genitalia. Laboratory studies reveal a potassium of 2.8 mEq/dL and a serum bicarbonate of 32 mEq/dL. Fasting blood glucose is 114 mg/dL. What is the likely diagnosis?

A.  Congenital adrenal hyperplasia
B.  Fibromuscular dysplasia
C.  Cushing's syndrome
D.  Conn's syndrome

**V-64.** *(Continued)*

E.    Pheochromocytoma

**V-65.** What is the best way to diagnose this disease?

A.    Renal vein renin levels
B.    24-h urine collection for metanephrines
C.    Magnetic resonance imaging of the renal arteries
D.    24-h urine collection for cortisol
E.    Plasma aldosterone/renin ratio

**V-66.** A 42-year-old female presents to your office for a routine visit. She is found to have a blood pressure of 152/94. Her past medical history is significant for gestational diabetes mellitus with the birth of her second child 8 years ago. She has a family history of hypertension. Her mother died of a myocardial infarction at age 68. Her father died from complications after a stroke at age 84. She does not smoke. Her body mass index is 27. Fasting blood glucose is 106 mg/dL, and creatinine is 0.5 mg/dL. All the following should be part of your initial recommendations to the patient *except*

A.    She should participate in regular aerobic activity for 30 min several times weekly.
B.    She should be encouraged to lose weight to decrease her body mass index to less than 25.
C.    She should limit her alcohol intake to no more than two drinks daily.
D.    She should limit her sodium intake to less than 2.4 g daily.
E.    She should return for follow-up within 3 months for repeat blood pressure measurement and consideration of drug therapy if blood pressure is not less than 140/90.

**V-67.** A 28-year-old male with type 1 diabetes mellitus is seen in the clinic for routine follow-up. The patient has hypertension. He is being maintained on an insulin pump and lisinopril 5 mg daily. He has been on this dose of antihypertensive medication for approximately 6 weeks. He has a creatinine of 1.0 mg/dL and no proteinuria. Blood pressure is 138/88. What do you recommend?

A.    Continue the current dose of lisinopril and return for follow-up in 3 months as the patient has achieved his target blood pressure of less than 140/90.
B.    Ask the patient to follow up for a return visit in 6 weeks; if his blood pressure remains at this level, increase the dose of lisinopril.
C.    Increase lisinopril to 10 mg daily to achieve a goal blood pressure of less than 130/80.
D.    Assure the patient that he is suffering from "white-coat" hypertension and plan no intervention.
E.    Switch the patient from lisinopril to losartan.

**V-68.** Which of the following antihypertensive drugs is incorrectly matched with the indication for therapy?

A.    ACE inhibitor—diabetic nephropathy
B.    Beta blocker—coronary artery disease
C.    Calcium channel blocker—angina
D.    Diuretics—heart failure
E.    Loop diuretic—gout

**V-69.** A 49-year-old female presents to you for an initial visit to establish health care. She has no past medical history and denies a family history of diabetes mellitus, early cardiovascular disease, or renal disease. Her blood pressure on presentation is 185/112. She denies headache or visual complaints. She has no chest pain, shortness of breath, or change in urine color. Her physical examination is normal with the exception of an $S_4$ gallop heard at the fourth intercostal space just to the left of the sternum. An electrocardiogram is significant for left ventricular hypertrophy and left axis deviation. There are no signs of cardiac ischemia. Urinalysis shows no red blood cells or proteinuria. What is your recommendation for therapy for this patient?

A.    Initiate therapy with hydrochlorothiazide in combination with a beta blocker.
B.    Initiate therapy with hydrochlorothiazide alone.
C.    Initiate therapy with an ACE inhibitor alone.
D.    Advise the patient to go to the nearest emergency department for further treatment for a hypertensive emergency.
E.    Advise the patient on lifestyle modifications and plan a return visit for 2 weeks.

**V-70.** A 63-year-old male with a history of diabetes, hypertension, and tobacco abuse is admitted after three episodes of anginal-type chest pain in the last 24 hours. He takes no medications besides occasional sublingual nitroglycerine. Physical exam is unremarkable. The initial electrocardiogram shows nonspecific T-wave changes, but troponin is elevated at 1.1 ng/mL. His risk of death, myocardial infarction, or urgent revascularization in the next 14 days can be estimated at

A.    4.7%
B.    8.3%
C.    13.2%
D.    19.9%
E.    26.2%

**V-71.** A 35-year-old male with no past medical history presents with severe substernal chest pain while at rest for 2 h with associated shortness of breath and vomiting. His only habit is tobacco abuse, and he takes no medications. Physical exam shows normal vital signs, and cardiac and pulmonary exams are normal. An electrocardiogram shows ST-segment elevation in leads $V_1$ through $V_4$. Car-

**V-71.** *(Continued)*

diac catheterization is performed and shows spasm in the left anterior descending artery that is relieved with intracoronary nitroglycerine. Which of the following statements is correct?

A. This patient with Prinzmetal's angina is unlikely to have any significant stenoses in the coronary arteries.

B. The left anterior descending artery is the most common site for focal spasm in patients with Prinzmetal's angina.

C. Hyperventilation can be used to provoke transient ST elevation and coronary spasm in patients with Prinzmetal's angina.

D. Medical management of this patient should include beta blockers.

E. Aspirin is indicated to decrease the severity of ischemic episodes.

**V-72.** A 59-year-old male is admitted to the hospital with 2 h of crushing substernal chest pain and ST-segment elevation in ECG leads $V_2$ to $V_4$. He undergoes cardiac catheterization with angioplasty and stent placement for a thrombotic lesion in the left anterior descending coronary artery. During the first 72 h of admission he should receive all the following medications *except*

A. abciximab
B. aspirin
C. clopidogrel
D. dexamethasone
E. enalapril

**V-73.** A 45-year-old female who immigrated to the United States 10 years ago from Peru presents with dyspnea on exertion for the last 4 months. She denies chest pain but has noted significant accumulation of fluid in her abdomen and lower extremity edema. She has a history of tuberculosis, which was treated with a four-drug regimen when she was a child. Electrocardiography shows normal sinus rhythm but no other abnormality. A CT of the chest is obtained and shows pericardial calcifications. In addition to an elevated jugular venous pressure and a third heart sound, which of the following is likely to be found on physical exam?

A. Rapid *y* descent in jugular venous pulsations
B. Double systolic apical impulse on palpation
C. Loud, fixed split $P_2$ on auscultation
D. Cannon *a* wave in jugular venous pulsations
E. An opening snap on auscultation

**V-74.** A 19-year-old male is referred for evaluation of a cardiac murmur before clearance to play collegiate sports. He has no symptoms, has never had syncope, and has no known family history of cardiac disease. A III/VI systolic

**V-74.** *(Continued)*

murmur is heard at the apex with no radiation. On squatting, the murmur decreases in intensity, and on sustained handgrip, the murmur also is decreased. The murmur probably is due to which of the following?

A. Aortic regurgitation
B. Mitral regurgitation
C. Aortic stenosis
D. Hypertrophic cardiomyopathy
E. Pulmonary stenosis

**V-75.** A 25-year-old male is seen in the clinic for a routine physical examination. He has no complaints and is asymptomatic with no episodes of syncope and has no family history of cardiac disease. A III/VI systolic murmur is heard at the apex. On Valsalva maneuver the murmur decreases in intensity, and the murmur is accentuated with sustained handgrip. His murmur probably is due to which of the following?

A. Aortic regurgitation
B. Mitral regurgitation
C. Aortic stenosis
D. Hypertrophic cardiomyopathy
E. Pulmonic stenosis

**V-76.** A 28-year-old male is seen in the clinic for a routine physical examination. He has no complaints and is asymptomatic with no episodes of syncope, and he has no family history of cardiac disease. A II/VI systolic murmur is heard best at the right lower sternal border. The murmur is accentuated with inspiration and decreases with Valsalva. The murmur most likely is due to which of the following?

A. Aortic regurgitation
B. Tricuspid regurgitation
C. Mitral regurgitation
D. Hypertrophic cardiomyopathy
E. Flow murmur

**V-77.** A 63-year-old male with end-stage ischemic cardiomyopathy is offered a heart transplant from a 20-year-old female with brain death after a skiing accident. Which of the following is not a risk that the patient should be advised about if he decides to accept the heart?

A. Increased risk of malignancy
B. Risk of rejection of transplanted organ
C. Coronary artery disease
D. Increased risk of infections
E. Increased risk of bradyarrhythmias

**V-78.** A 58-year-old female has a left ventricular assist device placed for end-stage idiopathic dilated cardiomyop-

**V-78.** *(Continued)*

athy. She does well postoperatively. Which of the following are risks associated with this device?

A.   Thromboembolism
B.   Infection
C.   Tachyarrhythmias
D.   A and B
E.   A, B, and C

**V-79.** A 55-year-old male is seen in the ophthalmology clinic to follow up on his glaucoma. Surprisingly, the following finding shown in Figure V-79 (Color Atlas) is seen in his left eye. Which of the following tests is most appropriate to evaluate this finding?

A.   CT of the chest, abdomen, and pelvis to rule out malignancy
B.   Bilateral carotid dopplers to evaluate stenosis
C.   Transesophageal echocardiogram to rule out vegetation from endocarditis
D.   Glycosylated hemoglobin to evaluate for diabetes mellitus
E.   Lipid profile to evaluate familial hyperlipidemia

**V-80.** Pulsus paradoxus can be described by which of the following statements?

A.   Pulsus paradoxus can be seen in patients with acute asthma exacerbations in which the negative intrathoracic pressure decreases afterload of the heart with a resultant increase in systolic pressure during inspiration.
B.   Pulsus paradoxus has not been described in patients with superior vena cava syndrome.
C.   Pulsus paradoxus describes the finding of diminished pulses during inspiration, when the peripheral pulse is normally augmented during inspiration.
D.   A drop in systolic pressure during inspiration of more than 5 mmHg indicates the presence of pulsus paradoxus.
E.   Pulsus paradoxus occurs during cardiac tamponade when there is an exaggeration of the normal decrease in the systolic blood pressure during inspiration.

**V-81.** A 48-year-old male presents to the emergency department with an alteration in consciousness after cocaine ingestion. On presentation, the patient's blood pressure is 254/162, with an oxygen saturation of 83% on room air. Physical examination is notable for depressed consciousness. The patient does not follow commands but purposely withdraws from pain in all extremities. His pupils are equal and reactive. The cardiovascular exam is notable for a hyperdynamic precordium with a loud $S_4$ gallop. There are no murmurs. Crackles are heard diffusely in

**V-81.** *(Continued)*

both lung fields. The chest radiograph is consistent with pulmonary edema. CT scan of the head reveals diffuse cerebral edema without hemorrhage. The electrocardiogram shows left ventricular hypertrophy with T-wave inversions in $V_3$ to $V_6$. Urinalysis shows 1+ proteinuria with 25- to 50 red blood cells per high-power field. Creatinine is 2.6 mg/dL. What is the most appropriate management for this patient?

A.   Administer a single dose of intravenous metoprolol.
B.   Initiate nitroprusside by continuous infusion.
C.   Administer a single dose of sublingual nifedipine and assess the response to therapy.
D.   Initiate enalaprilat by continuous infusion.
E.   Initiate fenoldopam by continuous infusion.

**V-82.** A 20-year-old female is seen in the emergency department with symptoms of severe periodic headaches, sweating, and nausea with vomiting. She also complains of feeling light-headed with standing. Her blood pressure on presentation is 240/136, with a heart rate of 92. On standing, the patient has a blood pressure of 204/98, with a heart rate of 136. On ophthalmologic examination the patient has mild blurring of the optic discs without hemorrhage. The examination is otherwise normal. What is the best medication for the management of this patient's hypertension?

A.   Phentolamine
B.   Fenoldopam
C.   Esmolol
D.   Nicardipine
E.   Diazoxide

**V-83.** What test would best determine the patient's diagnosis?

A.   Plasma catecholamines
B.   24-h urine collection for 5-hydroxy-indoleacetic acid
C.   Abdominal CT scan
D.   24-h urine collection for metanephrines and vanillylmandelic acid.
E.   Adrenal vein sampling for renin levels.

**V-84.** A 36-year-old male presents with the acute onset of severe chest pain that began after he lifted weights at the gym this afternoon. He describes the pain as sharp and tearing, radiating to the back. The patient has no other medical problems and takes no medications. He denies cocaine use. On physical examination the patient is in moderate distress from the pain. His blood pressure is 190/90 with a heart rate of 100. Cardiac examination reveals a normal $S_1$ and $S_2$. There is a blowing II/VI diastolic murmur heard at the right sternal border. The right radial

**V-84.** *(Continued)*

pulse is noted to be weakened. You suspect an acute aortic dissection, which is confirmed on spiral chest CT. Which of the following is the most appropriate next step in the management of this condition?

- A. Control hypertension with intravenous nitroprusside and esmolol to decrease systolic blood pressure below 120 mmHg
- B. Emergent cardiac surgery consultation
- C. Control hypertension with intravenous nitroprusside and hydralazine to decrease systolic blood pressure below 120 mmHg
- D. A and B
- E. B and C

**V-85.** Which of the following patients with aortic dissection can be managed without surgical or endovascular intervention?

- A. A 72-year-old male with a dissection of the descending aorta that begins just distal to the left subclavian artery and extends to below the left renal artery and with a baseline creatinine of 1.8 mg/dL that is not increasing
- B. A 41-year-old male with an ascending aortic dissection that extends past the left common carotid artery after an automobile accident
- C. A 42-year-old male with Marfan's syndrome with a distal aortic dissection beginning just below the left subclavian artery and an aortic root of 53 mm
- D. A 72-year-old male with a chronic type B dissection with a CT that shows advancement of the dissection at 6 months
- E. A 56-year-old male with a descending aortic dissection that encompasses the origin of the renal and iliac arteries with rest claudication

**V-86.** A 68-year-old male presents to your office for routine follow-up care. He reports that he is feeling well and has no complaints. His past medical history is significant for hypertension and hypercholesterolemia. He continues to smoke a pack of cigarettes daily. He is taking chlorthalidone 25 mg daily, atenolol 25 mg daily, and pravastatin 40 mg nightly. Blood pressure is 133/85, and heart rate is 66. Cardiac and pulmonary examinations are unremarkable. A pulsatile abdominal mass is felt just to the left of the umbilicus and measures approximately 4 cm. You confirm the diagnosis of abdominal aortic aneurysm by CT imaging. It is located infrarenally and measures 4.5 cm. All the following are true about the patient's diagnosis *except*

- A. The 5-year risk of rupture of an aneurysm of this size is 1 to 2%.
- B. Surgical or endovascular intervention is warranted because of the size of the aneurysm.

**V-86.** *(Continued)*

- C. Infrarenal endovascular stent placement is an option if the aneurysm experiences continued growth in light of the location of the aneurysm infrarenally.
- D. Surgical or endovascular intervention is warranted if the patient develops symptoms of recurrent abdominal or back pain.
- E. Surgical or endovascular intervention is warranted if the aneurysm expands beyond 5.5 cm.

**V-87.** A 32-year-old female is seen in the emergency department for acute shortness of breath. A helical CT shows no evidence of pulmonary embolus, but incidental note is made of dilatation of the ascending aorta to 4.3 cm. All the following are associated with this finding *except*

- A. syphilis
- B. Takayasu's arteritis
- C. giant cell arteritis
- D. rheumatoid arthritis
- E. systemic lupus erythematosus

**V-88.** A 50-year-old female is seen in the emergency department with complaints of shortness of breath for 2 weeks and bony pain, particularly in the hips, for several months. She has progressive dyspnea on exertion, orthopnea, and paroxysmal nocturnal dyspnea. She takes no medications and has no allergies. On physical exam she has elevated jugular venous pressure and peripheral edema as well as tachycardia without a third heart sound. Electrocardiography, besides sinus tachycardia, is normal. A chest radiograph shows mild pulmonary vascular congestion, and plain films of the hips show severe and diffuse bony changes consistent with Paget's disease. Which of the following statements could be made to counsel this patient on her disease?

- A. She has high-output heart failure as a result of Paget's disease, and with therapy for her bony disease, the heart failure symptoms will improve.
- B. She needs to undergo cardiac catheterization to evaluate for ischemic heart failure.
- C. She is at high risk for ventricular tachycardia.
- D. She should not require diuretic therapy for the heart failure symptoms.
- E. A fat pad biopsy is warranted.

**V-89.** A 60-year-old female is seen in the clinic for follow-up for ischemic dilated cardiomyopathy. She has no angina currently, and the most recent echocardiogram shows an ejection fraction of 20%. Besides mild pedal edema, the examination is normal. Which of the following agents will not confer a mortality benefit on this patient?

**V-89.** *(Continued)*
  A. Captopril
  B. Isosorbide mononitrite
  C. Metoprolol XL
  D. Aspirin
  E. An implantable defibrillator

**V-90.** A 66-year-old male presents with the chief complaint of leg pain. He reports that he has had right leg pain with ambulation for the last 5 years. Initially, the pain would occur after he walked three city blocks, but now the pain occurs upon walking only 50 ft. Occasionally at night the patient will have a similar pain while resting. He describes the pain as cramping, located in the back of the thigh, and relieved with rest. He has a past history of hypertension and continues to smoke two packs of cigarettes daily. He is taking lisinopril 30 mg daily. Blood pressure is 140/86, and heart rate is 78 beats per minute. Cardiac examination is unremarkable. The patient has no carotid bruits. A right femoral bruit is noted. The patient has strong radial and carotid pulses. His left femoral and popliteal pulses are 2+, but a diminished dorsalis pedis and posterior tibial pulse is noted on the left. On the right the femoral pulse is diminished with absent popliteal, dorsalis pedis, and posterior tibial pulses. There is delayed capillary refill in the right great toe to 5 seconds with slight cyanosis and coolness to touch. All the following may be useful in the management of this patient *except*

  A. adding clopidogrel to the regimen
  B. adding aspirin to the current regimen
  C. changing lisinopril to nifedipine sustained release to improve arterial dilation
  D. encouraging smoking cessation
  E. performing percutaneous intervention to the right femoral artery

**V-91.** The tumor that most commonly metastasizes to the heart is

  A. melanoma
  B. non-Hodgkin's lymphoma
  C. Hodgkin's lymphoma
  D. breast
  E. renal cell

**V-92.** A 48-year-old male is admitted to the coronary care unit with an acute inferior myocardial infarction. Two hours after admission blood pressure is 86/52 mmHg; heart rate is 40 beats per minute with sinus rhythm. Which of the following would be the most appropriate initial therapy?

  A. Immediate insertion of a temporary transvenous pacemaker
  B. Intravenous administration of atropine sulfate 0.6 mg

**V-92.** *(Continued)*
  C. Intravenous administration of normal saline 300 mL over 15 min
  D. Intravenous administration of dobutamine 0.35 mg/min
  E. Intravenous administration of isoproterenol 5.0 μg/min

**V-93.** A 68-year-old male with a history of hypertension, diabetes, and urinary retention awoke feeling nauseated and light-headed. He did not respond to questions from his wife. When the emergency medical technicians arrived, his blood pressure was 60 by palpation. IV fluids and oxygen were administered. Vital signs obtained in the emergency room were blood pressure 60, heart rate 120 and regular, temperature 38.9°C (102°F), and respiratory rate 30. A brief physical examination revealed coarse rales approximately halfway up the chest bilaterally and inaudible heart sounds. An indwelling urinary catheter was placed with drainage of 10 to 20 mL of dark urine. Chest x-ray revealed bilateral interstitial infiltrates; ECG was unremarkable except for sinus tachycardia. Antibiotics were administered, and the patient was transferred to the ICU, where a right heart catheterization was performed. Pulmonary capillary wedge pressure was 28 mmHg. Cardiac output was 1.9 L/min. Right atrial mean pressure was 10 mmHg. The most likely cause of this man's hypotension was

  A. left ventricular dysfunction
  B. right ventricular infarction
  C. gram-negative sepsis
  D. gastrointestinal bleeding
  E. pulmonary emboli

**V-94.** A 67-year-old male who has experienced recurrent episodes of dizziness over the last several months is admitted to the hospital because of a fainting episode. No evidence of acute myocardial infarction is documented. On the evening of admission the patient tells his nurse that approximately 10 min earlier he experienced several minutes of dizziness. The current rhythm appears to be normal sinus; however, a monitoring strip obtained at the time of this episode reveals absent QRS complexes every third beat. The PR interval, though slightly prolonged, is constant from beat to beat. P waves are present at regular intervals. Which of the following is the most appropriate therapeutic action?

  A. Insertion of a permanent cardiac pacemaker
  B. Insertion of a temporary cardiac pacemaker followed by insertion of a permanent cardiac pacemaker
  C. Administration of atropine 2 mg IV
  D. Administration of isoproterenol 2 mg/min IV
  E. No specific therapy for this benign arrhythmia

**V-95.** A 25-year-old male complains of light-headedness on exertion. Examination of the carotid pulse reveals two impulses or peaks during ventricular systole. Which of the following physical findings probably would be associated with this finding?

A.  Diastolic murmur beginning after an opening snap

**V-95.** *(Continued)*

B.  Decrease in systolic arterial pressure during inspiration
C.  Systolic murmur increasing during the Valsalva maneuver
D.  Right-sided third heart sound
E.  Left-sided third heart sound

**V-96.** The electrocardiogram is consistent with which of the following clinical situations?

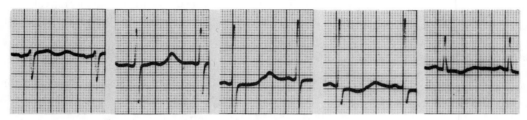

From Schlant, et al: *Hurst's The Heart*, 8/e. New York, McGraw-Hill, 1994, with permission.

A.  A 55-year-old male complaining of crushing substernal chest pain
B.  A 25-year-old female with acute renal failure resulting from lupus nephritis
C.  A 27-year-old male with prolonged neutropenia after induction therapy for acute myeloid leukemia who is receiving amphotericin B
D.  A 57-year-old female with metastatic breast cancer who is receiving etidronate
E.  A 72-year-old female receiving digitalis therapy for chronic congestive heart failure

**V-97.** A 15-year-old boy residing with his parents on a military base presents with a fever of 38.6°C (101.5°F) and complains of lower back, knee, and wrist pain. The arthritis is not localized to any single joint. He gives a history of a severe sore throat several weeks earlier. Physical examination of the skin reveals pea-sized swellings over the elbows and wrists. He also has two serpiginous, erythematous pink areas on the anterior trunk, each about 5 cm in diameter. Laboratory investigation includes negative blood cultures, negative throat culture, normal complete blood count (CBC), and an erythrocyte sedimentation rate (ESR) of 100. An antistreptolysin-O (ASO) titer is elevated. At this point appropriate therapy would consist of

A.  supportive care alone
B.  parenteral penicillin
C.  parenteral penicillin and glucocorticoids
D.  parenteral penicillin and aspirin
E.  parenteral penicillin, aspirin, and diazepam

**V-98.** Each of these patients is alert and oriented and has a blood pressure of 110/60. In which patient would adenosine constitute appropriate initial therapy?

A.  A 65-year-old male with no ischemic heart disease and wide complex tachycardia
B.  A 65-year-old female with known ischemic disease and narrow complex tachycardia
C.  A 25-year-old female with known preexcitation syndrome and narrow complex tachycardia

D.  A 28-year-old male with known preexcitation syndrome and wide complex tachycardia
E.  A 44-year-old male with atrial fibrillation without a prior history of heart disease

**V-99.** A 68-year-old male who had a recent syncopal episode is hospitalized with congestive heart failure. Blood pressure is 160/80 mmHg, pulse is 80 beats per minute, and there is a grade III/VI harsh systolic murmur. An echocardiogram shows a disproportionately thickened ventricular septum and systolic anterior motion of the mitral valve. Which of the following findings most likely would be present in this patient?

A.  Radiation of the murmur to the carotid arteries
B.  Decrease of the murmur with handgrip
C.  Delayed carotid upstroke
D.  Reduced left ventricular ejection fraction
E.  Signs of mitral stenosis

**V-100.** Which of the following congenital cardiac disorders will lead to a left-to-right shunt, generally with cyanosis?

A.  Anomalous origin of the left coronary artery from the pulmonary trunk
B.  Patent ductus arteriosus without pulmonary hypertension
C.  Total anomalous pulmonary venous connection
D.  Ventricular septal defect
E.  Sinus venosus atrial septal defect

**V-101.** A 22-year-old Michigan female presents to the local emergency room complaining of dizziness over the last several days, including two syncope episodes followed in each case by unresponsiveness for several minutes. She has always been in excellent health, having played varsity soccer in college. Her last illness occurred 4 months ago, when she developed fever, chills, and generalized weakness; those symptoms cut short a 2-week camping trip to the Cape Cod National Seashore. She uses oral contraceptives but no other prescription medications. She admits to inhaling cocaine over the last 4 months. Physical examination reveals blood pressure of 100/62 and pulse of 30 but is otherwise unremarkable. Chest x-ray and serum chemistries are unremarkable. ECG demonstrates complete heart block with nonspecific ST- and T-wave changes. There is no evidence of prior myocardial infarction. The most likely cause of her complete heart block is

A. Myocardial infarction from cocaine use
B. Myocardial infarction caused by a coronary artery embolus
C. Infection resulting from *Ixodes dammini*
D. Infection caused by *Borrelia burgdorferi*
E. Infection caused by HIV

**V-102.** A 70-year-old male is admitted to the hospital with chest pain for 8 h. Serum studies demonstrate elevation of troponin and CK-MB. ECG demonstrates anterior ST elevation, for which he is given tissue plasminogen activator, heparin, and intravenous nitroglycerin. His symptoms resolve after treatment. He is started on oral medications and transferred out of the cardiac intensive care unit on day 3. The subsequent hospital course is uneventful until day 4, when he develops severe shortness of breath. Blood pressure is 110/70, and pulse is 120. Examination reveals a new systolic murmur. The most appropriate therapeutic intervention would be

A. Emergent cardiac surgery consultation and transfer to the operating room
B. IV heparin
C. IV heparin and streptokinase
D. IV heparin and furosemide
E. IV sodium nitroprusside

**V-103.** A 68-year-old male with known aortic sclerosis was admitted with chest pain and ruled out for myocardial infarction but had recurrent symptoms during weaning from IV heparin and nitroglycerin over the ensuing 5 days. Cardiac catheterization revealed three-vessel disease with a normal ejection fraction, and he underwent coronary bypass grafting. On postoperative day 3 he complained of pain in the right arm and was found to have an absent right brachial pulse and a cold distal right arm. Laboratory work revealed a hematocrit of 38%, platelets 32,000, prothrombin time 15, INR 1.4, and partial throm-

**V-103.** *(Continued)*
boplastin time 65. What is the most likely explanation for this patient's absent brachial pulse?

A. Left ventricular thrombus caused by a myocardial infarction with a subsequent brachial artery embolus
B. Embolization from aortic sclerosis
C. Embolization from paradoxical emboli through a patent foramen ovale from a deep venous thrombosis (DVT) arising postoperatively
D. Thrombosis in situ caused by postoperative hypercoagulability
E. Heparin-induced thrombocytopenia

**V-104.** Cystic medial necrosis is prevalent in which of the following disorders?

A. Takayasu's arteritis
B. Ehlers-Danlos syndrome type IV
C. Congenital aortic aneurysms
D. Syphilitic aortitis
E. Giant cell arteritis

**V-105.** A 30-year-old male is transported to the emergency room after a motor vehicle accident. He is complaining of moderate chest pain. He becomes hypotensive, and his blood pressure pattern reveals a pulsus paradoxus. The heart sounds appear distant. An examination of the neck veins fails to reveal a Kussmaul's sign. An electrocardiogram is unremarkable, and a chest x-ray reveals an enlarged cardiac silhouette. A right heart catheter is placed. Which of the following values is consistent with this patient's diagnosis?

|   | Pressure, RA mmHg | Pressure, PA mmHg | Pressure, PCW mmHg |
|---|---|---|---|
| A | 16 | 75/30 | 11 |
| B | 16 | 34/16 | 16 |
| C | 16 | 100/30 | 28 |
| D | 16 | 45/22 | 20 |
| E | 16 | 22/12 | 10 |
| Normal values | 0–5 | 12–28/3–13 | 3–11 |

*Note*: RA, atrial pressure; PA, pulmonary arterial; PCW, pulmonary capillary wedge

**V-106.** You are asked to give medical clearance for a 75-year-old male before an elective carotid endarterectomy. His past medical history is significant for hypercholesteremia and hypertension. He also has diet-control diabetes mellitus. Current medications include simvastatin and hydrochlorothiazide. He denies any current or prior cardiac symptoms and has never had a myocardial infarction. Physical examination is unrevealing with the exception of a right carotid bruit. An electrocardiogram is unremarkable with the exception of premature ventricular contrac-

**V-106.**  *(Continued)*
tions (PVCs) at a rate of two to three per minute. Laboratory analysis is unremarkable, including normal renal
function and liver function tests. Oxygen saturations are
also normal. What would be the expected serious complication rate (perioperative MI, pulmonary edema, or
ventricular tachycardia) in this patient?

A.  <0.1%
B.  0.1–1.0%
C.  1.0–3.0%
D.  3.0–10%

**V-106.**  *(Continued)*
E.  10%

**V-107.**  Which of the following has been demonstrated to
reduce perioperative mortality in patients undergoing noncardiac surgery?

A.  Nitrates
B.  Beta blocker
C.  Calcium channel blocker
D.  $\alpha_2$ Agonist
E.  Diuretic therapy

**V-108.**  A 62-year-old male loses consciousness in the street, and resuscitative efforts are
undertaken. In the emergency room an electrocardiogram is obtained, part of which is
shown below. Which of the following disorders could account for this man's presentation?

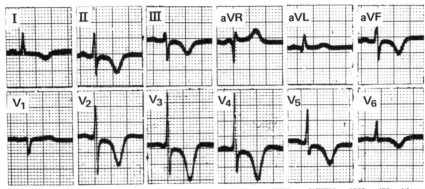

From Marriott HJL: *Practical Electrocardiography*, 7th ed. Baltimore, Williams & Wilkins, 1983, p 400, with permission.

A.  Hypokalemia
B.  Hyperkalemia
C.  Intracerebral hemorrhage
D.  Digitalis toxicity
E.  Hypocalcemic tetany

**V-109.**  Acute hyperkalemia is associated with which of the
following electrocardiographic changes?

A.  QRS widening
B.  Prolongation of the ST segment
C.  A decrease in the PR interval
D.  Prominent U waves
E.  T-wave flattening

**V-110.**  A 37-year-old male with Wolff-Parkinson-White
syndrome develops a broad-complex irregular tachycardia
at a rate of 200 beats per minute. He appears comfortable
and has little hemodynamic impairment. Useful treatment
at this point might include

A.  Digoxin
B.  Amiodarone
C.  Propranolol
D.  Verapamil
E.  Direct-current cardioversion

**V-111.**  In which of the following patients would you recommend a preoperative noninvasive functional assessment?

A.  An emergent repair of a ruptured appendix
B.  A 65-year-old male before undergoing a carotid
    endarterectomy who underwent a coronary artery
    bypass graft (CABG) 2 years earlier and has had
    no prior symptoms
C.  A 62-year-old male with hypertension, hypercho-
    lesterolemia, and diabetes mellitus who is having
    recurrent chest pain with only minimal exertion
    before a radical prostatectomy
D.  A 65-year-old male with a prior history of angina
    but no history of myocardial infarction who is
    planning to undergo an elective hip replacement
E.  A 52-year-old female with no cardiac symptoms
    and a normal physical exam before a breast biopsy
    for a newly identified mass

# V. DISORDERS OF THE CARDIOVASCULAR SYSTEM

## ANSWERS

**V-1. The answer is B.** *(Chap. 7)* The Revised Cardiac Risk Index was developed to assess perioperative cardiovascular risk in patients undergoing noncardiac surgery. It consists of six components derived from a multivariate analysis of patients undergoing elective noncardiac surgery. All six of the risk factors were associated with a similar odds ratio of complications. Risk increases with each point and substantially increases when more than two factors are present. Several traditional risk factors that are known to increase the risk of coronary artery disease *do not* increase the risk of postoperative cardiac complications. They include hypertension with a diastolic blood pressure less than 110, obesity, hypercholesterolemia, cigarette smoking, and bundle branch block.

The Revised Cardiac Risk Index

| Factor | Adjusted Odds Ratio (OR) for Cardiac Complications in Derivation Cohort |
|---|---|
| 1. High-risk surgery | 2.8 |
| 2. Ischemic heart disease | 2.4 |
| 3. History of congestive heart failure | 1.9 |
| 4. History of cerebrovascular disease | 3.2 |
| 5. Insulin therapy for diabetes mellitus | 3.0 |
| 6. Preoperative serum creatinine > 2.0 mg/dL | 3.0 |

| Class | Number of Factors | Cardiac Complication Rates, % | |
|---|---|---|---|
| | | Derivation Cohort | Validation Cohort |
| I | 0 | 0.5 | 0.4 |
| II | 1 | 1.3 | 0.9 |
| III | 2 | 3.6 | 6.6 |
| IV | 3–6 | 9.1 | 11.0 |

*Source*: Adapted from TH Lee et al. Circulation 100:1043, 1999; with permission.

**V-2. The answer is C.** *(Chap. 7)* Cardiac complications are the most important cause of perioperative morbidity and mortality, and primary care physicians are frequently asked to assess a patient's perioperative risk for cardiac events before cardiac procedures. Multiple clinical risk scores have been developed by various professional organizations, such as the American College of Physicians and the American Heart Association. Patients deemed to be at low risk may proceed to surgery without further intervention. The patient described above has only one major risk—intraperitoneal surgery—on the six-point revised cardiac risk index (see Table V-1). This puts the patient into an intermediate-risk classification by this scale; however, further testing is indicated only if the patient is undergoing vascular surgery. In addition, the patient has excellent functional status and can achieve greater than four metabolic equivalents with ease. Examples of activities that consume four metabolic equivalents are climbing one flight of stairs and walking two blocks on level ground. The risk of postoperative cardiovascular complications does not appear to be influenced by stable hypertension, elevated cholesterol, obesity, cigarette smoking, or bundle branch block. Perioperative beta blockade has been shown to decrease rates of postoperative myocardial infarction and cardiac death by at least 50% and is recommended for any patient who has cardiac risk factors or is at intermediate risk of cardiovascular complications after surgery. The patient's prior adverse reaction to beta blockade should not preclude its use in the perioperative period, as it consisted of only mild fatigue and decreased sexual functioning. Finally, the patient's pulmonary risk is likely to be low as he quit smoking more than 8 weeks before surgery and has good functional status without dyspnea.

**V-3.  The answer is A.**  *(Chap. 218)*   This patient is presenting with Eisenmenger's syndrome. This designation is applied to patients with communications between the right and left circulations, pulmonary hypertension, and a predominantly right-to-left shunt. Eisenmenger's syndrome can develop in patients with communication at the atrial, ventricular, or aortopulmonary level. These shunts are initially left to right and therefore do not present with cyanosis. Pulmonary hypertension develops over years as a result of increased pulmonary flow, increased vascular tone, and erythrocytosis. Cyanosis develops when the pulmonary hypertension becomes so severe that it reverses the shunt. Atrial septal defects are most common in adults presenting with Eisenmenger's syndrome. This patient had no evidence of pulmonary hypertension or cyanosis 10 years ago. Ebstein's anamoly, tetralogy of Fallot, and truncus arteriosis all cause cyanosis.

**V-4 and V-5.  The answers are C and A.**  *(Chap. 218)*   This patient has a coarctation of the aorta presenting with marked hypertension proximal to the lesion. The narrowing most commonly occurs distal to the origin of the left subclavian artery, explaining the equal pressure in the arms and reduced pressure in the legs. Coarctations account for approximately 7% of congenital cardiac abnormalities, occur more frequently (2×) in men than in women, and are associated with gonadal dysgenesis and bicuspid aortic valves. Adults will present with hypertension, manifestations of hypertension in the upper body (headache, epistaxis), or leg claudication. Physical examination reveals diminished and/or delayed lower extremity pulses, enlarged collateral vessels in the upper body, or reduced development of the lower extremities. Cardiac examination may reveal findings consistent with left ventricular (LV) hypertrophy. There may be no murmur, a midsytolic murmur over the anterior chest and back, or an aortic murmur with a bicuspid valve. Transthoracic (suprasternal/parasternal) or transesophageal echocardiography, contrast CT or MRI of the thorax, or cardiac catheterization can be diagnostic. MRI of the head would not be useful diagnostically. The clinical picture is not consistent with renal artery stenosis, pheochromocytoma, carcinoid, or Cushing's syndrome.

**V-6 and V-7.  The answers are D and A.**  *(Chaps. 109 and 229)*   This patient presented with a syndrome consistent with bacterial endocarditis with fever and a predisposing condition and no other localizing findings on examination. He probably has third-degree heart block caused by valve ring abscess. Appropriate initial management would include blood cultures, intensive care admission, and empirical intravenous antibiotics to cover gram-positive organisms in light of his poor clinical condition; serial cardiac markers may be helpful to ensure that ischemia is not the source of bradycardia. A temporary pacemaker is indicated with symptomatic heart block, but a permanent pacemaker is contraindicated with active infection. Furthermore, appropriate antibiotic therapy may improve conduction abnormalities and obviate the need for permanent pacemaker placement.

Blood cultures persistently positive for *S. aureus* strongly suggest bacterial endocarditis in a predisposed individual but do not meet sufficient Duke criteria to determine definitively that the patient has endocarditis. A transthoracic echocardiogram may be negative in up to 35% of patients with bacterial endocarditis, and the more sensitive test, the transesophageal echocardiogram, is indicated. Additionally, the transesophageal echocardiogram is the test of choice for the diagnosis of valve ring abscess as it allows better visualization of perivalvular structures. Ischemia is unlikely to be the source of bradycardia in this case without ST-segment abnormalities; therefore, dobutamine stress echocardi-ogram and cardiac catheterization are not indicated at this point. Although cardiac surgery may be indicated with valve ring abscess, cardiac surgical consultation is less urgent than the diagnostic study.

**V-8 and V-9.   The answers are B and C.**   *(Chaps. 109 and 219)*   The patient probably has endocarditis with persistent fevers, and no other clear etiology or predisposing condition of prosthetic cardiac valve has been identified. In prosthetic valve endocarditis the caus-ative organisms are linked to the temporal distance from the surgery. In patients who are less than 2 months postoperative, infection is acquired as a result of perioperative bacte-remia with nosocomial organisms, typically coagulase-negative *Staphylococcus* species, *S. aureus,* facultative gram-negative rods, diphtheroids, and fungi. Although coagulase-negative staphylococcal endocarditis has been observed up to 12 months postoperatively, the organisms associated with endocarditis beyond 2 months after the procedure are typ-ically those seen in community-acquired bacterial endocarditis. This patient could have either *S. epidermis* or *Pseudomonas aeruginosa* postoperatively, but given the benign clinical presentation, *S. epidermis* is more likely. At lease 85% of postoperative coagulase-negative staphylococcal infections are methicillin-resistant, and so the most appropriate initial therapy would be vancomycin.

**V-10.   The answer is A.**   *(Chaps. 109 and 219)*   Indications for endocarditis prophylaxis with procedures are assessed by taking into account the nature of the cardiac lesion and the risk posed by the procedure. High-risk cardiac lesions include prosthetic heart valves, a history of bacterial endocarditis, complex cyanotic congenital heart disease, patent ductus arteri-osus, coarctation of the aorta, and surgically constructed systemic portal shunts. Moderate-risk patients include those with congenital cardiac malformations other than high-risk or low-risk lesions, acquired aortic or mitral valve dysfunction, hypertrophic cardiomyopathy with asymmetric septal hypertrophy, and mitral valve prolapse with valve thickening or regurgitation. Low-risk lesions include isolated secundum atrial septal defect (ASD), a surgically repaired ASD, ventricular septal defect (VSD), patent ductus arteriosis (PDA), prior coronary bypass graft, mitral valve prolapse without regurgitation or thickened valves, a history of rheumatic fever without valvular dysfunction, and cardiac pacemakers or implantable defibrillators. This patient falls into the moderate-risk category. Her pro-cedure is an esophageal dilation, which, like dental procedures, calls for prophylaxis in the moderate- to high-risk groups. Amoxicillin 2 g PO 1 h before the procedure is the standard recommendation, but this patient may be penicillin-allergic. Acceptable alterna-tives include clarithromycin 500 mg PO 1 h before the procedure, clindamycin 600 mg PO 1 h before, or cephalexin 2 g PO 1 h before if the patient is able to tolerate cephalo-sporins.

**V-11.   The answer is A.**   *(Chaps. 214 and 256)*   The patient has a torsade de pointes arrhythmia probably induced by underlying hypokalemia and hypomagnesemia from diarrhea. Ad-ministration of intravenous magnesium may restore the patient to a normal sinus rhythm. However, in any case of unstable or pulseless rhythm, initiation of the advanced cardiac life support protocol should be done as well.

**V-12 and V-13.   The answers are A and B.**   *(Chaps. 219 and 228)*   The patient has developed acute mitral regurgitation as evidenced by the development of a new holosystolic murmur and the presence of large *v* waves noted on the pulmonary capillary wedge tracing. A similar murmur and tracing may be seen in patients with acute ventricular septal rupture, but the lack of increase in oxygen saturation between the right atrium and the pulmonary artery has ruled out this complication. Acute mitral regurgitation is associated with ische-mia of the posteromedial papillary muscle in 80% of cases. The posterior descending artery that was part of the territory at risk during the patient's acute inferior myocardial infarction supplies this papillary muscle. Ventricular septal rupture and left ventricular rupture occur more commonly after acute anterior myocardial infarction. Prolonged ischemic time and recurrent angina are predictors of patients more likely to develop these complications. Acute mitral regurgitation is rapidly fatal without surgical intervention. Placement of an intra-aortic balloon pump or the initiation of therapy with nitroprusside may be used as a temporizing measure before surgical intervention. Dobutamine often causes worsening of symptoms and clinical deterioration.

**V-14.** **The answer is E.** *(Chap. 210)* The limb lead aVR generally has a negative deflection as the primary vector for ventricular depolarization is directed down and away from this lead. Therefore, in the case of left ventricular hypertrophy the negative deflection, or S wave, would be expected to be larger without an effect on the R wave. There are multiple criteria for diagnosing left ventricular hypertrophy on ECG.

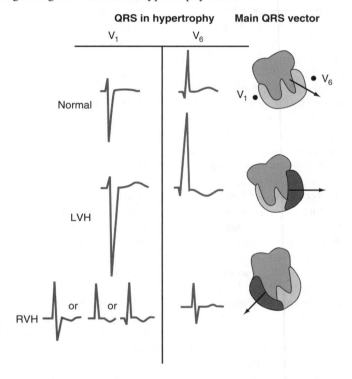

**V-15.** **The answer is C.** *(Chap. 219)* Over two-thirds of patients with mitral stenosis (MS) are female. Rheumatic heart disease is the cause in almost all cases. The choice among various management strategies for mitral stenosis is dependent on the symptoms of the patient and the characteristics of the mitral valve lesion. Penicillin prophylaxis and control of volume status are critical in the management of all patients with MS. However, in light of the degree of symptoms in this patient (hemoptysis and pulmonary edema), routine follow-up without more definitive therapy is inappropriate. Coronary angiography is useful when there is a discrepancy between the clinical and echocardiographic finings. It is also useful in patients with extensive risk factors for coronary artery disease. In this young female with no prior history of coronary artery disease an angiogram is unnecessary. Mitral valve replacement is indicated in patients with significant mitral regurgitation (MR), in those in whom the valve is not amenable to valvotomy, and in those whose valves have been damaged by prior procedures. The lack of significant MR, calcification, or leaflet thickening makes valvotomy the initial procedure of choice. In addition to the patient not requiring cardiopulmonary bypass, a percutaneous balloon approach has a lower morbidity and mortality rate than does the open procedure and would therefore be the most appropriate form of management.

**V-16.** **The answer is A.** *(Chap. 219)* Age-related degenerative calcific AS is now the most common cause of AS in adults in the Western world. Rheumatic heart disease remains an important entity in the developing world, but its significance has diminished with the advent of widespread antibiotic use. Up to 80% of adults with symptomatic AS are male. Increasing obstruction of the aortic valve may take place over years, with a gradual onset of symptoms. Reductions in cardiac output and left ventricular dilatation occur later in the natural history. Predominant symptoms include dyspnea, angina pectoris, exertional syncope, and congestive heart failure. Classic studies from Boston showed that the average time to death ranged from 3 years for angina or syncope to under 2 years with symptoms of congestive heart failure.

**V-17.   The answer is D.**   *(Chap. 219)*   The single most important decision in the management of AS is the advisability and timing of surgical therapy. In asymptomatic patients with normal left ventricular (LV) function it is advisable to hold off on surgical therapy as these patients may do well for many years. Close follow-up is recommended. In patients with symptoms or evidence of LV dysfunction, prompt surgical valve replacement is recommended. Operative risk is high in patients with late-stage LV failure. Therefore, in this patient with symptoms and an impaired ejection fraction, aortic valve replacment is recommended. Diuretics and nitrates have a role in the treatment of congestive heart failure but are not definitive therapies. Likewise, HMG-CoA reductase inhibitors may slow the progression of leaflet calcification, but this patient is already advanced enough that a surgical intervention is necessary. Balloon angioplasty has a high restenosis rate and is not as successful as it is in the case of mitral stenosis and should be reserved only as a "bridge" to operation or an option for patients too ill to tolerate surgery.

**V-18.   The answer is A.**   *(Chap. 219)*   Although nonsurgical management of patients with mitral regurgitation (MR) can improve symptoms significantly, consideration of the advisability and timing of surgical treatment is critical. MR may progress at a very slow rate, with minimal symptoms and preserved LV function. However, various observational studies demonstrate that patients with mild symptoms have better outcomes with mitral valve replacement (MVR) than do patients with severe symptoms and severe LV dysfunction. Indeed, patients with an LV ejection fraction below 30% do poorly with MVR, especially if chordal continuity cannot be preserved. Operation is contraindicated in these patients. Therefore, surgical repair or replacement of the mitral valve is considered in symptomatic patients and in asymptomatic patients with impairment in LV function demonstrated by either a declining ejection fraction below 60% and/or an end-systolic cavity dimension greater than 45 mm. The optimal treatment of choice for patients with symptomatic mitral stenosis includes balloon valvuloplasty, open valvotomy, and mitral valve replacement. However, in patients with mitral stenosis and concomitant mitral regurgitation, replacement is indicated.

**V-19.   The answer is E.**   *(Chaps. 219 and 231)*   Aortic aneurysm results from numerous mechanisms. The vast majority are associated with atherosclerosis. The risk factors for atherosclerosis (hypertension, hypercholesterolemia, etc.) are also risk factors for aneurysm formation. It is unclear if atherosclerosis is the primary cause or a result of the same pathophysiologic mechanisms that lead to dilatation. Other etiologies include congenital causes. Marfan's syndrome and Ehlers-Danlos syndrome are the most frequently noted. However, there is also an association with osteogenesis imperfecta. Turner's syndrome is associated with coarctation of the aorta. Repair of coarctation may predispose to later dilation and aneurysm formation. Klinefelter's syndrome, however, is not associated with aneurysm formation. Chronic infectious causes include syphilis and mycotic aneurysm from bacterial endocarditis. Chronic inflammatory states such as Takayasu's arteritis, giant cell arteritis, and seronegative spondyloarthropathies such as Reiter's syndrome and ankylosing spondylitis are also associated with aneurysms.

**V-20.   The answer is A.**   *(Chap. 219)*   Bioprosthetic valves are made from human, porcine, or bovine tissue. The major advantage of a bioprosthetic valve is the low incidence of thromboembolic phenomena, particularly 3 months after implantation. Although in the immediate postoperative period some anticoagulation may occur, after 3 months there is no further need for anticoagulation or monitoring. The downside is the natural history and longevity of the bioprosthetic valve. Bioprosthetic valves tend to degenerate mechanically. Approximately 50% will need replacement at 15 years. Therefore, these valves are useful in patients with contraindications to anticoagulation, such as elderly patients with co-morbidities and younger patients who desire to become pregnant. Elderly people may also be spared the need for repeat surgery as their life span may be shorter than the natural history of the bioprosthesis. Mechanical valves offer superior durability. Hemodynamic parameters are improved with double-disk valves compared with single-disk or ball-and-chain valves. However, thrombogenicity is high and chronic anticoagulation is mandatory. Younger patients with no contraindications to anticoagulation may be better served by mechanical valve replacement.

**V-21. The answer is E.** *(Chap. 256; N Engl J Med 346:877–883; 2002.)* Sudden cardiac death caused by arrhythmia is a major cause of morbidity and mortality in patients with a history of myocardial infarction (MI). Several trials have shown a benefit to placement of an ICD in patients with depressed left ventricular function. A recent study looked at patients with a history of MI and an ejection fraction of 30% or less who were randomized to either ICD placement or optimal medical management. The patients were not required to have an electrophysiologic study beforehand. There was a significant survival benefit for the individuals who had an ICD placed. ICD placement should be considered the standard of care for all individuals with a history of MI and an ejection fraction of 30% or less. Digoxin has not been shown to have a survival benefit in patients after an MI. It does reduce rehospitalization in patients with chronic heart failure, but since this patient is not having significant symptoms, digoxin is unnecessary. Amiodarone is a potent anti-arrhythmic, but the patient's depressed ejection fraction makes ICD placement the more important therapy. Repeat cardiac catheterization is unnecessary in the absence of new symptoms. CABG is not indicated in this individual with a history of single-vessel disease and no evidence of recurrent or more advanced disease.

**V-22. The answer is B.** *(Chap. 256)* Resuscitation of a patient with cardiac arrest is dependent on the rapidity of the initiation of resuscitative efforts, the clinical status of the patient before the arrest, and the mechanism of the event. The most appropriate management of an individual with pulseless ventricular tachycardia consists of an initial 200-J defibrillation. Follow-up shocks at 300 J and 360 J should be attempted if a normal rhythm is not reestablished. The current Advanced Cardiovascular Life Support (ACLS) guidelines call for the administration of either epinephrine or vasopressin, continued CPR, and repeat attempts at defibrillation. Furthermore, in patients with VT intravenous amiodarone has emerged as the optimal antiarrhythmic. Sodium bicarbonate may be given to an individual with a persistent acidosis, but there is no evidence to support this. Lidocaine is a second-line agent and may be given to patients in whom amiodarone has not been successful. Bretylium and procainamide have little or no role in modern ACLS guidelines.

**V-23. The answer is A.** *(Chaps. 208 and 230)* Essential hypertension causes 92 to 94% of cases of hypertension in the general population, and screening for secondary causes of hypertension is not cost-effective in most instances. The abrupt onset of severe hypertension or the onset of any hypertension before the age of 35 or after age 55 should prompt evaluation for renovascular hypertension. In addition, patients should be evaluated for secondary causes if previously well-controlled blood pressure suddenly becomes increasingly difficult to control as this may indicate the development of renovascular disease. Any symptoms or physical findings of concern should be investigated further as well. In the scenarios presented in Question 23, (B) should signal concern for adult-onset polycystic kidney disease and (E) describes a woman with possible Cushing's disease. Other causes of secondary hypertension include pheochromocytoma, primary hyperaldosteronism, medication-induced , and vasculitis.

**V-24. The answer is C.** *(Chap. 230)* Several factors have been shown to confer an increased risk of complications from hypertension. In the patient described here there is only one:

ongoing tobacco use. Epidemiologic factors that have poorer prognosis include African-American race, male sex, and onset of hypertension in youth. In addition, comorbid factors that independently increase the risk of atherosclerosis worsen the prognosis in patients with hypertension. These factors include hypercholesterolemia, obesity, diabetes mellitus, and tobacco use. Physical and laboratory examination showing evidence of end organ damage also may portend a poorer prognosis. This includes evidence of retinal damage or hypertensive heart disease with cardiac enlargement or congestive heart failure. Furthermore, electrocardiographic evidence of ischemia or left ventricular strain but not left ventricular hypertrophy alone may predict worse outcomes. A family history of hypertensive complications does not worsen the prognosis if diastolic blood pressure is maintained at less than 110 mmHg.

**V-25. The answer is B.** *(Chap. 213)* Although sinoatrial node dysfunction is seen most commonly in the elderly with no specific etiology identified, certain disease states are associated with sinoatrial dysfunction, including infiltrative diseases such as amyloid and sarcoidosis. Additionally, multiple systemic disorders are associated with sinus bradycardia, for instance, hypothyroidism, advanced liver disease, hypoxemia, hypercapnia, acidemia, and acute hypertension. Finally, several infectious diseases are classically associated with sinus bradycardia, notably typhoid fever and brucellosis. Leptospirosis is not associated with sinus bradycardia.

**V-26. The answer is C.** *(Chap. 213)* The atrioventricular node is supplied by the posterior descending coronary artery in 90% of the population. Furthermore, this artery in the majority of the population arises from the right coronary artery. Thus, a patient who presents as this one does with symptoms consistent with an acute coronary syndrome and who has a Mobitz type II second-degree block probably has significant ischemia in the right coronary artery. Right coronary artery transmural infarct is manifest most commonly by ST elevation in II, III, and aVF. Wellen's T waves are deep symmetric T-wave inversions that are seen in either significant left main coronary artery stenosis or proximal left anterior descending artery stenosis.

**V-27. The answer is A.** *(Chap. 213; Gregoratas G, Circulation 106:2145, 2002.)* In this case, it is of note that patients with supranodal third-degree heart block that resolves do not require permanent placement. Further, asymptomatic atrioventricular block with associated fasicular block does not warrant pacemaker placement. Additionally, asymptomatic intermittent third-degree atrioventricular block is a class III indication for a pacemaker. Patients with Lyme disease–associated third-degree block generally are reversible with antibiotic therapy, in which case a permanent pacemaker is not indicated. Carotid sinus hypersensitivity syndrome is defined as a greater than 3-s ventricular asystole after carotid sinus massage. Patients with this syndrome who have recurrent syncope warrant permanent pacemaker placement. Of note, many elderly patients also have ventricular asystole greater than 3 seconds without symptoms. In these patients pacemakers are not always indicated.

**V-28. The answer is D.** *(Chap. 214)* The patient is a young woman with no cardiac disease. In this population asymptomatic premature ventricular contractions (PVCs) require no specific therapy as they are not associated with increased mortality. In patients with symptoms such as palpitations, the primary therapy should be patient reassurance. If this is unsuccessful, beta blockers can be helpful, especially in patients whose symptoms are more prominent during stressful situations and patients with hyperthyroidism. Even in patients with myocardial infarction and PVCs there is no benefit to administering antiarrhythmic therapy with the goal of decreasing the PVC rate. Trials such as CAST comparing ectopy suppression by encainide, flecainide, moricizine, or placebo showed that mortality was increased in all the drug groups compared with placebo at 2 years. Thus, it has become clear that PVC reduction cannot be used as a surrogate endpoint for reduction of risk from sudden cardiac death.

**V-29.  The answer is B.**  *(Chap. 214)*   Atrial fibrillation is characterized by disorganized atrial activity with an irregular ventricular response to atrial activity. This lack of organization results in stasis of blood in the atria and puts the patient at risk for cardioembolic stroke. Several factors associated with increased stroke risk have been identified, including diabetes mellitus, hypertension, age over 65, rheumatic heart disease, a prior stroke or transient ischemic attack, congestive heart failure, and a transesophageal echocardiogram showing spontaneous echo contrast in the left atrium, left atrial atheroma, or left atrial appendage velocity <20 cm/s. Hypercholesterolemia is not associated with an increased risk of stroke in patients with atrial fibrillation.

**V-30 and V-31.  The answers are D and D.**  *(Chap. 214)*   The patient's preoperative electrocardiogram is notable for the shortened PR interval, a delta wave, and a widened QRS. These findings suggest that there is ventricular preexcitation via a bypass tract. Patients with Wolff-Parkinson-White (WPW) syndrome have both preexcitation on the electrocardiogram and paroxysmal tachycardias, as this patient has. Atrial fibrillation is common in these patients, and as the atrial impulse can be conducted along the bypass tract that has no decremental conducting properties like the AV node, the rate can be unusually rapid and can result in ventricular fibrillation. Patients with bypass tracts and atrial fibrillation require special caution in their care. Patients who are unstable should have direct-current cardioversion performed immediately. As this patient was mentating and had a normal blood pressure, pharmacologic therapy should be attempted first. Digoxin and calcium channel blockers should be avoided in these patients as they occasionally can shorten the refractory period of the bypass tract and precipitate ventricular fibrillation. Beta blockers are similarly unhelpful in decreasing the conduction rate. Lidocaine and procainamide are the most commonly applied pharmacotherapy, and there is recent evidence that ibutilide may be helpful. Chronic management of patients with WPW syndrome should include referral to an electrophysiologist for ablation of the bypass tract. This procedure is in most cases curative. Anticoagulation can be considered if the patient was in atrial fibrillation for more than 48 hours. Pacemakers occasionally induce atrial fibrillation and consequently are not recommended for patients with WPW.

**V-32.  The answer is B.**  *(Chap. 214)*   The differentiation of ventricular tachycardia from supraventricular tachycardia with an aberration of intraventricuar conduction can be challenging and has important implications for management. By definition, however, ventricular tachycardia is associated with atrioventricular (AV) dissociation. Cannon *a* waves are found in the jugular venous pulsations when the atria are contracting against a closed tricuspid valve. This can occur only with AV dissociation, thus proving ventricular tachycardia. Hypotension, irregular rhythm, and syncope can all be seen in both ventricular tachycardia and supraventricuar tachycardia with aberrancy.

**V-33 and V-34.  The answers are C and C.**  *(Chap. 214)*   The patient's rhythm is torsade de pointes, with polymorphic ventricular tachycardia and QRS complexes with variations in amplitude and cycle length giving the appearance of oscillation about an axis. Torsades de pointes is associated with a prolonged QT interval; thus, anything that is associated with a prolonged QT can potentially cause torsade. Most commonly, electrolyte disturbances such as hypokalemia and hypomagnesemia, phenothiazines, fluoroquinolones, antiarrhythmic drugs, tricyclic antidepressants, intracranial events, and bradyarrhythmias are associated with this malignant arrhythmia. Management, besides stabilization, which may require electrical cardioversion, consists of removing the offending agent. In addition, success in rhythm termination or prevention has been reported with the administration of magnesium as well as overdrive atrial or ventricular pacing, which will shorten the QT interval. Beta blockers are indicated for patients with congenital long QT syndrome but are not indicated in this patient.

**V-35.  The answer is D.**  *(Chap. 222)*   The ECG shows widespread ST elevation in $V_2-V_6$ with reciprocal changes in aVR. These changes are typical of acute pericarditis. The clinical presentation of acute pericarditis can mimic acute myocardial infarction (MI), aortic dissection, pulmonary embolism, or gastroesophageal reflux disease (GERD). The classic history of acute pericarditis includes sharp substernal pain that is worse supine and improved upright. However, the pain may be dull, pleuritic, or precordial. Serum biomarkers of acute myocardial injury may be modestly elevated, especially in light of the widespread ECG abnormalities. A three-component friction rub is the classic physical finding of acute pericarditis and may be heard best in the sitting position during expiration. The rub is often inconsistent and variable. Most causes of acute pericarditis are viral in origin (echovirus and coxsackievirus are the most common) and are best treated with nonsteroidal anti-inflammatory drugs.

**V-36.  The answer is B.**  *(Chap. 222)*   This tracing demonstrates equalization of diastolic pressures and the characteristic "dip and plateau" or "square root" morphology of constrictive pericarditis. Kussmaul's sign occurs when the jugular venous pressure increases (rather than having the normal decrease) during inspiration. Patients will also have a prominent "y" descent. The holodiastolic low-pitched murmur at the cardiac apex is characteristic of mitral stenosis. A pansystolic murmur at the lower sternal border is typical of a ventricular septal defect (VSD). Pericardial friction rubs are seen in patients with pericarditis. Pulsus paradoxus, an enhanced fall in systolic blood pressure during inspiration, may be found in approximately a third of patients with constrictive pericarditis but is more typical of pericardial tamponade. Kussmaul's sign is usually absent in pericardial tamponade. Patients with constrictive pericardial disease typically present with fatigue, dyspnea on exertion, increased abdominal girth, hepatomegaly, jugular venous distention, and dependent edema. Most cases result from healing of an acute fibrinous or serofibrinous pericarditis (tuberculosis, systemic lupus erythematosus, after radiation) or from the long-term presence of a pericardial effusion (neoplasia, myxedema, uremia). The "dip and plateau" pattern on catheterization may also be seen in restrictive cardiomyopathy.

**V-37.  The answer is D.**  *(Chap. 214)*   Several drugs are associated with QT interval prolongation and the development of polymorphic ventricular tachycardia (torsades de pointes). They include antiarrhythmic agents (quinidine, sotalol, ibutilide, procainamide, amiodarone), antiinfective agents (quinolones, erythromycin, clarithromycin, pentamidine), antiemetics (droperidol, domperidone), antipsychotics (haloperidol, thioridazine), and other drugs (cisapride, methadone). Prologation of the QT interval to more than 500 ms should prompt consideration of drug alternatives. Unlike other antipsychotic medications, olanzapine does *not* contribute significantly to QT prolongation, although caution is recommended during concomitant treatment with drugs that do prolong the QT interval.

**V-38.  The answer is B.**  *(Chaps. 220 and 221)*   This patient presents with classic findings of right-sided heart failure. The differential diagnosis includes pulmonary vascular disease, restrictive cardiomyopathy, constrictive pericarditis, cor pulmonale, and any cause of long-standing left-sided heart failure. A CT or MRI of the chest would assess for pericardial calcifications or parenchymal lung disease not visualized on radiography. Iron studies are a component of the evaluation for hemochromatosis, and fat pad biopsy is a component of the evaluation for amyloidosis, both of which may cause restrictive cardiomyopathy. The tuberculin test is useful for ascertaining the presence of prior infection with *Mycobacterium tuberculosis,* which is associated with the development of constrictive pericarditis. A coronary angiogram would not be helpful in a young patient with no physical signs or echocardiographic findings of left-sided heart failure.

**V-39.  The answer is C.**  *(Chap. 225)*   The National Cholesterol Education Program (NCEP) has developed guidelines for the detection, evaluation, and treatment of high blood cholesterol in adults. The most recent NCEP recommendations, the Adult Treatment Panel III (ATP III) guidelines, were released in May 2001 and reiterate the importance of LDL-C reduction to modify the risk of congestive heart failure (CHF). New features of the guidelines include the identification of CHD risk equivalents; lower treatment target goals; an emphasis on conditions conferring a higher risk for CHD, such as the metabolic syndrome; and a scoring system for calculating CHD risk. High-risk patients are recommended to have a goal LDL-C <100 and include those with established coronary artery disease (stable angina, unstable angina, prior myocardial infarction); coronary heart disease equivalents, which include diabetes; peripheral vascular disease; abdominal aortic disease; carotid artery disease (carotid stroke, over 50% carotid obstruction); multiple risk factors; and a greater than 20% 10-year risk of CHD (Framingham scoring). Intermediate-risk patients, like the patient in (C), should have a goal LDL-C below 130.

**V-40.** **The answer is F.** *(Chap. 20)* Neurocardiogenic syncope is a term that includes both vasovagal syncope and vasodepressor syncope. In both cases the patient loses sympathetic tone with subsequent vasodilation. Vasovagal syncope also adds increased vagal tone with resultant bradycardia. Neurocardiogenic syncope is the most common cause of syncope and presents often with a characteristic history. Generally the event occurs in certain situations, especially hot or crowded spaces, stressful situations, after long periods of standing, after alcohol ingestion, with hunger, or with pain. A prodrome is often present that may last from seconds to minutes and generally consists of light-headedness, diaphoresis, nausea, weakness, visual changes sometimes with transient blindness, and frequently the sensation of a forceful heartbeat. Patient often appear gray or ashen when they lose consciousness and, generally because of the prodrome, are able to avoid falls with significant injury. The period when the patient has lost consciousness may last from several seconds to a few minutes. Occasional clonic jerks of the face and limbs can be seen, and the pulse is often noted to be thready or absent. Loss of continence is not typical for neurocardiogenic syncope and often suggests seizure.

**V-41.** **The answer is D.** *(Chap. 20)* The patient presents with carotid hypersensitivity syndrome in which pressure on the carotid sinus baroreceptors results in activation of the sympathetic nervous system with subsequent bradycardia caused by sinus arrest or atrioventricular block, vasodilation, or both. Generally, men older than 50 are at risk for this condition, and it classically presents with syncope in the setting of shaving, wearing a tight collar, or turning the head to one side. Diagnosis is suggested by carotid sinus massage with prolonged (more than 3 s) asystole.

**V-42.** **The answer is E.** *(Chap. 20)* Orthostatic syncope accounts for 30% of syncope in the elderly. Although dehydration may be a contributor, often polypharmacy with antihypertensives in combination with antidepressants is underlying. In this case the patient was adequately hydrated, with persistent symptoms. At this point it is appropriate to discontinue the likely offenders. Beta blockers will blunt the normal response of tachycardia when venous return drops when the patient is transitioning from lying to standing and thus will contribute to orthostatis. As the antidepressant may be contributing to the symptoms, it is reasonable to stop this medication as well.

**V-43.** **The answer is C.** *(Chap. 20)* Although ventricular tachycardia is classically associated with ischemic heart disease, in which scarred myocardium provides a substrate for reentrant tachyarrhythmias, other cardiac lesions put a patient at risk for ventricular tachycardia. Notably, hypertrophic obstructive cardiomyopathy, aortic stenosis, and long QT syndrome carry an increased risk for ventricular tachycardia. Atrial myxoma, which can cause syncope by obstructing blood flow with resultant decreased cardiac output, is not associated with ventricular tachycardia.

**V-44.** **The answer is C.** *(Chap. 20)* Cough syncope is thought to be due to elevated intrathoracic pressure that is transmitted to the inferior and superior vena cavae. Because of the increased pressure on the venous systems, there is a drop in venous return with a concomitant drop in cardiac output. Bradycardia also can contribute to the syncope with increased vagal tone during the event.

**V-45.   The answer is E.**   *(Chap. 229)*   Initial stabilization for patients with an unstable angina variant of acute coronary syndrome should include beta blockers, nitrates, heparin, and antiplatelet therapy, including at a minimum aspirin and in many cases a platelet glyco-protein IIb/IIIa receptor blocker. Trials of medical management alone versus early attempts at revascularization using cardiac catheterization have shown that the latter approach re-sults in a more rapid return to work, fewer readmissions, and late revascularizations and may offer a reduction in late events compared with medical therapy alone.

**V-46.   The answer is D.**   *(Chap. 229; N Engl J Med 335:217–225, 1996.)*   The standard in-dications for coronary artery bypass graft surgery are severe three-vessel disease (patient A) and significant left main stenosis (patient B) or, more recently, patients with diabetes mellitus and two-vessel coronary disease per the BARI trial, as in patient C. In these patients a clear mortality benefit has been demonstrated compared with medical manage-ment and percutaneous coronary revascularization. Many patients with other indications for cardiac surgery, such as symptomatic valvular disease, also undergo bypass surgery at the time of their procedure; thus patient E would undergo bypass surgery as well. Patient D with normal left ventricular function and single-vessel disease and a probably clinically insignificant rugurgitant murmur is not a candidate for bypass surgery.

**V-47.   The answer is D.**   *(Chap. 222)*   The echocardiogram shows a large pericardial effusion with right ventricular collapse. This echocardiogram in conjunction with the clinical pre-sentation is consistent with pericardial tamponade. Tamponade occurs when there is a sufficient amount of fluid in the pericardium to impede ventricular filling. The most com-mon causes of pericardial tamponade include neoplastic disease (lung and breast most common), idiopathic pericarditis, uremia, trauma, and postsurgical patients. Pulsus para-doxus greater than 10 mmHg may also be present clinically. Treatment requires prompt drainage of the pericardial fluid. The echocardiogram that is shown is not consistent with mitral valve prolapse, mitral stenosis, postpartum cardiomyopathy, or aortic stenosis.

**V-48.   The answer is E.**   *(Chap. 210)*   The ECG shows a junctional rhythm with an atrioven-tricular (AV) block and ST-segment elevation in leads II, III, and aVF. There are also reciprocal changes in I and aVL. These changes are consistent with an acute inferior wall myocardial infarction. The ECG is more useful in localizing regions of ischemia in ST elevation than in non-ST elevation MI. Anteroseptal ischemia causes changes in $V_1 - V_3$ and apical/lateral ischemia in $V_4 - V_6$. The right coronary artery (RCA) generally supplies blood flow to the right ventricle and the AV node. The inferior-posterior region of the left ventricle is supplied by the right coronary artery or the left circumflex coronary artery. In approximately 60 to 70% of people it is supplied by the RCA (right dominant). In this case the presence of AV nodal dysfunction and inferior ischemia makes disease of the RCA most likely.

**V-49.   The answer is D.**   *(Chaps. 103 and 228; Tenaglia AN et al, Am J Cardiol 68:1015–1019, 1991.)*   Among these patients, the only absolute contraindication to thrombolytic therapy is a cerebrovascular event within the preceding 3 months. A history of a hemor-rhagic CVA any time in the past, recent head trauma, intracerebral neoplasm, blood pres-sure greater than 200/120, trauma or significant surgery within the preceding 2 weeks, pregnancy, and suspected aortic dissection are also absolute contraindications to throm-bolytic therapy. The other patients have relative contraindications. Trained nontraumatic CPR of less than 10 minutes' duration is not associated with an increased risk of bleeding and should be considered a relative contraindication.

**V-50.   The answer is B.**   *(Chaps. 212 and 216)*   The Swan-Ganz catheter readings show a marked reduction in cardiac index with low left ventricular filling pressure, pulmonary hypertension, and right-sided heart failure. These findings are consistent with cor pulmon-ale. These results would also be consistent with a pulmonary embolism. Aortic stenosis with left ventricular (LV) failure, mitral stenosis, or acute myocardial infarction (MI) would cause an increase in the PCW pressure. Cardiac tamponade causes equalization of the PA diastolic pressure, PCW pressure, and right atrial pressure.

**V-51.  The answer is C.**  *(Chaps. 228 and 253)*   This patient has a right ventricular infarction. The combination of findings consistent with bradycardia, cardiogenic shock, low normal left ventricular and PA pressures, and markedly elevated right atrial pressure is consistent with acute right ventricular (RV) failure. An acute pulmonary embolus may also cause acute RV failure, but the PA pressure is usually elevated. RV infarction is usually due to occlusion of the right coronary artery; the bradycardia is due to sinus or AV node ischemia. Right-sided precordial ECG will show ST-segment elevation. Occlusion of the left main artery will cause cardiogenic shock, but the PCW pressure will be elevated. Perforated duodenal ulcer and ruptured aortic aneurysm will cause hypovolemic shock with low RA and PCW pressures. Gram-negative sepsis will generally have an normal or increased cardiac index with normal filling pressures and low blood pressure.

**V-52.  The answer is C.**  *(Chap. 210)*   The ECG shows convex elevation of the J point at the end of the QRS and the beginning of the ST segment in multiple leads (Osborne waves, easily visible in II, III, aVF, and $V_4-V_6$). These changes along with QT-interval prolongation develop when the core body temperature drops to approximately 30°C (86°F). They will resolve with appropriate rewarming. Acute pericarditis causes more diffuse and extensive ST-segment elevation that mimics acute MI. Hypokalemia causes U waves and QT-interval prolongation. Hypocalcemia also prolongs the QT interval.

**V-53.  The answer is C.**  *(Chaps. 210 and 221)*   The ECG shows slight right axis deviation and low voltage. These changes are typical of emphysema when the thorax is hyperinflated with air and the flattened diaphragm pulls the heart inferiorly and vertically. An acute central nervous system (CNS) event such as a subarachnoid hemorrhage may cause QT prolongation with deep, wide inverted T waves. Hyperkalemia will cause peaked narrowed T waves or a wide QRS complex. Patients with hypertrophic cardiomyopathy will have left ventricular hypertrophy and widespread deep, broad Q waves

**V-54.  The answer is D.**  *(Chap. 229)*   With improved techniques and the advent of drug-eluting stents, complications from percutaneous coronary revascularization are decreasing in frequency. However, the most common complications include hematoma at the catheter insertion site, balloon deployment can result in coronary dissection and in-stent restenosis, and, rarely, the artery at the insertion site (usually femoral) can be damaged during the procedure with the subsequent formation of a pseudoaneurysm. The jugular vein is not cannulated during cardiac catheterization and subsequently is not prone to thrombosis.

**V-55.  The answer is E.**  *(Chap. 229)*   The patient has undergone a myocardial infarction, and clear benefit has been demonstrated in this patient population with angiotension converting-enzyme (ACE) inhibitors, aspirin, and beta blockers. After stent placement clopidogrel is indicated for at least 3 months to prevent in-stent thrombosis. Warfarin was commonly prescribed in the early days of percutaneous revascularization, but increased bleeding complications and the advent of platelet ADP-receptor blockers have obviated the need for this medication.

**V-56.  The answer is D.**  *(Chap. 227)*   Although troponin is a commonly used biomarker for myocardial necrosis in the setting of acute myocardial infarction, it is also associated with and caused by a number of other clinical entities, including pulmonary embolism, myocarditis, and congestive heart failure. Troponin elevations are not known to be caused by pneumonia in the absence of myocardial necrosis.

**V-57.  The answer is B.**  *(Chap. 227)*   The patient has a presentation consistent with unstable angina, including new electrocardiographic changes without elevations in cardiac biomarkers. Although it generally is true that T-wave changes do not predict the angiographic location of culprit lesions, the one exception is the eponymous Wellen's T waves. In this case deep symmetric T-wave inversions in the early precordial leads suggest either significant left main stenosis or high left anterior descending stenosis.

**V-58.  The answer is D.**   *(Chap. 225)*   HMG-CoA reductase inhibitors ("statins") clearly reduce cardiovascular events in patients with atherosclerosis. The mechanism appears to be more complex than simply the reduction of serum LDL. Lipid-lowering drugs do not appear to cause significant regression of fixed coronary lesions. The benefit of statins appears to be related to stabilization of plaques, long-term egress of lipids, and/or improved vasodilatory tone. The improved vasodilatory tone appears to be mediated by modulation of endothelial-dependent vasodilators such as nitric oxide. Thus, the beneficial effect of the statins probably consists of an early effect on vasomotion (or other mechanisms) and a long-term effect on serum and plaque lipids.

**V-59.  The answer is B.**   *(Chaps. 225 and 335)*   This patient meets the criteria for the metabolic syndrome. These patients with type 2 diabetes and an abnormal lipid profile have insulin resistance and a marked increase in cardiovascular risk. The LDL in these patients may not be markedly elevated, but the particles are smaller and denser. These small LDL particles are thought to be more atherogenic than are normal LDL particles. Patients with the metabolic syndrome have reduced HDL levels. Elevated serum endothelin levels may contribute to hypertension, and elevated homocysteine levels have been suggested as a cardiovascular risk factor.

Clinical Identification of the Metabolic Syndrome—Any Three Risk Factors

| Risk Factor | Defining Level |
| --- | --- |
| Abdominal obesity[a] | |
| Men (waist circumference)[b] | >102 cm (>40 in.) |
| Women | >88 cm (>35 in.) |
| Triglycerides | >1.7 mmol/L (>150 mg/dL) |
| HDL cholesterol | |
| Men | <1.0 mmol/L (<40 mg/dL) |
| Women | <1.3 mmol/L (<50 mg/dL) |
| Blood pressure | ≥130/≥85 mmHg |
| Fasting glucose | >6.1 mmol/L (>110 mg/dL) |

[a] Overweight and obesity are associated with insulin resistance and the metabolic syndrome. However, the presence of abdominal obesity is more highly correlated with the metabolic risk factors than is an elevated body-mass index (BMI). Therefore, the simple measure of waist circumference is recommended to identify the BMI component of the metabolic syndrome.

[b] Some male patients can develop multiple metabolic risk factors when the waist circumference is only marginally increased, e.g., 94–102 cm (37–39 in.). Such patients may have a strong genetic contribution to insulin resistance. They should benefit from life-style changes, similarly to men with categorical increases in waist circumference.

**V-60.  The answer is E.**   *(Chap. 225)*   Although tight glycemic control clearly decreases the risk of the microvascular complications of diabetes (renal function, retinopathy), demonstration of a benefit for myocardial infarction or stroke is less compelling. However, other factors in the management of these patients have been shown to decrease risk. These factors include the use of HMG-CoA reductase inhibitors over all ranges of LDL cholesterol; gemfibrazil, particularly in patients with the metabolic syndrome; strict control of hypertension; and the use of an antihypertensive agent that inhibits the actions of angiotensin II, such as an ACE inhibitor or an angiotensin receptor blocker.

**V-61.  The answer is A.**   *(Chap. 225; JAMA 228:321, 2002.)*   Although hormone replacement therapy (HT) has been demonstrated to have beneficial effects on lipid profiles, including a reduction in LDL cholesterol and an increase in HDL cholesterol, recent clinical trials have not demonstrated a reduction in cardiovascular events in primary or secondary prevention. In fact, some trials have demonstrated an increased risk of cardiovascular events, particularly in the first 2 years of treatment. These events may be related to a prothrombotic effect of estrogen. However, HT has been shown to decrease vasomotor symptoms and vaginal dryness. It also has been shown to reduce bone loss and decrease the risk of osteoporotic fractures in the hip, spine, and wrist.

**V-62.   The answer is B.**   *(Chap. 225)*   Recent studies have demonstrated that markers of inflammation correlate with coronary risk and that inflammation plays a role in atheromatous plaque instability. Elevations of C-reactive protein (CRP) identify patients at increased risk of myocardial infarction (MI) and poor outcome of acute coronary syndromes. Measurement of CRP adds information regarding risk stratification to standard risk factors such as hypertension, diabetes, smoking, and lipids. Elevations in homocysteine, lipoprotein A, and plasminogen activator factor 1 have all been associated with an increased risk of cardiovascular events; however, at this time none have been shown to be useful in populations to improve risk stratification. Recent studies have suggested that infection with agents such as *C. pneumoniae* and cytomegalovirus may play a role in the development of atherosclerosis. To date no studies have demonstrated a conclusive association, and early studies looking at the utility of antibiotic treatment in coronary artery disease have shown no benefit.

**V-63.   The answer is C.**   *(Chap. 228)*   Myoglobin is released from ischemic myocardial cells and appears in serum within hours. It has a very short half-life in serum as it is excreted rapidly in the urine. Serum myoglobin returns to normal within 24 h after an infarction. Therefore, in this patient a new elevation of myoglobin would be helpful in distinguishing new myocardial necrosis. Troponin-I and troponin-T are more specific markers of myocardial necrosis but have a long half-life in the circulation. They may remain elevated for over a week after an acute MI. Therefore, they are not as useful for detecting new or recurrent injury. In the presence of a preexisting left bundle branch ECG is of limited utility in detecting new ischemia. Serial echocardiograms may detect new wall motion abnormalities that suggest new ischemia or infarction, but in the absence of a prior study a single echocardiogram would have limited utility in this patient.

**V-64 and V-65.   The answers are D and E.**   *(Chap. 230)*   This patient presents at a young age with hypertension that is difficult to control, raising the question of secondary causes of hypertension. The most likely diagnosis in this patient is primary hyperaldosteronism, also known as Conn's syndrome. The patient has no physical features that suggest congenital adrenal hyperplasia or Cushing's syndrome. In addition, there is no glucose intolerance as is commonly seen in Cushing's syndrome. The lack of episodic symptoms and the labile hypertension make pheochromocytoma unlikely. The findings of hypokalemia and metabolic alkalosis in the presence of difficult to control hypertension yield the likely diagnosis of Conn's syndrome. Diagnosis of the disease can be difficult, but the preferred test is the plasma aldosterone/renin ratio. This test should be performed at 8 A.M., and a ratio above 30 to 50 is diagnostic of primary hyperaldosteronism. Caution should be made in interpreting this test while the patient is on ACE inhibitor therapy as ACE inhibitors can falsely elevate plasma renin activity. However, a plasma renin level that is undetectable or an elevated aldosterone/renin ratio in the presence of an ACE inhibitor therapy is highly suggestive of primary hyperaldosteronism. Selective adrenal vein renin sampling may be performed after the diagnosis to help determine if the process is unilateral or bilateral. Although fibromuscular dysplasia is a common secondary cause of hypertension in young females, the presence of hypokalemia and metabolic alkalosis should suggest Conn's syndrome. Thus, magnetic resonance imaging of the renal arteries is unnecessary in this case. Measurement of 24-h urine collection for potassium wasting and aldosterone secretion can be useful in the diagnosis of Conn's syndrome. The measurement of metanephrines or cortisol is not indicated.

**V-66.   The answer is C.**   *(Chap. 230; JAMA 289:2560–2572, 2003; Ann Intern Med 135: 1019–1028, 2001.)*   This patient is presenting with stage I hypertension as defined by the guidelines of the Joint National Committee on the Prevention, Detection, Evaluation, and Treatment of High Blood Presssure. The guidelines have adopted new targets for the treatment and diagnosis of hypertension. Normal blood pressure is defined as less than 120/80, with a new category of prehypertension being introduced to describe patients with a blood pressure of 120–139/80–89. These patients are defined as a group of individuals who are likely to develop hypertension in the future and should be closely followed. This patient falls into the category of stage I hypertension with a blood pressure of 140–159/90–99. The final category is stage II hypertension, defined as greater than 160/100. Based on these guidelines, this patient should be encouraged to pursue lifestyle modifications and have frequent follow-ups at 3- to 6-month intervals to determine if drug therapy should be initiated. Drug therapy should be initiated earlier in patients with concomitant diabetes mellitus or chronic kidney disease. This patient's history of gestational diabetes mellitus is not a compelling indication to initiate therapy currently, although she should be followed for the development of glucose intolerance more closely.

Several lifestyle modifications have been demonstrated to lower blood pressure in randomized trials. Weight reduction to a normal body mass index (18.5 to 24.9) is recommended, with expected reductions in systolic pressure from 5 to 20 mmHg for each 10 kg of weight loss. Other dietary modifications include recommendations for adopting the DASH diet, which is high in fruits, vegetables, and low-fat dairy products while avoiding saturated and total fats. This diet was proved in the Dietary Approaches to Stop Hypertension study to decrease systolic blood pressure by as much as 14 mmHg. Adopting a low-sodium diet with no more than 2.4 g of sodium daily also improves blood pressure by 2 to 8 mmHg. Further lifestyle modifications include recommendations for physical activity for a minimum of 30 min several days weekly and limitation of alcohol beverages to one drink daily in women and two in men.

**V-67.   The answer is C.**   *(Chap. 230)*   Angiotensin converting-enzyme inhibitors are considered first-line agents for the treatment of hypertension in diabetic patients. These agents have been shown to decrease the progression of diabetic nephropathy and albuminuria. The goal blood pressure in diabetic patients and patients with chronic kidney disease is lower than that for patients with essential hypertension alone. The blood pressure target should be less than 130/90 in these individuals. This patient should have his dose of lisinopril increased at the current visit as the effects of the lisinopril should be seen within 6 weeks. There is no indication to switch the patient from an ACE inhibitor to an angiotensin receptor blocker unless the patient develops intolerance to the ACE inhibitor, with the most frequent adverse effect being cough. The issue of "white-coat" hypertension is frequently revisited in the medical literature. If this is an ongoing concern of the treating physician, ambulatory blood pressure monitoring may be warranted. However, in this young individual with diabetes mellitus the problems associated with untreated hypertension warrant further attention.

**V-68.   The answer is E.**   *(Chaps. 230, 313)*   Gout may be precipitated by the use of any diuretic agent, and diuretics should be used with caution in patients with a history of gout. ACE inhibitors are the drug of choice in patients with diabetic nephropathy. Angiotensin receptor blockers may be used if a patient is intolerant of ACE inhibitors. In patients with known coronary artery disease or heart failure ACE inhibitors and beta blockers are useful in preventing death. Diuretics will improve symptoms in patients with heart failure, and calcium channel blockers are indicated for refractory angina, particularly vasospastic angina.

**V-69.   The answer is A.**   *(Chap. 230; JAMA 289:2560–2572, 2003.)*   The most recent recommendation for the treatment of hypertension is for the initiation of combination therapy as first-line treatment if blood pressure is higher than 160/100 mmHg. A thiazide diuretic should be a part of all combination regimens and can be combined with an ACE inhibitor, calcium channel blocker, angiotensin receptor blocker, or beta blocker. The patient has no symptoms of hypertensive emergency and has no evidence of end organ damage on physical and laboratory examination. Thus, the patient does not need intravenous administration of antihypertensive medications and can safely be managed as an outpatient on oral medications with close follow-up. Lifestyle modifications have at best been shown to lower systolic pressure by 10 to 20 mmHg and would not alone be sufficient for treatment of this degree of hypertension.

**V-70.** **The answer is C.**
*(Chap. 227)* The patient has a presentation consistent with the diagnosis of non-ST elevation myocardial infarction with anginal chest pain and elevated cardiac biomarkers. To determine his risk for future cardiac events, including death, myocardial infarction, and urgent revasculariza-

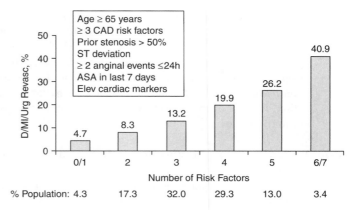

tion, in the next 14 days, the TIMI risk score has been used. This score can be applied to patients with unstable angina or non-ST elevation myocardial infarction and was validated among patients from the Thrombolysis in Myocardial Ischemia Trial (TIMI). It includes seven risk factors: age over 65, three or more risk factors for coronary artery disease, documented stenosis of more than 50% at catheterization, aspirin use 7 days before an episode, two or more episodes of pain within 24 hours, ST-segment deviation, and elevated serum cardiac markers. By adding up the risk factors, one can generate a likelihood of an adverse outcome in the ensuing 14 days, as here. Clinicians can use this risk stratification tool to guide further management decisions.

**V-71.** **The answer is C.** *(Chap. 227)* Prinzmetal's, or variant, angina is defined by transient epicardial coronary artery vasospasm with subsequent electrocardiographic abnormalities that include ST-segment elevation or depression. In the majority of patients with this disorder, there is significant coronary stenosis within at least one major vessel and the spasm occurs within 1 cm of the obstruction. The most common site of focal spasm is the right coronary artery. Epidemiologically, patients with variant angina are younger and have fewer coronary risk factors and lack preceding chronic stable angina. Patients with this as a suspected diagnosis can undergo provocative maneuvers to elicit the electrocardiographic or angiographic changes. Of note, hyperventilation ergonovine, acetylcholine, and other vasoconstrictors have been used. The mainstays of therapy are nitrates and calcium channel blockers to promote vasodilation and prevent spasm. Aspirin is thought to increase the severity of ischemic episodes and is relatively contraindicated.

**V-72.** **The answer is D.** *(Chap. 228)* Glucocorticoid and nonsteroidal anti-inflamatory medications (except aspirin) are contraindicated in patients with an acute ST elevation myocardial infarction (MI). These medications may impede healing, increase the risk of myocardial rupture, and result in a larger infarct scar. Aspirin should be given initially to all patients suspected of having myocardial ischemia to block platelet function and reduce ischemia. After primary percutaneous angioplasty and stent placement, clopidogrel and abciximab reduce the incidence of stent restenosis. They may also be beneficial in limiting infarct size in the absence of percutaneous intervention. ACE inhibitors should be started in all hemodynamically stable patients with ST elevation MI within 24 h to reduce mortality and chronic ventricular remodeling. Beta blockers should also be prescribed acutely when possible to reduce in-hospital mortality and chronically to reduce the incidence of reinfarction and recurrent ischemia.

**V-73.** **The answer is A.** *(Chap. 209)* The patient presents with signs and symptoms consistent with congestive heart failure. Her history of tuberculosis puts her at risk for constrictive pericarditis, and indeed, chest CT shows the classic pericardial calcifications of this disorder. As she is relatively young and does not have enlarged chambers or ischemic changes on the electrocardiogram, dilated or ischemic cardiomyopathy is unlikely. Constrictive pericarditis has certain suggestive physical findings, notably the prominent and rapid $y$ descent in the jugular venous pulsations that represents early and rapid filling of the right ventricle during early diastole. Other findings that have been associated include rapid $x$ descent, pericardial knock that is similar to a third heart sound, and impressive ascites, edema, and occasionally Kussmaul's sign (lack of inspiratory decline in jugular venous pressure). A double systolic apical impulse has been described in patients with hypertrophic cardiomyopathy. A loud and fixed split $P_2$ suggests pulmonary hypertension. Cannon $a$ waves are most commonly seen in arrhythmias that cause atrioventricular dissociation. Finally, opening snaps are brief, high-pitched diastolic sounds that usually are due to mitral stenosis.

**V-74, V-75, and V-76.   The answers are D, B, and B.**   *(Chap. 209)*   Differentiating between the etiologies of systolic murmurs can be challenging, and in this situation using maneuvers to change cardiac physiology can be quite helpful. Inspiration increases flow through the right side of the heart and subsequently increases the sound of tricuspid regurgitation, as in Question 76. The Valsalva maneuver will decrease the sound of most murmurs by decreasing preload; the primary exceptions are hypertrophic cardiomyopathy and the late systolic murmur of mitral valve prolapse, which paradoxically are augmented by this maneuver. Standing, which decreases preload, behaves similarly in response to the Valsalva maneuver. Squatting, however, increases both venous return and systemic afterload, which will increase the intensity of most murmurs except hypertrophic cardiomyopathy and mitral valve prolapse. Finally, sustained handgrip increases afterload and heart rate with subsequent accentuation of mitral regurgitation, aortic regurgitation, and mitral stenosis but decreased intensity of the murmur of hypertrophic cardiomyopathy.

**V-77.   The answer is E.**   *(Chap. 217)*   Approximately 3000 heart transplants are performed each year in the United States. Generally the recipients do well, with survival rates of 76% at 3 years and an average transplant "half-life" of 9.3 years. However, certain complications are common with the necessary immunosupression, including an increased risk of malignancy and infections. Additionally, patients are at risk of rejection of the transplanted organ that can be acute or chronic. Chronic cardiac transplant rejection manifests as coronary artery disease, with characteristic long, diffuse, and concentric stenosis seen on angiography. It is thought that these changes represent chronic rejection of the transplanted organ. The only definitive therapy is retransplantation. Bradyarrhythmias are not known to occur more frequently in transplant recipients.

**V-78.   The answer is D.**   *(Chap. 217)*   Prolonged assisted circulation with left ventricular assist devices is used primarily as a temporary bridge to cardiac transplantation in patients who cannot survive with medical therapy alone while they wait for a cadaveric heart. These devices in general include a power source and a mechanical pump that is connected to the heart via a drain. The pump propels blood to the systemic circulation. There are generally external portions of these devices. The three U.S. Food and Drug Administration (FDA)-approved devices all share a risk of infection because of the external components and the presence of hardware as well as a risk of thromboembolism with blood passing over hardware. Mechanical pump failure has also been described. Tachyarrhythmias, though common in patients with underlying end-stage congestive heart failure, are not known to be increased by the presence of these devices. In fact, in some cases left ventricular assist devices can be used in the treatment of refractory ventricular tachycardia.

**V-79.   The answer is B.**   *(Chap. 209)*   Examination of the retina is essential in the evaluation of the cardiovascular system as it the only vascular bed visible to the examiner with minimal equipment and can give clues to the health of the entire cardiovascular system. Common findings include hypertensive and diabetic retinopathy, but occasionally retinal emboli can be seen. Retinal emboli can be made up of platelets, cholesterol (Hollenhorst plaque as shown in the question), or calcium. Hollenhorst plaques are generally identified at vessel bifurcation, and their presence suggests that the patient has atherosclerotic plaque proximal to the retinal artery, commonly aortic, heart, great vessel, or carotid. Carotid dopplers are indicated in this case to evaluate for stenosis caused by plaque buildup. Roth spots are seen in the retinal vessels as well, but they generally do not appear to be situated in the blood vessel and may be distant from any vessel. Diabetic retinopathy more commonly presents with microaneurysms and cotton-wool spots.

**V-80.** **The answer is E.** *(Chap. 209)* During normal inspiration there is a small, less than 10 mmHg decrease in systolic pressure. In several disease states, notably severe obstructive lung disease, pericardial tamponade, and superior vena cava obstruction, an accentuation of this normal finding can occur. Indeed, in the most pronounced cases the peripheral pulse may not be palpable during inspiration.

**V-81.** **The answer is E.** *(Chap. 230; Chest 118:214–227, 2000)* The patient is suffering from the hypertensive effects of cocaine ingestion with a hypertensive emergency manifested as cerebral edema, congestive heart failure, and renal failure. The first goal of therapy is to decrease the mean blood pressure quickly by 20 to 25%. This should be accomplished by means of continuous intravenous infusion. Sublingual calcium channel blockers are no longer used, as they were demonstrated to cause increased adverse events as a result of a rapid and unpredictable decline in mean arterial pressure. Many agents are available as intravenous preparations for the treatment of a hypertensive emergency. Among the options presented, fenoldopam is the best choice. Fenoldopam is an intravenous selective dopamine-1 agonist that has been newly introduced in the treatment of hypertensive emergency. It is highly specific for dopamine-1 receptors at 10 times greater affinity than dopamine and does not bind to $\alpha_1$ or $\beta_1$ receptors. Because of its actions at the dopamine-1 receptor, fenoldopam increases renal blood flow and natriuresis. It has an onset of action within 5 minutes, and no rebound is associated with discontinuation of the continuous infusion. No oral preparation is available. Nitroprusside is relatively contraindicated in this patient because it increases intracranial pressure, and this patient already has evidence of neurologic compromise caused by elevated intracranial pressures. The intravenous ACE inhibitor enalaprilat should not be used because the patient has evident renal dysfunction that may be worsened by the efferent arteriolar constriction caused by ACE inhibitors. Finally, beta blockers are contraindicated in the setting of cocaine use as there is a risk of unopposed alpha stimulation in the setting of cocaine use, thus worsening the hypertension.

**V-82 and V-83.** **The answers are A and D.** *(Chaps. 320 and 322)* The scenario describes a young patient with severe hypertension and should prompt consideration of secondary causes of hypertension. The episodic symptoms and orthostasis despite marked hypertension are suggestive of pheochromocytoma. Thus, the most appropriate management of this patient should include an $\alpha$-adrenergic receptor blocker. Phentolamine and nitroprusside are two agents that can be used intravenously in the setting of hypertensive crises. This patient should be managed as such as she has evidence of increased intracranial pressure on ophthalmologic examination. An oral $\alpha$-adrenergic blocker is available in the form of phenoxybenzamine. The diagnosis of pheochromocytoma is best made by 24-h urine collection for metanephrines and vanillylmandelic acid. Plasma catecholamines are elevated in patients with pheochromocytoma, but the routine measurement of these levels for diagnosis is confounded by the wide variation in levels associated with various stressors. If plasma catecholamines are to be used, the levels must be drawn with the patient at rest for at least 30 minutes and drawn through an indwelling intravenous catheter. False-positive results are common. Abdominal CT imaging can also be adjunctive to assess for an adrenal or periaortic mass associated with pheochromocytoma but is not diagnostic without concurrent demonstration of elevated catecholamines. Measurement of 5-HIAA and renin levels is done for diagnosis of carcinoid syndrome and primary hyperaldosteronism, respectively.

**V-84. The answer is D.** *(Chap. 231)* The patient has an acute ascending aortic dissection, which is a surgical emergency. The immediate medical management before surgical intervention consists of intensive care unit hemodynamic monitoring and blood pressure control. The management of hypertension should be aimed at decreasing cardiac contractility and thus decreasing the shear stresses that the aorta experiences. Therefore, intravenous beta blockers are the drug of choice in this situation. They should be combined with nitroprusside to bring systolic blood pressure below 120 mmHg. The use of hydralazine or other direct arterial vasodilators is contraindicated as they may increase the shear forces in the aorta.

**V-85. The answer is A.** *(Chap. 231)* Ascending aortic dissections require surgical intervention, whereas descending aortic dissections that are uncomplicated may be managed medically. Indications for intervention for descending dissections acutely include occlusion of a major aortic branch with symptoms. For example, paralysis may occur with occlusion of the spinal artery or worsening renal failure may occur in the case of dissection that involves the renal arteries. Once a descending dissection has been found, intensive medical management of blood pressure is imperative and should include agents that decrease cardiac contractility and aortic shear force. Follow-up with CT or MRI imaging every 6 to 12 months is recommended, and surgical intervention should be considered if there is continued advancement despite medical therapy. Finally, patients with Marfan's syndrome have increased complications with descending dissections and should be considered for surgical repair, especially if there is concomitant disease in the ascending aorta as demonstrated by aortic root dilation to greater than 50 mm.

**V-86. The answer is B.** *(Chap. 231)* Abdominal aortic aneurysms (AAAs) affect 1 to 2% of men older than age 50. Most AAAs are asymptomatic and are found incidentally on physical examination. The predisposing factors for AAA are the same as those for other cardiovascular disease, with over 90% being associated with atherosclerotic disease. Most AAAs are located infrarenally, and recent data suggest that an uncomplicated infrarenal AAA may be treated with endovascular stenting instead of the usual surgical grafting. Indications for proceeding to surgery include any patient with symptoms or an aneurysm that is growing rapidly. Serial ultrasonography or CT imaging is imperative, and all aneurysms larger than 5.5 cm warrant intervention becaue of the high mortality associated with repair of ruptured aortic aneurysms. The rupture rate of an AAA is directly related to size, with the 5-year risk of rupture being 1 to 2% with aneurysms less than 5 cm and 20 to 40% with aneurysms more than 5 cm. Mortality of patients undergoing elective repair is 1 to 2% and is greater than 50% for emergent treatment of a ruptured AAA. Preoperative cardiac evaluation before elective repair is imperative as coexisting coronary artery disease is common.

**V-87. The answer is E.** *(Chap. 231)* Aortitis and ascending aortic aneurysms are commonly caused by cystic medial necrosis and mesoaortitis that result in damage to the elastic fibers of the aortic wall with thinning and weakening. Many infectious, inflammatory, and inherited conditions have been associated with this finding, including syphilis, tuberculosis, mycotic aneurysm, Takayasu's arteritis, giant cell arteritis, rheumatoid arthritis, and the spondyloarthropathies (ankylosing spondylitis, psoriatic arthritis, Reiter's syndrome, Behçet's disease). In addition, it can be seen with the genetic disorders Marfan's syndrome and Ehlers-Danlos syndrome.

**V-88. The answer is A.** *(Chap. 216)* The patient presents with high-output heart failure in the setting of Paget's disease. In addition to this disorder, several other conditions have been associated with high-output states, including anemia, arteriovenous fistulas, pregnancy, hyperthyroidism, and beriberi. In this case, in light of the lack of clinical risk factors, ischemic cardiomyopathy is very unlikely, as is amyloid. Patients with high-output heart failure in general respond well to treatment of the underlying condition, with subsequent improvement of heart failure symptoms. Diuretics are helpful for symptomatic relief. Although sinus tachycardia is common in this patient population, ventricular tachycardia is not.

**V-89.    The answer is B.**  *(Chap. 216)*   The patient has an ischemic cardiomyopathy with an ejection fraction below 35%. In this patient population mortality benefit has clearly been demonstrated with ACE inhibitors and beta blockers, namely, metoprolol XL and carvedilol. Because of her history of myocardial infarction, aspirin is indicated. In patients with ischemic cardiomyopathy and a depressed ejection fraction, there is now good evidence that implantable defibrillators confer a mortality benefit. No data suggest a mortality benefit with the long-acting oral nitrate isosorbide mononitrite. There is a mortality benefit of isosorbide dinitrite and hydralizine versus placebo, but this regimen is still not as beneficial as ACE inhibitors.

**V-90.    The answer is C.**  *(Chap. 232)*   The patient has worsening claudication caused by atherosclerotic peripheral vascular disease. The most useful therapy for treatment of peripheral vascular disease is to repair the obstructing lesion if possible. After appropriate investigation, percutaneous intervention could be attempted, with an initial success rate of percutaneous intervention (PCI) to the femoral area approximately 80%. Often reocclusion occurs, and medical management of risk factors is important, including smoking cessation and management of hypertension and hypercholesterolemia. Medical therapy is often unsuccessful in treating the symptoms of disease. In particular, arterial vasodilators such as calcium channel blockers, hydralazine, and $\alpha$-adrenergic blockers may worsen symptoms as they cause peripheral vasodilation distal to the occlusion, causing perfusion pressure to drop. Other adjunctive therapy for symptom relief includes pentoxifylline, which presumably works by increasing red blood cell deformability, and cilostazol, which has both antiplatelet and vasodilatory properties. Antiplatelet agents such as aspirin and clopidogrel have also been shown to be useful adjunctive agents to decrease the incidence of associated cardiovascular morbidity.

**V-91.    The answer is A.**  *(Chap. 223)*   Melanoma is the tumor most likely to metastasize to the heart, although the most common primaries originating from tumors of the heart are breast and lung owing to the high incidence of these tumors.

**V-92.    The answer is B.**  *(Chaps. 213 and 228)*   The combination of hypotension and bradycardia suggests a vagal response in the setting of an acute myocardial infarction. Administration of the anticholinergic agent atropine is the treatment of choice. If the bradyarrhythmia and hypotension persist after 2.0 mg of atropine has been administered in divided doses, the insertion of a temporary pacemaker is indicated. Isoproterenol should be avoided in patients with acute myocardial infarction since it may greatly increase myocardial oxygen consumption and thus intensify ischemia. Volume replacement and inotropic support may be required if hypotension persists after correction of the bradyarrhythmia, but they are not indicated as initial therapies.

**V-93.    The answer is A.**  *(Chaps. 221 and 253)*   A patient presenting with hypotension and oliguria is critically ill and requires urgent definition of the etiology of the condition. The clinical presentation with shock, fever, and pulmonary infiltrates is consistent with either noncardiogenic or cardiogenic pulmonary edema. The elevated pulmonary capillary wedge pressure strongly suggests failure of left ventricular output as a result of primary myocardial dysfunction or obstruction caused by pericardial tamponade. Pulmonary emboli, septic shock, and hypovolemia from gastrointestinal blood loss would all cause the pulmonary capillary wedge pressure to be decreased. Although pericardial tamponade could produce elevated pulmonary capillary wedge pressure, the obstruction to right ventricular inflow should be associated with equally abnormal right atrial mean, right ventricular end-diastolic, and pulmonary artery end-diastolic pressures. Therefore, this patient has cardiogenic shock caused by left ventricular myocardial dysfunction on the basis of myocardial infarction, severe cardiomyopathy, or myocarditis. In light of the relatively normal electrocardiogram and the fever, the last condition is a distinct possibility.

**V-94. The answer is A.** *(Chap. 213)* The electrocardiogram discloses sudden failure of atrial ventricular conduction without a preceding change in the PR interval, termed *Mobitz type II second-degree AV block*, which usually reflects significant disease of the conduction system. It may occur after a significant anterior myocardial infarction or in Lev's disease, which involves calcification and sclerosis of the fibrous cardiac skeleton (frequently involving the aortic and mitral valves), or Lenègre's disease, which involves only the conducting system. Mobitz type II block is inherently unstable and tends to progress to complete heart block with a slow, lower-escape pacemaker. Therefore, pacemaker implantation is necessary in this condition, particularly if the patient is symptomatic, as in this case.

**V-95. The answer is C.** *(Chaps. 209, 219, and 221)* Assessment of the central aortic pulse wave is best carried out by examination of the carotid pulsations. Normally, the carotid pulse is characterized by a fairly rapid rise to a somewhat rounded peak. If two such peaks are found, diagnostic considerations include aortic regurgitation and hypertrophic cardiomyopathy. In the latter condition obstruction to outflow usually occurs in midsystole. Moreover, obstruction is more manifest in the presence of reduced left ventricular size, such as after a Valsalva maneuver with subsequent decreased venous return. A brief decline in pressure follows the sudden decrease in the rate of left ventricular ejection during midsystole because of the development of obstruction. The second peak is caused by a smaller positive pulse wave produced by the remainder of ventricular ejection and by reflected waves from peripheral sources. The so-called bisferiens pulse should be distinguished from pulsus alternans, in which there is a regular alteration of the pressure pulse amplitude from beat to beat, usually associated with severe impairment of left ventricular function and therefore occurring in the setting of a third heart sound. Pulsus paradoxus, which is found in pericardial tamponade, severe airway disease, and superior vena cava obstruction, reflects an exaggerated decrease in systolic arterial pressure during inspiration.

**V-96. The answer is C.** *(Chap. 210)* This ECG reveals an abnormal increase in the amplitude of the U wave, a small deflection after the T wave that usually has the same polarity as the T wave. Recognition of a pronounced U wave is important, for it may represent increased susceptibility to a torsades de pointes type of ventricular tachycardia. Prominent U waves are most commonly seen after the use of antiarrhythmic drugs such as quinidine, procainamide, and disopyramide or are due to hypokalemia. The latter condition would be typical of a patient receiving amphotericin B, which typically produces severe renal potassium wasting as a result of renal tubular damage. A patient with acute renal failure and hyperkalemia would display peaked T waves or an increased QRS duration on ECG. Hypercalcemia, such as that which occurs in patients with metastatic breast cancer, and digitalis intoxication tend to produce short QT intervals. Inverted U waves are sometimes a subtle sign of myocardial ischemia.

**V-97. The answer is D.** *(Chaps. 121 and 219)* Acute rheumatic fever is a nonsuppurative complication of infection with group A streptococci. Although the incidence of rheumatic fever has been declining, there have been recent domestic outbreaks on military bases. In those outbreaks the attack rate of rheumatic fever after streptococcal pharyngitis may be as high as 3%. The diagnosis of rheumatic fever requires two of the following major manifestations of the illness: carditis, migratory polyarthritis, chorea, erythema marginatum, and subcutaneous nodules. The patient in question has three of those features. In addition to fever, he has evidence of a recent history of streptococcal infection by virtue of an elevated ASO titer. Even if streptococci cannot be isolated, it is preferable to administer a therapeutic course of parenteral penicillin (a single injection of 1.2 million units of benzathine penicillin IM for 10 days). Prophylactic therapy with penicillin should be administered indefinitely to prevent recurrent attacks. Glucocorticoid therapy is probably unnecessary, especially in patients without carditis. Arthritis can be managed entirely with salicylates. Prophylactic therapy for the associated movement disorder is unnecessary.

**V-98.   The answer is B.**   *(Chap. 214; Camm, Garratt, N Engl J Med 325:1621–1629, 1991.)* Adenosine is currently approved for the termination of paroxysmal supraventricular tachycardias at a dose of 6 mg or, if 6 mg fails, 12 mg. The primary mechanism of adenosine is to decrease conduction velocity through the atrioventricular (AV) node. Thus, it is an ideal drug for acute termination of regular reentrant supraventricular tachycardia involving the AV node. Side effects may include chest discomfort and transient hypotension. The half-life is extremely short, and the side effects tend to be brief. Patients with wide complex tachycardia suggestive of ventricular tachycardia or known preexcitation syndrome should be treated with agents that decrease automaticity, such as quinidine and procainamide. However, in patients with apparent ventricular tachycardia who have neither a history of ischemic heart disease nor preexcitation syndrome, adenosine may be a useful diagnostic agent to determine whether a patient has a reentrant tachycardia, in which case the drug may terminate it; an atrial tachycardia, in which case the atrial activity may be unmasked; or a true, preexcited tachycardia, in which case adenosine will have no effect. Although adenosine is not the recommended primary therapy for patients with wide complex tachyarrhythmia, patients with junctional tachycardia who have evidence of poor ventricular function or concomitant $\beta$-adrenergic blockade may be reasonable candidates for its use.

**V-99.   The answer is B.**   *(Chaps. 209, 219, and 221)*   Echocardiographic evidence of a disproportionately thickened ventricular septum and systolic anterior motion of the mitral valve strongly suggest idiopathic hypertrophic subaortic stenosis (IHSS). The typical harsh systolic murmur usually does not radiate to the carotid arteries and decreases when ventricular volume enlarges with isometric exercise (e.g., handgrip). The carotid upstroke is brisk and often bifid. Congestive failure often occurs because of reduced ventricular compliance despite normal ventricular systolic function. Malposition of the mitral apparatus, a result of the distorted septum, often leads to some degree of mitral regurgitation.

**V-100.   The answer is C.**   *(Chap. 218; Brickner et al, N Engl J Med 342:252–263, 334–342, 2000.)*   Left-to-right shunts occur in all types of atrial and ventricular septal defects but generally do not result in cyanosis, whereas large right-to-left shunts frequently do. The magnitude of the shunt depends on the size of the defect, the diastolic properties of both ventricles, and the relative impedance of the pulmonary and systemic circulations. Defects of the sinus venosus type occur high in the atrial septum near the entry of the superior vena cava or lower near the orifice of the inferior vena cava and may be associated with anomalous connection of the right inferior pulmonary vein to the right atrium. In the case of anomalous origin of the left coronary artery from the pulmonary artery, as pulmonary vascular resistance declines immediately after birth, perfusion of the left coronary artery from the pulmonary trunk ceases and the direction of flow in the anomalous vessel reverses. Twenty percent of patients with this defect can survive to adulthood because of myocardial blood supply flowing totally through the right coronary artery. In the absence of pulmonary hypertension blood will flow from the aorta to the pulmonary artery throughout the cardiac cycle, resulting in a "continuous" murmur at the left sternal border. In total anomalous pulmonary venous connection all the venous blood returns to the right atrium; therefore, an interatrial communication is required and right-to-left shunts with cyanosis are common.

**V-101.   The answer is D.**   *(Chaps. 157 and 213)*   This patient's clinical scenario is consistent with secondary manifestations of Lyme disease, which is caused by the spirochete *Borrelia burgdorferi*. Her exposure presumably occurred on Cape Cod, a high-risk area of New England. Lyme disease occurs in three stages: the initial infection shortly after the tick bite, manifested by a skin rash (erythema chronica migrans) and often flulike symptoms; a secondary stage with cardiac and/or neurologic signs and symptoms; and a tertiary stage with arthritis.

Lyme carditis most often is manifested by AV nodal conduction disturbances, including first-, second-, or third-degree heart block. Antibiotic therapy, typically high-dose penicillin, usually leads to resolution of the heart block without the need for permanent pacing, although a temporary pacemaker may be necessary. Spirochetes can be detected within cardiac tissue, suggesting that the carditis is due to the presence of the organism. Other cardiac manifestations include nonspecific ECG changes, myocardial inflammation, and left ventricular dysfunction.

Cocaine can result in myocardial ischemia and infarction, but this more likely would be an acute complication, making the timing incorrect in this case. *Ixodes dammini* is the deer tick whose bite transmits the infection to humans. This patient's presentation is inconsistent with an acute coronary embolus. Complete heart block is not commonly seen with HIV carditis.

**V-102. The answer is E.** *(Chap. 228)* This patient most likely is having a ventricular septal rupture and a subsequent defect, a not uncommon complication of myocardial infarction (MI) that explains the need to auscultate the heart on a daily basis during the early period after an MI. Myocardial rupture after an MI can occur either in the free wall, with bleeding into the pericardium, tamponade, and a high incidence of fatality, or in the ventricular septum, with a greater potential for successful therapy despite the fact that this is a critical complication. Therapy is geared toward decreasing afterload and systemic vascular resistance. Interventions to be considered include IV nitroglycerin, IV sodium nitroprusside, and/or intra-aortic balloon counterpulsation. Often cardiac surgery with septal repair is the only viable long-term intervention; however, this is best undertaken when the patient has stabilized and ideally once the infarction has healed. In many cases the patient does not stabilize, at which point acute surgical intervention is indicated.

**V-103. The answer is E.** *(Chap. 103)* Heparin-induced thrombocytopenia (HIT) syndrome occurs in 1 to 5% of patients treated with heparin and probably is due to platelet aggregation caused by heparin-induced antibodies. Therapy usually consists of discontinuation of the heparin and the use of other anticoagulants, in particular warfarin, with several days of overlap if possible. If the platelet count falls beneath 50,000/$\mu$L, heparin should be discontinued. If proximal DVT is present, consideration may have to be given to the placement of an inferior vena caval filter. Arterial thrombosis also may be a manifestation of the HIT syndrome and represents a separate indication for the discontinuation of heparin. The thrombosis is thought to be due to antibody-mediated platelet activation, which can lead to platelet aggregation.

**V-104. The answer is D.** *(Chap. 231)* Cystic medial necrosis is a descriptive term for pathologic changes seen in the aorta. This entity consists of degeneration of collagen and elastin fibers in the tunica media of the aorta as well as cell loss in the medial layer. A mucoid material replaces the space occupied by the degenerated cells. This abnormality typically is seen in the proximal aorta and the sinuses of Valsalva, leading to weakness and aneursym formation. Cystic medial necrosis is a risk factor for aortic dissection. This condition is particularly prevalent in patients with Marfan's syndrome and Ehlers-Danlos syndrome type IV. Cystic medial necrosis also occurs in pregnant women, patients with hypertension, and patients with a history of valvular heart disease.

**V-105. The answer is B.** *(Chap. 222)* This patient presents with pericardial tamponade. These patients often have distant heart sounds and on examination typically have pulsus paradoxus. Jugular veins are distended and typically show a prominent *x* descent and an absent *y* descent, as opposed to patients with constrictive pericarditis. In addition, Kussmaul's sign is absent in tamponade but present in constrictive pericarditis. The electrocardiogram is normal or shows low voltage. Rarely, electrical alternans may be present. Echocardiographic findings typically reveal right atrial collapse and right ventricular diastolic collapse. Cardiac catheterization will reveal equalization of diastolic pressures across the cardiac chambers. Therefore, the pulmonary capillary wedge pressure will be equal to the diastolic pulmonary arterial pressure, and this will be equal to the right atrial pressure. These catheterization findings are also present in a patient with constrictive pericarditis.

**V-106.** **The answer is B.** *(Chap. 208)* Cardiovascular disease is the leading cause of death in the United States. Many patients have undiagnosed cardiovascular disease and therefore are at unsuspected risk for perioperative cardiac morbidity, defined as perioperative MI, pulmonary edema, or ventricular tachycardia. Multivariable analysis first proposed by Goldman and colleagues identified several risk factors, including age over 70 years, an MI within the last 6 months, evidence of aortic stenosis or pulmonary edema on exam, and abnormalities within the electrocardiogram or laboratory analysis, as well as the type of surgical procedure being performed, with an emergency surgery being more highly associated with complication risk. In this patient the only risk is age over 70 years. The presence of two to three PVCs per minute is within the normal range. His hypertension, hypercholesterolemia, and diabetes mellitus, although significant, were not identified as independent risk factors. Therefore, this patient's risk of serious complication is ~0.6%.

**V-107.** **The answer is B.** *(Chap. 208; Mangano, Goldman, N Engl J Med 335:1713–1720, 1996.)* In patients who have or are at risk for coronary artery disease and who must undergo noncardiac surgery, treatment with atenolol during hospitalization can significantly reduce mortality as well as the incidence of cardiovascular complications. This benefit may last as long as 2 years after surgery.

**V-108.** **The answer is C.** *(Chap. 210)* The electrocardiographic T wave represents myocardial repolarization, and its configuration can be altered nonspecifically by metabolic abnormalities, drugs, neural activity, and ischemia through a dispersion effect on the activation or repolarization of action potentials. Although myocardial ischemia and subendocardial infarction can produce deep, symmetric T-wave inversions which would result in tachyarrhythmias and syncope, noncardiac phenomena such as intracerebral hemorrhage can similarly affect ventricular repolarization. Hyperkalemia is manifested by tall peaked T waves, not inverted ones. Hypocalcemia is manifested by prolonged QT intervals.

**V-109.** **The answer is A.** *(Chap. 210)* Hyperkalemia leads to partial depolarization of cardiac cells. As a result, there is slowing of the upstroke of the action potential as well as reduced duration of repolarization. The T wave becomes peaked, the RS complex widens and may merge with the T wave (giving a sine-wave appearance), and the P wave becomes shallow or disappears. Prominent U waves are associated with hypokalemia; ST-segment prolongation is associated with hypocalcemia.

**V-110.** **The answer is E.** *(Chap. 214)* Persons who have Wolff-Parkinson-White syndrome are predisposed to develop two major types of atrial tachyarrhythmias. The first, which resembles paroxysmal supraventricular tachycardia (SVT) with reentry, involves the atrioventricular node in anterograde conduction and the bypass tract in retrograde conduction. This tachycardia typically has a narrow QRS complex and can be treated similarly to other forms of SVT. The other, more dangerous tachyarrhythmia (present in the patient described in this question) is atrial fibrillation, which usually is conducted anterograde down the bypass tract and has a wide QRS configuration. The ventricular rate in this situation is quite rapid, and cardiovascular collapse or ventricular fibrillation may result. The usual treatment is direct-current cardioversion, though quinidine may slow conduction through the bypass tract. Verapamil and propranolol have little effect on the bypass tract and may further depress ventricular function, which already is compromised by the rapid rate. Digoxin may accelerate conduction down the bypass tract and lead to ventricular fibrillation.

**V-111.** **The answer is D.** *(Chap. 208; Mangano, Goldman, N Engl J Med 333:1750–1756, 1995)* Preoperative noninvasive assessment can be useful in patients with suspected coronary disease. Patients who require emergent surgical procedures are unable to undergo the elective preoperative assessment. In addition, patients who have had coronary revascularization either through surgery or percutaneously within the last 5 years and have had no further symptoms should not undergo routine preoperative noninvasive assessment. The patient described in (C) is having active coronary symptoms and should proceed to coronary angiography before his elective surgical procedure. The patient in (E) is undergoing a low-risk surgical procedure and has no coronary risk factors and no current symptoms, and therefore routine preoperative noninvasive testing is not required. The patient in (D), however, does have suspected coronary disease with intermittent angina and is undergoing an elective hip procedure. He would be best served by undergoing an outpatient noninvasive functional assessment, and the recommendation is dependent on the analysis of this test before the elective surgery to minimize perioperative cardiac morbidity.

# VI. DISORDERS OF THE RESPIRATORY SYSTEM

## QUESTIONS

**DIRECTIONS:** Each question below contains four or five suggested responses. Choose the **one best** response to each question.

**VI-1.** A 45-year-old female with known rheumatoid arthritis complains of a 1-week history of dyspnea on exertion and dry cough. She had been taking hydroxychloroquine and prednisone 7.5 mg until 3 months ago, when low-dose weekly methotrexate was added because of active synovitis. The patient's temperature is 37.8°C (100°F), and her room air oxygen saturation falls from 95% to 87% with ambulation. Chest-x-ray shows new bilateral alveolar infiltrates.

Pulmonary function tests reveal the following:

$FEV_1$, 3.1 L (70% of predicted)
TLC, 5.3 L (60% of predicted)
FVC, 3.9 L (68% of predicted)
VC, 3.9 L (58% of predicted)
$FEV_1$/FVC, 79%
Diffusion capacity for carbon monoxide (DLCO), 62% of predicted

She had a normal pulmonary function test (PFT) 1 year ago. All but which of the following would be an appropriate next step?

A. Start broad-spectrum antibiotics.
B. Increase the methotrexate dose.
C. Perform bronchoalveolar lavage with transbronchial lavage.
D. Increase prednisone to 60 mg/d.
E. Discontinue methotrexate.

**VI-2.** A 72-year-old male with a long history of tobacco use is seen in the clinic for 3 weeks of progressive dyspnea on exertion. He has had a mild nonproductive cough and anorexia but denies fevers, chills, or sweats. On physical examination, he has normal vital signs and normal oxygen saturation on room air. Jugular venous pressure is normal, and cardiac examination shows decreased heart sounds but no other abnormality. The trachea is midline, and there is no associated lymphadenopathy. On pulmonary examination, the patient has dullness over the left lower lung field, decreased tactile fremitus, decreased breath sounds, and no voice transmission. The right lung examination is

**VI-2.** *(Continued)*
normal. After obtaining chest plain film, appropriate initial management at this point would include which of the following?

A. Intravenous antibiotics
B. Thoracentesis
C. Bronchoscopy
D. Deep suctioning
E. Bronchodilator therapy

**VI-3 to VI-6.** Among the following pulmonary function test results, pick those which are the most likely finding in each of the following respiratory disorders:

A. Increased total lung capacity (TLC), decreased vital capacity (VC), decreased $FEV_1$/FVC ratio
B. Decreased TLC, decreased VC, decreased residual volume (RV), increased $FEV_1$/FVC ratio, normal maximum inspiratory pressure (MIP)
C. Decreased TLC, decreased RV, normal $FEV_1$/FVC ratio, decreased MIP
D. Normal TLC, normal RV, normal $FEV_1$/FVC ratio, normal MIP

**VI-3.** Myasthenia gravis

**VI-4.** Idiopathic pulmonary fibrosis

**VI-5.** Familial pulmonary hypertension

**VI-6.** Chronic obstructive pulmonary disease

**VI-7.** In a patient with severe bullous emphysema, the most appropriate method for measuring lung volumes is

A. body plethysmography
B. diffusing capacity of carbon monoxide
C. spirometry
D. helium dilution
E. transdiaphragmatic pressure

167

**VI-8.** Which of the following organisms is unlikely to be found in the sputum of a patient with cystic fibrosis?

A. *Haemophilus influenzae*
B. *Acinetobacer baumannii*
C. *Burkholderia cepacia*
D. *Aspergillus fumigatus*
E. *Staphylococcus aureus*

**VI-9.** A 45-year-old female is seen in the clinic for evaluation of a chronic cough. She reports a cough that began in her early twenties that is occasionally productive of yellow or green thick sputum. She has been treated with innumerable courses of antibiotics, all with brief improvements in the symptoms. The patient has been told that she has asthma, and her only medications are fluticasone and albuterol metered-dose inhalers (MDIs). Physical examination is notable for normal vital signs and an oxygen saturation of 92% on room air. The patient's lungs have dullness in the upper lobes bilaterally and diffuse expiratory wheezing. She has mild digital clubbing. The remainder of the physical examination is normal. Pulmonary function testing shows airflow obstruction. Review of the sputum culture data shows that she has had multiple positive cultures for *Pseudomonas aeruginosa* and *Staphylococcus aureus*. Posteroanterior (PA) and lateral chest radiography shows bilateral upper lobe infiltrates. Which of the following tests is the most important first step in diagnosing the underlying disease?

A. Chest computed tomogram (CT)
B. Bronchoscopy with transbronchial biopsy
C. Sweat chloride testing
D. Blood polymerase chain reaction (PCR) for ΔF508 mutation
E. Sputum cytology

**VI-10.** A 45-year-old male is evaluated in the clinic for asthma. His symptoms began 2 years ago and are characterized by an episodic cough and wheezing that responded initially to inhaled bronchodilators and inhaled corticosteroids but now require nearly constant prednisone tapers. He notes that the symptoms are worst on weekdays but cannot pinpoint specific triggers. His medications are an albuterol MDI, a fluticasone MDI, and prednisone 10 mg PO daily. The patient has no habits and works as a textile worker. Physical examination is notable for mild diffuse polyphonic expiratory wheezing but no other abnormality. Which of the following is the most appropriate next step?

A. Exercise physiology testing
B. Measurement of $FEV_1$ before and after work
C. Methacholine challenge testing
D. Skin testing for allergies
E. Sputum culture for *Aspergillus fumigatus*

**VI-11.** A 60-year-old male is seen in the clinic for counseling about asbestos exposure. He is well and has no symptoms. He also has hypertension, for which he takes hydrochlorothiazide. The patient smokes one pack of cigarettes a day but has no other habits. He is currently retired but worked for 30 years as a pipefitter and says he was around "lots" of asbestos, often without wearing a mask or other protective devices. Physical examination is normal except for nicotine stains on the left second and third fingers. Chest radiography shows pleural plaques but no other changes. Pulmonary function tests, including lung volumes, are normal. Which of the following statements should be made to this patient?

A. He must quit smoking immediately as his risk of emphysema is higher than that of other smokers because of asbestos exposure.
B. He does not have asbestosis.
C. His risk of mesothelioma is higher than that of other patients with asbestos exposure because he has a history of tobacco use.
D. He has no evidence of asbestos exposure on chest radiography.
E. He should undergo biannual chest radiography screening for lung cancer.

**VI-12.** A 53-year-old male is seen in the emergency department with sudden-onset fever, chills, malaise, and shortness of breath but no wheezing. He has no significant past medical history and is a farmer. Of note, he worked earlier in the day stacking hay. PA and lateral chest radiography shows bilateral upper lobe infiltrates. Which organism is most likely to be responsible for this presentation?

A. *Nocardia asteroides*
B. *Histoplasma capsulatum*
C. *Cryptococcus neoformans*
D. *Actinomyces*
E. *Aspergillus fumigatus*

**VI-13.** Secondhand tobacco smoke has been associated with which of the following?

A. Increased risk of lung cancer
B. Increased prevalence of respiratory illness
C. Excess cardiac mortality
D. A and B
E. All of A, B, and C

**VI-14.** A 54-year-old female presents to the hospital because of hemoptysis. She has coughed up approximately 1 teaspoon of blood for the last 4 days. She has a history of cigarette smoking. A chest radiogram shows diffuse bilateral infiltrates predominantly in the lower lobes. The hematocrit is 30%, and the serum creatinine is 4.0 mg/dL.

**VI-14.**  *(Continued)*

Both were normal previously. Urinalysis shows 2+ protein and red blood cell casts. The presence of autoantibodies directed against which of the following is most likely to yield a definitive diagnosis?

A. Glomerular basement membrane
B. Glutamic acid decarboxylase
C. Phospholipids
D. Smooth muscle
E. U1 ribonucleoprotein (RNP)

**VI-15.**  A 32-year-old male is brought to the emergency department after developing sudden-onset shortness of breath and chest pain while coughing. He reports a 3-month history of increasing dyspnea on exertion, nonproductive cough, and anorexia with 15 lb of weight loss. He has no past medical history and takes no medications. The patient smokes one or two packs of cigarettes a day, uses alcohol socially, and has no risk factors for HIV infection. A chest radiogram shows a right 80% pneumothorax, and there are nodular infiltrates in the left base that spare the costophrenic angle. After placement of a chest tube, a chest CT shows bilateral small nodular opacities in the lung bases and multiple small cystic spaces in the lung apex. Which of the following interventions is most likely to improve the symptoms and radiograms?

A. Intravenous $\alpha_1$ antitrypsin
B. Isoniazid, rifampin, ethambutol, and pyrazinamide
C. Prednisone and cyclophosphamide
D. Smoking cessation
E. Trimethoprim-sulfamethoxazole

**VI-16.**  A 21-year-old female tells her physician that she has had 5 days of increasing shortness of breath, right-sided chest pain, fevers, and chills. She is a college student who works evenings caring for an elderly woman who was recently diagnosed with cavitary tuberculosis and is receiving treatment. On physical examination the patient has a temperature of 38.3°C (100.9°F) and normal vital signs. There is dullness to percussion at the right lung base with focal egophony and a pleural friction rub. A chest radiogram demonstrates a free-flowing pleural effusion approximately one-third up the right lung. Thoracentesis reveals a protein of 5.2 mg/dL with a white cell count of 2000/$\mu$L (80% lymphocytes, 20% neutrophils, 0% macrophages), and the patient's glucose concentration is 40 mg/dL. Which of the following statements regarding this woman's case is most likely to be true?

A. Her intermediate-strength purified protein derivative (PPD) will be negative.
B. Pleural biopsy will show noncaseating granulomas.
C. Pleural fluid cultures will grow *Mycobacterium tuberculosis.*

**VI-16.**  *(Continued)*

D. She probably will require tube thoracostomy.
E. This disease represents reactivation of latent disease.

**VI-17.**  A 23-year-old hospital worker is evaluated for a known contact with a patient with active tuberculosis. One year ago his intermediate-strength PPD had 3 mm of induration; now it has 13 mm of induration at 48 h. He has no significant past medical history and is on no medications. Subsequent management should include

A. chest radiography
B. isoniazid 300 mg/d for 3 months
C. measurement of baseline liver function tests
D. measurement of liver function tests every 3 months
E. repeated intermediate-strength PPD testing in 2 weeks

**VI-18.**  Which of the following contacts with a patient infected with tuberculosis is most likely to develop the disease?

A. The child of a parent with smear-negative, culture-positive pulmonary tuberculosis
B. The co-worker in a small office of a patient with laryngeal tuberculosis
C. The HIV-negative partner of an HIV-infected patient with pulmonary tuberculosis
D. The parent of a young child in diapers with renal tuberculosis
E. The spouse of a patient with miliary tuberculosis

**VI-19.**  Which of the following statements about tuberculosis in an HIV-infected patient is true?

A. A person with a prior positive PPD who subsequently acquires HIV is no more likely to develop active tuberculosis than is an HIV-uninfected individual.
B. Extrapulmonary tuberculosis is an unusual manifestation of tuberculosis.
C. HIV-infected patients with pulmonary tuberculosis are usually diagnosed with positive sputum smears.
D. Tuberculosis meningitis is more common in HIV-infected individuals than in HIV-uninfected individuals.
E. Upper lobe pulmonary cavitary disease is an unusual manifestation of tuberculosis.

**VI-20.**  All the following patients should be considered to have a positive intermediate-strength PPD and should be evaluated for the treatment of latent disease *except*

A. a 19-year-old male with type 1 diabetes mellitus with 12 mm of induration

**VI-20.**   *(Continued)*

  B.  a 21-year-old college student from Peru who received bacillus Calmette-Guerin (BCG) vaccination as a child with 8 mm of induration

  C.  a 38-year-old male recently diagnosed with HIV infection with 8 mm of induration

  D.  a 45-year-old female whose husband was recently diagnosed with active pulmonary tuberculosis with 8 mm of induration

  E.  a 66-year-old female with apical fibrosis on chest radiography and 8 mm of induration

**VI-21.**   A 50-year-old female receives an uncomplicated double lung transplant for a history of primary pulmonary hypertension. She was cytomegalovirus (CMV)-seropositive and received CMV prophylaxis immediately after the transplant. On postoperative day 7 she developed fever and a new infiltrate in the right lung. Which of the following organisms is most likely to be the causative agent of these findings?

  A.  Cytomegalovirus
  B.  *Listeria monocytogenes*
  C.  *Nocardia asteroides*
  D.  *Pneumocystis carinii*
  E.  *Pseudomonas aeruginosa*

**VI-22.**   A 59-year-old male is evaluated for worsening shortness of breath for 1 week. Fourteen months ago he received a single right lung transplant for a history of idiopathic pulmonary fibrosis. The posttransplant course was complicated by three episodes of acute rejection in the first year. His current immunosuppressive medications include prednisone, tacrolimus, and mycophenolate. On physical examination the patient is afebrile with normal vital signs except for a respiratory rate of 20/min. There are diffuse crackles on the left and diminished breath sounds on the right with dullness to percussion. A chest radiogram reveals a moderate to large right pleural effusion that was not present 2 months ago. Evaluation of the pleural fluid shows malignant T lymphocytes that are consistent with primary lymphoma. Which of the following is most likely to be responsible for the malignant pleural effusion?

  A.  Cytomegalovirus
  B.  Epstein-Barr virus
  C.  Human herpesvirus 8
  D.  Parvovirus B19
  E.  Respiratory syncytial virus

**VI-23.**   Which of the following is the most appropriate therapy for a 60-year-old male with 2 weeks of productive cough, fever, shortness of breath, and the chest radiogram as shown in the following figure?

**VI-23.**   *(Continued)*

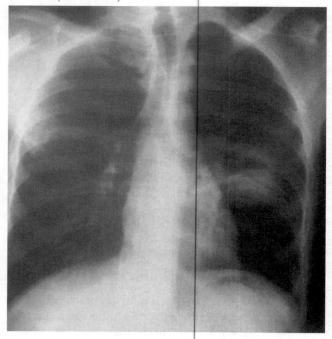

  A.  Cephalexin
  B.  Ciprofloxacin
  C.  Clindamycin
  D.  Penicillin
  E.  Vancomycin

**VI-24.**   A 17-year-old boy is admitted to the intensive care unit with fever, jaundice, renal failure, and respiratory failure. Ten days ago he was part of a community service group from his school that cleaned up a rat-infested alley. Two of his colleagues developed a flulike illness with headache, fever, myalgias, and nausea that has begun to resolve. He developed similar symptoms with the addition of jaundice. On the day of admission he developed shortness of breath. The physical examination is notable for a temperature of 38.4°C (101.1°F), blood pressure of 95/65 mmHg, heart rate of 110/min, respiratory rate of 25/min, and oxygen saturation of 92% on 100% face mask. He has notable jaundice and icterus as well as bilateral conjunctival suffusion. A chest radiogram shows bilateral diffuse infiltrates. Laboratory studies are notable for creatinine 2.5 mg/dL, total bilirubin 12.3 mg/dL, and normal aspartate aminotransferase (AST), alanine aminotransferase (ALT), and prothrombin time. Which of the following antibiotics should be included in his therapy?

  A.  Cefipime
  B.  Ciprofloxacin
  C.  Clindamycin
  D.  Penicillin
  E.  Vancomycin

**VI-25.** Which of the following is the most common cause of ambulatory care visits in the United States?

A. Bacterial upper respiratory tract infection
B. Enterovirus upper respiratory tract infection
C. Influenza
D. Respiratory syncytial virus (RSV) upper respiratory infection
E. Rhinovirus upper respiratory infection
F. Streptococcal pneumonia

**VI-26.** A 36-year-old male comes to his primary care physician complaining of 3 days of worsening headache, left frontal facial pain, and yellow nasal discharge. The patient reports that he has had nasal stuffiness and coryza for about 5 days. Past medical history is notable only for seasonal rhinitis. The physical examination is notable for a temperature of 37.9°C (100.2°F) and tenderness to palpation over the left maxillary sinus. The oropharynx has no exudates, and there is no lymphadenopathy. Which of the following is the most appropriate next intervention?

A. Aspiration of the maxillary sinus
B. Nasal fluticasone
C. Oral amoxicillin
D. Serum antineutrophil cytoplasmic antibodies (ANCA)
E. Sinus CT scan

**VI-27.** A 45-year-old man is seen in the clinic for evaluation of bronchiectasis. Among the following disorders, which is not likely to be the potential underlying cause of this bronchiectasis?

A. Allergic bronchopulmonary aspergillosis
B. Endobronchial carcinoid tumor
C. Panhypogammaglobulinemia
D. Kartagener's syndrome
E. *Mycoplasma* infection

**VI-28.** Chest CT of this patient shows bronchiectasis of the airway leading to the right lower lobe only. Review of previous chest plain radiograms shows that he has had recurrent pneumonia of the right lower lobe seven times in the last 3 years. Which of the following disorders is the likely culprit?

A. Allergic bronchopulmonary aspergillosis
B. Endobronchial carcinoid tumor
C. Panhypogammaglobulinemia
D. Kartagener's syndrome
E. *Mycoplasma* infection

**VI-29.** A 35-year-old male is seen in the clinic for evaluation of infertility. He has never fathered any children, and after 2 years of unprotected intercourse his wife has not achieved pregnancy. Sperm analysis shows a normal

**VI-29.** *(Continued)*
number of sperm, but they are immotile. Past medical history is notable for recurrent sinopulmonary infections, and the patient recently was told that he has bronchiectasis. Chest radiography is likely to show which of the following?

A. Bihilar lymphadenopathy
B. Bilateral upper lobe infiltrates
C. Normal findings
D. Situs inversus
E. Water balloon–shaped heart

**VI-30.** A 65-year-old man with a past history of bronchiectasis presents to the emergency department with hemoptysis. He reports increased cough and sputum production over the last week with low-grade fevers. There is often blood streaking his sputum, but in the last day he has noted that he is coughing up tablespoons of clotted blood, approximately 1 cup total over 24 h. Physical examination shows normal vital signs, with oxygen saturation of 98% on room air. The patient is mildly dyspneic and has diffuse expiratory wheezing. Radiography of the chest, besides showing bronchiectasis, is normal. What is the most likely etiology of the hemoptysis?

A. Alveolar hemorrhage
B. *Aspergillus* colonization
C. Bronchial artery erosion
D. Endobronchial neoplasia
E. Necrotizing gram-negative infection

**VI-31.** What is the most appropriate immediate treatment for this hemoptysis?

A. Bronchoscopy
B. Bronchial artery embolization
C. Chest CT
D. Lung transplantation
E. Surgical resectioning

**VI-32.** A 54-year-old male presents to your clinic complaining of dyspnea on exertion. The patient notes that he previously was quite active despite having had poliomyelitis at age 14. He was left with no chronic motor impairments, although he remembers being confined to an "iron lung" for 6 months. One year ago the patient played tennis three time weekly and jogged 3 miles a day; now he cannot jog a mile. He also notes that he is unable to sleep flat at night because of dyspnea. On physical examination, the patient appears well developed and has no obvious difficulty with speech. When the patient lies flat, paradoxical abdominal motion is seen. On chest examination there are no crackles, wheezes, or rhonchi. However, usual thoracic expansion with inspiration is not seen and diaphragmatic excursion is not appreciated. Which of

**VI-32.** *(Continued)*

the following statements about the patient's condition is true?

A. An elevation in the alveolar-arterial (A-a) gradient is expected.

B. The patient's baseline $Pa_{co_2}$ while awake is invariably elevated.

C. A cuirass is a form of positive-pressure ventilation that may be used to assist the patient with nocturnal ventilation.

D. The patient's maximal voluntary ventilation is normal.

E. The presence of respiratory muscle dysfunction during the original presentation of polio increases the likelihood that the patient will develop chronic respiratory difficulties with postpolio syndrome.

**VI-33.** A 42-year-old female presents to the emergency department with excessive somnolence noted by her family. She is morbidly obese with a body mass index of 52 kg/m². In addition, the patient has smoked one pack of cigarettes a day for the last 25 years. She has a past medical history of asthma and intermittently uses albuterol metered-dose inhalers. She has never been diagnosed with a sleep-related breathing disorder or chronic obstructive pulmonary disease. Recently the patient has been complaining of a cough with increased sputum production. On initial presentation, the patient is somnolent but oriented to person, place, and time. She is able to give her full history. The initial respiratory rate is 14 breaths/min, with an oxygen saturation of 76% on room air. She is noted to have basilar crackles with scattered expiratory wheezes. The cardiac examination is remarkable for an accentuation of the second heart sound at the upper left sternal border. She has woody edema to the thighs bilaterally. In the emergency department she is placed on a nonrebreather mask. Fifteen minutes later you are called to a respiratory arrest as the patient is now apneic and unresponsive. The patient is orally intubated. An arterial gas obtained before the intubation revealed a pH of 7.01, a $Pa_{co_2}$ of 120 mmHg, and a $Pa_{o_2}$ of 98 mmHg. A chemistry panel reveals a baseline serum bicarbonate of 34 meq/L, and hematocrit is 54% on presentation. The patient is weaned from the ventilator over 48 h, and her arterial blood gases (ABG) before extubation revealed a pH of 7.35, a $Pa_{co_2}$ of 72 mmHg, and a $Pa_{o_2}$ of 61 mmHg. Which of the following statements best characterizes the patient's underlying condition?

A. At baseline, the patient has normal compliance of the lungs and chest wall.

B. As a result of long-standing cigarette use, the patient is expected to have an increased functional residual capacity.

**VI-33.** *(Continued)*

C. Leptin deficiency probably is playing a role in the pathogenesis of this condition.

D. The patient's initial decline on presentation was due to overcorrection of hypoxemia with a subsequent decline in respiratory drive.

E. The patient by definition must have concurrent obstructive sleep apnea.

**VI-34.** Which of the following may be considered for the long-term management of this patient?

A. Weight loss

B. Smoking cessation

C. Correction of obstructive sleep apnea, if present

D. Progesterone

E. All of the above

**VI-35.** A 54-year-old male presents to your office complaining of sleepiness. He states that he invariably naps after dinner and normally is in bed for 8 to 10 h nightly. He does report, however, that he feels that his sleep is fragmented. When the patient awakens in the morning, he rarely feels refreshed. His wife has complained for years of his snoring to the extent that she now sleeps in a different room. The patient notes that he frequently has difficulty staying awake during the late afternoon at work. He is seeking evaluation now because his job performance has been impaired and he has been put on probation at work. Past medical history is significant for hypertension since age 38 that has recently worsened despite medication. Body mass index is 36 kg/m². He is noted to have central obesity and a thick neck. You suspect obstructive sleep apnea (OSA). All the following are long-term consequences of untreated OSA *except*:

A. personality disturbance

B. worsening of congestive heart failure

C. increased risk of proteinuria and chronic kidney disease

D. increased risk of systemic hypertension

E. increased risk of motor vehicle accidents

**VI-36.** A 38-year-old female with seasonal allergic rhinitis presents in early September for evaluation of snoring. She has multiple documented allergies, including cats, ragweed, and grass. The patient has noted that the allergy symptoms have been worse recently. She is currently using desloratadine as needed and continues to get weekly immunotherapy. She denies poor sleep quality or excessive daytime somnolence. The patient states that the only reason for the evaluation for snoring is the fact that her bed partner complains that it is disturbing her sleep. On physical examination she appears well. Body mass index is 24 kg/m². She has boggy enlarged nasal turbinates and

**VI-36.** *(Continued)*
cobblestoning of the posterior nasopharynx. What do you advise next in the evaluation and treatment of this patient?

A. Nasal corticosteroids
B. Polysomnography
C. Nocturnal pulse oximetry
D. Uvulopalatopharyngoplasty
E. Nasal polypectomy

**VI-37.** All the following are components of polysomnography *except*

A. electrocardiography
B. electromyography
C. electrooculography
D. pulse oximetry
E. arterial carbon dioxide monitoring

**VI-38.** A 64-year-old male presents with a history of cough with rusty-colored sputum for 4 days. In addition, he has had fevers and chills. Past medical history is significant for alcohol abuse and hypertension. He currently is taking no medications. The physical examination reveals a disheveled man with acetone breath. He is febrile to 39.7°C (103.4°F), with an oxygen saturation of 86% on room air. Heart rate is 112, with blood pressure of 136/78. Dentition is poor. Lung examination reveals dullness to percussion with decreased tactile fremitus of approximately half the lung field on the right. Breath sounds are markedly decreased in this area, with crackles and egophony appreciated in the right midlung field. A chest radiogram shows right lower lobe and right middle lobe consolidation with a moderate right-sided effusion. A right lateral decubitus shows that the fluid is not loculated and layers at 1.5 cm along the right chest wall. The patient has a white blood cell count of 24,300/mm³ with 14% bands and 80% polymorphonucleocytes. A sputum Gram stain shows gram-positive diplococci. What is the most appropriate next step?

A. Treatment with ceftriaxone and azithromycin and thoracentesis in 48 h if the fluid does not resolve
B. Immediate thoracentesis after the initiation of antibiotics
C. Computed tomography of the chest to look for an abscess
D. Tube thoracostomy
E. Initiation of therapy with ceftriaxone and clindamycin and consultation with surgery for decortication as the patient probably has an anaerobic pleural infection

**VI-39.** A 52-year-old female presents with a community-acquired pneumonia complicated by pleural effusion. A thoracentesis is performed, with the following results:

**VI-39.** *(Continued)*

| | |
|---|---|
| Appearance | Viscous, cloudy |
| pH | 7.11 |
| Protein | 5.8 g/dL |
| LDH | 285 IU/L |
| Glucose | 66 mg/dL |
| WBC | 3800/mm³ |
| RBC | 24,000/mm³ |
| PMNs | 93% |
| Gram stain | Many PMNs; no organism seen |

Bacterial cultures are sent, but the results are not currently available. Which characteristic of the pleural fluid is most suggestive that the patient will require tube thoracostomy?

A. Presence of more than 90% polymorphonucleocytes (PMNs)
B. Glucose less than 100 mg/dL
C. Presence of more than 1000 white blood cells
D. pH less than 7.20
E. Lactate dehydrogenase (LDH) more than two-thirds of the normal upper limit for serum

**VI-40.** A 42-year-old female presents to the emergency room complaining of dyspnea on exertion for 3 weeks. She has not been febrile but does have a dry cough. Past medical history is significant for chronic active hepatitis B with cirrhosis. Her current medications include furosemide 20 mg daily, spironolactone 50 mg daily, and lactulose 30 g twice daily. On physical examination the patient appears dyspneic. Oxygen saturation is 87% on room air, with a respiratory rate of 32 breaths/min. Chest examination is notable for absent breath sounds throughout the right lung field with dullness to percussion. The patient also has moderate ascites on abdominal examination. A chest radiogram confirms a large right-sided pleural effusion. Thoracentesis reveals a protein of 1.4 g/dL, an LDH of 68 IU/L, a white blood cell count of 32/mm³, and a red blood cell count of 50/mm³. What is the most appropriate management of this patient?

A. Tube thoracostomy for drainage
B. Increased dosage of diuretics
C. Placement of a transjugular intrahepatic portosystemic shunt
D. Liver transplantation
E. Tube thoracostomy followed by pleurodesis

**VI-41.** A 25-year-old male presents to the emergency department complaining of shortness of breath and fevers for 2 weeks. He has a nonproductive cough. The patient is a native of Mexico but has been living in the United States for 3 years. He reports having received BCG vaccination as a child. He has no past medical history and denies tuberculosis or HIV risk factors. The physical examination is remarkable for a temperature of 38.2°C

**VI-41.**   *(Continued)*

(100.8°F). Respiratory rate is 24 breaths/min. He has dullness to percussion with decreased tactile fremitus over the lower third of the right hemithorax. Breath sounds are also decreased in this area. Chest radiography confirms a right pleural effusion without evidence of pneumonia or mediastinal lymphadenopathy. A thoracentesis is performed and reveals the following:

| | |
|---|---|
| WBC | 3329/mm³ |
| Differential | 99% mononuclear cells, 1% polymorphonucleocytes |
| RBC | 24,000/mm³ |
| pH | 7.00 |
| LDH | 620 IU/L |
| Protein | 6 g/dL |
| Glucose | 82 mg/dL |
| Gram stain | No PMNs; no organisms seen |
| AFB stain | Negative |

Which of the following tests is least sensitive for the diagnosis of tuberculous pleural effusion?

A.   Mycobacterial culture of pleural fluid
B.   Pleural fluid adenosine deaminase more than 45 IU/L
C.   Pleural fluid interferon γ above 140 pg/mL
D.   Pleural biopsy showing caseating granuloma formation
E.   Polymerase chain reaction for tuberculous DNA on pleural fluid

**VI-42.**   A 24-year-old male presents with shortness of breath and pleuritic chest pain of 1 week's duration. The pain started while the patient was at rest. He had no antecedent coughing, fevers, or chills. The patient denies trauma or a prior history of lung disease. He currently smokes one pack of cigarettes a day. On physical examination the patient is a thin man who appears to be in no distress. Oxygen saturation is 95% on room air, with a respiratory rate of 20 breaths/min. Heart rate is 110 beats/min, and blood pressure is 116/72. Lung examination reveals decreased lung expansion of the left chest with decreased breath sounds on the left side. A chest radiogram shows a right 30 to 40% pneumothorax. What is the most appropriate next step in the management of this patient?

A.   Tube thoracostomy
B.   Consultation with thoracic surgery for video thorascopy and pleurodesis
C.   Observation
D.   Aspiration of the pleural space
E.   Chest CT to evaluate for underlying lung disease

**VI-43.**   A 32-year-old female presents with subjective complaints of paresthesias and weakness. She reports that she was well until 4 weeks ago, when she had a self-

**VI-43.**   *(Continued)*

limited diarrheal illness that lasted 4 days. For the last week she has noted tingling in the fingers and toes. More recently she feels as if she is developing weakness to the extent where she has difficulty walking because she is unable to lift her toes. Additionally, she feels that she has lost significant grip strength. You suspect Guillain-Barré syndrome after a *Campylobacter* infection, and the patient is hospitalized and started on intravenous immunoglobulin. After the hospitalization, the patient's symptoms worsen so that she now is unable to lift her legs against gravity and is complaining of shortness of breath with a decreased voice. Which of the following is an indication for the initiation of mechanical ventilation in this patient with suspected diaphragmatic weakness?

A.   Vital capacity below 20 mL/kg
B.   Elevated $Pa_{co_2}$
C.   Maximum inspiratory pressure less than 30 cm $H_2O$
D.   Maximum expiratory pressure less than 40 cm $H_2O$
E.   All of the above

**VI-44.**   A 72-year-old female with severe osteoporosis presents for evaluation of shortness of breath. She is a lifetime nonsmoker and has had no exposures. On physical examination you note marked kyphoscoliosis. All the following pulmonary abnormalities are expected *except*

A.   restrictive lung disease
B.   alveolar hypoventilation
C.   obstructive lung disease
D.   ventilation-perfusion abnormalities with hypoxemia
E.   pulmonary hypertension

**VI-45.**   The immune response generated in hypersensitivity pneumonitis is best described as a(n)

A.   allergic reaction
B.   cytotoxic T cell reaction
C.   delayed-type hypersensitivity
D.   immune complex–mediated response

**VI-46.**   A 34-year-old female seeks evaluation for a complaint of cough and dyspnea on exertion that has gradually worsened over 3 months. The patient has no past history of pulmonary complaints and has never had asthma. She started working in a pet store approximately 6 months ago. Her duties there include cleaning the reptile and bird cages. She reports occasional low-grade fevers but has had no wheezing. The cough is dry and nonproductive. Before 3 months ago the patient had no limitation of exercise tolerance, but now she reports that she gets dyspneic climbing two flights of stairs. On physical examina-

**VI-46.** *(Continued)*

tion the patient appears well. She has an oxygen saturation of 95% on room air at rest but desaturates to 91% with ambulation. Temperature is 37.7°C (99.8°F). The pulmonary examination is unremarkable. No clubbing or cyanosis is present. The patient has a normal chest radiogram. A high-resolution chest CT shows diffuse ground-glass infiltrates in the lower lobes with the presence of centrilobular nodules. A transbronchial biopsy shows an interstitial alveolar infiltrate of plasma cells, lymphocytes, and occasional eosinophils. There are also several loose noncaseating granulomas. All cultures are negative for bacterial, viral, and fungal pathogens. What is the diagnosis?

A. Sarcoidosis
B. Psittacosis
C. Hypersensitivity pneumonitis
D. Nonspecific interstitial pneumonitis related to collagen vascular disease
E. Aspergillosis

**VI-47.** What treatment do you recommend?

A. Glucocorticoids
B. Doxycycline
C. Glucocorticoids plus azathioprine
D. Glucocorticoids plus removal of antigen
E. Amphotericin

**VI-48.** All the following drugs can cause eosinophilic pneumonia *except*

A. nitrofurantoin
B. sulfonamides
C. nonsteroidal anti-inflammatory drugs (NSAIDs)
D. isoniazid
E. amiodarone

**VI-49.** A 42-year-old female presents with a 3-month history of cough with fevers and chills. She describes the cough as nonproductive. She has lost 15 lb over this period. The patient has no wheezing or sinus disease. A previous workup failed to yield a diagnosis. Induced sputum cultures for mycobacteria, fungi, bacteria, parasites, and viruses have been negative on four occasions. The only notable laboratory finding is a peripheral blood eosinophilia of 13% with an absolute eosinophil count of 940/mm$^3$. Antinuclear and antineutrophil cytoplasmic antibodies are negative. Chest radiography shows peripherally distributed infiltrates in a pattern of reverse pulmonary edema. What is the diagnosis?

A. Allergic bronchopulmonary aspergillosis
B. Chronic eosinophilic pneumonia
C. Churg-Strauss disease
D. Hypereosinophilic syndrome
E. Tropical eosinophilic pneumonia

**VI-50.** Which of the following interstitial lung diseases is not associated with smoking?

A. Desquamative interstitial pneumonitis
B. Respiratory bronchiolitis – interstitial lung disease
C. Idiopathic pulmonary fibrosis
D. Bronchiolitis obliterans organizing pneumonia
E. Pulmonary Langerhans cell histiocytosis

**VI-51.** A 56-year-old male presents to his primary medical doctor for evaluation of progressive dyspnea and fatigue. The man states that he has felt that he cannot do as much activity as he once could but attributes that to aging. He thinks he first noticed feeling dyspnea with exertion 1 year ago. At that time the patient could no longer carry his golf bag and started to use a golf cart on the course. The patient now reports that he cannot play golf anymore because of shortness of breath. The dyspnea has progressed to the point where the patient feels breathless when he climbs the two flights of stairs in his home from the basement to the bedroom. He frequently has to stop after one flight to catch his breath. There is no past medical history. He smoked cigarettes for 30 years but quit 10 years ago. He takes no medications. The patient has experienced no fevers, chills, or weight loss. On physical examination the patient appears his stated age and does not get dyspneic during conversation. Resting oxygen saturation is 94% on room air; with walking, it declines to 82%. Blood pressure is 128/38, and heart rate is 98 beats/min. The pulmonary examination is remarkable for normal expansion and percussion. On inspiration, fine, dry crackles are heard bilaterally at the bases. The patient has clubbing. No edema or cyanosis is present. What is the best test for definitively making the diagnosis in this patient?

A. Pulmonary function testing
B. High-resolution computed tomography
C. Bronchoscopy with transbronchial biopsy
D. Surgical lung biopsy
E. Ventilation-perfusion scan

**VI-52.** A diagnosis of idiopathic pulmonary fibrosis is made. What do you tell the patient about the treatment and prognosis?

A. His survival and quality of life will be improved with the combined use of prednisone and cyclophosphamide.
B. His 5-year survival is less than 10%.
C. Single-lung transplantation should be considered if he continues to exhibit clinical deterioration while on medical therapy.
D. Interferon $\gamma$ has been shown to improve survival in all patients with this disease.
E. Glucocorticoids alone are the best therapy.

**VI-53.** All the following are pulmonary manifestations of systemic lupus erythematosus *except*

A. pleuritis
B. progressive pulmonary fibrosis
C. pulmonary hemorrhage
D. diaphragmatic dysfunction with loss of lung volumes
E. pulmonary vascular disease

**VI-54.** A 42-year-old male presents with progressive dyspnea on exertion, low-grade fevers, and weight loss over 6 months. He also is complaining of a primarily dry cough, although occasionally he coughs up a thick mucoid sputum. There is no past medical history. He does not smoke cigarettes. On physical examination, the patient appears dyspneic with minimal exertion. The patient's temperature is 37.9°C (100.3°F). Oxygen saturation is 91% on room air at rest. Faint basilar crackles are heard. On laboratory studies, the patient has polyclonal hypergammaglobulinemia and a hematocrit of 52%. A CT scan reveals bilateral alveolar infiltrates that are primarily perihilar in nature with a mosaic pattern. The patient undergoes bronchoscopy with bronchoalveolar lavage. The effluent appears milky. The cytopathology shows amorphous debris with periodic acid-Schiff (PAS)-positive macrophages. What is the diagnosis?

A. Bronchiolitis obliterans organizing pneumonia
B. Desquamative interstitial pneumonitis
C. Nocardiosis
D. *Pneumoncystis carinii* pneumonia
E. Pulmonary alveolar proteinosis

**VI-55.** What treatment is most appropriate at this time?

A. Prednisone and cyclophosphamide
B. Trimethoprim-sulfamethoxazole
C. Prednisone
D. Whole-lung saline lavage
E. Doxycycline

**VI-56.** A 25-year-old African-American male is seen in the clinic for evaluation of cough of 6 months' duration. He reports paroxysms of coughing lasting several minutes that occur at any time of the day or night and in all seasons of the year. He has no sputum production and no associated fever, chills, or weight loss. There is no wheezing. He takes no medications besides guaifenesin and has no allergies. He denies tobacco use. Physical examination shows cobblestoning of the oropharyngeal mucosa, normal breath sounds, and a normal cardiac examination. Which of the following findings is likely on a chest radiogram?

A. Bronchiectasis
B. Bilateral hilar adenopathy

**VI-56.** *(Continued)*
C. Bilateral alveolar infiltrates
D. Normal findings
E. Cardiomegaly

**VI-57.** A 68-year-old male is seen in the clinic for evaluation of chronic cough that has lasted 4 months. He reports that the cough is dry and occurs at any time of the day. He denies hemoptysis or associated constitutional symptoms. Further, there is no wheezing, acid reflux symptoms, or postnasal drip. Past medical history is notable for a well-compensated ischemic cardiomyopathy that was diagnosed 6 months ago. His current medications include aspirin, carvedilol, furosemide, ramipril, amlodipine, and digoxin. He has no history of tobacco or alcohol abuse and denies occupational exposure. Physical examination shows a normal upper airway, clear lungs, and a normal cardiac examination with the exception of an enlarged point of maximal impulse. Plain radiography of the chest is normal with the exception of cardiomegaly. Which of the following is the most appropriate next step in his management?

A. Bronchoscopy
B. Changing furosemide to bumetanide
C. Discontinuing digoxin
D. Changing ramipril to valsartan
E. Giving azithromycin for 5 days

**VI-58.** A patient is admitted to the intensive care unit with massive hemoptysis from an area of bronchiectasis in the right upper lobe airway. Which of the following interventions is indicated for acute managment?

A. Antitussive admininistration
B. Dual-lumen intubation
C. Positioning the patient right side down
D. A and B
E. A, B, and C

**VI-59.** A 78-year-old male is seen for evaluation of cough. He has had a cough for over 3 months that he reports is productive of blood-streaked yellow sputum. The patient has received several courses of antibiotics without any improvement. His other medical problems include atrial fibrillation, hypertension, and benign prostatic hypertrophy. His medications include lisinopril, warfarin, and prazosin. The patient has a history of smoking more than 100 packs a year. Physical examination is normal, as is PA and lateral chest film. Which of the following is the most appropriate next step?

A. Acid-fast stain and culture of sputum
B. Initiation of omeprazole
C. Initiation of inhaled ipratropium bromide
D. Bronchoscopy
E. Discontinuation of lisinopril

**VI-60.** Which of the following is not a physiologic response to hypoxia?

A. Erythrocytosis
B. Hyperventilation
C. Increased cardiac output
D. Lactic acidosis
E. Systemic arterial vasoconstriction

**VI-61.** A patient is evaluated in the emergency department for peripheral cyanosis. Which of the following is not a potential etiology?

A. Cold exposure
B. Deep venous thrombosis
C. Methemoglobinemia
D. Peripheral vascular disease
E. Raynaud's phenomenon

**VI-62.** Which of the following is the most common cause of mortality in patients who survive more than 1 year after lung transplantation?

A. Acute rejection
B. Bronchomalacia
C. Chronic rejection
D. CMV infection
E. Ischemia–reperfusion injury

**VI-63.** A 63-year-old female is seen in the pulmonary clinic for evaluation of progressive dyspnea. She underwent single-lung transplantation 4 years ago for idiopathic pulmonary fibrosis and did well until the last 6 months, when she noted that her exercise tolerance had decreased as a result of shortness of breath. She denies fevers, chills, weight loss, or medication noncompliance. The patient does have an occasional dry cough. Her current medications include tacrolimus, prednisone, trimethoprim-sulfamethoxazole (TMP-SMX), pantoprazole, diltiazem, and mycophenolate mofetil. She denies any current habits but has a remote history of tobacco use. Physical examination is notable for dry crackles on the side of the native lung and decreased breath sounds on the side of the transplanted lung but no adventitious sounds. Review of pulmonary function testing shows an $FEV_1/FVC$ ratio of 50% of the predicted value and an $FEV_1$ of 0.91 L. Additionally, $FEV_1$ has fallen by 30% progressively over the last year. Which of the following can ameliorate the fall in $FEV_1$ in this patient?

A. Augmented immunosuppression
B. Reduced immunosuppression
C. Antifungal therapy
D. Antiviral therapy
E. Administration of $\alpha_1$ antitrypsin
F. None of the above

**VI-64.** A 55-year-old female is seen in the clinic with a recent diagnosis of idiopathic pulmonary fibrosis. Her dyspnea on exertion is stable. She is currently not taking any medications. Besides evaluating the need for supplemental oxygen and appropriate vaccinations, which of the following interventions should be done?

A. Initiation of *Pneumocystis carinii* prophylaxis
B. Initiation of inhaled glucocorticoids
C. Referral for lung transplantation
D. B and C
E. A, B, and C

**VI-65.** A 23-year-old male is climbing Mount Kilimanjaro. He has no medical problems and takes no medications. Shortly after beginning the climb, he develops severe shortness of breath. Physical examination shows diffuse bilateral inspiratory crackles. Which of the following is the most likely etiology?

A. Acute interstitial pneumonitis
B. Acute respiratory distress sydrome
C. Cardiogenic shock
D. Community-acquired pneumonia
E. High-altitude pulmonary edema

**VI-66.** Which of the following statements about this condition is true?

A. Acetazolamide is indicated for the treatment of this disorder.
B. Older patients are more at risk for this disorder than are younger patients because hypoxic vasoconstriction is more pronounced as patients age.
C. Oxygen is an ineffective therapy for this disorder.
D. Persons who live at high altitudes are not at risk for this disorder even when they return to a high altitude after time spent at sea level.
E. Prevention can be achieved by means of gradual ascent.

**VI-67.** A 58-year-old male is seen in the clinic for evaluation of dyspnea on exertion. He has a history of myocardial infarction 5 years ago and a tobacco use history of 75 packs a year, though he quit after the myocardial infarction. A pulmonary function test shows mild obstruction but no other abnormality. To determine if the patient's dyspnea results from cardiac or pulmonary dysfunction, cardiopulmonary exercise testing is ordered. Which of the following findings suggests that his symptoms are due to pulmonary dysfunction?

1. Blood pressure drop with maximum exercise
2. Heart rate more than 85% of the predicted rate
3. Increased ratio of dead space to tidal volume
4. Oxygen desaturation

**VI-67.** *(Continued)*

A.  1
B.  1 and 2
C.  1, 3, and 4
D.  3 and 4
E.  1, 2, 3, and 4

**VI-68.**  A patient is evaluated for an abnormal respiratory pattern noted by his wife. The patient denies dyspnea at rest, though he is short of breath with exertion. On observation, he is noted to have a Cheyne-Stokes respiratory pattern. Which of the following is likely to be found on physical examination?

A.  Diffuse wheezing
B.  Depressed jugular venous pressure
C.  Fruity odor on the breath
D.  Morbid obesity
E.  Third heart sound

**VI-69.**  A 65-year-old male is seen for evaluation of cough and fever. The symptoms developed 24 h ago and are notable for yellow phlegm, right-sided pleuritic chest pain, and fevers of 38.5°C (101.3°F). Physical examination shows fever and dullness to percussion in the right lower lung field with crackles and egophony. Chest radiography shows a right lower lobe infiltrate. What is the most likely method of acquisition of the organism causing this disorder?

A.  Aerosol inhalation
B.  Direct extension from a contiguous infected site
C.  Gross aspiration
D.  Hematogenous spread
E.  Microaspiration

**VI-70.**  With regard to therapy for community-acquired pneumonia, which of the following statements is true?

A.  In therapy for community-acquired pneumonia, the lowest mortality rate is associated with combination therapy with an aminoglycoside and another antibiotic.
B.  Mortality is higher in patients with penicillin-nonsusceptible pneumococcus than in patients who have susceptible isolates of pneumococcus.
C.  Patients who have been treated with fluoroquinolone in the last 3 months are eligible to receive fluoroquinolone therapy again for community-acquired pneumonia.
D.  Patients who receive antibiotics within 8 h of arrival in the emergency department have lower mortality than do those who receive antibiotic more than 8 h after arrival.

**VI-70.**  *(Continued)*

E.  The percentage of penicillin-nonsusceptible pneumococci is negligible and should not be taken into account in choosing initial therapy for community-acquired pneumonia.

**VI-71.**  A 59-year-old African-American female is admitted to the hospital with community-acquired pneumonia. She has a past medical history notable for COPD and hypertension. Her current medications are albuterol and chlorthalidone. Although she quit tobacco use 5 years ago, her husband continues to smoke. Blood cultures rapidly grow *S. pneumoniae.* Which of the following are her risk factors for invasive pneumococcal disease?

A.  African-American ethnicity
B.  History of chronic illness
C.  Passive tobacco exposure
D.  A and B
E.  A, B, and C

**VI-72.**  A 58-year-old male is evaluated after several weeks of night sweats and cough productive of putrid sputum. He also reports about a 10-lb weight loss. He takes no medications and has no allergies. The patient drinks alcohol daily: approximately 12 beers per day. Physical examination is notable for a temperature of 37.8°C (100°F), poor dentition, clear lung fields, and mild clubbing; the remainder of the examination is normal. His sputum is noted to be yellow and foul-smelling. Chest radiography shows a thick-walled abscess in the right middle lobe. Which of the following is appropriate initial therapy for this patient?

A.  Ceftazidime
B.  Clindamycin
C.  Levofloxacin
D.  Surgical resection
E.  Trimethoprim-sulfamethoxizole

**VI-73.**  A 63-year-old female is in the intensive care unit for urosepsis. She required intubation and mechanical ventilation early in the course. Blood and urine cultures initially grew *Escherichia coli* and sterilized within 2 days of admission. However, she was unable to be extubated because of depressed mental status. The patient is started on enteral nutrition through a nasogastric tube. On the seventh hospital day the patient has increasing respiratory secretions and a fever. A chest radiogram is obtained and shows a new infiltrate in the right lower lobe. Current medications include cefazolin, omeprazole, and acetaminophen. Which of the following interventions has been shown to prevent this complication?

A.  Elevation of the head of the bed to 30°
B.  Frequent ventilator circuit changes

**VI-73.** *(Continued)*

C. Prophylactic antibiotics

D. Selective digestive decontamination

E. Stomach placement of an enteral feeding tube

**VI-74.** Appropriate antibiotic therapy for this patient would be

A. ceftazidime

B. ceftriaxone and azithromycin

C. levofloxacin

D. vancomycin and ceftazidime

E. vancomycin

**VI-75.** A 67-year-old female is admitted to the hospital with a hip fracture after a fall. Which of the following regimens constitutes appropriate venous thromboembolism prophylaxis for this patient?

A. Intermittent pneumatic compression devices

B. Subcutaneous unfractionated heparin

C. Subcutaneous low-molecular-weight heparin

D. Warfarin, with a target international normalized ratio (INR) of 1.5 to 2.0

E. A and B

**VI-76.** A 63-year-old male with a long history of cigarette smoking comes to see you for a 4-month history of progressive shortness of breath and dyspnea on exertion. The symptoms have been indolent, with no recent worsening. He denies fever, chest pain, or hemoptysis. He has a daily cough of 3 to 6 tablespoons of yellow phlegm. The patient says he has not seen a physician for over 10 years. Physical examination is notable for normal vital signs, a prolonged expiratory phase, scattered rhonchi, elevated jugular venous pulsation, and moderate pedal edema. Hematocrit is 49%. Which of the following therapies is most likely to prolong his survival?

A. Atenolol

B. Enalapril

C. Oxygen

D. Prednisone

E. Theophylline

**VI-77.** A patient who is being evaluated for shortness of breath is found to have an arterial $P_{o_2}$ of 7.9 kPa (59 mmHg) while breathing room air at sea level and an arterial $P_{o_2}$ of 8.1 kPa (61 mmHg) while breathing 40% inspired $O_2$. The arterial $P_{co_2}$ is normal. Which of the following conditions is most likely to account for these findings?

A. Idiopathic pulmonary fibrosis

B. Chronic obstructive pulmonary disease

C. Severe asthma exacerbation

D. $\alpha_1$-Antitrypsin deficiency

E. Osler-Rendu-Weber syndrome

**VI-78.** Although asthma is a heterogeneous disease, an individual with asthma would be most likely to

A. relate a personal or family history of allergic diseases

B. conform to a characteristic personality type

C. display a skin-test reaction to extracts of airborne allergens

D. demonstrate nonspecific airway hyperirritability

E. have supranormal serum immunoglobulin E

**VI-79.** A 22-year-old female with a history of intermittent wheezing in response to exercise presents to the emergency room with shortness of breath. The attack occurred during an aerobics class. At this point she is having obvious difficulty breathing and has diffuse wheezes on pulmonary examination. $O_2$ saturation is 95% by pulse oximetry. The most effective treatment at this point would be

A. intravenous aminophylline

B. inhaled cromolyn sodium

C. inhaled albuterol

D. intravenous hydrocortisone

E. inhaled beclomethasone

**VI-80.** A 23-year-old female complains of dyspnea and substernal chest pain on exertion. Evaluation for this complaint 6 months ago included arterial blood gas testing, which revealed pH 7.48, $P_{o_2}$ 79 mmHg, and $P_{co_2}$ 31 mmHg. Electrocardiography then showed a right axis deviation. Chest x-ray now shows enlarged pulmonary arteries but no parenchymal infiltrates, and a lung perfusion scan reveals subsegmental defects that are thought to have a "low probability for pulmonary thromboembolism." Echocardiography demonstrates right heart strain but no evidence of primary cardiac disease. The most appropriate diagnostic test now would be

A. open lung biopsy

B. Holter monitoring

C. right-heart catheterization

D. transbronchial biopsy

E. serum $\alpha_1$-antitrypsin level

**Questions VI-81 to VI-82.** A 35-year-old male seeks medical attention for breathlessness on exertion. He has never smoked cigarettes and has not been coughing. One sibling died of respiratory failure at 40 years of age. His three children are healthy. Physical examination reveals the patient to be tachypneic as he exhales through pursed lips. His chest is tympanitic to percussion, and breath sounds are poorly heard on auscultation. Chest x-ray shows flattened diaphragms with peripheral attenuation of bronchovascular markings that is most noticeable at the lung bases.

**VI-81.** Expected results of pulmonary function testing of this patient would include

  A. increased lung elastic recoil
  B. increased total lung capacity
  C. reduced functional residual capacity
  D. increased vital capacity
  E. increased diffusing capacity

**VI-82.** Which of the following would be the most reasonable next step in the assessment of this patient?

  A. Measurement of serum $\alpha_1$-antitrypsin activity
  B. Measurement of sweat chloride concentration
  C. High-resolution CT scan

**VI-82.** *(Continued)*
  D. Exercise stress test
  E. Echocardiogram

**VI-83.** A 19-year-old normal nonsmoking female has a moderately severe pulmonary embolism while on oral contraceptive pills. Which of the following is the most likely predisposing factor?

  A. Abnormal factor V
  B. Abnormal protein C
  C. Diminished protein C level
  D. Diminished protein S level
  E. Diminished antithrombin III level

# VI. DISORDERS OF THE RESPIRATORY SYSTEM

## ANSWERS

**VI-1. The answer is B.** *(Chap. 243)* This patient's clinical-radiologic presentation, in addition to the lung function information, which revealed a moderate restrictive defect and a moderate gas transfer defect, suggests an acute pneumonitis. The differential diagnosis includes various causes of diffuse alveolar hemorrhage, idiopathic bronchiolitis obliterans organizing pneumonia, acute eosinophilic pneumonia, interstitial lung disease secondary to connective tissue disorders [systemic lupus erythematosus (SLE), rheumatoid arthritis, polymyositis], and diffuse alveolar damage secondary to other causes (sepsis, drugs, toxins, infections, etc.). Methotrexate has been associated with an idiosyncratic drug reaction, with particular risk in the elderly and in patients with decreased creatinine clearance. Discontinuing the medicine and in some cases adding high-dose steroids constitute the initial management. Initiating empirical broad-spectrum antibiotics until a more definite result could be obtained via a bronchoscopy would be a reasonable approach.

**VI-2. The answer is B.** *(Chap. 233)* This patient presents with subacute-onset dyspnea and an examination consistent with pleural effusion. Dullness to percussion can be seen with consolidation, atelectasis, and pleural effusion. With consolidation, voice transmission is increased during expiration so that one may hear whispered pectoriloquy or egophony. However, in both pleural effusion and atelectasis, breath sounds are diminished and there is no augmentation of voice transmission. Although this patient could have either atelectasis or pleural effusion, the lack of tracheal deviation points to pleural effusion. Atelectasis would have to be of many segments to account for these findings, and such significant airway collapse would generally cause ipsilateral tracheal deviation. The clinician would expect to find pleural effusion on chest film, and the most appropriate next management step would be thoracentesis to aid in the diagnosis of the etiology and for symptomatic relief. With a lack of symptoms to suggest infection, antibiotics are not indicated. Similarly, in the absence of wheezing or significant sputum production, bronchodilators and deep suctioning are unlikely to be helpful. Bronchoscopy may be indicated ultimately in the management of this patient, particularly if malignancy is suspected; however, the most appropriate first attempt at diagnosis is by means of thoracentesis.

**VI-3, VI-4, VI-5, and VI-6. The answers are C, B, D, and A.** *(Chap. 234)* Ventilatory function can be easily measured with lung volume measurement and the $FEV_1/FVC$ ratio. A decreased $FEV_1/FVC$ ratio diagnoses obstructive lung disease. Alternatively, low lung volumes, specifically decreased TLC, and occasionally decreased RV diagnose restrictive lung disease. With extensive air trapping in obstructive lung disease, TLC is often increased and RV may also be increased. VC is proportionally decreased. MIP measures respiratory muscle strength and is decreased in patients with neuromuscular disease. Thus, myasthenia gravis will produce low lung volumes and decreased MIP, whereas patients with idiopathic pulmonary fibrosis will have normal muscle strength and subsequently a normal MIP but decreased TLC and RV. In some cases of pulmonary parenchymal restrictive lung disease, the increase in elastic recoil results in an increased $FEV_1/FVC$ ratio. The hallmark of obstructive lung disease is a decreased $FEV_1/FVC$ ratio; thus, the correct answer for QVI-6 is A.

**VI-7. The answer is A.** *(Chap. 234)* Spirometry does not measure total lung capacity because it cannot account for residual volume. The most frequently used and accurate measures of lung volumes are steady-state helium dilution lung volumes and body plethysmography. In helium dilution the patient inspires a known concentration of helium from a closed circuit of known volume. After the patient rebreathes in the closed circuit for a period of time, the concentration of helium equilibrates, and subsequently the lung volumes can be calculated by using Avogadro's law. This calculation assumes that gas in the circuit will rapidly equilibrate with the ventilated portions of the lung. However, if there are slowly emptying areas of the lung, as in cystic fibrosis patients, or parts of the lung that do not participate in gas exchange at all, as in bullous emphysema patients, helium dilution will underestimate true lung volumes. Subsequently, body plethysmography is the preferred method for lung volume measurement in these disease states. To perform body plethysmography, the patient sits in a sealed box and pants against a closed mouthpiece. Panting results in changes in the pressure of the box that, when compared with changes at the mouthpiece, can be used to calculate lung volumes. This method measures total thoracic gas volume and is more accurate than helium dilution. Helium lung volumes are easier to perform for patients and staff and give reliable results in most circumstances. Many centers measure a single-breath helium dilution lung volume when measuring the diffusing capacity of carbon monoxide, which has the same or greater limitations as the rebreathing method. Transdiaphragmatic pressure is used to measure respiratory muscle strength, not lung volumes.

**VI-8.  The answer is B.**  *(Chap. 241)*  Patients with cystic fibrosis are at risk for colonization and/or infection with a number of pathogens, and in general these infections have a temporal relationship. In childhood, the most frequently isolated organisms are *Haemophilus influenzae* and *Staphylococcus aureus*. As patients age, *Pseudomonas aeruginosa* becomes the predominant pathogen. Interestingly, *Aspergillus fumigatus* is found in the airways of up to 50% of cystic fibrosis patients. All these organisms merely colonize the airways but occasionally can also cause disease. *Burkholderia* (previously called *Pseudomonas*) *cepacia* can occasionally be found in the sputum of cystic fibrosis patients, where it is always pathogenic and is associated with a rapid decline in both clinical parameters and pulmonary function testing. Atypical myocobacteria can occasionally be found in the sputum but are often merely colonizers. *Acinetobacter baumannii* is not associated with cystic fibrosis; rather, it is generally found in nosocomial infections.

**VI-9.  The answer is C.**  *(Chap. 241)*  This patient has a history suggestive of cystic fibrosis, with the exception of her age. The persistent asthma, airflow obstruction, and sputum cultures growing *P. aeruginosa* and *S. aureus* coupled with bilateral upper lobe infiltrates should prompt further investigation for this disease. The diagnosis of cystic fibrosis is based on clinical criteria plus laboratory evidence. The laboratory test of choice remains analysis of sweat chloride values. Patients with mutations in the cystic fibrosis transmembrane regulator (CFTR) will have increased amounts of chloride in their sweat, and a chloride value over 70 meq/L will generally be found. Approximately 1 to 2% of patients with cystic fibrosis will have normal results of sweat chloride testing, and in these cases the nasal transepithelial potential difference has been used for diagnosis. While the ΔF508 mutation accounts for the majority of patients with cystic fibrosis, more than 1000 other mutations that can cause this disorder have been described. Thus, the absence of this mutation does not rule out cystic fibrosis. Bronchoscopy with transbronchial biopsy probably will show bronchiectasis and chronic airway inflammation but will not be diagnostic. Similar findings probably will be found on a chest CT but are not diagnostic.

**VI-10.  The answer is B.**  *(Chap. 238)*  The patient presents with typical asthma symptoms; however, the symptoms are escalating and now require nearly constant use of oral steroids. It is of note that the symptoms are worse during weekdays and better on weekends. This finding suggests that there is an exposure during the week that may be triggering the patient's asthma. Often textile workers have asthma resulting from the inhalation of particles. The first step in diagnosing a work-related asthma trigger is to check $FEV_1$ before and after the first shift of the workweek. A decrease in $FEV_1$ would suggest an occupational exposure. Skin testing for allergies would not be likely to pinpoint the work-related exposure. Although *A. fumigatus* can be associated with worsening asthma from allergic bronchopulmonary aspergillosis, this would not have a fluctuation in symptoms throughout the week. The patient does not require further testing to diagnose that he has asthma; therefore, a methacholine challenge is not indicated. Finally, the exercise physiology test is generally used to differentiate between cardiac and pulmonary causes or deconditioning as etiologies for shortness of breath.

**VI-11. The answer is B.** *(Chap. 238)* Asbestos was a commonly used insulating material from the 1940s to the mid-1970s, after which it was largely replaced by fiberglass and slag wool. Workers in many occupations had significant exposure and often did not use protective equipment. There are several pulmonary manifestations of asbestos exposure in the lungs, the most important of which are pleural plaques, benign asbestos pleural effusions, asbestosis, lung cancer, and mesothelioma. Pleural plaques, which appear as calcifications or thickening along the parietal pleura, simply suggest exposure and not pulmonary impairment. Benign pleural effusions can occur and are often bloody. They may regress or progress spontaneously. Asbestosis refers to interstitial lung disease, generally with fibrosis, seen in the lower lung fields of a chest radiogram or chest CT and an associated restrictive ventilatory defect. This patient does not have interstitial changes on chest radiography and has no restriction on pulmonary function tests; therefore, he does not have asbestosis. The risk of lung cancer, including squamous cell cancer and adenocarcinoma, is elevated in all patients with asbestos exposure but is amplified further by cigarette smoking. In contrast, mesothelioma risk, though elevated in patients with asbestos exposure, is not increased by cigarette smoking. Interestingly, despite the high risk of malignancies in this group of patients, no benefit has been ascribed to screening techniques, including biannual chest radiograms.

**VI-12. The answer is D.** *(Chap. 238)* The patient presents with acute-onset pulmonary symptoms, including wheezing, with no other medical problems. He is a farmer and was recently handling hay. The clinical presentation and radiogram are consistent with farmer's lung, a hypersensitivity pneumonitis caused by *Actinomyces*. In this disorder moldy hay with spores of actinomycetes are inhaled and produce a hypersensitivity pneumonitis. The disorder is seen most commonly in rainy periods, when the spores multiply. Patients present generally 4 to 8 h after exposure with fever, cough, and shortness of breath without wheezing. Chest radiograms often show patchy bilateral, often upper lobe infiltrates. The exposure history will differentiate this disorder from other types of pneumonia.

**VI-13. The answer is E.** *(Chap. 238)* Passive cigarette smoking, or secondhand smoking, has been associated in the last 15 years with many adverse outcomes. A correlation has been demonstrated between the number of smokers in a house and the concentration of respirable particulate load. Furthermore, meta-analyses of the best data have shown that persons who receive passive cigarette smoke have a 25% increase in mortality associated with lung cancer, respiratory illness, and cardiac disease compared with persons without such an exposure. Children with smoking parents have been shown to have an increased prevalence of respiratory illness and decreased lung function compared with nonexposed children.

**VI-14. The answer is A.** *(Chaps. 30, 243, and 299)* A variety of autoimmune diseases may cause pulmonary/renal disease, including Wegener's granulomatosis, microscopic polyangiitis, SLE, and cryoglobulinemia. Goodpasture's syndrome is characterized by the presence of anti–glomerular basement antibodies that cause glomerulonephritis with concurrent diffuse alveolar hemorrhage. The disease typically presents in patients over 40 years old with a history of cigarette smoking. These patients usually do not have fevers or joint symptoms. Among the listed options, antibodies to glutamic acid decarboxylase are seen in patients with type 1 diabetes or stiff-man syndrome, anti–smooth muscle antibodies in patients with autoimmune hepatitis, and anti–U1 RNP in those with mixed connective tissue disease. Antiphospholipid antibody syndrome may cause renal disease and alveolar hemorrhage, but this usually occurs in the context of a systemic illness with prominent thrombosis in other organ systems [extremities, central nervous system (CNS)].

**VI-15.   The answer is D.**   *(Chap. 243)*   This patient's presentation is typical of pulmonary Langerhans cell histiocytosis (eosinophilic granulomas). Cigarette smoking is virtually universal among these patients. The disease may be found incidentally on radiograms or may present with respiratory and systemic complaints. Spontaneous pneumothorax is a common presentation and occurs in approximately 25% of these patients. The radiographic combination of small reticular/nodular opacities in the bases (with sparing of the costophrenic angle) and apical cysts is characteristic and virtually diagnostic. Pulmonary function testing will show a reduced DLCO. Lung volumes may be normal or reduced, depending on the severity. Approximately 33% of these patients improve with smoking cessation, but most develop progressive interstitial disease. Immunosuppressive agents do not appear to influence the course of disease. Intravenous $\alpha_1$ antitrypsin may benefit patients with deficiency, who will present with lower lobe emphysema. Miliary tuberculosis radiographically appears with multiple small nodules, but cysts are not typical. *Pneumocystic carinii* pneumonia (PCP) may present with spontaneous pneumothorax in patients with HIV infection; however, this patient has no apparent risk factors, and the small nodules on CT are not typical.

**VI-16.   The answer is B.**   *(Chap. 150)*   Pleural tuberculosis is a form of primary infection that occurs when a small number of tubercle bacilli penetrate from the primary lung infection into the pleura and evoke a vigorous immune reaction. These infections may resolve spontaneously but when diagnosed should be treated because of the risk of dissemination or reactivation. The PPD will be positive in over two-thirds of cases because the pleural disease is partially mediated by a hypersensitivity response similar to the PPD skin response. Because of the paucity of organisms, pleural fluid cultures are seldom positive. Pleural biopsy demonstrates noncaseating granulomas and tissue cultures are positive in approximately 70% of cases. Tube thoracostomy is seldom necessary in patients without empyema.

**VI-17.   The answer is A.**   *(Chap. 150)*   This patient has evidence of recent tuberculosis infection with the change from a negative to a positive PPD. A chest radiogram should be performed to rule out active disease and the presence of latent disease. If there is no abnormality, isoniazid should be prescribed to prevent subsequent development of active disease. The optimal duration of therapy is 6 to 12 months, with most recommending 9 months to achieve maximal protection from active disease. The major complication of this therapy is hepatitis. Isoniazid should not be given to patients with active liver disease. All these patients should be educated about the signs or symptoms of hepatitis and should be instructed to discontinue the medication if those symptoms develop. Patients should be questioned about symptoms monthly. Baseline liver function tests need be obtained only in patients with a history of liver disease or daily alcohol use. Serial measurement of liver function is not necessary in the absence of a history of liver disease or alcohol use.

**VI-18.   The answer is B.**   *(Chap. 150)*   *M. tuberculosis* is spread by droplet nuclei that are aerosolized by coughing, sneezing, or speaking. The droplets dry quickly and may stay airborne and subject to inhalation for hours. The probability of acquiring tuberculosis is related to the degree of infectiousness and the intimacy and duration of contact. Smear-positive patients have the greatest infectivity. Patients with cavitary, laryngeal, or endobronchial disease produce the most infectious organisms. Patients with smear-negative/culture-positive or disseminated disease are less infectious. Patients with culture-negative (treated) or extrapulmonary tuberculosis are essentially noninfectious. Patients with tuberculosis who are HIV-infected also appear to be less infectious because of the lower frequency of cavitary disease. These factors emphasize the importance of public health measures to control the transmission of tuberculosis.

**VI-19.    The answer is D.**    *(Chap. 150)*    HIV infection is an important factor in the recent rise in the worldwide incidence of tuberculosis. A person with latent tuberculosis who acquires HIV infection is estimated to have a 3 to 15% annual risk of developing active tuberculosis, which is substantially higher than the risk in HIV-uninfected individuals. Active tuberculosis may develop at any point in the course of HIV infection. The clinical presentation varies with the degree of immune suppression. Typical upper lobe cavitary disease is common early in the course of HIV infection, when immune suppression is least. As the degree of immune suppression becomes more advanced, extrapulmonary or atypical presentations such as mediastinal lymph node, disseminated, and meningeal disease become more common. HIV-infected patients have a decreased frequency of sputum smear–positive disease that in conjunction with the atypical presentations makes diagnosis often more difficult than is the case in HIV-uninfected individuals.

**VI-20.    The answer is B.**    *(Chap. 150)*    Skin testing with PPD is still widely used as a screening tool for latent tuberculosis, although newer methods utilizing cytokine release have been approved by the U.S. Food and Drug Administration (FDA) and are being refined. In quantifying the PPD response it is important to measure the diameter of induration, not inflammation. False-negative reactions are most common in immune-suppressed patients and those with overwhelming active tuberculosis. The interpretation of a positive PPD response is dependent on the patient being tested. Infection with nontuberculosis strains of mycobacterium and prior vaccination with BCG may cause a false-positive reaction. Patients with HIV infection, close contacts of patients with active tuberculosis, and individuals with fibrotic lesions on chest radiography have a threshold of 5 mm for a positive PPD test. Patients with high-risk medical conditions, including diabetes mellitus, or with occupations with potential exposure have a threshold of 10 mm for a positive PPD test. Individuals with a low risk of prior tuberculosis exposure have a threshold of 15 mm for a positive PPD test.

**VI-21.    The answer is E.**    *(Chap. 117)*    Patients with lung transplants have the highest risk of pneumonia among all recipients of solid organ transplants. The pathogens causing pulmonary infections vary with the time after transplantation. The most common pathogens in the first 2 weeks (early period) after surgery are the gram-negative bacteria, particularly Enteriobacteriaceae and *Pseudomonas, Staphylococcus, Aspergillus,* and *Candida.* Between 1 and 6 months (middle period), most infections are due to either primary activation or reactivation of CMV. CMV pneumonia is often difficult to distinguish from acute transplant rejection. More than 6 months after a transplant (late period), the chronic suppression of cell-mediated immunity places patients at risk of infection from *Pneumocystis, Nocardia, Listeria,* other fungi, and intracellular pathogens. Pretransplant lung donor cultures often guide posttransplant empirical antibiotic choices. Prophylaxis against CMV in seropositive donors or recipients and *Pneumocystis* is routine after lung transplantation.

**VI-22.    The answer is C.**    *(Chap. 117)*    Human herpesvirus type 8 (HHV-8) is causally associated with primary effusion lymphoma as well as Kaposi's sarcoma and multicentric Castleman's disease. Primary effusion lymphoma is composed of T lymphocytes. Patients with chronic profound impairment of cell-mediated immunity such as HIV infection, solid organ transplantation, and bone marrow transplantation are at risk of disease. Epstein-Barr virus can cause posttransplant B cell lymphoproliferative disease in transplant recipients. Parvovirus B19 infection does not cause lymphoma but may lead to a pure red blood cell aplasia. Cytomegalovirus causes acute pneumonitis and has been associated with an increased risk of chronic rejection or bronchiolitis obliterans syndrome after lung transplantation. Respiratory syncytial virus may cause an acute pneumonitis after lung transplantation.

**VI-23.    The answer is C.**    *(Chaps. 148 and 239)*    The radiogram shows a left lower lobe lung abscess that most likely is due to anaerobic infection. The anaerobes involved are most likely oral, but *Bacteroides fragilis* is isolated in up to 10% of cases. Vancomycin, ciprofloxacin, and cephalexin have no significant activity against anaerobes. Most oral anaerobic strains have the capacity to produce β-lactamase. For many years penicillin was considered the standard treatment for anaerobic lung infections. However, clinical studies have demonstrated the superiority of clindamycin over penicillin in the treatment of lung abscess. When there are contraindications to clindamycin, penicillin plus metronidazole is likely to be as effective as clindamycin.

**VI-24.  The answer is D.**  *(Chap. 155)*  This patient presents with the classic findings of severe leptospirosis (Weil's syndrome). Leptospires are spirochetes that persist in the renal tubules of a variety of animal reservoirs. The most important reservoir is the rat, and humans are infected after exposure to rat urine. Exposure to rodent urine followed by a flulike illness approximately 1 week later is typical for anicteric leptospirosis. Many of these patients with mild disease have resolution of their symptoms within a week and then develop a recurrence after 1 to 3 days during the immune phase. It is during the immune phase that patients develop aseptic meningitis. A minority of patients with leptospirosis develop Weil's syndrome, which is characterized by severe jaundice without evidence of hepatocellular damage, acute renal failure, and respiratory failure. Conjunctival suffusion is a classic physical finding. Rhabdomyolysis, hemolysis, shock, and adult respiratory distress syndrome may develop. The diagnosis is usually established by serology; culture is performed in reference laboratories and takes weeks. In cases of presumptive severe leptospirosis, therapy with penicillin, amoxicillin, erythromycin, or doxycycline should be initiated. Newer-generation cephalosporins have in vitro activity, but no clinical studies have evaluated in vivo efficacy. Severe leptospirosis is epidemiologically and clinically similar to hantavirus infection.

**VI-25.  The answer is D.**  *(Chap. 27)*  Upper respiratory tract infections (URIs) are the leading cause of ambulatory care visits in the United States and have a major impact on public health. Nonspecific URIs include rhinitis, rhinopharyngitis, coryza, and the common cold. Approximately 30 to 40% of these infections are caused by one of the over 100 immunotypes of rhinovirus. Influenza, adenovirus, parainfluenza, and coronavirus are also common causes. RSV accounts for only a small percentage of cases, particularly in adults. Enteroviruses, rubella virus, and varicella virus usually do not cause URIs. Bacterial URIs represent less than 25% of cases, yet this is the leading diagnosis for the prescription of antibiotics in the United States. This practice has led to enormous unnecessary costs and contributed to the rapid rise in the prevalence of antibiotic-resistant *S. pneumoniae,* the most common cause of bacterial pneumonia.

**VI-26.  The answer is B.**  *(Chap. 27)*  Antibiotics are tremendously overprescribed for the presumptive diagnosis of acute sinusitis. Acute bacterial sinusitis is uncommon in patients with symptoms of less than 7 days' duration even in the presence of purulent discharge. Most cases are due to viral infections. Decongestants and nasal lavage should be prescribed initially. In a patient with a known history of allergic rhinitis, nasal corticosteroids may be added. Empirical antibiotic therapy may be prescribed for patients whose symptoms do not improve with conservative therapy after 1 week and patients with a known predisposition to sinus infection (e.g., cystic fibrosis). Imaging of the sinuses should not be performed in routine cases. For recurrent or persistent sinusitis, CT is preferred to standard sinus radiography. Aspiration should be performed when there is known opacification of a sinus and empirical therapy has not been effective or the patient is at risk of opportunistic infection. In the absence of nasal perforation, lung symptoms or signs, or renal disease that raises suspicion of vasculitis or Wegener's granulomatosis, measurement of serum ANCA is not warranted.

**VI-27 and VI-28.  The answers are E and B.**  *(Chap. 240)*  Bronchiectasis is an abnormal and permanent dilation of the airway resulting from a number of insults. The most common cause is severe viral infection or bacterial pneumonia with subsequent airway destruction. The most commonly associated organisms include *Staphylococcus aureus, Klebsiella,* and anaerobes. *Mycobacterium tuberculosis* can cause bronchiectasis; similarly, *Mycobacterium avium* complex has been described as both causing bronchiectasis and colonizing already bronchiectatic airways. These diseases result in focal bronchiectasis. Allergic bronchopulmonary aspergillosis is associated with central bronchiectasis from chronic airway inflammation and mucus inspissation. Impaired host defense mechanisms such as cystic fibrosis, immunodeficiency such as with panhypogammaglobulinemia and HIV, and ciliary dysfunction as in Kartagener's syndrome are associated with diffuse bronchiectasis. Focal bronchiectasis is usually caused by other disorders that lead to localized airway obstruction, such as enlarged lymph nodes, carcinoid tumors, and endobronchial lung cancer.

**VI-29.  The answer is D.**  *(Chap. 240)*   The combination of infertility and recurrent sinopulmonary infections should prompt consideration of an underlying disorder of ciliary dysfunction that is termed primary ciliary dyskinesia. These disorders account for approximately 5 to 10% of cases of bronchiectasis. A number of deficiencies have been described, including malfunction of dynein arms, radial spokes, and microtubules. All organ systems that require cilary function are affected. The lungs rely on cilia to beat respiratory secretions proximally and subsequently to remove inspired particles, especially bacteria. In the absence of this normal host defense, recurrent bacterial respiratory infections occur and can lead to bronchiectasis. Otitis media and sinusitis are common for the same reason. In the genitourinary tract, sperm require cilia to provide motility. Kartagener's syndrome is a combination of sinusitis, bronchiectasis, and situs inversus. It accounts for approximately 50% of patients with primary ciliary dyskinesia. Although cystic fibrosis is associated with infertility and bilateral upper lobe infiltrates, it causes a decreased number of sperm or absent sperm on analysis because of the congenital absence of the vas deferens. Sarcoidosis, which is often associated with bihilar adenopathy, is not generally a cause of infertility. Water balloon–shaped heart is found in those with pericardial effusions, which one would not expect in this patient.

**VI-30 and VI-31.  The answers are C and B.**  *(Chap. 240)*   This patient has underlying bronchiectasis and is admitted with worsening sputum production and significant hemoptysis. The most common cause of minor hemoptysis in patients with bronchiectasis is inflammation of the bronchial wall from baterial infection. However, when patients report this degree of hemoptysis, it more commonly represents erosion of the bronchial artery with subsequent bleeding that is generally large-volume as a result of the presence of systemic circulatory arterial pressures in the bronchial artery. Although *Aspergillus* may produce localized fungus balls that can result in hemoptysis, the radiogram did not confirm this finding. Generally, airway colonization does not result in hemoptysis. Alveolar hemorrhage, because the blood comes from the pulmonary circulation, is generally small-volume and thus produces pink sputum if it produces any. Finally, endobronchial neoplasia is less likely to have such an acute presentation but may also cause small-volume hemoptysis. The most appropriate initial treatment after clinical stabilization is bronchial arterial embolization. This allows direct visualization of the bleeding source and localized treatment. In refractory cases, surgical resection can be considered. Bronchoscopy can localize bleeding, which is especially important in patients with generalized bronchiectasis in which the bleeding airway is unknown. However, bronchoscopy offers no treatment options. Chest CT similarly can localize bleeding but provides no therapeutic benefit. Lung transplantation is not acutely indicated for the management of hemoptysis from bronchiectasis but can be a treatment modality for patients with significant disability despite maximal medical therapy for dyspnea and sputum and infections or colonization.

**VI-32.  The answer is E.**  *(Chap. 246)*   Patients who develop postpolio syndrome tend to have affliction of the same muscle groups that were affected in the original presentation. This patient presents with symptoms of diaphragmatic muscle weakness 40 years after the initial presentation with poliomyelitis. The initial presentation was complicated by respiratory muscle weakness as evidenced by his need for negative-pressure ventilation in an "iron lung." Diaphragmatic muscle weakness can present insidiously with dyspnea on exertion and orthopnea as primary complaints as a result of the actions of accessory muscles. Physical examination may reveal accessory muscle use, paradoxical abdominal motion, and lack of diaphragmatic excursion with inspiration. The diagnosis can be confirmed by electromyography of the diaphragm with nerve conduction studies of the phrenic nerve, measurement of maximum inspiratory and expiratory pressures, fluoroscopy of the diaphragm during sniff maneuver, or measurement of transdiaphragmatic pressure with esophageal and gastric balloons. Maximum voluntary ventilation shows early fatigability. Early in the process, symptoms are most pronounced at night because the accessory muscles contract with less vigor during sleep. $Pa_{CO_2}$ usually rises nocturnally but may normalize during the daytime hours early in the disease. The ability for gas exchange is not affected, and the alveolar-arterial oxygen gradient should be normal although hypoxemia may be present if significant hypoventilation occurs. Lung mechanics are altered, and there is decreased vital capacity and lung compliance. Most patients with postpolio syndrome ultimately become dependent on ventilation at least nocturnally, although some require continuous mechanical ventilatory support. A cuirass is a form of negative-pressure ventilation that is used infrequently. More commonly patients receive positive-pressure support ventilation through a nasal mask or tracheostomy.

**VI-33 and VI-34.  The answers are D and E.**  *(Chap. 246)*   This patient has symptoms consistent with obesity-hypoventilation syndrome, also known as Pickwickian syndrome. Massive obesity causes decreased compliance of the chest wall, with a subsequent decline in functional residual capacity. Thus, the patient breathes at lower lung volumes and often fails to expand the lung bases at tidal breathing. Over time, this results in increases in an A-a gradient and $CO_2$ retention. Additionally, a small proportion of these patients also develop a decrease in central respiratory drive, allowing a further rise in $CO_2$. These patients become dependent on hypoxemic respiratory drive, and rapid increases in arterial oxygen tension may result in hypoxemia. This patient's apneic event on presentation was related to overcorrection of hypoxemia. The long-term effects of obesity-hypoventilaton syndrome are related to right heart dysfunction and hypoxemia. Many of these patients ultimately become dependent on mechanical ventilatory support. The pathogenesis of obesity-hypoventilation syndrome is unclear, but a resistance to serum leptin concentrations is postulated because leptin levels are high in patients with this condition. Obstructive sleep apnea is often present concurrently, but this is not always the case. Management of patients with obesity-hypoventilation syndrome should include weight loss, smoking cessation, and assessment for and treatment of concurrent obstructive sleep apnea. These patients should also be screened for hypothyroidism. Enhancement of respiratory drive with medications such as progesterone may also be tried, although the usefulness of this treatment is debated.

**VI-35.  The answer is C.**  *(Chap. 247)*   Obstructive sleep apnea is an increasingly common disorder that affects 4% of middle-aged men and 2% of middle-aged women. As the population is becoming more obese, with 50% of the population categorized as overweight or obese, the incidence of OSA will increase in the ensuing years. The critical event in OSA is occlusion of the upper airway during sleep, usually at the level of the oropharynx. This occurs when the negative pressure generated on inspiration exceeds the ability of the airway dilator and abductor muscles to maintain airway stability. Alcohol exacerbates the disease because it further decreases upper respiratory muscle tone. The primary pathophysiologic consequences of this dynamic airway obstruction are twofold, relating to fragmented sleep architecture and the effects of this on cardiopulmonary function and increased sympathomimetic activity. The most common manifestations are those related to fragmentation of sleep and loss of slow-wave sleep. These manifestations include personality disturbance, memory loss, impaired job performance, and excessive daytime somnolence with a twofold to sevenfold increased incidence of motor vehicle accidents. The cardiopulmonary abnormalities seen in OSA patients are related to nocturnal hypoxemia and increased negative intrathoracic pressure. Many of these patients demonstrate bradycardia during apneic or hypopneic episodes. In addition, there is lack of a normal nocturnal drop in blood pressure presumably as a result of the effects of increased afterload caused by

OSA. Studies have also demonstrated that these effects are not limited to nocturnal hours, with an increased incidence of daytime hypertension as well. In addition, emerging data suggest that worsening heart failure, myocardial ischemia, and cerebrovascular accidents can be precipitated by OSA.

**VI-36. The answer is A.** *(Chap. 247)* This patient is experiencing increased symptoms related to her seasonal allergic rhinitis, including snoring. She does not report symptoms of obstructive sleep apnea and is not overweight. At this point, treatment of her nasal allergies alone should alleviate the snoring. The best treatment of seasonal allergies is the addition of intranasal corticosteroids. No surgical intervention is needed, as no nasal polyps were demonstrated on examination. In light of the low suspicion for obstructive sleep apnea, further evaluation with polysomnography or nocturnal oximetry is not warranted.

**VI-37. The answer is E.** *(Chap. 247)* The definitive investigation for obstructive and central sleep apnea is polysomnography. This is a detailed overnight sleep study that measures many variables, including sleep stage, oxygen saturation, and heart rate variability. The electrographic measurements include an electroencephalogram, an electromyogram, and an electrooculogram. These measurements allow the observer to determine the stages of the sleep cycle and the time spent in each stage. In addition, ventilatory variables may be measured, including end-tidal carbon dioxide concentrations and transcutaneous carbon dioxide concentrations. Arterial blood gas monitoring is not routinely performed. Oxygen saturation is followed continuously by pulse oximetry. Finally, heart rate variability is most often followed by electrocardiography to determine concurrent arrhythmias, although in some instances oximetry alone is used.

**VI-38. The answer is B.** *(Chap. 245)* The patient is presenting with an acute illness with symptom onset within 4 days of presentation, suggesting an acute bacterial illness. History and physical examination are consistent with community-acquired pneumonia, and the Gram stain suggests *Streptococcus pneumoniae* as the pathogenic organism. The presenting course is complicated by the presence of a pleural effusion that is not loculated. A diagnostic thoracentesis is therefore indicated. Delaying thoracentesis for 48 h while treating a patient with antibiotics will not resolve a complicated parapneumonic effusion or empyema, as both require more aggressive treatment with tube thoracostomy. Computed tomography of the chest is not indicated currently, although it may be useful after thoracentesis to evaluate the underlying lung parenchyma better. Finally, although anaerobic abscess and empyema are more common among patients with alcohol abuse, this patient's history does not suggest anaerobic infection. Anaerobic infection of the pleural space presents with a subacute course of fevers, weight loss, anemia, and leukocytosis.

**VI-39. The answer is D.** *(Chap. 245)* Thoracentesis is indicated for any patient presenting with pneumonia and a pleural effusion more than 10 mm thick on lateral decubitus imaging because a significant percentage of these patients will show evidence of bacterial invasion and require further intervention. Other indications for thoracentesis for pleural effusions that complicate pneumonias include loculation of the pleural fluid and evidence of thickened parietal pleura on chest CT. The pleural fluid should be sent for cell count, differential, pH, protein, LDH, glucose, and culture with Gram stain. This will allow one to differentiate a simple parapneumonic effusion from a complicated one or from empyema. All effusions complicating pneumonia should be exudative, meeting at least one of Light's criteria: (1) pleural fluid protein/serum protein over 0.5, (2) pleural fluid LDH/serum LDH over 0.6, and (3) pleural fluid LDH more than two-thirds of the normal upper limit for serum. Factors that increase the likelihood that tube thoracostomy will have to be performed include loculated pleural fluid, pH below 7.20, pleural fluid glucose below 60 mg/dL, positive Gram stain or culture of pleural fluid, and presence of gross pus on aspiration.

**VI-40. The answer is B.** *(Chap. 245)* This patient presents with a large transudative effusion in the setting of cirrhosis with ascites consistent with the diagnosis of hepatic hydrothorax.

Usually right-sided, hepatic hydrothorax may cause massive pleural effusion and frequently presents with shortness of breath. The pathophysiology for the development of hepatic hydrothorax is translocation of fluid through small diaphragmatic holes influenced by the negative pressures generated through the respiratory cycle. The management of hepatic hydrothorax can be difficult, and initial management should be similar to that for massive ascites. Diuretics and salt restriction are the cornerstones of treatment. If this fails, there should be consideration of liver transplantation or transjugular intrahepatic portosystemic shunting. Although large-volume thoracentesis may be necessary in the setting of respiratory compromise, tube thoracostomy should not be performed because it promotes continued drainage of fluid and will worsen nutritional status as protein and albumin are continuously lost through the fluid. Video thorascopy to correct diaphragmatic defects with talc pleurodesis may be considered an alternative for a patient with refractory hepatic hydrothorax.

**VI-41. The answer is A.** *(Chaps. 150 and 245; N Engl J Med 346:1971–1977, 2002.)* Tuberculosis should be considered in any exudative pleural effusion with lymphocytic predominance. However, positive pleural fluid AFB cultures are present in less than 40% of these patients. Consequently, other markers of tuberculosis infections have been developed and have been shown to have much higher sensitivity for the detection of tuberculous pleural effusion. Elevations in pleural fluid adenosine deaminase to more than 45 IU/L have been shown to be 99% sensitive and 97% specific. In addition, interferon-$\gamma$ levels higher than 140 pg/mL perform similarly. Demonstration of tuberculous DNA by polymerase chain reaction and demonstration of caseating granulomas on pleural biopsy are alternative sensitive means for making the diagnosis. Treatment for pleural tuberculosis is the same as that for pulmonary tuberculosis.

**VI-42. The answer is D.** *(Chap. 245)* This patient presents with a primary spontaneous pneumothorax, which occurs most commonly in young men who are smokers. A primary spontaneous pneumothorax probably represents rupture of a small subpleural bleb. The pneumothorax is usually small and rarely is life-threatening. Presentation is often subacute, with most patients presenting with more than 1 week of symptoms, most commonly pleuritic chest pain and dyspnea with exertion. On physical examination, the most common finding is tachycardia. Lung examination may reveal hyperresonance to percussion, decreased tactile fremitus, decreased expansion, and decreased or absent breath sounds. Management depends on the size of the pneumothorax. Pneumothoraces less than 15% can often be managed with supplemental oxygen therapy alone, although observation only is not recommended because resorption by this method is quite slow. For a pneumothorax greater than 15% simple aspiration is a recommended treatment if the patient is hemodynamically stable. Tube thoracostomy can be placed if the lung fails to reexpand. Approximately half these individuals will have a recurrence. If this occurs, thorascopy with stapling of blebs and/or mechanical abrasion will prevent further recurrence in almost 100% of patients.

**VI-43. The answer is E.** *(Chap. 245; Arch Neurol 58(6):893–898, 2001.)* Patients with Guillain-Barré syndrome (acute inflammatory demyelinating polyneuropathy) are at high risk of developing respiratory failure, with up to 30% requiring mechanical ventilation during the course of their illness. Patients with this syndrome should be hospitalized and followed for evidence of respiratory failure. The most common means of doing this is serial measurements of vital capacity and maximum inspiratory pressure. Once the vital capacity has fallen to less than 20 mL/kg body weight, mechanical ventilation is indicated. Other measures of impending ventilatory failure include a maximum inspiratory pressure less than 30 cmH$_2$O and a maximum expiratory pressure less than 40 cmH$_2$O. Although rising Pa$_{\text{CO}_2}$ provides clear evidence of ventilatory failure and is an indication for the initiation of mechanical ventilation, ideally these other measures will identify these individuals before their progression to overt ventilatory failure.

**VI-44.  The answer is C.**  *(Chap. 245)*   Severe kyphoscoliosis causes pulmonary symptoms in up to 3% of patients with this condition. The physical abnormalities caused by the forward and lateral curvature of the spine result in abnormal pulmonary mechanics. This is manifested primarily as restrictive lung disease with chronic alveolar hypoventilation. This in turn leads to ventilation-perfusion imbalances that result in hypoxic vasoconstriction and may cause the eventual development of pulmonary hypertension.

**VI-45.  The answer is C.**  *(Chap. 243)*   Early studies of hypersensitivity pneumonitis explored the possibility of immune complex–mediated injury as causative because precipitating antibodies to mold extracts could be demonstrated in patients with farmer's lung. However, subsequent studies in both human and animal models provided support for the idea that delayed-type hypersensitivity plays the primary role. In the acute reaction, an increase in airway polymorphonuclear leukocytes is seen in the alveoli and small airways. This is followed by an influx of mononuclear cells into the lung, with the formation of the classic loose granulomas that are seen in hypersensitivity pneumonitis. Interferon $\alpha$ and interleukin 12 are felt to be contributors to the immune response in patients with hypersensitivity pneumonitis.

**VI-46 and VI-47.  The answers are C and D.**  *(Chap. 237)*   The patient has a subacute presentation of hypersensitivity pneumonitis related to exposure to bird droppings and feathers at work. Hypersensitivity pneumonitis is a delayed-type hypersensitivity reaction that has a variety of presentations. Some people develop acute onset of shortness of breath, fevers, chills, and dyspnea within 6 to 8 h of antigen exposure. Others may present subacutely with worsening dyspnea on exertion and dry cough over weeks to months. Chronic hypersensitivity pneumonitis presents with more severe and persistent symptoms with clubbing. Progressive worsening is common with the development of chronic hypoxemia, pulmonary hypertension, and respiratory failure. The diagnosis relies on a variety of tests. Peripheral eosinophilia is not a feature of this disease, although neutrophilia and lymphopenia are frequently present. Other nonspecific markers of inflammation may be elevated, including the erythrocyte sedimentation rate, C-reactive protein, rheumatoid factor, and serum immunoglobulins. If a specific antigen is suspected, serum precipitins directed toward that antigen may be demonstrated. Chest radiography may be normal or show a diffuse reticulonodular infiltrate. High-resolution chest CT is the imaging modality of choice and shows ground-glass infiltrates in the lower lobes. Centrilobular infiltrates are often seen as well. In the chronic stages patchy emphysema is the most common finding. Histopathologically, interstitial alveolar infiltrates predominate, with a variety of lymphocytes, plasma cells, and occasional eosinophils and neutrophils seen. Loose, noncaseating granulomas are typical.

Treatment depends on removing the individual from exposure to the antigen. If this is not possible, the patient should wear a mask that prevents small-particle inhalation during exposure. In patients with mild disease, removal from antigen exposure alone may be sufficient to treat the disease. More severe symptoms require therapy with glucocorticoids at an equivalent prednisone dose of 1 mg/kg daily for 7 to 14 days. The steroids are then gradually tapered over 2 to 6 weeks.

**VI-48.  The answer is E.**  *(Chap. 237)*   Multiple drugs have been associated with eosinophilic pulmonary reactions. They include nitrofurantoin, sulfonamides, NSAIDs, penicillins, thiazides, tricyclic antidepressants, hydralazine, and chlorpropramide, among others. Amiodarone can cause an acute respiratory distress syndrome with the initiation of the drug as well as a syndrome of pulmonary fibrosis. Eosinophilic pneumonia is not caused by amiodarone.

**VI-49.  The answer is D.**  *(Chap. 237)*   The patient has chronic eosinophilic pneumonia. This presents in a subacute course over weeks to months with symptoms of cough and dyspnea on exertion. In addition, fevers, chills, night sweats, anorexia, and weight loss are common.

An extensive workup is done to exclude other causes, including fungal and parasitic diseases. Peripheral eosinophilia suggests the underlying diagnosis. Chest radiography shows characteristic peripheral lung infiltrates that have been described as the photographic negative of pulmonary edema. The combination of typical clinical and radiographic findings with peripheral blood eosinophilia can be used to make the diagnosis. Rapid improvement in symptoms occurs within 48 h of the initiation of glucocorticoids.

**VI-50. The answer is D.** *(Chap. 243)* Desquamative interstitial pneumonitis, respiratory bronchiolitis–interstitial lung disease, pulmonary Langerhans cell histiocytosis, Goodpasture's disease, and pulmonary alveolar proteinosis are almost always associated with cigarette smoking. In addition, 67 to 75% of patients with idiopathic pulmonary fibrosis also have a history of cigarette use. Bronchiolitis obliterans organizing pneumonia (BOOP), or cryptogenic organizing pneumonia, is often an idiopathic syndrome that presents in the fifth to sixth decade of life with dyspnea on exertion, cough, fevers, malaise, and weight loss. The cause in most instances is unknown, although BOOP may occur concomitantly with primary pulmonary disorders as a nonspecific reaction to lung injury. BOOP usually responds to steroid therapy, which induces clinical recovery in two-thirds of patients. It is not associated with previous tobacco use.

**VI-51 and VI-52. The answers are D and C.** *(Chap. 243; N Engl J Med 350:125–133, 2004.)* Idiopathic pulmonary fibrosis (IPF) is the most common form of idiopathic interstitial pneumonia. This patient presents with the usual clinical manifestation of slowly progressive dyspnea on exertion. As the age of onset of IPF is most commonly above age 50, many patients attribute their initial symptoms to aging alone. Thus, by the time of presentation most patients have had symptoms for a prolonged period, sometimes for longer than a year. A dry cough is often also present. Additionally, up to 75% of patients with IPF give a history of cigarette smoking. The typical findings on physical examination are fine, dry inspiratory crackles that often are described as "Velcro"-like. Another common physical finding is digital clubbing. Oxygen desaturation with ambulation may be the only physiologic consequence early in the disease, although all these patients will progress to needing oxygen at rest over the course of their illness. A definitive diagnosis can be made only on surgical lung biopsy. However, high-resolution CT imaging of the lung can be highly suggestive, and if the clinical presentation is typical, surgical lung biopsy may not be needed. Findings on high-resolution CT imaging that are typical of IPF are patchy, predominantly basilar, subpleural reticular opacities and honeycombing that is worse at the bases. The histopathologic correlate of IPF is usual interstitial pneumonia (UIP) and requires surgical lung biopsy for identification. Transbronchial biopsies are not helpful in diagnosing UIP. The hallmark of UIP is a heterogeneous pattern at low-power magnification with alternating areas of normal lung, dense collagen proliferation with fibroblast foci, interstitial inflammation, and honeycombing.

Even with the best medical therapy, the prognosis for patients with UIP is poor, with a 5-year survival of only 20 to 40%. Recommendations for initial therapy are prednisone at a dose of 1 mg/kg combined with a cytotoxic agent such as azathioprine or cyclophosphamide. However, there is no firm evidence that any treatment prolongs survival or improves quality of life in IPF patients. Recently, interferon γ has been tried as an antifibrotic therapy. After encouraging initial results in a small study, a recent large trial failed to show any change in mortality or rate of decline in lung function. In subgroup analysis, there may be a benefit from the use of interferon γ in patients with preserved lung function at baseline, but further trials are necessary before this can be recommended. Single-lung transplantation should be considered early in the disease process for anyone who experiences declining lung function despite medical therapy.

**VI-53. The answer is B.** *(Chap. 243)* Pulmonary complications are common in patients with systemic lupus erythematosus (SLE). The most common manifestation is pleuritis with or without effusion. Other possible manifestations include pulmonary hemorrhage, diaphragmatic dysfunction with loss of lung volumes (the so-called shrinking lung syndrome), pulmonary vascular disease, acute interstitial pneumonitis, and bronchioltis obliterans organizing pneumonia. Other systemic complications of SLE also cause pulmonary complications, including uremic pulmonary edema and infectious complications. Chronic progressive pulmonary fibrosis is not a complication of SLE.

**VI-54 and VI-55. The answers are E and D.** *(Chap. 243)* Pulmonary alveolar proteinosis (PAP) is a rare disorder with an incidence of approximately 1 in 1 million. The disease usually presents between ages 30 and 50 and is slightly more common in men. Three distinct subtypes have been described: congenital, acquired, and secondary (most frequently caused by acute silicosis or hematologic malignancies). Interestingly, the pathogenesis of the disease has been associated with antibodies to granulocyte-macrophage colony-stimulating factor (GM-CSF) in most cases of acquired disease in adults. The pathobiology of the disease is failure of clearance of pulmonary surfactant. These patients typically present with subacute dyspnea on exertion with fatigue and low-grade fevers. Associated laboratory abnormalities include polycythemia, hypergammaglobulinemia, and increased LDH levels. Classically, the CT appearance is described as "crazy pavement" with ground-glass alveolar infiltrates in a perihilar distribution and intervening areas of normal lung. Bronchoalveolar lavage is diagnostic, with large amounts of amorphous proteinaceous material seen. Macrophages filled with PAS-positive material are also frequently seen. The treatment of choice is whole-lung lavage through a double-lumen endotracheal tube. Survival at 5 years is higher than 95%, although some patients will need a repeat whole-lung lavage. Secondary infection, especially with *Nocardia,* is common, and these patients should be followed closely.

**VI-56. The answer is B.** *(Chap. 30)* The patient presents with chronic cough as his symptoms have lasted more than 3 weeks. The common causes of chronic cough are cough-variant asthma, gastroesophageal reflux disease, and postnasal drip. However, history and physical examination occasionally point to different etiologies of cough. In this case the patient has a "cobblestoned" airway. This finding suggests granulomatous disease, specifically sarcoidosis. Often when sarcoidosis involves the airways, including the trachea, the inflammation triggers cough. Chest radiography would most commonly show bilateral hilar adenopathy. Less likely would be a normal radiogram with only airway involvement. Sarcoidosis generally causes interstitial, not alveolar, infiltrates. Cardiomegaly is uncommon without a dilated cardiomyopathy from sarcoidosis from which the patient would generally be symptomatic. Bronchiectasis, if found at all in patients with sarcoidosis, is a very late finding that generally results from end-stage fibrotic lung disease.

**VI-57. The answer is D.** *(Chap. 30)* The patient presents with chronic cough as it has lasted for more than 3 weeks. He denies symptoms of the most common causes of chronic cough, such as asthma, gastroesophageal reflux disease, and postnasal drip. However, he does take an angiotensin-converting enzyme (ACE) inhibitor, which is known to cause chronic cough in 5 to 20% of the patients who take this class of medications. Cough that is due to ACE inhibitors generally begins between 1 week and 6 months after medication initiation. The most appropriate diagnostic and therapeutic step at this point is to discontinue the ramipril. Angiotensin receptor blockers can be used instead of the ACE inhibitor to improve cardiac outcomes but are generally not recommended as first-line therapy. In light of this patient's lack of risk factors for malignancy and lack of sputum production, bronchoscopy would not be helpful in this case. Furosemide and digoxin are not associated with cough. As the patient denies having infectious or constitutional symptoms, empirical courses of antibiotics are not warranted.

**VI-58. The answer is E.** *(Chap. 30)* Although mild hemoptysis (generally less than 250 mL in 24 h) can be managed either on an outpatient basis or on a regular medical floor, a patient with massive hemoptysis should be admitted to an intensive care unit. The focus of care should be on airway protection and prevention of blood reaching the normal lung and resulting in asphyxiation. This is generally achieved by means of dual-lumen intubation so that the bleeding side can be isolated and the normal side can be protected. The patient can be positioned with the bleeding side down to encourage pooling of blood in the already abnormal lung. Finally, measures to maximize clot formation and stabilization should be undertaken, including correction of coagulopathy and attempts to keep the patient still, often with antitussives or sedatives as needed when the airway is protected.

**VI-59.   The answer is D.**   *(Chaps. 30 and 235)*   This patient presents with chronic cough but has features that raise concern about etiologies other than the common asthma, postnasal drip, and gastroesophageal reflux disease. The history of extensive tobacco abuse and hemoptysis suggests endobronchial cancer. Another etiology might be chronic bronchitis, but the patient has not responded well to previous courses of antibiotics, and it is appropriate at this point to investigate the possibility of endobronchial neoplasia. Sputum cytology is helpful when it is positive for cancerous cells; unfortunately, its sensitivity is only approximately 5%. The gold standard for evaluation of the airways is bronchoscopy; this modality allows visualization of the bleeding source and biopsy for diagnosis. Empirical courses of ipratropium or omeprazole are not warranted before endobronchial neoplasia is ruled out. Although lisinopril may cause chronic cough, it is not associated with sputum production or hemoptysis. Although tuberculosis is unlikely with a normal chest radiogram, atypical mycobacteria can colonize abnormal airways. However, they rarely cause hemoptysis with no infiltrate; again, in this high-risk patient, endobronchial cancer must be investigated.

**VI-60.   The answer is E.**   *(Chap. 31)*   Hypoxia has many physiologic consequences that generally serve as attempts to compensate for the abnormalities that have been created. As oxygen is essential for aerobic metabolism, during times of hypoxia anaerobic metabolism becomes a more prominent source of adenosine triphosphate (ATP) generation. Because of this shift, pyruvate, which is generated from glucose, is preferentially degraded to lactic acid, with resultant lactic acidosis. Hypoxia stimulates chemoreceptors in the carotid bodies and brainstem to trigger increased ventilation. Tissue hypoxia results in vasodilation in all vascular beds except the pulmonary arteries. As a result of widespread vasodilation, cardiac output increases. Finally, the kidneys sense hypoxia and increase the production of erythropoietin. With chronically elevated erythropoietin levels, polycythemia, or erythrocytosis, develops.

**VI-61.   The answer is C.**   *(Chap. 31)*   In the evaluation of cyanosis, the first step is to differentiate central from peripheral cyanosis. In central cyanosis, because the etiology is either reduced oxygen saturation or abnormal hemoglobin, the physical findings include bluish discoloration of both mucous membranes and skin. In contrast, peripheral cyanosis is associated with normal oxygen saturation but slowing of blood flow and an increased fraction of oxygen extraction from blood; subsequently, the physical findings are present only in the skin and extremities. Mucous membranes are spared. Peripheral cyanosis is commonly caused by cold exposure with vasoconstriction in the digits. Similar physiology is found in Raynaud's phenomenon. Peripheral vascular disease and deep venous thrombosis result in slowed blood flow and increased oxygen extraction with subsequent cyanosis. Methemoglobinemia causes abnormal hemoglobin that circulates systemically. Consequently, the cyanosis associated with this disorder is systemic. Other common causes of central cyanosis include severe lung disease with hypoxemia, right-to-left intracardiac shunting, and pulmonary arteriovenous malformations.

**VI-62.   The answer is C.**   *(Chap. 248)*   In patients who undergo lung transplantation, the complications to which they are susceptible are distributed by time after the procedure. Immediately postoperatively, these patients are at risk for graft dysfunction, or ischemia–reperfusion injury, as well as anatomic complications related to the surgical procedure. Less commonly, hyperacute rejection occurs. During the first year after transplantation acute rejection and CMV infection are the most important sources of morbidity and mortality. After the first year chronic rejection, or bronchiolitis obliterans syndrome, is the major cause of declining respiratory function and mortality. Infections other than CMV, such as *Aspergillus* and *Pseudomonas,* are common in patients with chronic rejection. Chronic allograft rejection results from diffuse small airway narrowing and fibrosis without acute inflammation. Other large airway complications, such as bronchomalacia and stenosis at anastamotic sites, occur but rarely result in significant mortality.

**VI-63.   The answer is F.**   *(Chap. 248)*   The most common cause of mortality in patients who have undergone lung transplantation is chronic allograft rejection, also known as bronchiolitis obliterans syndrome (BOS). This disorder results from fibroproliferation of the small airways with resultant airflow obstruction. Histologically, there is an absence of acute inflammation. Clinically, the diagnosis is made by a sustained fall of 20% or more in $FEV_1$ in the setting of airflow limitation. Alternatively, the diagnosis can be made on lung biopsy. Risk factors for the development of BOS include acute rejection episodes and lymphocytic bronchiolitis. CMV pneumonitis has inconsistently been named as a risk factor as well. With a prevalence in lung transplant recipients of 50% at 3 years, this disorder is the main limitation on long-term survival after lung transplantation. These patients often have concurrent bacterial infection or colonization that may improve with therapy. When identified, chronic rejection or BOS generally is treated with increased immunosuppression. However, no controlled trials have shown consistent efficacy of this approach, and anecdotally the results appear to be poor.

**VI-64.   The answer is C.**   *(Chaps. 243 and 248)*   Patients with idiopathic pulmonary fibrosis have a very poor survival rate, and treatment results are generally disappointing. Unfortunately, there are not enough cadaveric lungs available in the United States to meet the needs of patients with indications for lung transplantation. In 1997 the median waiting time for patients to receive lung transplantation was 1053 days, and approximately 10% of patients on the waiting list die each year. Patients with idiopathic pulmonary fibrosis have a higher mortality on the wait list for lung transplantation than do patients with other indications. In light of these findings, the recommendation currently is to refer suitable patients with idiopathic pulmonary fibrosis for lung transplantation immediately after the diagnosis is made. Suitable patients include generally those with no significant systemic illness, those less than 65 years old, and those with no uncured malignancy. There is no known benefit to initiating *Pneumocystis carinii* prophylaxis in patients with idiopathic pulmonary fibrosis without immunosuppressive therapy. Similarly, inhaled glucocorticoids are not useful in patients with idiopathic pulmonary fibrosis.

**VI-65 and VI-66.   The answers are E and E.**   *(Chap. 29)*   The mountain climber is at risk for two well-described altitude-related conditions: high-altitude cerebral edema and high-altitude pulmonary edema. High-altitude pulmonary edema is a well-described subset of pulmonary edema. Other causes of pulmonary edema include cardiogenic, neurogenic, and noncardiogenic (as seen in acute respiratory distress syndrome). Although the exact mechanism of this disorder is unclear, one commonly accepted hypothesis suggests that increased cardiac output and hypoxic vasoconstriction with resultant pulmonary hypertension combine to cause high-pressure pulmonary edema. Persons less than 25 years old are more likely than are older persons to develop this condition, probably because hypoxic vasoconstriction of the pulmonary arteries is more pronounced in this population. Persons who regularly live at high altitudes are still at risk for high-altitude pulmonary edema when they descend to a lower altitude and then return to higher areas. Prevention can be achieved by means of prophylactic administration of acetazolamide and gradual ascent to higher altitudes. Once this condition develops, the most important therapy is to descend to a lower altitude. Other therapies include oxygen to decrease hyopoxic pulmonary vasoconstriction and diuretic therapy as needed.

**VI-67.   The answer is D.**   *(Chap. 29)*   Cardiopulmonary exercise testing is an important modality that is used frequently to determine whether dyspnea originates from a cardiac or a pulmonary source. Generally, patients ride a stationary bicycle or walk on a treadmill with graduated difficulty while exhaled gas is collected for analysis, blood pressure, and electrocardiography and optionally arterial blood gases are closely monitored. Certain features of the test results suggest the underlying etiology of dyspnea. In patients with cardiovascular dysfunction, findings include a heart rate more than 85% of the maximum heart rate, a low anaerobic threshold, reduced maximum oxygen consumption, arrhythmia or ischemia on electrocardiography, and a drop in blood pressure without desaturation or achievement of the maximal predicted ventilation. Conversely, pulmonary dysfunction is suggested by achieving or exceeding maximal ventilation, desaturation, a drop in $FEV_1$ with exercise, and stability or an increase in the ratio of dead space to tidal volume without reaching 85% of the maximal heart rate or ischemic changes on electrocardiography.

**VI-68.   The answer is E.**   *(Chap. 29)*   Cheyne-Stokes respirations, in which tidal volume and frequency wax and wane alternately, is indicative of cardiac dysfunction. Frequently this respiratory pattern is found in patients with decompensated heart failure. Physical examination confirms this pattern with elevated jugular venous pressure, an enlarged cardiac impulse, third and fourth heart sounds, and peripheral edema. The exact mechanism of Cheyne-Stokes respirations in heart failure is not known; however, current hypotheses suggest that increased circulatory time in heart failure leads to alterations in acid-base status that subsequently affect the brainstem chemoreceptors that govern the respiratory pattern. Treatment with a return to euvolemia and occasionally nocturnal noninvasive positive-pressure ventilation can reverse this condition. This respiratory pattern is not associated with asthma or obesity hypoventilation. A fruity odor on the breath is usually found in patients with diabetic ketoacidosis, which is associated with Kussmaul's respirations, or tachypnea with large tidal volumes.

**VI-69.   The answer is E.**   *(Chap. 239)*   For bacteria to cause pneumonia, they must enter the lower respiratory tract and evade the natural host defenses in doing so. Natural defense mechanisms include the sinuses and contours of the upper airway, cilia and mucus that normally trap particles and protect the distal airway, and immune cells that inhabit the lower and upper airways to survey and fight pathogenic organisms. There are several ways in which organisms can gain entry to the lower respiratory tract and cause pneumonia; they include large volume or gross aspiration, microaspiration of already colonized oropharyngeal secretions, hematogenous spread, aerosol inhalation, and direct extension from a contiguously infected site. The most common mode of contracting community-acquired pneumonia is microaspiration of colonized oropharyngeal contents. Macroaspiration generally occurs only in those with a neurologic embarrassment, such as during a seizure or after a stroke. Hematogenous spread occurs in the setting of bacteremia of another source, often bacterial endocarditis with septic emboli. Aerosol inhalation is the primary method of entry for endemic fungi such as *Histoplasma* and *Coccidiodes* as well as mycobacteria. Direct extension from a contiguously infected site is a rare mode of acquisition.

**VI-70.   The answer is D.**   *(Chap. 239)*   Initial therapy for community-acquired pneumonia is most often empirical and thus must cover both the typical and the atypical organisms that are likely to be causative in an individual patient. Coverage for *Legionella* can be obtained only with macrolides, fluoroquinolones, and, in the outpatient setting, doxycycline. Furthermore, with regard to therapy with typical agents, the pneumococcus is developing increasing resistance to penicillin. In the late 1990s, it was noted that 35% of isolates in a multicenter trial were resistant to penicillin. It is important to note that higher mortality has not been shown in patients with nonsusceptible pneumococcus isolates. These findings and data from retrospective trials have prompted national organizations such as the Infectious Diseases Society of America and the American Thoracic Society to recommend that initial therapy for community-acquired pneumonia in hospitalized patients begin with second- or third-generation cephalosporin plus a macrolide or a second- or third-generation fluoroquinolone antibiotic. Indeed, higher mortality has been seen in patients whose initial therapy consisted of an aminoglycoside and another antibiotic. Emerging resistance to fluoroquinolones among pneumococci has been rarely reported. Risk factors include chronic obstructive pulmonary disease (COPD), age >64 years, and recent fluoroquinolone exposure. Current recommendations are to avoid fluoroquinolones for treating community-acquired pneumonia when patients have received these agents within the last 3 months.

**VI-71. The answer is E.** *(Chap. 239)* This patient presents with invasive pneumococcal disease manifest by positive blood cultures. Risk factors for pneumococcal pneumonia are dementia, seizures, congestive heart failure, tobacco smoking, alcoholism, COPD, and cerebrovascular disease. Risk factors for invasive pneumococcal disease are male gender, African-American ethnicity, current tobacco use, passive tobacco exposure, and chronic illness. This patient is African American, has COPD, and also has had chronic passive tobacco exposure. Certainly she would warrant a pneumococcal vaccination before discharge from the hospital in light of her risk factors and underlying lung disease.

**VI-72. The answer is B.** *(Chaps. 148 and 239)* Lung abscesses classically present with a delayed progression of constitutional symptoms and a productive cough that is occasionally foul-smelling. Clubbing can be found in about 10% of these patients, especially when the duration of symptoms is more than 3 weeks. Clinical suspicion is confirmed with either plain chest film or a CT of the chest. Generally the abscess is in the dependent lung fields when aspiration is the underlying cause. Risk factors for this disorder are those which are associated with an impaired cough reflex, which normally prevents aspiration. Thus, increased incidence is found in patients with alcohol and drug abuse, epilepsy, stroke, and anesthesia. Lesser risk factors are dental caries, bronchiectasis, bronchial carcinoma, and pulmonary infarction. Most commonly the infection is polymicrobial with a predominance of *Bacteroides* sp., *Peptostreptococcus* sp., *Prevotella* sp., and fusobacterium in patients with anaerobic infection. Other organisms include S*treptococcus milleri, Klebsiella pneumoniae,* and *Staphylococcus aureus.* The presence of putrid sputum suggests an anaerobic infection. In this patient, the putrid sputum and the risk factors for aspiration and anaerobic infection make the appropriate initial therapy clindamycin. Surgical resection and percutaneous drain placement are rarely indicated. Therapy should be continued for at least 6 weeks and should be guided by radiographic improvement. Certainly one must be aware that other disorders can cavitate, namely, mycobacterial disease and neoplasia, and be vigilant to exclude these diagnoses as much as is possible with culture, cytologic, and radiographic data.

**VI-73 and VI-74. The answers are A and D.** *(Chap. 239)* Hospital-acquired pneumonia (HAP) remains a common problem, affecting 5 to 10% of all medical and surgical discharges, with an associated mortality of 30 to 70%. The most common microbe is *Staphylococcus aureus,* including methicillin-resistant strains; however, enteric gram-negatives also are important pathogens. Risk factors include impaired host defenses, including nasogastric and endotracheal intubation and enteral feedings, which increase the risk of microaspiration and macroaspiration. In critically ill patients, elevated gastric pH resulting from antacids, proton pumps, and $H_2$ inhibitors and enteral feedings are associated with gastric bacterial overgrowth. This bacterial burden can in turn be aspirated. Current recommendations suggest weighing the benefits of gastrointestinal prophylaxis against the risk of bacterial overgrowth and potential aspiration and/or pneumonia. To minimize HAP risk, placement of enteral feeding tubes ideally should be postpyloric and the tube should be the smallest caliber possible. Ventilator circuit manipulations are associated with an increased risk of HAP, and thus circuit changes should be minimized. Neither prophylactic antibiotics nor selective gastrointestinal decontamination has been shown to decrease the risk of HAP. Importantly, elevation of the head of the bed to 30° has been shown in randomized trials to decrease the risk of HAP. Initial therapy is empirical and should cover the most likely pathogens: *S. aureus* and enteric gram-negative bacilli. In light of the frequency of methicillin-resistant *S. aureus,* it would be most appropriate to use vancomycin and a third-generation cephalosporin or penicillin with antipseudomonal activity.

**VI-75.** **The answer is C.** *(Chap. 244)* In determining the appropriate regimen for venous thromboembolism prophylaxis, one must consider the risk associated with the patient and/ or the procedure. High-risk patients include those who undergo orthopedic procedures involving the knee or pelvis, those with a hip or pelvis fracture, and those who have undergone gynecologic cancer surgery. Generally, these patients should receive an aggressive approach to thromboembolism prophylaxis, including warfarin with a goal INR of 2.0 to 2.5 for 4 to 6 weeks, twice-daily subcutaneous low-molecular-weight heparin, or intermittent pneumatic compression devices plus warfarin. Moderate-risk patients, including those undergoing gynecologic, urologic, thoracic, or abdominal surgery, and medically ill patients can be appropriately treated with subcutaneous unfractionated heparin plus graded compression stockings or intermittent pneumatic compression devices. Low-risk patients do not require medications or devices for prophylaxis but should be encouraged to ambulate frequently.

**VI-76.** **The answer is C.** *(Chap. 242)* The only therapy that has been proved to improve survival in patients with COPD is oxygen in the subset of patients with resting hypoxemia. This patient probably has resting hypoxemia resulting from the presence of an elevated jugular venous pulse, pedal edema, and an elevated hematocrit. Theophylline has been shown to increase exercise tolerance in patients with COPD through a mechanism other than bronchodilation. Glucocorticoids are not indicated in the absence of an acute exacerbation and may lead to complications if they are used indiscriminately. Atenolol and enalapril have no specific role in therapy for COPD but are often used when there is concomitant illness.

**VI-77.** **The answer is E.** *(Chap. 250)* The general mechanisms responsible for hypoxemia include alveolar hypoventilation, impaired diffusion, ventilation-perfusion inequality, and shunting (blood bypassing ventilated areas of the lung). In each of these cases except for shunting, the arterial $P_{O_2}$ increases significantly when the inspired $P_{O_2}$ is raised. Examples of shunts (which could account for the lack of response to oxygen therapy in this patient) include congenital heart disease that produces direct right-to-left intracardiac flow (usually associated with pulmonary hypertension), intrapulmonary vascular shunting (i.e., congenital telangiectatic disorders such as Osler-Rendu-Weber syndrome), and, most commonly, perfused alveoli that are not ventilated because of atelectasis or fluid buildup (pneumonia or pulmonary edema). Because impaired diffusion usually is not severe enough to lead to disordered gas exchange except during exercise, most cases of normocapnic hypoxemia are due to ventilation-perfusion mismatch. Many processes that affect the lungs (alveolar disease, interstitial lung disease, pulmonary vascular disease, airway disease) do so unevenly, leading to some areas with adequate perfusion and poor ventilation and some with good ventilation and poor perfusion.

**VI-78.** **The answer is D.** *(Chap. 236; Larsen, N Engl J Med 326:1540–1542, 1992; Goldstein et al, Ann Intern Med 121:698–708, 1994.)* The importance of immune mechanisms in the pathogenesis of asthma is suggested by the common association between the disease and the presence of allergic diseases, skin-test sensitivity, and increased serum IgE levels. In addition, many susceptible persons develop bronchospasm after inhalation challenge with airborne allergens. A large proportion of asthmatic subjects, however, have none of these markers of immunologic activity and are classified as having idiosyncratic asthma. When tested for bronchial hyperirritability with various nonantigenic bronchoprovocational agents (e.g., histamine and cold air), asthmatic subjects are found to be more sensitive than normal, and the bronchoconstriction is generally reversible after exposure to a β-adrenergic agonist; the reason for this airway hyperirritability, which is a common feature in all asthmatic persons, is unknown. Although psychological factors certainly influence the expression of asthma, no single personality type is considered "asthmatic."

**VI-79.** **The answer is C.** *(Chap. 236; McFadden, Am J Med 99:651, 1995.)* Asthmatic patients who present with an acute attack and lack signs of impending ventilatory collapse should be treated with an inhaled aerosolized $\beta_2$ agonist such as albuterol or isoproterenol. Such medicines can be given up to every 20 min by inhaled nebulizer for three doses, with the frequency reduced afterward. Those drugs are five times more effective than intravenous aminophylline. Intravenous or inhaled steroids have a delayed onset of action, if they are destined to be beneficial at all. Patients should be reassured that mortality from asthma is unlikely; however, it is nonetheless advisable to respect an acute asthmatic attack, especially one accompanied by $CO_2$ retention.

---

Nomenclature and Classification of Pulmonary Hypertension

---

### Diagnostic Classification

1. Pulmonary arterial hypertension
   Primary pulmonary hypertension: sporadic and familial
   Related to
   a. Collagen-vascular disease
   b. Congenital systemic to pulmonary shunts
   c. Portal hypertension
   d. HIV infection
   e. Drugs/toxins: anorexigens and other
   f. Persistent pulmonary hypertension of the newborn
   g. Other
2. Pulmonary venous hypertension
   Left-side atrial or ventricular heart disease
   Left-side valvular heart disease
   Extrinsic compression of central pulmonary veins: fibrosing mediastinitis and adenopathy/tumors
   Pulmonary veno-occlusive disease
   Other
3. Pulmonary hypertension associated with disorders of the respiratory system and/or hypoxemia

   | Chronic obstructive pulmonary disease | Chronic exposure to high altitude |
   |---|---|
   | Interstitial lung disease | Neonatal lung disease |
   | Sleep-disordered breathing | Alveolar-capillary dysplasia |
   | Alveolar hypoventilatory disorders | Other |

4. Pulmonary hypertension due to chronic thrombotic and/or embolic disease
   Thromboembolic obstruction of proximal pulmonary arteries
   Obstruction of distal pulmonary arteries
   a. Pulmonary embolism (thrombus, tumor, ova and/or parasites, foreign material)
   b. In-situ thrombosis
   c. Sickle cell disease
5. Pulmonary hypertension due to disorders directly affecting the pulmonary vasculature
   Inflammatory: Schistosomiasis; Sarcoidosis; other
   Pulmonary capillary hemangiomatosis

---

**VI-80. The answer is C.** *(Chap. 260)* Primary pulmonary hypertension is an uncommon disease that usually affects young females. Early in the illness affected persons often are diagnosed as psychoneurotic because of the vague nature of the presenting complaints, for example, dyspnea, chest pain, and evidence of hyperventilation without hypoxemia on arterial blood gas testing. However, progression of the disease leads to syncope in approximately one-half of cases and signs of right heart failure on physical examination. Chest x-ray typically shows enlarged central pulmonary arteries with or without attenuation of peripheral markings. The diagnosis of primary pulmonary hypertension is made by documenting elevated pressures by right heart catheterization and excluding other pathologic processes. Lung disease of sufficient severity to cause pulmonary hypertension would be evident by history and on examination. Major differential diagnoses include thromboemboli and heart disease; outside the United States, schistosomiasis and filariasis are common causes of pulmonary hypertension, and a careful travel history should be taken.

**VI-81. The answer is B.** *(Chap. 242)* This patient presents with physical signs (pursed lip breathing, chest hyperexpansion) and radiographic evidence (flattened diaphragms, attenuated markings) suggestive of obstructive lung disease with loss of lung tissue. Reduced expiratory airflow rates are produced by narrowing of airways (e.g., in asthma), loss of airways (e.g., in bronchiolitis obliterans), or loss of elastic tissue (e.g., in emphysema). Pathophysiologically, these conditions cause increased resistance as airways are narrowed or collapse as well as decreased driving pressure that represents loss of elastic recoil. Air trapping and reduced lung recoil lead to an increase in both total lung capacity (TLC) and functional residual capacity (FRC), which is the volume at which the tendency of the lung to recoil inward is just balanced by the tendency of the chest to recoil outward. Although TLC is increased, vital capacity, the maximum amount of gas that can be exhaled from the lungs with a single breath, is reduced owing to the great increase in residual volume produced by gas trapping. Not only is vital capacity reduced, it takes longer to empty the lungs; thus, forced expiratory volume in 1 s (FEV$_1$) is reduced as a percentage of vital capacity. When alveolar capillaries are destroyed by emphysema, the diffusing capacity, which reflects in part the surface area of alveolar membrane available for gas exchange, is reduced.

**VI-82.   The answer is A.**   *(Chap. 242)*   To establish baseline information in persons who have emphysema, spirometry should be performed, and for persons with significant complaints or physical findings, arterial blood gases also should be checked. Although cigarette smoking accounts for the vast majority of cases of emphysema, a small percentage of persons who develop this illness have had no exposure to tobacco products. A subset of this nonsmoking, emphysematous population is deficient in $\alpha_1$ antitrypsin, which is a protease inhibitor that normally is found in serum. It is currently believed that release of proteolytic enzymes from inflammatory cells accounts for the lung destruction that typifies emphysema, and $\alpha_1$-antitrypsin deficiency, a familial disorder the genotype of which is acid starch gel and immunoelectrophoresis, permits this destruction to occur unimpeded. Exercise testing is not necessary as an initial screening test for emphysema but should be considered before oxygen therapy is prescribed. A male who has emphysematous respiratory failure, gives no history of respiratory infections, and has children would not have cystic fibrosis (affected men are sterile); therefore, a sweat chloride test would not be a useful procedure. High-resolution CT scan would be unlikely to add any significant alteration to the differential diagnosis, and an exercise stress test and an echocardiogram are not necessary in the evaluation of this patient.

**VI-83.   The answer is A.**   *(Chap. 244; Ridker, N Engl J Med 332:912, 1995.)*   Many patients who develop pulmonary thromboembolism have an underlying inherited predisposition that remains clinically silent until they are subjected to an additional stress, such as the use of oral contraceptive pills, surgery, or pregnancy. The most frequently inherited predisposition to thrombosis is so-called activated protein C resistance. The inability of a normal protein C to carry out its anticoagulant function is due to a missense mutation in the gene coding for factor V in the coagulation cascade. This mutation, which results in the substitution of a glutamine for an arginine residue in position 506 of the factor V molecule, is termed the factor V Leiden gene. Based on the Physicians Health Study, about 3% of healthy male physicians carry this particular missense mutation. Carriers are clearly at an increased risk for deep venous thrombosis and also for recurrence after the discontinuation of warfarin. The allelic frequency of factor V Leiden is higher than that of all other identified inherited hypercoagulable states combined, including deficiencies of protein C, protein S, and antithrombin III and disorders of plasminogen.

# VII. CRITICAL CARE MEDICINE

## QUESTIONS

**DIRECTIONS:** Each question below contains five suggested responses. Choose the **one best** response to each question.

**VII-1.** All of the following statements about sepsis are true, except for which one?

A. Sepsis is defined as evidence of the systemic inflammatory response syndrome (SIRS) with proven or suspected microbial infection.
B. For sepsis to be classified as severe, two or more organ systems must show evidence of dysfunction
C. SIRS can be caused by inflammation other than infection.
D. SIRS is defined by the presence of tachypnea, tachycardia, fever or hypothermia, and leukocytosis, leukopenia, or more than 10% bands.
E. Septic shock is defined as persistent hypotension after fluid resuscitation or the need for vasopressors to maintain a systolic blood pressure above 90 mmHg or a mean arterial blood pressure above 70 mmHg.

**VII-2.** A 65-year-old male presents to the emergency department with cough, shortness of breath, and fevers for 2 days. On presentation, he is obtunded with an oxygen saturation of 72% on a nonrebreather mask. Blood pressure is 92/45, heart rate is 130, respiratory rate is 42, and temperature is 39.8°C (103.6°F). The patient's weight is 70 kg. He has alveolar infiltrates on chest radiography throughout the lungs with dense consolidation of the right lower and middle lobes. He is intubated, paralyzed, and brought to the medical intensive care unit. Initial blood gas performed before intubation revealed a pH of 7.32, a $Pa_{co_2}$ of 28 mmHg, a $Pa_{o_2}$ of 44 mmHg, and a bicarbonate of 16. Blood cultures grow *Streptococcus pneumoniae* within 12 h. Which of the following are the most appropriate initial ventilator settings for this patient (A/C, assist control; PS, pressure support; SIMV, synchronized intermittent mechanical ventilation)?

**VII-2.** *(Continued)*

| Mode | Rate | $FI_{o_2}$ | Tidal Volume | PEEP | Pressure Support |
|------|------|------|--------|------|------------------|
| A. A/C | 12 | 1.0 | 750 | 5 | N/A |
| B. A/C | 24 | 1.0 | 420 | 12 | N/A |
| C. PS | N/A | 1.0 | N/A | 5 | 15 |
| D. SIMV | 12 | 1.0 | 300 | 15 | 5 |
| E. SIMV | 24 | 1.0 | 700 | 15 | 5 |

**VII-3.** A 68-year-old male with known chronic obstructive pulmonary disease presents with fevers, increasing shortness of breath, and cough. He was using an ipratropium metered-dose inhaler every 2 h without relief before coming to the emergency department. He is noted to be quite dyspneic on presentation, with use of accessory muscles. He is unable to speak in full sentences. Oxygen saturation is 84% on room air. Respiratory rate is 34 breaths/min. Lung examination is notable for markedly diminished breath sounds on inspiration with a prolonged expiratory phase and expiratory wheezing. Initial arterial blood gas shows a pH of 7.28, a $Pa_{co_2}$ of 72 mmHg, and a $Pa_{o_2}$ of 60 mmHg on 4 L oxygen by nasal cannula. Which of the following is the most appropriate next management step?

A. Initiate therapy with nasal continuous positive airway pressure at 5 cmH$_2$O.
B. Intubate the patient and place on assist-control ventilation.
C. Continue nebulized albuterol and repeat and arterial blood gas in 2 h.
D. Initiate therapy with bilevel positive airway pressure with an inspiratory pressure of 12 cmH$_2$O and an expiratory pressure of 4 cmH$_2$O.
E. Change the patient to high-flow oxygen therapy by 50% Venturi mask.

**VII-4.** A 45-year-old male is brought to the emergency department after hydrochloric acid ingestion at his workplace. The physical examination is notable for respiratory distress, diffuse crackles, and tachycardia. Jugular venous

**VII-4.**    *(Continued)*

pressure is normal. The oropharynx shows no significant lesions. $Pa_{O_2}$ on 100% nonrebreather is 56. A chest radiogram shows diffuse bilateral alveolar infiltrates. He is emergently intubated. The patient weighs 70 kg. Which of the following are appropriate initial settings for mechanical ventilation?

A.    Tidal volume 420 mL, respiratory rate 24, $FI_{O_2}$ 100%, PEEP 5

B.    Tidal volume 700 mL, respiratory rate 20, $FI_{O_2}$ 100%, PEEP 5

C.    Tidal volume 420 mL, respiratory rate 24, $FI_{O_2}$ 50%, PEEP 5

D.    Tidal volume 700 mL, respiratory rate 20, $FI_{O_2}$ 50%, PEEP 5

E.    Tidal volume 840 mL, respiratory rate 20, $FI_{O_2}$ 100%, PEEP 5

**VII-5.**    A patient is admitted to the intensive care unit with sudden-onset shortness of breath and chest pain followed by pulseless electrical activity arrest. After cardiopulmonary resuscitation, the patient is dependent on vasopressors. The patient is 45 years old and is undergoing therapy for metastatic breast cancer. She complained to her husband 3 days earlier that her left leg was slightly more swollen than her right. Current medications, aside from the chemotherapy regimen, include furosemide, tamoxifen, pantoprazole, and diazepam. Physical examination is notable for cool extremities, tachycardia, elevated jugular venous pressure, and a right ventricular heave. Lungs are clear. Which of the following is indicated for this patient now?

A.    Fondaparinux
B.    Intra-aortic balloon pump
C.    Intravenous tissue plasminogen activator (tPA)
D.    Subcutaneous enoxaparin
E.    None of the above

**VII-6.**    The patient in Question IX-5 survives and is ready for discharge from the hospital. Which of the following medications should be discontinued?

A.    Diazepam
B.    Furosemide
C.    Pantoprazole
D.    Tamoxifen
E.    None of the above

**VII-7.**    A 58-year-old female was intubated and placed on mechanical ventilation in the setting of pneumococcal pneumonia and bacteremia. She is treated with moxifloxacin based on sensitivities and improves over the course of 5 days. She required vasopressors for the initial 3 days but now has a stable blood pressure of 130/72. The patient's sedative medications have been halved. The patient remains mildly sedated but is following commands and

**VII-7.**    *(Continued)*

has a strong cough. Vital signs reveal a heart rate of 90 beats/min, a blood pressure of 130/72, a respiratory rate of 16, and an $SaO_2$ of 96%. The ventilator settings currently are SIMV rate 12, $FI_{O_2}$ 0.4, PEEP 5 $cmH_2O$, and pressure support 5 $cmH_2O$. The respiratory therapist initiates a spontaneous breathing trial on continuous positive airway pressure (CPAP) 5 $cmH_2O$ for 1 min. During that time the patient has a spontaneous respiratory rate of 20 breaths/min with a tidal volume of 450 mL. The patient has a negative inspiratory pressure of −40 $cmH_2O$. At this time the patient continues on CPAP 5 $cmH_2O$ with an $FI_{O_2}$ of 0.4. After 30 min of spontaneous breathing, the patient's heart rate has increased to 136, but blood pressure remains stable. The patient's respiratory rate has increased to 24 with a tidal volume that has declined to 375 mL. Oxygen saturation has fallen to 92%. Arterial blood gas is pH 7.42, $Pa_{CO_2}$ is 45 mmHg, and $Pa_{O_2}$ is 66 mmHg. Which of the following statements about liberation of the patient from mechanical ventilation is true?

A.    Liberation is unlikely to be successful because of an abnormally high rapid shallow breathing index (respiratory rate/tidal volume ratio) at 30 min.

B.    The patient's negative inspiratory pressure of −40 $cmH_2O$ indicates significant diaphragmatic weakness.

C.    The rise in the patient's heart rate by more than 20 beats/min is a concern because it may represent fatigue from increased work of breathing.

D.    The patient's mental state is prohibitive for extubation.

E.    The patient is unlikely to maintain adequate oxygenation after extubation as predicted by the fall in oxygen saturation during the spontaneous breathing trial.

**VII-8.**    A 48-year-old male is admitted to the cardiac intensive care unit after undergoing an uncomplicated coronary artery bypass and aortic valve replacement. He is sedated and is receiving mechanical ventilation with assist control with a tidal volume of 500 mL and a respiratory rate of 14/min. Twelve hours later the nurse calls you because the patient's peak airway pressures have suddenly risen from 25 $cmH_2O$ to 60 $cmH_2O$. All the following could explain the increase in airway pressure *except*

A.    acute pulmonary edema
B.    auto-PEEP
C.    bronchospasm
D.    endotracheal tube cuff leak
E.    mucus plugging

**VII-9.**    A 32-year-old female presents to the emergency department complaining of acute shortness of breath and wheezing. She has a history of severe persistent asthma with multiple allergic triggers. The patient has had increased symptoms of nasal allergies for the last month

**VII-9.** *(Continued)*

with the onset of the ragweed season. For the last 2 days she has felt as if she had a "cold" with a sore throat, low-grade fevers, and increased cough. The baseline peak flow is 400 L/s. This morning, this value fell to 125 L/s. By the time of presentation, she is in severe respiratory distress despite using an albuterol metered-dose inhaler every 15 min. She is using accessory muscles and is unable to speak more than one word at a time. Initial arterial blood gas reveals a pH of 7.28, a $Pa_{co_2}$ of 68 mmHg, and a $Pa_{o_2}$ of 89 mmHg on 50% face mask. The patient is intubated and taken to intensive care. The patient's initial ventilator settings are

| Mode | Assist control |
|---|---|
| Rate | 20 breaths/min |
| Tidal volume | 550 mL |
| $FI_{o_2}$ | 0.5 |
| PEEP | 0 cmH$_2$O |

Twenty minutes later you are called to evaluate the patient for hypotension. Blood pressure is 85/40, with a heart rate of 120 beats/min. The respiratory rate is 28 breaths/min, and oxygen saturation is 89%. She has equal breath sounds with inspiratory and expiratory wheezes throughout expiration. The extremities are warm, but pulses are rapid and thready. All but which of the following changes in ventilatory management could be made to prevent further episodes of hypotension?

A. Add 10 cmH$_2$O positive end-expiratory pressure (PEEP).
B. Change the ventilatory mode to synchronized intermittent mandatory ventilation.
C. Decrease the respiratory rate to 14 breaths/min.
D. Decrease the tidal volume to 450 mL.
E. Increase the inspiratory flow rate to achieve an inspiratory/expiratory ratio of 1:6 or higher.

**VII-10.** A 62-year-old female is brought to the emergency department by ambulance for altered mental status. She was well until 3 days ago, when she complained of fatigue and right flank pain. She subsequently developed nausea and vomiting. The patient's oral intake also decreased. Her family reports that she went to bed early last night and was unarousable this morning. The past medical history is notable for hypertension and diabetes mellitus. She normally takes chlorthalidone 25 mg daily and metformin 500 mg twice daily. She stopped taking those medications 2 days ago because of a generalized feeling of malaise. On presentation, the patient has a blood pressure of 65/35. Heart rate is 130 beats/min, and temperature is 39.7°C (103.4°F). Respiratory rate is 36 breaths/min, and oxygen saturation is 89% on room air. The patient's weight is 64 kg. She is minimally responsive to sternal rub with purposeful withdrawal to pain. Her mucous membranes are dry. A cardiovascular examination reveals a regular tachycardia with an S$_4$ gallop. The chest examination reveals

**VII-10.** *(Continued)*

no crackles or wheezes. The abdominal examination is unremarkable. A Foley catheter is placed, and minimal amounts of thick, cloudy urine are obtained. Laboratory studies are as follows:

| | |
|---|---|
| Sodium: | 148 meq/L |
| Potassium: | 5.2 meq/L |
| Chloride: | 118 meq/L |
| Bicarbonate: | 10 meq/L |
| BUN: | 68 mg/dL |
| Creatinine: | 3.6 mg/dL |
| Glucose: | 532 mg/dL |
| pH: | 6.98 |
| $Pa_{co_2}$: | 36 mmHg |
| $Pa_{o_2}$: | 59 mmHg |
| Hemoglobin: | 9.4 g/dL |
| Hematocrit: | 28.5% |
| WBC: | 16,785/mm$^3$ |
| Platelets: | 76,000/mm$^3$ |
| Differential: | 9% PMNs; 10% bands; 1% lymphocytes |
| PT: | 15.4 s |
| aPTT: | 40.2 s |

Blood cultures grow gram-negative bacilli within 6 h. Which of the following is an appropriate intervention at this time?

A. Intubation and mechanical ventilation for hypoxemic respiratory failure
B. Intravenous volume resuscitation with rapid infusion of 1 to 2 L of normal saline in the first hour
C. Initiation of dopamine at a dose of 10 $\mu$g/kg per minute
D. Intravenous bicarbonate administration
E. Intravenous hydrocortisone and fludrocortisone

**VII-11.** The patient in Question VII-10 is diagnosed with pyelonephritis and urosepsis. She is initiated on the therapy described above and receives gatifloxacin and ceftriaxone. Despite this management, she continues to be hypotensive on two vasopressors. In addition, her mental status remains poor. The patient is intubated and has had only 150 mL of urine output in the first 8 h. All the following are criteria for the initiation of therapy with activated protein C for sepsis *except*

A. presence of the systemic inflammatory response syndrome
B. use of vasopressors to maintain a systolic blood pressure greater than 90 mmHg
C. urine output less than 0.5 mL/kg per hour for more than 1 h
D. platelet count less than 80,000/mm$^3$
E. elevation of prothrombin and activated partial thromboplastin time

**VII-12.** A 45-year-old female is admitted to the intensive care unit with several days of dysuria and recent confu-

**VII-12.** *(Continued)*

sion. She has no other medical problems and takes no medications regularly. Physical examination on admission shows a temperature of 40°C (104°F), a pulse of 140 beats/min, a respiratory rate of 30, and blood pressure of 70/30 mmHg. The patient is confused, but aside from tachypnea and tachycardia, cardiac and pulmonary examinations are normal. Abdominal examination is unremarkable. Catheterization-obtained urinalysis shows numerous white blood cells and many bacteria. White blood cell count is 25,000/mm³. Blood pressure is unchanged after adequate fluid administration. After the initiation of vasopressors, which of the following tests is indicated to evaluate the low blood pressure?

A. Cosyntropin stimulation test
B. Metyrapone test
C. Salivary cortisol measurement
D. Serum ACTH measurement
E. None of the above

**VII-13.** A 60-year-old male with chronic obstructive pulmonary disease is brought to the emergency department with altered consciousness. His family reports a 2-day history of increasing shortness of breath that requires nebulized albuterol every 2 h. In addition, the patient has had increasing sputum production with a change in the sputum color from white to green. On presentation, the patient was breathing eight times per minute and was unarousable. Initial arterial blood gas revealed a pH of 6.98, a $Pa_{co_2}$ of 110 mmHg, and a $Pa_{o_2}$ of 100 mmHg while the patient was on a nonrebreather mask. The patient is emergently intubated and brought to the intensive care unit. The initial ventilatory settings are as follows:

**VII-13.** *(Continued)*

| | |
|---|---|
| Mode | Assist control |
| Rate | 12 breaths/min |
| Tidal volume | 500 mL |
| PEEP | 0 cmH₂O |
| $FI_{o_2}$ | 0.5 |

Initially, the patient does well with improvement in arterial blood gases (ABG) to pH 7.20, a $Pa_{co_2}$ of 82 mmHg, and a $Pa_{o_2}$ of 215 mmHg. You are called emergently to the patient's bedside 2 h later to deal with hypotension. The patient currently is breathing 14 times per minute, but his oxygen saturation has decreased from 100% to 84%. Blood pressure is 66/42. Heart rate is 130 beats/min with sinus tachycardia. Temperature is 38.2°C (100.8°F). The patient is sedated, and his respirations do not appear labored. Breath sounds are markedly decreased on the right side with tracheal deviation to the left. The patient has thready peripheral pulses and is cool to touch. You notice that the patient's peak inspiratory pressure has risen from 40 cmH₂O to more than 75 cmH₂O. What is the most important next step in stabilizing this patient?

A. Disconnect the patient from the ventilator to relieve intrinsic positive end-expiratory pressure (PEEP).
B. Perform deep suctioning to relieve mucus plugging.
C. Initiate fluid resuscitation and vasopressor support for sepsis syndrome.
D. Insert a large-bore needle into the right pleural space to relieve a pneumothorax.
E. Administer a paralytic agent because the patient's decompensation can be attributed to dyssynchrony with mechanical ventilation.

# VII. CRITICAL CARE MEDICINE

## ANSWERS

**VII-1. The answer is C.** *(Chap. 254)* A consensus conference in 1992 established definitions for the spectrum of disease that clinically manifests as systemic inflammatory response syndrome (SIRS) and sepsis. SIRS is an inflammatory response that does not have to be caused by infection. Clinically it manifests as tachypnea with a respiratory rate more than 24 breaths/min and tachycardia with a heart rate above 90 beats/min. Either fever [above 38.0°C (100.4°F)] or hypothermia [below 36°C (96.8°F)] is seen. Finally, leukocytosis greater than 12,000/$\mu$L and leukopenia less than 4,000/$\mu$L or more than 10% are required for a diagnosis of SIRS. Sepsis is diagnosed when there is suspected or proven infection in the setting of SIRS. Severe sepsis is present if at least one organ system distant from the site of infection is involved. For example, hypotension, oliguria, acute lung injury, acidosis, and thrombocytopenia or coagulopathy are examples of organ dysfunctions that are seen frequently. Septic shock is identified when hypotension develops that requires vasopressors and occurs despite adequate fluid resuscitation with systolic blood pressure less than 90 or more than 40 points below the patient's usual systolic pressure.

**VII-2. The answer is B.** *(Chap. 252; Brower R et al, N Engl J Med 343:812–814, 2000.)* This patient presents with acute hypoxemic respiratory failure in the setting of *Streptococcus pneumoniae* bacteremia. With bilateral lung infiltrates, a $Pa_{o_2}/FI_{o_2}$ ratio below 200, and no evidence of heart failure, the patient is developing acute respiratory distress syndrome (ARDS) in the setting of community-acquired pneumonia. This disorder is marked by dramatic decreases in lung compliance, and recent data suggest that ventilation at high lung volumes ($\geq$10 mL/kg ideal body weight) may induce further ventilator-associated lung injury. A ventilator management strategy that employs higher levels of positive end-expiratory pressure while limiting lung volumes and plateau pressure has been shown to be protective against further lung injury and leads to better outcomes in patients with ARDS. In this patient, the most appropriate mode of ventilation is assist control with initial tidal volumes of approximately 6 to 8 mL/kg. The best option to provide this is choice B. Further decreases in tidal volume may be necessary to prevent ventilator-associated lung injury; however, starting with a tidal volume of 4 mL/kg is not advised because this limits minute ventilation and causes a rise in $Pa_{co_2}$. In this patient, the usual mode of ventilation is assist control, although synchronized intermittent mandatory ventilation is also used. Pressure support is not an appropriate mode of ventilation in a paralyzed patient because spontaneous breathing is required.

**VII-3. The answer is D.** *(Chap. 252; N Engl J Med 333:817–822, 1995.)* Patients with chronic obstructive pulmonary (COPD) disease have frequent flares. Many ultimately succumb to respiratory failure or become dependent on mechanical ventilatory support. In patients with COPD who present with hypercarbic respiratory failure, noninvasive positive-pressure ventilation (NIPPV) has been shown to decrease the need for mechanical ventilation, hospital days, and mortality. NIPPV for the treatment of COPD conventionally uses bilevel pressure support to assist with ventilation through a tightly fitting face or nasal mask. When a patient initiates an inspiratory effort, the machine applies a designated pressure to assist with inspiratory flow. The pressure will continue to be applied until inspiratory flow has fallen to a level determined by the machine, usually 25% of maximal inspiratory flow. An expiratory pressure may also be set that acts similarly to positive end-expiratory pressure to assist with recruitment of small airways. Indications for use of

NIPPV in patients with COPD include increasing symptoms of dyspnea and fatigue despite medical therapy and rising $Pa_{CO_2}$. Specific criteria for the initiation of NIPPV have not been clearly established. There are several contraindications for the use of NIPPV, including facial trauma or fracture, depressed mental status or inability to cooperate, upper airway obstruction, nonrespiratory organ failure, and after cardiac or respiratory arrest. Similarly, there are no clear guidelines for the discontinuation of NIPPV, although most experts agree that patients should show evidence of improved ventilatory status and $Pa_{CO_2}$ before discontinuation.

**VII-4. The answer is A.** *(Chaps. 251 and 253; Acute Respiratory Distress Syndrome Network, N Engl J Med 342:1301–1308, 2000.)* This patient presents with acute respiratory distress syndrome (ARDS), and the question asks for the most appropriate initial settings for the mechanical ventilator. Traditional settings for the ventilator are a tidal volume of 10 to 12 mL/kg; however, a trial published in the *New England Journal of Medicine* by the Acute Respiratory Distress Syndrome Network compared this approach with a lung protective strategy using lower tidal volume ventilation. The lower tidal volume arm used initial settings of 6 mL/kg for tidal volume and adjusted the tidal volume down as needed to keep the plateau pressure below 30. Patients in the lower tidal volume group had decreased mortality. Thus, the most appropriate tidal volume is 70 kg × 6 mL/kg = 420 mL. Initial $FI_{O_2}$ should be 100% in light of the patient's profound hypoxemia before intubation.

**VII-5 and VII-6. The answers are C and D.** *(Chap. 244; Matisse Investigators, N Engl J Med 1695–1702, 2003; Duggan C et al, J Clin Oncol 19:3588–3593, 2003.)* The patient presents with a classic history for acute pulmonary embolism with acute onset of shortness of breath and chest pain in the setting of risk factors for malignancy and tamoxifen use. Although most patients with a submassive pulmonary embolism can be managed with unfractionated or low-molecular-weight heparins, this patient has a life-threatening pulmonary embolism. In light of the recent arrest and vasopressor-requiring hypotension, which are manifestations of obstructive shock, thrombolytic therapy is indicated. Although recent trials have shown that fondaparinux is safe and effective in the treatment of hemodynamically stable pulmonary embolism compared with intravenous unfractionated heparin, that finding does not apply to this patient. Similarly, subcutaneous low-molecular-weight heparins are not indicated in therapy for a massive pulmonary embolism. Intra-aortic balloon pump placement is used for cardiogenic shock, not for obstructive shock. Upon discharge, medications that potentially cause thrombophilia should be discontinued. Tamoxifen has been associated with an increased risk of thromboembolic disease.

**VII-7. The answer is C.** *(Chap. 252; Hall J et al, Principles of Critical Care Medicine, 2d ed., Chap. 39, 1998.)* Several factors must be taken into account when one is considering discontinuation of mechanical ventilation and extubation. In addition, there are several approaches to deciding who is appropriate for extubation. Before one considers respiratory variables for extubation, an initial first step is to evaluate whether the patient's mental status is appropriate for extubation. All sedatives should be halved or discontinued, and the patient should be following commands. A strong cough and a strong gag response are also desirable to prevent accumulation of abnormal secretions. Frequently upper airway patency is also assessed by the respiratory therapist to ensure that air is able to move through the airway when the endotracheal tube cuff is deflated. Measures of ventilatory function are also important before extubation to assess whether the patient will be able to maintain spontaneous respiration. The most commonly used tool to determine whether a patient is an appropriate candidate for extubation is the rapid-shallow-breathing index. This is calculated by dividing the respiratory rate by the tidal volume in liters. A value above 105 breaths/min per liter is highly predictive of failure to be successfully extubated, with a sensitivity between 72 and 97%. However, a ratio less than 105 does have many false positives, and this index alone should not be used to decide on extubation. Many experts recommend using this as a guide for who should undergo a spontaneous breathing trial for 30 to 60 min. An inspiratory pressure greater than $-30$ cmH$_2$O and a vital capacity greater than 10 mL/kg are also good indicators of diaphragmatic and chest wall function and are desirable before extubation. Alveolar ventilation is generally adequate for extubation when pH can be maintained between 7.35 and 7.40. However, a minute ventilation above 20 L/min is worrisome. Similarly, oxygenation should be maintained during a spontaneous breathing trial and can be predicted by maintenance of an SaO$_2$ above 90% or a Pa$_{O_2}$ below 60 mmHg while the patient is on an FI$_{O_2}$ less than 0.5 and a PEEP less than 5 cmH$_2$O. Other markers of increased work of breathing should be monitored as well. A rise in heart rate greater than 20 beats/min or in systolic blood pressure more than 20 mmHg may signify prohibitive work of breathing and indicate that the patient should be carefully evaluated before extubation.

**VII-8.** **The answer is C.** *(Chap. 252)* The peak airway pressure will increase as a result of any factor that increases the positive end-expiratory airway pressure (PEEP or auto-PEEP), decreases lung compliance (pulmonary edema, pneumothorax), or increases airway resistance (bronchospasm, mucus, biting the tube). An endotracheal tube cuff leak will decrease peak airway pressure by decreasing the effective delivered tidal volume.

**VII-9.** **The answer is A.** *(Chap. 252)* In patients with asthma, airflow obstruction does not allow full exhalation, and these patients feel dyspnea related to respiration at higher lung volumes. When respiratory failure develops in the setting of an asthma flare, ventilator management can be quite difficult. The rise in Pa$_{CO_2}$ stimulates ventilatory drive in patients with normal central nervous system function. This can lead to what is commonly called breath stacking while a patient is on a ventilator. *Breath stacking* is a term used to describe the situation when a patient triggers another ventilator-delivered breath although the previous breath has not been fully exhaled. The positive pressure that develops when this occurs is called intrinsic positive end-expiratory pressure. If this pressure accumulates to a high level, venous return can be impeded, resulting in hypotension. The immediate management in this case consists of disconnecting the patient from the ventilator for several seconds to allow full exhalation. Multiple other variables can be manipulated through the mechanical ventilator to prevent this pressure from reaccumulating. The main principle of management is to increase the time for exhalation. Maneuvers that can accomplish this include decreasing the tidal volume delivered, decreasing the respiratory rate, changing the inspiratory flow rate, and changing the inspiratory wave form to one that delivers a breath most rapidly. Additionally, the assist-control mode of ventilation delivers a full breath at the designated tidal volume for each patient-triggered breath over the set rate. In this setting, synchronized intermittent mandatory ventilation is used to decrease minute ventilation in a patient who may be breathing quite rapidly. Finally, deep sedation or paralysis may be needed to prevent the patient from triggering additional breaths and prevent the development of intrinsic PEEP. All these strategies for manipulating the ventilator in the setting of obstructive lung disease rely on permissive hypercapnia, meaning that the elevated Pa$_{CO_2}$ is allowed to be elevated above normal to prevent the complications of mechanical ventilation.

**VII-10 and VII-11.** **The answers are B and E.** *(Chap. 254; Bernard GR et al, N Engl J Med 344:699–709, 2001.)* This patient has evidence of severe sepsis syndrome as manifested by evidence of a source of infection, hypotension, metabolic acidosis, low platelet count, and abnormal renal function. The initial step in managing hypotension in a patient with sepsis is the administration of intravenous fluids because effective intravascular volume is low as a result of the vasodilatory effects of endotoxin with a subsequent fall in systemic vascular resistance. This initially requires the administration of a minimum of 1 to 2 L of intravenous normal saline over the first 1 or 2 h. Additional fluids may be necessary, and some studies suggest that up to 9 L of fluid are needed in the first 24 h of a sepsis syndrome. Maintaining central venous pressure between 8 and 12 cmH$_2$O or pulmonary capillary wedge pressure between 12 and 16 cmH$_2$O makes it possible to assess the adequacy of volume resuscitation. In one-third of these patients adequate blood pressure can be maintained with volume resuscitation alone. If vasopressors are required, the goal for titration is a systolic blood pressure above 90 mmHg or a mean arterial pressure above 65 mmHg. In this patient, intubation and mechanical ventilation will be required as the patient shows evidence of an inadequate ventilatory response to metabolic acidosis as predicted by Winter's formula [predicted $Pa_{CO_2}$ 1.5(measured $HCO_3$) + 8 ± 2]. Thus, the patient has concurrent respiratory acidosis indicative of impending ventilatory failure as well as metabolic acidosis. In addition, endotracheal intubation should be considered because of the patient's poor mental state. At present the patient does not show evidence of hypoxemic respiratory failure, although the patient is at high risk of developing ARDS. Intravenous bicarbonate may be considered in patients with a pH less than 7.2 but is not the first step in the management of this patient.

Recombinant activated protein C (aPC) is the first U.S. Food and Drug Administration (FDA)-approved treatment for severe sepsis syndrome and septic shock. This therapy is directed at the pathogenesis of sepsis because sepsis syndrome and its complications are caused by intravascular thrombosis. Clotting is favored by impairment in function of the protein C–protein S inhibitory pathway as well as depletion of protein C and antithrombin. Further, there is increased plasminogen-activator inhibitor-1. The PROWESS investigators demonstrated a decreased 28-day mortality versus placebo (24.7% versus 30.8%) in patients who received aPC within the first 48 h of the onset of sepsis-related organ dysfunction. However, this improvement is not without problems associated with increased bleeding events, and a survival advantage was evident only in patients with an APACHE II score ≥25. Patients who should be considered for therapy are those with the criteria for severe sepsis (see the table below) with evidence of the involvement of one or more organ systems.

---

Definitions Used to Describe the Condition of Septic Patients

| | |
|---|---|
| Bacteremia | Presence of bacteria in blood, as evidenced by positive blood cultures |
| Septicemia | Presence of microbes or their toxins in blood |
| Systemic inflammatory response syndrome (SIRS) | Two or more of the following conditions: (1) fever (oral temperature >38°C) or hypothermia (<36°C); (2) tachypnea (>24 breaths/min); (3) tachycardia (heart rate > 90 beats/min); (4) leukocytosis (>12,000/μL), leukopenia (<4,000/μL), or >10% bands; may have a noninfectious etiology |
| Sepsis | SIRS that has a proven or suspected microbial etiology |
| Severe sepsis (similar to "sepsis syndrome") | Sepsis with one or more signs of organ dysfunction—for example: <br> 1. *Cardiovascular:* Arterial systolic blood pressure ≤90 mmHg or mean arterial pressure ≤ 70 mmHg that responds to administration of intravenous fluid <br> 2. *Renal:* Urine output < 0.5 mL/kg per hour for 1 h despite adequate fluid resuscitation <br> 3. *Respiratory:* $Pa_{O_2}/FI_{O_2}$ ≤ 250 or, if the lung is the only dysfunctional organ, ≤200 <br> 4. *Hematologic:* Platelet count < 80,000/μL or 50% decrease in platelet count from highest value recorded over previous 3 days <br> 5. *Unexplained metabolic acidosis:* A pH ≤ 7.30 or a base deficit ≥ 5.0 mEq/L and a plasma lactate level > 1.5 times upper limit of normal for reporting lab <br> 6. *Adequate fluid resuscitation:* Pulmonary artery wedge pressure ≥ 12 mmHg or central venous pressure ≥ 8 mmHg |
| Septic shock | Sepsis with hypotension (arterial blood pressure <90 mmHg systolic, or 40 mmHg less than patient's normal blood pressure) for at least 1 h despite adequate fluid resuscitation; <br> *or* <br> Need for vasopressors to maintain systolic blood pressure ≥ 90 mmHg *or* mean arterial pressure ≥ 70 mmHg |
| Refractory septic shock | Septic shock that lasts for >1 h and does not respond to fluid or pressor administration |
| Multiple-organ dysfunction syndrome (MODS) | Dysfunction of more than one organ, requiring intervention to maintain homeostasis |

*Source:* Adapted from the American College of Chest Physicians/Society of Critical Care Medicine Consensus Conference Committee.

Elevation of coagulation parameters is not included in the diagnosis of severe sepsis. Patients with an increased risk of bleeding should not receive a PC. These factors include a platelet count below 30,000/mm³, recent surgery, stroke, gastrointestinal bleeding, or cerebral aneurysm and recent treatment with anticoagulant therapy. Other patients who have been excluded from trials include those with a known life expectancy less than 28 days, organ transplants or bone marrow transplants, cirrhosis, chronic renal failure, and acute pancreatitis without evidence of infection.

**VII-12.** **The answer is A.** *(Chap. 254; Annane et al, JAMA 288:862–871, 2002.)* The patient presents with urosepsis and fails to increase blood pressure after the administration of intravenous fluid. Vasopressors are indicated at this point. In addition, recent data have suggested that there is an increased prevalence of relative adrenal insufficiency in the critically ill patient population. Furthermore, treatment of this relative adrenal insufficiency with hydrocortisone and fludrocortisone is associated with a mortality benefit. Current recommendations are to assess adrenal function in critically ill patients with 250 $\mu$g cosyntropin and replete with hydrocortisone and fludrocortisone in patients whose serum cortisol levels rise 9 $\mu$g/dL or less. Serum ACTH, salivary cortisol, and metyrapone testing have not been used for this purpose.

**VII-13.** **The answer is D.** *(Chaps. 245 and 252)* Patients with chronic obstructive pulmonary disease (COPD) are at increased risk of several complications associated with mechanical ventilation, and physicians must be alert for the development of those complications. This patient has evidence of spontaneous tension pneumothorax related to the rupture of a preexisting bulla in the presence of positive-pressure ventilation. Clinically, the manifestations are decreased blood pressure, tachycardia, and decreased breath sounds on the affected hemithorax with a shift of the trachea to the contralateral side. Additionally, increased inspiratory pressures are noted on the mechanical ventilator. Immediate decompression of the pneumothorax followed by tube thoracostomy is indicated to prevent electromechanical dissociation as the patient is demonstrating evidence of shock with hypotension and peripheral hypoperfusion.

Other complications of mechanical ventilation in COPD include the development of intrinsic positive end-expiratory pressure and mucus plugging. Intrinsic PEEP develops when insufficient time for exhalation is given and is particularly important in patients with obstructive lung disease. If intrinsic PEEP accumulates, a high intrathoracic pressure may develop, causing hypotension from decreased venous return. Disconnecting the patient from the ventilator temporarily allows full exhalation and relieves the positive pressure and hypotension. Many options are available to prevent intrinsic PEEP from recurring, including slowing the respiratory rate, decreasing the tidal volume, and maximizing the inspiratory/expiratory ratio by changing the ventilator mechanics. Mucus plugging can also cause sudden-onset hypoxemia, decreased breath sounds, and elevated ventilatory pressures, as seen in this patient. Hypotension, however, is rarely seen. Furthermore, mucus plugging should cause deviation of the trachea toward the side of the lung, with the decreased breath sounds resulting from volume loss.

Ventilatory dyssynchrony is a common problem that causes hypoxemia but is not apparent clinically here as the patient is not described as appearing agitated or tachypneic. Sepsis syndrome should be considered if the patient develops refractory hypotension after alleviation of the pneumothorax and adequate fluid resuscitation.

# VIII. DISORDERS OF THE KIDNEY AND URINARY TRACT

## QUESTIONS

**DIRECTIONS:** Each question below contains five suggested responses. Choose the **one best** response to each question.

**VIII-1.** A 56-year-old male is evaluated in the clinic after complaining of inability to maintain an erection. He reports good sexual function until 4 months ago. Since that time he has noted that he cannot maintain erections. The patient awakens three times weekly with an erection that is unchanged compared with his previous status. He states that his libido is unchanged but that he loses his erection within minutes. He has been married for 25 years and denies any extramarital affairs. He does not smoke. Recently the patient has had increased stressors in his life when he was laid off his job as a worker in an oil refinery. Past medical history is significant for hypertension, which is being treated with atenolol. On physical examination, blood pressure is 136/76 mmHg and heart rate is 64/min. The patient has normal secondary sexual characteristics without gynecomastia. There is no liver enlargement. The testes are firm and rubbery without masses and have an estimated volume of 35 mL by orchiometry. The penis is circumcised and without fibrotic plaques. Rectal examination reveals a normal prostate and normal anal sphincter tone. The bulbocavernosus reflex is intact. Prostate-specific antigen (PSA) is 4.12 ng/mL. The testosterone level is 537 ng/dL. What is the best way to treat this patient's erectile dysfunction?

A. Discontinue atenolol.
B. Start sildenafil.
C. Initiate therapy with transdermal testosterone.
D. Initiate therapy with intraurethral injection of alprostadil.
E. Further explore the patient's psychosocial history for evidence of anxiety and depression and consider referral for psychotherapy.

**VIII-2.** A 34-year-old male presents with acute onset of right flank pain radiating to the groin. He is not febrile but appears to be very uncomfortable. He is writhing in his bed. The physical examination is otherwise unremarkable. Urinalysis shows 25 to 35 red blood cells per high-power field. Which of the following is the diagnostic test of choice?

A. Noncontrast helical computed tomography (CT)
B. Contrast-enhanced computed tomography

**VIII-2.** *(Continued)*
C. Intravenous pyelography
D. Plain radiograms of the abdomen and pelvis
E. Ultrasound

**VIII-3.** A 35-year-old male with a history of hypertension presents to the emergency room with fever, left flank pain, dysuria, and hematuria. He had one episode of calcium oxalate nephrolithiasis in the past. Family history is significant for a mother with diabetes mellitus, hypertension, and end-stage renal disease (ESRD). The examination is otherwise normal. Urine culture is positive for gram-negative bacilli. Renal ultrasound is significant for enlarged kidneys and more than five renal cysts bilaterally without any hydronephrosis or evidence of stones. What is the most likely underlying diagnosis?

A. Tuberous sclerosis
B. Von Hippel–Lindau disease
C. Autosomal recessive polycystic kidney disease
D. Autosomal dominant polycystic kidney disease-1
E. Autosomal dominant polycystic kidney disease-2

**VIII-4.** What is the recommended treatment?

A. Ciprofloxacin
B. Ampicillin
C. Vancomycin
D. Gentamicin
E. Clindamycin

**VIII-5.** A clinic patient who has a diagnosis of polycystic kidney disease has been doing research on the Internet. She is asymptomatic and has no significant family history. She asks you for screening for intracranial aneurysms. You recommend which of the following?

A. Head CT scan without contrast
B. CT angiogram
C. Cerebral angiogram
D. Magnetic resonance angiogram
E. No further testing

**VIII-6.** A 16-year-old female star gymnast presents to your office complaining of fatigue, diffuse weakness, and

**VIII-6.** *(Continued)*

muscle cramps. She has no previous medical history and denies tobacco, alcohol, or illicit drug use. There is no significant family history. Examination shows a thin female with normal blood pressure. Body mass index (BMI) is 18 kg/m$^2$. Oral examination shows poor dentition. Muscle tone is normal, and neurologic examination is normal. Laboratory studies show hematocrit of 38.5%, creatinine of 0.6 mg/dL, serum bicarbonate of 30 meq/L, and potassium of 2.7 meq/L. Further evaluation should include which of the following?

A. Urinalysis and urine culture
B. Plasma renin and aldosterone levels
C. Urine toxicology screen for opiates
D. Urine toxicology screen for diuretics
E. Serum magnesium level

**VIII-7.** A patient with a history of Sjögren's syndrome has the following laboratory findings: plasma sodium 139 meq/L, chloride 112 meq/L, bicarbonate 15 meq/L, and potassium 3.0 meq/L; urine studies show a pH of 6.0, sodium of 15 meq/L, potassium of 10 meq/L, and chloride of 12 meq/L. The most likely diagnosis is

A. type I renal tubular acidosis (RTA)
B. type II RTA
C. type III RTA
D. type IV RTA
E. chronic diarrhea

**VIII-8.** Which of the following is the most appropriate treatment for a patient with Hartnup disease?

A. Folate
B. Niacin
C. Nicotinamide
D. Pyridoxine
E. Vitamin B$_{12}$

**VIII-9.** In the emergency room a male patient presents with complaints of right flank pain without radiation during micturition and intermittent polyuria with other periods of decreased urine output. The patient denies having dysuria, hematuria, and fever. He denies any significant past medical history, and a review of all other symptoms is negative. Examination shows normal vital signs, and there is a normal abdominal examination except for mild costophrenic angle tenderness on the right. Rectal examination shows no tenderness, and there is a normal prostate examination. There is no edema in the lower extremities. Urinalysis is bland without pyuria, bacteria, or casts. Serum blood urea nitrogen (BUN) and creatinine are 50 mg/dL and 2.0 mg/dL, respectively. Renal ultrasound shows bilateral hydronephrosis. What is the most likely diagnosis?

A. Acute cystitis
B. Genitourinary tuberculosis

**VIII-9.** *(Continued)*

C. Nephrolithiasis
D. Transitional cell carcinoma of the bladder
E. Vesicoureteral reflux disease

**VIII-10.** A 35-year-old female presents with complaints of bilateral lower extremity edema, polyuria, and moderate left-sided flank pain that began approximately 2 weeks ago. There is no past medical history. She is taking no medications and denies tobacco, alcohol, or illicit drug use. Examination shows normal vital signs, including normal blood pressure. There is 2+ edema in bilateral lower extremities. The 24-h urine collection is significant for 3.5 g of protein. Urinalysis is bland except for the proteinuria. Serum creatinine is 0.7 mg/dL, and ultrasound examination shows the left kidney measuring 13 cm and the right kidney measuring 11.5 cm. You are concerned about renal vein thrombosis. What test do you choose for the evaluation?

A. Computed tomography of the renal veins
B. Contrast venography
C. Magnetic resonance venography
D. $^{99}$Tc-labeled pentetic acid (DPTA) imaging
E. Ultrasound with Doppler evaluation of the renal veins

**VIII-11.** A 62-year-old female with a history of coronary artery disease with previous myocardial infarction, hypertension, and diabetes mellitus presents to your office for evaluation. She is asymptomatic; however, despite therapy with hydrochlorothiazide, metoprolol, and lisinopril, her blood pressure remains elevated at 185/100 mmHg. Examination of the abdomen reveals a soft bruit in the right upper quadrant. Laboratory evaluation is significant for normal electrolytes, a BUN of 30 mg/dL, and a creatinine of 1.8 mg/dL. What is your recommendation?

A. Abdominal magnetic resonance angiography with gadolinium
B. Renal contrast-enhanced angiography
C. Renal ultrasonography
D. $^{99}$Tc-labeled pentetic acid (DPTA) imaging
E. No imaging evaluation

**VIII-12.** A 40-year-old African-American male with a history of hypertension presents to the emergency room with complaints of headache and blurred vision. His family reports that the patient has been intermittently confused over the last 48 h. He reports adherence to antihypertensive medications. On examination the patient is found to be afebrile with a blood pressure of 220/130 mmHg and a heart rate of 74/min. Eye examination reveals papilledema. He is admitted to the cardiac intensive care unit. Over the next 36 h with control of blood pressure, he has a rapid decline in urine output and an acute rise in BUN and creatinine. Urinalysis shows microscopic hematuria, proteinuria, and red and white blood cell casts. He is di-

**VIII-12.** *(Continued)*
agnosed with malignant hypertension. Medical therapy successfully controls the blood pressure, and he recovers with a creatinine of 2.0 mg/dL. What is this patient's 5-year survival rate?

A. 10%
B. 25%
C. 50%
D. 75%
E. 90%

**VIII-13.** A patient with a diagnosis of scleroderma who has diffuse cutaneous involvement presents with malignant hypertension, oliguria, edema, hemolytic anemia, and renal failure. You make a diagnosis of scleroderma renal crisis (SRC). What is the recommended treatment?

A. Captopril
B. Carvedilol
C. Clonidine
D. Diltiazem
E. Nitroprusside

**VIII-14.** The posterior pituitary secretes arginine vasopressin (antidiuretic hormone) under which of the following stressors?

A. Hyperosmolarity
B. Hypernatremia
C. Volume depletion
D. A and B
E. A and C

**VIII-15.** A 26-year-old female who competed in a marathon earlier in the day presents with symptoms consistent with hypovolemia, including thirst and light-headedness with standing. All the following laboratory results would be expected *except*

A. blood urea nitrogen/creatinine ratio >20
B. urine sodium <20 mmol/L
C. urine osmolarity <300 mosmol/L
D. urine specific gravity >1.015
E. elevation above baseline in hematocrit

**Questions VIII-16 to VIII-19.** Acute Renal Failure: For each of the following questions, choose the pathophysiologic mechanism of reduced glomerular filtration rate (GFR).

A. Acute tubular necrosis
B. Decreased relaxation of afferent arterioles
C. Glomerulonephritis
D. Hypovolemia
E. Increased relaxation of efferent arterioles

**VIII-16.** A 55-year-old male has a history of hypertension and myocardial infarction. He is seen in the clinic to fol-

**VIII-16.** *(Continued)*
low up on his blood pressure. There are no symptoms. The patient's current medical regimen includes amlodipine, hydrochlorothiazide, and atenolol. Blood pressure is measured at 165/83 in both arms. The remainder of the physical examination is notable for an abdominal bruit. Lisinopril is added to the regimen. One week later blood work shows a creatinine that has risen from 1.3 mg/dL to 5.0 mg/dL.

**VIII-17.** An 88-year-old female is admitted to the hospital after being found in her apartment with altered mental status by family members. Physical examination is notable for delirium, poor skin turgor, and dry mucous membranes. BUN is 63 mg/dL, and creatinine is 1.3 mg/dL.

**VIII-18.** A 62-year-old female with hypertension is seen in the clinic with acute-onset pain in the right great toe. Her current medications include clopidogrel and ramipril. The patient's primary care physician diagnoses gout and prescribes indomethacin. Routine laboratories 3 days later show that her creatinine has increased from 0.7 mg/dL to 3.7 mg/dL.

**VIII-19.** A 35-year-old female is admitted to the intensive care unit with pneumococcal pneumonia and hypotension. Despite adequate volume resuscitation she remains hypotensive, and vasopressors are started. Creatinine on admission is 1.5 mg/dL and rises to 5.1 mg/dL on the third hospital day. Urinalysis shows muddy brown granular casts.

**VIII-20.** A 79-year-old male with a history of dementia is brought to the emergency department because of an 8-h history of lethargy. For the last 2 days he has been complaining of lower abdominal pain. His oral intake was normal until the last 8 h. The patient takes no medications. Temperature is normal, blood pressure is 150/90 mmHg, heart rate is 105/min, and respirations are 20/min. Physical examination is notable for elevated neck veins and diffuse lower abdominal pain with normal bowel sounds. The bladder is percussed to the umbilicus, and there is an enlarged prostate. He is lethargic but responsive. Serum chemistries are notable for sodium of 128 meq/L, potassium of 5.7 meq/L, BUN of 100 mg/dL, and creatinine of 2.2 mg/dL. Two months ago his laboratory studies were normal. A Foley catheter is placed, yielding 1100 mL of urine. Which of the following statements regarding his clinical condition is true?

A. His renal function probably will return to normal within the next week.
B. He will need aggressive volume resuscitation over the next 24 h.
C. He will have oliguria over the next 24 h.
D. Immediate dialysis is indicated.
E. Urinalysis will reveal hypertonic urine.

**VIII-21.** A 33-year-old male is brought for medical attention after completing an ultramarathon. Upon finishing he was disoriented and light-headed. His normal weight is 60 kg. Physical examination reveals a body temperature of 38.3°C (100.9°F), blood pressure of 85/60 mmHg, and heart rate of 125/min. The patient's neck veins are flat, and skin turgor is poor. Laboratory studies are notable for a serum sodium of 175 meq/L. The patient's estimated free water deficit is

A. 0.75 L
B. 1.5 L
C. 7.5 L
D. 15 L
E. 22.5 L

**VIII-22.** Which of the following statements is true regarding the measurement of the glomerular filtration rate?

A. Urea clearance overestimates GFR because urea is reabsorbed by the tubules.
B. Serum creatinine can increase after the ingestion of cooked meat.
C. For similar age- and weight-matched individuals, a woman's plasma creatinine clearance will be 75% of the matched male value according to the Cockcroft-Gault equation.
D. Inulin clearance is a flawed measure of GFR because of renal secretion in the tubules.
E. Symptomatic uremia can be expected with a GFR <20 mL/min.

**VIII-23.** A 68-year-old male is seen in the clinic by his oncologist for the management of multiple myeloma. Laboratories show a creatinine of 5.6 mg/dL. Which of the following is a possible mechanism of his renal failure?

A. Intravascular volume depletion
B. Cast nephropathy
C. Light chain deposition
D. B and C
E. A, B, and C

**VIII-24.** A 25-year-old female with nephrotic syndrome from minimal-change disease is seen in the emergency department with increased right leg swelling. Ultrasound of the leg shows thrombosis of the superficial femoral vein. Which of the following is not a mechanism of hypercoagulability in this disorder?

A. Increased platelet aggregation
B. Low serum levels of protein C and protein S
C. Chronic disseminated intravascular coagulation
D. Hyperfibrinogenemia
E. Low serum levels of antithrombin III

**VIII-25.** A 50-year-old male is admitted to the hospital with pneumonia. He does well after the administration of antibiotics, but his sodium is noted to rise from 140 to 154 meq/L over 2 days. He reports thirst and has had a urine output of approximately 5 L per day. Which of the following is the most appropriate next step to evaluate the patient's disorder?

A. Measurement of serum osmolality
B. Measurement of serum vasopressin level
C. 24-h measurement of urinary sodium
D. Trial of arginine vasopressin
E. Trial of free water restriction

**VIII-26.** Which of the following would not be expected in a patient with chronic kidney disease?

A. Increased number of 1,25-dihydroxyvitamin D receptors in parathyroid gland
B. Hypertrophy of normal nephrons
C. Isosthenuria when GFR is less than 25 mL/min
D. Decreased serum 1,25-dihydroxyvitamin D level
E. Increased serum intact parathyroid hormone level

**VIII-27.** Which of the following is the most potent stimulus for hypothalamic production of arginine vasopressin?

A. Hypertonicity
B. Hyperkalemia
C. Hypokalemia
D. Hypotonicity
E. Intravascular volume depletion

**VIII-28.** All the following are associated with increased AVP secretion at a normal plasma osmolality *except*

A. ethanol
B. fluoxetine
C. HIV infection
D. nausea
E. stroke

**VIII-29.** A 36-year-old male undergoes knee surgery to repair torn ligaments. Postoperatively he is prescribed acetaminophen for pain. One day later he reports worsening pain. Physical examination reveals blood pressure 120/75 mmHg, heart rate 80/min, respiratory rate 14/min, and temperature 37°C (98.6°F). He has severe pain at the knee but no redness or signs of infection. Serum electrolytes are as follows:

| | |
|---|---|
| Sodium | 128 meq/L |
| Potassium | 4.0 meq/L |
| Chloride | 95 meq/L |
| Bicarbonate | 25 meq/L |
| BUN | 12 mg/dL |
| Creatinine | 1.0 mg/dL |

**VIII-29.** *(Continued)*
Which of the following therapies is most appropriate at this time?

A. Hypertonic saline
B. Furosemide
C. Morphine
D. Normal saline
E. Vancomycin

**VIII-30.** A 20-year-old college student seeks medical attention for light-headedness. He just completed a rigorous tennis match and did not drink any water or fluids. Supine blood pressure is 110/70 mmHg, and heart rate is 105/min. Upright, the blood pressure is 95/60 mmHg with a heart rate of 125/min. Temperature and mental status are normal. Which of the following laboratory results is most likely in this patient?

A. Serum BUN/creatinine ratio <20
B. Serum sodium <140 meq/L
C. Urine potassium <20 meq/L
D. Urine sodium <20 meq/L
E. Urine red blood cell casts

**VIII-31.** A 34-year-old male is brought to the hospital with altered mental status. He has a history of alcoholism. He is somnolent and does not answer questions. Physical examination reveals blood pressure 130/80, heart rate 105/min, respiratory rate 24/min, and temperature 37°C (98.6°F). The remainder of the physical examination is unremarkable. Microscopic analysis of urine is shown below. Which of the following most likely will be found on further diagnostic evaluation?

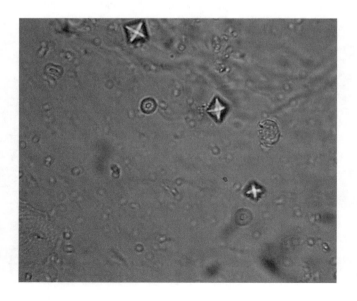

**VIII-31.** *(Continued)*

A. More than 10,000 bacterial colonies on urine culture
B. Anion gap metabolic acidosis
C. Hydronephrosis on ultrasound
D. Nephrolithiasis on CT scan
E. Positive antinuclear antibodies (ANA)

**VIII-32.** A 74-year-old female sees her physician for a follow-up visit for hypertension. One week ago she was started on an oral medication for hypertension. She takes no other medications. Blood pressure is 125/80 mmHg, and heart rate is 72/min. Serum chemistries reveal a sodium of 132 meq/L. Two weeks ago serum chemistries were normal. Which of the following medications most likely was initiated 1 week ago?

A. Enalapril
B. Furosemide
C. Hydrochlorothiazide
D. Metoprolol
E. Spironolactone

**VIII-33.** A 63-year-old male is brought to the emergency department after having a seizure. He has a history of an unresectable lung mass treated with palliative radiation therapy. He is known to have a serum sodium of 128 meq/L chronically. The patient's wife reports that on the night before admission he was somnolent. This morning, while she was trying to awaken him, he developed a generalized tonic-clonic seizure lasting approximately 1 min. In the emergency room he is unresponsive. Vital signs and physical examination are otherwise normal. Serum sodium is 111 meq/L. He is treated with 3% saline and transferred to the intensive care unit. One day later serum sodium is 137 meq/L. He has had no further seizures since admission and is awake but is barely able to move his extremities and is dysarthric. Which of the following studies is most likely to explain his current condition?

A. Arteriogram showing a vertebral artery thrombus
B. CT of the head showing metastases
C. EEG showing focal seizures
D. MRI of the brainstem showing demyelination
E. Transesophageal echocardiogram showing left atrial thrombus

**VIII-34.** A 28-year-old female with a history of intravenous drug use is being treated with oxacillin and gentamicin for *Staphylococcus aureus* endocarditis. Baseline renal and hepatic functions are normal, and she is afebrile 5 days after the initiation of antibiotics. Ten days into treatment she develops new fever and a macular nonpruritic rash over the legs, trunk, and arms. Laboratory examination reveals a BUN of 35 mg/dL and a creatinine of 2.2 mg/dL. Urinalysis reveals 2+ protein with positive red blood cells and white blood cells. Renal ultrasound shows mild bilaterally enlarged kidneys. Which of the following best explains the new renal failure?

**VIII-34.** *(Continued)*

    A.   Acute tubular necrosis

    B.   Allergic interstitial nephritis

    C.   Membranous glomerulonephritis

    D.   Nephrolithiasis

    E.   Septic emboli to the kidney

**VIII-35.** All the following are complications during hemodialysis *except*

    A.   anaphylactoid reaction

    B.   fever

    C.   hyperglycemia

    D.   hypotension

    E.   muscle cramps

**VIII-36.** A 63-year-old male with a history of diabetes mellitus is found to have a lung nodule on chest radiography. To stage the disease further he undergoes a contrast-enhanced CT scan of the chest. One week before the CT scan, his BUN is 26 mg/dL and his creatinine is 1.8 mg/dL. Three days after the study he complains of dyspnea, pedal edema, and decreased urinary output. Repeat BUN is 86 mg/dL and creatinine is 4.4 mg/dL. The most likely mechanism of the acute renal failure is

    A.   acute tubular necrosis

    B.   allergic hypersensitivity

    C.   cholesterol emboli

    D.   immune-complex glomerulonephritis

    E.   ureteral outflow obstruction

**VIII-37.** In the patient in Question X-36 the urinalysis is most likely to show

    A.   granular casts

    B.   red blood cell casts

    C.   urinary eosinophils

    D.   urinary neutrophils

    E.   white blood cell casts

**VIII-38.** A 50-year-old male presents to the emergency room complaining of cough without sputum production, mild fever, leg swelling, and hematuria. Past history is significant only for allergic rhinitis, and he is taking only aspirin 81 mg/d. Examination shows a temperature of 37.2°C (99°F), blood pressure of 150/70 mmHg, 2+ symmetric swelling of the lower extremities, and a purpuric rash on the extremities. Chest x-ray was normal. Laboratory was significant for a BUN of 70 mg/dL and a creatinine of 4.5 mg/dL. On repeat evaluation 12 h later serum creatinine is 5.0 mg/dL. Microscopic analysis of fresh urine shows many of the casts as shown in the following figure. Urine spot protein/creatinine ratio is 1.5. Your recommendation at this time is

**VIII-38.** *(Continued)*

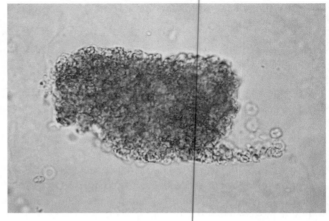

    A.   renal biopsy

    B.   serum antineutrophil cytoplasmic antibodies (ANCA) measurement

    C.   captopril 50 mg PO tid

    D.   solumedrol 1 mg/kg IV qd

    E.   cyclophosphamide 100 mg PO qd

**VIII-39.** All the following forms of glomerulonephritis (GN) have associated normal serum complement C4 levels *except*

    A.   lupus nephritis stage IV

    B.   poststreptococcal GN

    C.   hemolytic-uremic syndrome

    D.   membranoproliferative GN type II

    E.   endocarditis-associated GN

**VIII-40.** All the following are indications for the initiation of hemodialysis *except*

    A.   acute renal failure with potassium of 8.0 mmol/L and ECG abnormalities

    B.   acute renal failure, anuric, with evidence of pulmonary edema

    C.   chronic kidney disease with an estimated creatinine clearance of 20 mL/min per 1.73 m$^2$

    D.   salicylate ingestion with mental status changes

    E.   chronic kidney disease with asterixis on examination and mental status changes

**VIII-41.** A patient with lymphoma who is known to excrete 1.5 g urinary protein per day has a negative dipstick evaluation for urinary protein. Which of the following is the reason for this seeming inconsistency?

    A.   The excreted protein is too small to be picked up by the test strip.

    B.   The urine is not concentrated enough.

    C.   Only heavy chain sequences are recognized by the test strip.

**VIII-41.**  *(Continued)*

D.   Tamm-Horsfall protein blocks the reaction between the secreted protein and the test strip
E.   Dipsticks preferentially detect albumin compared with immunoglobulin because albumin is negatively charged.

**VIII-42.**   Laboratory evaluation of a 19-year-old male who is being worked up for polyuria and polydipsia yields the following results:

Serum electrolytes (mmol/L): $Na^+$ 144, $K^+$ 4.0, $Cl^-$ 107, $HCO_3^-$ 25
BUN: 6.4 mmol/L (18 mg/dL)
Blood glucose: 5.7 mmol/L (102 mg/dL)
Urine electrolytes (mmol/L): $Na^+$ 28, $K^+$ 32
Urine osmolality: 195 mosmol/kg water

After 12 h of fluid deprivation, body weight has fallen by 5%. Laboratory testing now reveals the following:

Serum electrolytes (mmol/L): $Na^+$ 150, $K^+$ 4.1, $Cl^-$ 109, $HCO_3^-$ 25
BUN: 7.1 mmol/L (20 mg/dL)
Blood glucose: 5.4 mmol/L (98 mg/dL)
Urine electrolytes (mmol/L): $Na^+$ 24, $K^+$ 35
Urine osmolality: 200 mosmol/kg water

One hour after the subcutaneous administration of 5 units of arginine vasopressin urine values are as follows:

Urine electrolytes (mmol/L): $Na^+$ 30, $K^+$ 30
Urine osmolality: 199 mosmol/kg water

The likely diagnosis is

A.   nephrogenic diabetes insipidus
B.   osmotic diuresis
C.   salt-losing nephropathy
D.   psychogenic polydipsia
E.   none of the above

**VIII-43.**   A 45-year-old female who has had slowly progressive renal failure begins to complain of increasing numbness and prickling sensations in the legs. Examination reveals loss of pinprick and vibration sensation below the knees, absent ankle jerks, and impaired pinprick sensation in the hands. Serum creatinine concentration, checked during the most recent clinic visit, is 790 μmol/L (8.9 mg/dL). The woman's physician should now recommend

A.   a therapeutic trial of phenytoin
B.   a therapeutic trial of pyridoxine (vitamin $B_6$)
C.   a therapeutic trial of cyanocobalamin (vitamin $B_{12}$)
D.   initiation of renal replacement therapy
E.   neurologic referral for nerve conduction studies

**VIII-44.**   In patients with chronic renal failure, which of the following is the most important contributor to renal osteodystrophy?

A.   Impaired renal production of 1,25-dihydroxyvitamin $D_3$ [$1,25(OH)_2D_3$]
B.   Hypocalcemia
C.   Hypophosphatemia
D.   Loss of vitamin D and calcium via dialysis
E.   The use of calcitriol

**VIII-45.**   A 50-year-old male is hospitalized for treatment of enterococcal endocarditis. He has been receiving ampicillin and gentamicin for the last 2 weeks but is persistently febrile. Laboratory results are as follows:

Serum electrolytes (mmol/L): $Na^+$ 145, $K^+$ 5.0, $Cl^-$ 110, $HCO_3^-$ 20
BUN: 14.2 mmol/L (40 mg/dL)
Serum creatinine: 300 μmol/L (3.5 mg/dL)
Urine sodium: 20 mmol/L
Urine creatinine: 3000 mmol/L (35 mg/dL)

Which of the following is the most likely cause of this patient's acute renal failure?

A.   Tubular necrosis
B.   Insensible skin losses
C.   Renal artery embolism
D.   Cardiac failure
E.   Nausea and vomiting

**VIII-46.**   The condition of a 50-year-old obese female with a 5-year history of mild hypertension controlled by a thiazide diuretic is being evaluated because proteinuria was noted during her routine yearly medical visit. Physical examination disclosed a height of 167.6 cm (66 in.), weight of 91 kg (202 lb), blood pressure of 130/80 mmHg, and trace pedal edema. Laboratory values are as follows:

Serum creatinine: 106 μmol/L (1.2 mg/dL)
BUN: 6.4 mmol/L (18 mg/dL)
Creatinine clearance: 87 mL/min
Urinalysis: pH 5.0; specific gravity 1.018; protein 3+; no glucose; occasional coarse granular cast
Urine protein excretion: 5.9 g/d

A renal biopsy demonstrates that 60% of the glomeruli have segmental scarring by light microscopy, with the remainder of the glomeruli appearing unremarkable (see following figure).

**VIII-46.** *(Continued)*

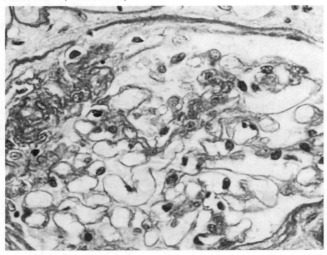

The most likely diagnosis is

A. hypertensive nephrosclerosis
B. focal and segmental sclerosis
C. minimal-change (nil) disease
D. membranous glomerulopathy
E. crescentic glomerulonephritis

**VIII-47.** A 45-year-old female with long-standing systemic lupus erythematosus (SLE) who has had intermittent bouts of acute renal failure over the last 6 years presents with anorexia. Physical examination is noncontributory. Laboratory evaluation includes hematocrit 29%, white blood cell count 5000 with a normal differential, and platelet count 27,500/$\mu$L. Renal biopsy shows sclerosis of 14/15 glomeruli, tubular atrophy, and interstitial fibrosis. The following values are also found:

Serum electrolytes (mmol/L): Na$^+$ 136, K$^+$ 6, Cl$^-$ 90, HCO$_3^-$ 20

**VIII-47.** *(Continued)*
BUN: 35.5 mmol/L (100 mg/dL)
Serum creatinine: 665 $\mu$mol/L (7.5 mg/dL)

Anti-double-strand DNA and C3 levels have been stable. Renal biopsy shows obliterative sclerosing glomerular lesions. The most appropriate management strategy would be

A. high-dose intravenous methylprednisolone
B. high-dose intravenous methylprednisolone and azathioprine
C. high-dose intravenous methylprednisolone and intravenous cyclophosphamide (500 mg/m$^2$)
D. intravenous cyclophosphamide (500 mg/m$^2$) plus low-dose prednisone
E. dialysis

**VIII-48.** A 10-year-old girl complaining of profound weakness, occasional difficulty walking, and polyuria is brought to the pediatrician. Her mother is sure the girl has not been vomiting frequently. The girl takes no medicines. She is normotensive, and no focal neurologic abnormalities are found. Serum chemistries include Na$^+$ 142 mmol/L, K$^+$ 2.5 mmol/L, HCO$_3^-$ 32 mmol/L, and Cl$^-$ 100 mmol/L. A 24-h urine collection on a normal diet reveals Na$^+$ 200 mmol/d, K$^+$ 50 mmol/d, and Cl$^-$ 30 mmol/d. Renal ultrasound demonstrates symmetrically enlarged kidneys without hydronephrosis. A stool phenolphthalein test and a urine screen for diuretics are negative. Plasma renin levels are found to be elevated. Which of the following conditions is most consistent with these data?

A. Conn's syndrome
B. Chronic ingestion of licorice
C. Bartter's syndrome
D. Wilms' tumor
E. Proximal renal tubular acidosis

**VIII-49.** A 53-year-old female with long-standing depression and a history of rheumatoid arthritis is brought in by her daughter, who states that she found an empty bottle of acetylsalicylic acid by her mother's bedside. The patient is found to be confused and lethargic and is unable to provide a definitive history. What is the most likely set of laboratory values?

| | Na$^+$ | K$^+$ | Cl$^-$ | HCO$_3^-$ | Serum Creatinine $\mu$mol/L (mg/dL) | Room Air ABG | | |
| | | | | | | P$_{O_2}$ | P$_{CO_2}$ | pH |
|---|---|---|---|---|---|---|---|---|
| | | (Serum, mmol/L) | | | | | | |
| A | 140 | 3.9 | 85 | 26 | 141 (1.6) | 100 | 40 | 7.40 |
| B | 140 | 3.9 | 85 | 16 | 141 (1.6) | 100 | 20 | 7.40 |
| C | 140 | 5.8 | 100 | 20 | 141 (1.6) | 100 | 34 | 7.38 |
| D | 150 | 2.9 | 100 | 36 | 141 (1.6) | 80 | 46 | 7.50 |
| E | 116 | 3.7 | 85 | 22 | 141 (1.6) | 80 | 46 | 7.50 |

**VIII-50.** A 72-year-old male develops acute renal failure after cardiac catheterization. Physical examination is notable for diminished peripheral pulses, livedo reticularis, epigastric tenderness, and confusion. Laboratory studies include (mg/dL) BUN 131, creatinine 5.2, and phosphate 9.5. Urinalysis shows 10 to 15 white blood cells (WBC), 5 to 10 red blood cells (RBC), and one hyaline cast per high-power field (HPF). The most likely diagnosis is

A. acute interstitial nephritis caused by drugs
B. rhabdomyolysis with acute tubular necrosis
C. acute tubular necrosis secondary to radiocontrast exposure
D. cholesterol embolization
E. renal arterial dissection with prerenal azotemia

**VIII-51.** A 45-year-old male with a diagnosis of ESRD secondary to diabetes mellitus is being treated with peritoneal dialysis. This is being carried out as a continuous ambulatory peritoneal dialysis (CAPD). He undergoes four 2-L exchanges per day and has been doing so for approximately 4 years. Complications of peritoneal dialysis include which of the following?

A. Hypotension after drainage of dialysate
B. Hypoalbuminemia
C. Hypercholesterolemia
D. Hypoglycemia
E. Left pleural effusion

# VIII. DISORDERS OF THE KIDNEY AND URINARY TRACT

## *ANSWERS*

**VIII-1.** **The answer is E.** *(Chap. 43)* The presence of unchanged nocturnal tumescence suggests psychogenic factors as the cause of the patient's erectile dysfunction (ED). Nocturnal tumescence occurs during REM sleep, and intact neurologic and circulatory systems are necessary for this to occur. Erectile dysfunction is reported in 52% of men between ages 40 and 70. The incidence of ED is higher in men with diabetes mellitus, heart disease, and hypertension and in tobacco users. Additionally, medications are frequently involved, especially many antihypertensive agents, including beta blockers, thiazide diuretics, calcium channel blockers, and angiotensin converting-enzyme (ACE) inhibitors. A thorough history and physical examination with limited laboratory testing usually yields the appropriate diagnosis.

**VIII-2.** **The answer is A.** *(Chap. 268)* For many years intravenous pyelography was the diagnostic procedure of choice for the diagnosis of a renal stone. In recent years it has been replaced by helical CT scan without intravenous contrast. Administration of radiodense intravenous contrast that is excreted in the urine may obscure ureteral stones. The advantages of this diagnostic tool include lack of exposure to contrast dye, ability to visualize uric acid stones, and possible visualization of other causes of abdominal pain. Plain radiograms and ultrasound are not sensitive for the detection of nephrolithiasis.

**VIII-3 and VIII-4.** **The answers are D and A.** *(Chap. 265)* Autosomal dominant polycystic kidney disease (ADPKD)–1 presents at any age but most frequently appears with symptoms in the third or fourth decade. Hematuria and infection are common. Additionally, calcium oxalate or uric acid stones occur in 15 to 20% of these patients. A family history of ESRD is important in identifying ADPKD. Eight-five percent of cases are ADPKD-1; however, ADPKD-2 presents similarly. Genetic linkage analysis is available for a definitive diagnosis. Autosomal recessive polycystic kidney disease is diagnosed within the first year of life. Tuberous sclerosis often presents with other findings, such as benign skin tumors. Von Hippel–Lindau disease is an autosomal dominant disease associated with hemangioblastomas of the retina and central nervous system. Patients with ADPKD are at high risk for developing infections within the cysts, or pyocysts. Specific antibiotics—ciprofloxacin, trimethoprim-sulfamethoxazole, and chloramphenicol—have been demonstrated to have high penetration into the pyocysts, and when ADPKD is suspected, these drugs should be chosen as the initial therapy.

**VIII-5.** **The answer is E.** *(Chap. 265)* Intracranial aneurysms are present in 5 to 10% of asymptomatic patients with ADPKD. Screening of all ADPKD patients is not recommended. Any presenting symptoms or a family history of subarachnoid hemorrhage or sudden death should prompt further screening with magnetic resonance angiography (MRA) or CT angiography or consideration of cerebral angiography.

**VIII-6.** **The answer is D.** *(Chap. 265)* In any patient with hypokalemia the use of diuretics must be excluded. This patient has multiple warning signs for the use of agents to alter her weight, including her age, gender, and participation in competitive sports. Her BMI is low, and the oral examination may suggest chronic vomiting. Chronic vomiting may be associated with a low urine chloride level. Once diuretic use and vomiting are excluded, the differential diagnosis of hypokalemia and metabolic alkalosis includes magnesium deficiency, Liddle's syndrome, Bartter's syndrome, and Gittleman's syndrome. Liddle's syndrome is associated with hypertension and undetectable aldosterone and renin levels. It is a rare autosomal dominant disorder. Classic Bartter's syndrome has a presentation similar to that of this patient. It may also include polyuria and nocturia because of hypo-kalemia-induced diabetes insipidus. Gittleman's syndrome can be distinguished from Bart-ter's syndrome by hypomagnesemia and hypocalciuria.

**VIII-7. The answer is A.** *(Chap. 265)* This patient has a normal anion gap metabolic acidosis (anion gap = 12). The calculated urine anion gap ($Na^+ + K^+ - Cl^-$) is +3; thus, the acidosis is unlikely to be due to gastrointestinal bicarbonate loss. In this patient the diag-nosis is type I renal tubular acidosis, or distal RTA. This is a disorder in which the distal nephron does not lower pH normally. It is associated with a urine pH > 5.5, hypokalemia, and lack of bicarbonaturia. This condition may be associated with calcium phosphate stones and nephrocalcinosis. Type II RTA, or proximal RTA, includes a pH < 5.5, hy-pokalemia, a positive urine anion gap, bicarbinaturia, hypophosphatemia, and hypercal-ciuria. This condition results from defective resorption of bicarbonate. Type III RTA is rare and most commonly is seen in children. Type IV RTA is also referred to as hyper-kalemic distal RTA. Hyporeninemic hypoaldosteronism is the most common cause of type IV RTA and is usually associated with diabetic nephropathy.

**VIII-8. The answer is C.** *(Chap. 265)* Hartnup disease is a disorder of reduced intestinal ab-sorption and renal resorption of neutral amino acids. The effect involves the jejunum and the proximal tubule. It is an autosomal recessive trait with an incidence of 1 in 24,000 live births. The majority of these patients are asymptomatic. The symptoms are similar to those seen in pellagra. The symptoms are thought to be due to a deficiency in the essential amino acid tryptophan, resulting in inadequate synthesis of nicotinamide. In patients the two conditions may be distinguished because Hartnup disease patients also have aminoaciduria (neutral acids) but have normal excretion of proline. Treatment consists of oral nicotin-amide 40 to 200 mg/d and a high-protein diet.

**VIII-9. The answer is E.** *(Chap. 270)* This patient probably has acute renal failure caused by urinary tract obstruction. Ultrasonography is 90% sensitive and specific for the detection of hydronephrosis. Although urinary tract obstruction can be due to many disease pro-cesses, including congenital abnormalities and acquired intrinsic and extrinsic defects of the urinary tract, this patient's symptoms are classic for vesicoureteral reflux disease. Infection must be ruled out as it is often superimposed, but this patient's urinalysis and examination are not consistent with an infectious etiology. Nephrolithiasis would present more typically with a constant pattern of pain with radiation to the lower abdomen, testes, or labia. Although genitourinary tumors may also result in obstruction, the pattern of pain is often less acute and other structural abnormalities may be seen on imaging. Diagnosis of vesicoureteral reflux disease may be confirmed with voiding cystourethrography.

**VIII-10. The answer is C.** *(Chap. 267)* Renal vein thrombosis occurs in 10 to 15% of patients with nephrotic syndrome accompanying membranous glomerulopathy and oncologic dis-ease. The clinical manifestations can be variable but may be characterized by fever, lumbar tenderness, leukocytosis, and hematuria. Magnetic resonance venography is the most sen-sitive and specific noninvasive form of imaging to make the diagnosis of renal vein throm-bosis. Ultrasound with Doppler is operator-dependent and therefore may be less sensitive. Contrast venography is the gold standard for diagnosis, but it exposes the patient to a more invasive procedure and contrast load. Nuclear medicine screening is not performed to make this diagnosis.

**VIII-11. The answer is B.** *(Chap. 267)* This patient has multiple risk factors and an examination consistent with renal artery stenosis (RAS) that probably is due to arteriosclerosis or renal vascular disease. Ischemic renal disease underlies end-stage renal disease in 15 to 20% of patients over age 50 years. Among all patients with hypertensive disease RAS accounts for 2 to 5%. Among the patients affected, bilateral involvement is present in 50%. Risk factors include atherosclerotic arterial disease, either cardiac or peripheral vascular disease, hypertension (especially if it is resistant to medical therapy, including a diuretic), and diabetes. In younger women a diagnosis of fibromuscular dysplasia may be considered. In this patient the suspicion for RAS in light of the clinical presentation and examination is very high. Therefore, despite mild chronic kidney disease the definitive diagnosis may be established during renal artery angiography with the use of minimal contrast. Definitive therapy (renal artery angioplasty and stenting) may be performed at the time of angiography. If there is uncertainty about the diagnosis, for example, no bruits on abdominal examination, the recommended test is gadolinium-enhanced three-dimensional magnetic resonance angiography, which has a sensitivity of over 90% and a specificity of 95%. Ultrasonography may raise your suspicion of a significant difference in renal size; however, Doppler evaluation is less sensitive because of interoperator variation and differences in technical experience.

**VIII-12.** **The answer is C.** *(Chap. 267)* Malignant arteriolar nephrosclerosis is a very damaging and deadly disease. Typical renal abnormalities are as described in this case. Nephrotic syndrome may also be present, and if it progresses, uremia and hyperkalemia often will develop. The kidneys are characterized by a "flea-bitten" appearance resulting from hemorrhages in the surface capillaries. Two distinct lesions are seen histologically: (1) fibrinoid necrosis, which is infiltration of the arteriolar wall with eosinophilic material, thickening of the vessel wall, and inflammatory infiltrate (or necrotizing arteriolitis); and (2) hyperplastic arteriolitis (onion-skin lesion), which is concentric hyperplastic proliferation of the vascular wall with deposition of collagen. The natural course of malignant hypertension includes a death rate of 80 to 90% in 1 year, usually as a result of uremia. However, even with medical therapy, the current estimated 5-year survival is 50%.

**VIII-13.** **The answer is A.** *(Chap. 267)* The prognosis for patients with scleroderma renal disease is poor. In SRC patients prompt treatment with an ACE inhibitor may reverse acute renal failure. In recent studies the initiation of ACE inhibitor therapy resulted in 61% of patients having some degree of renal recovery and not needing chronic dialysis support. The survival rate is estimated to be 80 to 85% at 8 years. Among patients who needed dialysis, when treated with ACE inhibitors, over 50% were able to discontinue dialysis after 3 to 18 months. Therefore, ACE inhibitors should be used even if the patient requires dialysis support.

**VIII-14.** **The answer is D.** *(Chap. 41)* Arginine vasopression is a neurohormone released from the posterior pituitary gland to help maintain water balance in the body. Also known as antidiuretic hormone, vasopressin is primarily released under conditions of hyperosmolarity and volume depletion. Although sodium is the main determinant of hyperosmolarity, sodium is not the only stimulus that affects the secretion of vasopressin. Other, less potent stimuli of vasopressin release include pregnancy, nausea, pain, stress, and hypoglycemia. In addition, many drugs can cause stimulation of the inappropriate secretion of vasopressin. This hormone acts on the principal cell in the distal convoluted tubule of the kidney to cause resorption of water. This occurs through nuclear mechanisms encoded by the aquaporin-2 gene that cause water channels to be inserted into the luminal membrane. The net effect is to cause the passive resorption of water along the osmotic gradient in the distal convoluted tubule.

**VIII-15.** **The answer is C.** *(Chap. 41)* In cases of hypovolemia the appropriate responses of the body are to reabsorb sodium and preserve water. Clinically this manifests as low urine sodium excretion and elevated urine osmolarity and specific gravity. Serum osmolarity is also increased. Also, there is a decreased glomerular filtration rate as a result of low intravascular volume. On laboratory examination this is represented as an elevated BUN/creatinine ratio of 20:1. The loss of free water and solute from the intravascular volume will cause hemoconcentration that resolves with rehydration.

**VIII-16, VIII-17, VIII-18, and VIII-19.   The answers are E, D, B, and A.** *(Chap. 40)* Decreased renal perfusion, or prerenal failure, is a common cause of renal failure and is often rapidly reversible. Frequently encountered causes include decreased circulating volume from volume loss, sequestration, or ineffective pump function or an alteration in renal autoperfusion as is commonly encountered with drug use. GFR is maintained at a constant state by prostaglandin-mediated relaxation of afferent arterioles and angiotensin II–triggered constriction of efferent arterioles. Drugs that interrupt this homeostatic mechanism can cause renal failure. Nonsteroidal anti-inflammatory drugs (NSAIDs) block prostaglandin synthesis and thus prevent normal relaxation of afferent arterioles. The resulting afferent arteriolar constriction causes a reduction in GFR as a result of decreased inflow. Conversely, ACE inhibitors decrease levels of angiotensin II with subsequent increased relaxation of the efferent arterioles. The resulting efferent arteriolar dilation decreases the pressure in the glomerulus and decreases GFR. The patient in Question X-16 has a history suggestive of renal artery stenosis with multiple antihypertensives and an abdominal bruit. Renal failure is common when these patients are given an ACE inhibitor. The patient with gout is on an ACE inhibitor and has lost her angiotensin II contribution to renal autoperfusion. When an NSAID is added to this regimen, her kidneys no longer have control of the afferent or efferent arteriolar tone, and renal failure ensues. The 88-year-old female with delirium has a classic presentation of dehydration with poor skin turgor and dry mucous membranes. In light of her advanced age, a creatinine of 1.3 mg/dL reflects very poor renal function. Indeed, her modification of diet in renal disease (MDRD)-calculated GFR is 50 mL/min per 1.72 m$^2$. Finally, the patient with pneumococcal pneumonia has normal volume status and progressive renal failure with associated hypotension and muddy brown granular casts on urinalysis. The most likely cause is acute tubular necrosis, which can often result from a sudden fall in GFR or exposure to tubular toxins (hypotension, sepsis, medication, contrast agents).

**VIII-20.   The answer is A.** *(Chap. 270)* The prognosis for the return of normal renal function is excellent in patients with acute bilateral renal obstruction, such as an obstruction that is due to prostate enlargement. With relief of the obstruction, the prognosis depends on whether irreversible renal damage has occurred. Return of GFR usually follows relief of obstruction lasting 1 to 2 weeks provided that there has been no intercurrent infection. After 8 weeks of obstruction recovery is unlikely. Acute relief of bilateral obstruction commonly results in polyuria. An osmotic diuresis caused by excretion of retained urea and resolution of volume expansion contributes to the diuresis. The urine is hypotonic. The diuresis usually abates with resolution of normal extracellular volume, and so aggressive volume resuscitation is generally not necessary unless hypotension or overt volume depletion develops. Indications for acute hemodialysis are those for the usual complications of acute renal failure, including electrolyte disturbances, uremia, and inability to control volume.

**VIII-21.   The answer is C.** *(Chap. 41)* In addition to correction of hypernatremia, patients such as this who are volume-depleted require restoration of extracellular fluid volume. The quantity of water required to correct a free water deficit in hypernatremic patients can be estimated from the following equation:

$$\text{Water deficit} = [(\text{plasma Na} - 140)/140] * \text{total body water}$$

Total body water is approximately 50% of lean body mass in men and 40% of lean body mass in women. In calculating the rate of water replacement, ongoing losses should be accounted for and plasma Na$^+$ should be lowered by no more than 0.5 meq/L an hour over the first 24 h. More rapid administration of water and normalization of serum sodium concentration may result in a rapid influx of water into cells that have already undergone osmotic normalization. The resulting cellular edema in the central nervous system (CNS) may cause seizures or neurologic damage.

**VIII-22.   The answer is B.** *(Chap. 40)* Monitoring glomerular filtration rate (GFR) is essential in many patient care settings. A number of methods for measuring or estimating the GFR are used clinically. Often creatinine clearance is used as a surrogate marker for GFR, as GFR is directly related to the urinary creatinine excretion and inversely related to the serum creatinine. Perhaps the most commonly used estimate of GFR is the Cockcroft-Gault equation:

$$\text{Creatinine clearance (mL/min)} = (140 - \text{age}) \times \text{lean body wt (kg)}$$
$$(\times\ 0.85 \text{ for women}) \text{ plasma creatinine (mg/dL)} \times 72$$

The equation must be adjusted for women, who have a decreased amount of muscle for a given body weight. Serum creatinine is affected by a number of factors, such as ingestion of cooked meat (which can raise this value), chronic illness, malnutrition, and age. More direct measures of GFR include urea clearance, inulin clearance, and radionuclide-labeled markers such as [125]I. Urea clearance is flawed as urea is reabsorbed in the tubules and thus can underestimate GFR. Inulin and [125]I, which are filtered at the glomerulus, are neither secreted nor absorbed and thus are highly accurate measures of GFR. It is very rare for a patient to develop symptomatic uremia until the GFR is less than 15.

**VIII-23. The answer is E.** *(Chap. 40)* Multiple myeloma commonly is associated with renal failure through multiple mechanisms. Immunoglobulins are filtered at the glomerulus and can be reabsorbed at the proximal tubule until the reabsorptive capacity is overwhelmed. At this point proteinuria will occur. These immunoglobulins can deposit in the tubules, causing cast nephropathy. Additionally, light chains can deposit in the glomeruli with resultant light chain deposition disease. Furthermore, hypercalcemia is frequently seen in patients with multiple myeloma from bony destruction. Calcium, which is an osmotic diuretic, can result in prerenal azotemia and even acute tubular necrosis.

**VIII-24. The answer is C.** *(Chap. 40)* It is important to note that nephrotic syndrome with any cause can be associated with hypercoagulability. Antithrombin III and proteins C and S are lost in the urine, with concomitantly decreased serum levels. Increased platelet aggregation has been described, and hyperfibrinogenemia is thought to result from an inflammatory response and increased liver synthetic activity caused by urinary protein losses. Additionally, IgG is lost in the urine, and occasionally these patients develop low serum levels with associated immunocompromise. Chronic disseminated intravascular coagulation is not a mechanism of hypercoagulability in patients with the nephrotic syndrome.

**VIII-25. The answer is B.** *(Chap. 40)* The patient's polyuria and thirst with rising sodium suggest diabetes insipidus. Although primary polydipsia can present similarly with thirst and polyuria, it does not cause hypernatremia; instead, hyponatremia results from increased extracellular water. Often patients with diabetes insipidus are able to compensate as outpatients when they have ready access to free water, but once hospitalized and unable to receive water freely, they develop hypernatremia. The first step in the evaluation of diabetes insipidus is to determine if it is central or nephrogenic. This is easily accomplished through measurement of the vasopressin level. In central diabetes insipidus it is low because of a failure of secretion from the posterior pituitary gland, whereas it is elevated in nephrogenic disease, in which the kidneys are insensitive to vasopressin. After measurement of the vasopressin level, a trial of nasal arginine vasopressin may be attempted. Generally nephrogenic diabetes insipidus will not improve significantly with this drug. Free water restriction, which will help with primary polydipsia, will cause worsening hypernatremia in patients with diabetes insipidus. Serum osmolality and 24-h urinary sodium excretion will not help in the diagnosis or management of this patient at this time.

**VIII-26. The answer is A.** *(Chap. 259)* Chronic renal failure is associated with a number of compensatory changes both within the kidney and throughout the body. The first change to occur with loss of functional kidney mass, either surgical or resulting from medical disease, is hypertrophy of the remaining normal nephrons. This can account for the near normalization in GFR that often is seen after single kidney resection. With continued nephron loss, ultimately the GFR will drop. Despite a prolonged period of compensation through many mechanisms, when the GFR is less than 25 mL/min, the kidney loses the ability to concentrate urine and subsequently isothenuria, or urine with the same osmolality as plasma, develops. One of the primary endocrine functions of the kidney is to complete the final hydroxylation of vitamin D to 1,25-dihydroxyvitamin D; thus, active vitamin D levels drop in patients with chronic kidney disease. As a consequence, less calcium is absorbed from the gut and serum calcium levels drop. Sensing lowered serum calcium levels, the intact parathyroid hormone levels rise in an attempt to normalize serum calcium with bony reabsorption. It is interesting to note that there is a decrease in 1,25-dihydroxyvitamin D receptors in the parathyroid gland in patients with chronic renal failure. Normally vitamin D is inhibitory on the parathyroid gland via these receptors. Thus, in chronic kidney disease the effect of vitamin D on the parathyroid gland is attenuated, leading to an additional factor that contributes to increased serum intact parathyroid hormone levels.

**VIII-27.   The answer is A.** *(Chap. 41)*   Excretion of water is tightly regulated at the collecting duct by arginine vasopressin (AVP, formerly antidiuretic hormone). An increase in plasma tonicity is sensed by hypothalamic osmoreceptors, causing AVP secretion from the posterior pituitary. AVP binding to the collecting duct leads to insertion of water channels (aquaporin-2) into the luminal membrane, promoting water reabsorption. Serum sodium is the principal extracellular solute, and so effective osmolality is determined predominantly by the plasma sodium concentration. Plasma osmolality normally is regulated within 1 to 2% of normal (280 to 290 mosmol/kg). The sensitivity of the baroreceptors for AVP release is far less than that of the osmoreceptors. Depletion of intravascular volume sufficient to decrease mean arterial pressure is necessary to stimulate AVP secretion.

**VIII-28 and VIII-29.   The answers are A and C.** *(Chap. 41; Endocrinol Metab Clin North Am 32:459–481, 2003.)*   Many nonosmotic factors may increase AVP secretion from the pituitary or its effect at the collecting duct. Pain, nausea, any intracranial event (e.g., stroke, hemorrhage, seizure, or infection), a pulmonary infection or an infiltrative process, stress, hypoglycemia, pregnancy, or drugs may cause hyponatremia with a normal intravascular volume. Recent reports have implicated selective serotonin reuptake inhibitors as a cause of the syndrome of inappropriate antidiuretic hormone secretion (SIADH). Postoperative patients may have increased secretion of AVP for "appropriate" (e.g., hyperosmolality, hypovolemia) or "inappropriate" (nonosmotic) reasons. Pain and nausea are among the most potent stimuli for AVP secretion. This patient has no evidence of intravascular volume depletion requiring normal or hypertonic saline or infection requiring antibiotics. Furosemide probably would worsen the hyponatremia and precipitate volume depletion. Improved pain control with free water restriction probably will correct the serum sodium. Ethanol inhibits the secretion of AVP from the pituitary and its effect at the collecting duct.

**VIII-30.   The answer is D.** *(Chap. 41)*   This patient has a reduction in extracellular fluid (ECF) volume as evidenced by the resting tachycardia and orthostatic fall in blood pressure. In response (to maintain ECF volume), there is renal arteriolar vasoconstriction that causes a decrease in the glomerular filtration rate and filtered sodium. Tubular reabsorption of sodium increases as a result of the decreased filtered load and the effects of angiotensin II. These changes result in low (<20 meq/L) urine sodium excretion. There will also be an *increase* in the ratio of BUN to creatinine because of increased BUN reabsorption. As a result of the effects of aldosterone and the avid sodium reabsorption, urine potassium will be higher than urine sodium. Sweat is hypotonic relative to serum, and so patients with excessive sweating are more likely to be hypernatremic than hyponatremic. Red blood cell casts indicate glomerular disease. Prolonged hypotension caused by ECF contraction may cause tubular injury, leading to granular or epithelial cell casts.

**VIII-31.   The answer is B.** *(Chaps. 40 and 42)*   The octahedral, or envelope-shaped, crystals are due to the presence of calcium oxalate in the urine. Calcium oxalate crystals are classically seen in ethylene glycol ingestion, which also causes a high anion gap metabolic acidosis.

White blood cell casts indicate an upper urinary tract infection associated with a positive urine culture. Uric acid (rhomboid shapes) or struvite ("coffin lids") crystals may be seen in cases of nephrolithiasis that causes hydronephrosis. Red blood cell casts are indicative of glomerular disease, often associated with a positive ANA.

**VIII-32.   The answer is C.**   *(Chap. 41)*   Diuretic-induced hyponatremia almost always is due to thiazide diuretics. It occurs mostly in the elderly. The reduction in serum sodium may be severe and cause symptoms. Loop diuretics such as furosemide cause hyponatremia far less often than do thiazide diuretics. Thiazide diuretics inhibit sodium and potassium reabsorption in the distal tubule, leading to $Na^+$ and $K^+$ depletion and AVP-mediated water retention. In contrast, loop diuretics impair maximal urinary concentrating capacity, limiting AVP-mediated water retention. Many drugs may cause hyponatremia by promoting AVP secretion or action at the collecting duct; however, metoprolol and enalapril are not significant causes of SIADH. Spironolactone is a competitive antagonist of aldosterone at the mineralocorticoid receptor. It has weak natriuretic activity and is most likely to cause hyperkalemia.

**VIII-33.   The answer is D.**   *(Chaps. 41 and 319)*   Rapid correction (or overcorrection) of hyponatremia may lead to the development of the osmotic demyelination syndrome. The relative hypertonicity of the extracellular fluid without time for intracellular compensation or osmotic compensation causes osmotic shrinkage of brain cells and demyelination. This syndrome usually occurs in patients with chronic hyponatremia who have osmotically equilibrated the intracellular space. These patients have flaccid paralysis, dysarthria, and dysphagia. Brain MRI will show demyelination, particularly in the brainstem (central pontine myelinolysis). Head CT scans will not demonstrate these lesions. The presence of bilateral extremity with minimal cranial nerve abnormalities would make a posterior circulation stroke less likely.

**VIII-34.   The answer is B.**   *(Chap. 266)*   Allergic interstitial nephritis results from hypersensitivity to numerous drugs, including penicillins, sulfonamides, cephalosporins, flouroquinolones, isoniazid, rifampin, diuretics, and NSAIDs. Most patients develop the nephritis after prolonged drug exposure. Renal biopsy will show normal glomeruli with edema and inflammation (neutrophils, lymphocytes, plasma cells, eosinophils) of the interstitium. In severe cases tubular injury will be present. The kidneys are enlarged because of the edema and inflammation. Renal failure develops in conjunction with fever and a skin rash consistent with a systemic process. Hematuria, pyuria, and mild to moderate proteinuria are typical. Peripheral eosinophilia and urine eosinophilia are highly suggestive of the diagnosis if present. Discontinuation of the offending drug usually leads to resolution of the renal failure. Aminoglycosides often cause acute tubular injury but will not be accompanied by rash and fever. The differential diagnosis should include glomerulonephritis; however, this clinical picture is typical of an allergic reaction.

**VIII-35.   The answer is C.**   *(Chap. 262)*   Hypotension is the most common complication during hemodialysis. The risk factors for developing hypotension during hemodialysis include excessive ultrafiltration, reduced intravascular volume before dialysis, impaired autonomic responses, osmolar shifts, food intake before dialysis, impaired cardiac function, and use of antihypertensive agents. The hypotension is usually managed with fluid administration and by decreasing the ultrafiltration rate. Muscle cramps are a decreasingly common complication of hemodialysis as a result of improvements in dialysis technique. Anaphylactoid reactions to the dialyzer once were common but are also decreasing in frequency with the use of newer-generation dialysis membranes. Fever is not a usual complication of hemodialysis but suggests the presence of an infection of the dialysis access site. Blood cultures should be obtained. Hyperglycemia is a complication of peritoneal dialysis, not of hemodialysis.

**VIII-36 and VIII-37.   The answers are A and A.**   *(Chap. 260; Solomon R, Kidney Int 53:230, 1998.)*   Radiocontrast agents are a common cause of acute renal failure and may result in acute tubular necrosis (contrast nephropathy). It is common for patients receiving intravenous contrast to develop a transient increase in serum creatinine. These agents cause renal failure by inducing intrarenal vasoconstriction and reducing renal blood flow, mimicking prerenal azotemia, and by directly causing tubular injury. The risk of contrast nephropathy may be reduced by initiating newer isoosmolar agents and minimizing the dose of contrast. When the reduction in renal blood flow is severe or prolonged, tubular injury develops, causing acute renal failure. Patients with intravascular volume depletion, diabetes, congestive heart failure, multiple myeloma, or chronic renal failure have an increased risk of contrast nephropathy. The urine sediment is bland in mild cases, but with acute tubular necrosis, muddy brown granular casts may be seen. Saline hydration plus $N$-acetylcysteine may decrease the risk and severity of contrast nephropathy. Red cell casts indicate glomerular disease, and white cell casts suggest upper urinary tract infection. Urinary eosinophils are seen in allergic interstitial disease caused by many drugs.

**VIII-38.  The answer is D.**  *(Chap. 264)*   This patient has a history and findings consistent with rapidly progressive glomerulonephritis (RPGN). This occurs when there is rapidly progressing acute renal failure over days to weeks. This is a clinical diagnosis. On the basis of these findings initiation of immunosuppressive therapy with steroids is indicated in an attempt to prevent the need for the initiation of renal replacement therapy. Ultimately the laboratory assessment and renal biopsy will secure the diagnosis; however, in rapidly worsening cases the initiation of therapy is indicated before renal biopsy results are available. This patient probably has Wegener's glomerulomatosis, which is p-ANCA-positive. ACE inhibitor therapy is not indicated in the acute setting for this acute glomerulonephritis. Cyclophosphamide is utilized for induction treatment after the diagnosis is confirmed by either additional laboratory findings or biopsy results.

**VIII-39.  The answer is A.**  *(Chap. 264)*   In different disease processes the complement pathway is activated either by classical pathway activation or by alternative pathway activation. If the classical pathway is activated, as in lupus nephritis, the serum complement measures of C3, C4, and CH50 are low. If the alternative pathway is activated, C3 and CH50 may be low but C4 is at normal levels. When acute GN is suspected, measurement of serum complement levels will often limit the differential diagnosis. Other conditions with normal C4 include ANCA-associated diseases. Low C4 may be seen with membranoproliferative GN types I and III. Type I disease also may be associated with cryoglobulinemia.

**VIII-40.  The answer is C.**  *(Chap. 262)*   Initiation of hemodialysis is recommended in any patient who develops evidence of the uremic syndrome, hyperkalemia unresponsive to conservative measures, extracellular volume expansion or pulmonary edema unresponsive to diuretics, acidosis refractory to medical therapy, and intoxication to drugs such as aspirin or for the management of hyperkalemia in digitalis intoxication. The recommended creatinine clearance for chronic kidney disease stage V if there is no evidence of the clinical syndromes listed above is 10 mL/min in the general population and 15 mL/min for patients with diabetes mellitus. The creatinine clearance may be based on estimates such as the Cockcroft-Gault equation or the modification of diet in renal disease (MDRD) equation when the patient's serum creatinine is in a steady state.

**VIII-41.  The answer is E.**  *(Chap. 40)*   Up to 150 mg/d of protein may be excreted by a normal person. The bulk of normal daily excretion is made up of the Tamm-Horsfall mucoprotein. Urine dipsticks may register a trace result in response to as little as 50 mg of protein per liter and are definitively positive once the urine protein exceeds 300 mg/L. A false negative may occur if the proteinuria is due to immunoglobulins, which are positively charged. If proteinuria is suspected or documented, a 24-h urine collection should be undertaken to measure the absolute protein excretion. Urine immunoelectrophoresis also may identify the particular immunoglobulin that is produced in excess.

**VIII-42.  The answer is A.**  *(Chaps. 41 and 319)*   Failure to concentrate urine despite substantial hypertonic dehydration suggests a diagnosis of diabetes insipidus. A nephrogenic origin will be postulated if there is no increase in urine concentration after exogenous vasopressin. The only useful mode of therapy is a low-salt diet and the use of a thiazide or amiloride, a potassium-sparing distal diuretic agent. The resultant volume contraction presumably enhances proximal reabsorption and thereby reduces urine flow.

**VIII-43.   The answer is D.**   *(Chap. 262)*   Development of advancing peripheral neuropathy is an indication for dialysis. Delaying dialysis could allow the development of irreversible motor deficits such as footdrop. Prompt institution of dialysis, by contrast, usually prevents the progression of uremic peripheral neuropathy and may ameliorate early sensory defects. No pharmacologic agent would confer a significant benefit in the clinical situation described here.

**VIII-44.   The answer is A.**   *(Chap. 270; Ifudu, N Engl J Med 339:1054–1062, 1998.)*   Renal osteodystrophy is a common complication of chronic renal disease and the most common complication secondary to impaired renal production of $1,25(OH)_2D_3$. This leads to a decreased calcium absorption in the gut as well as impaired renal phosphate excretion. The resulting hyperphosphatemia causes a secondary hyperparathyroidism. The hyperparathyroidism is subsequently worsened by hypocalcemia, which is present because of the hyperphosphatemia and the decreased enzymatic conversion of 25-hydroxyvitamin D to $1,25(OH)_2D_3$. Finally, $1,25(OH)_2D_3$ deficiency worsens hyperparathyroidism as the former is a direct inhibitor of parathyroid hormone secretion into the bone. The resultant decreased serum calcium concentration leads to secondary hyperparathyroidism. In addition, other causes of renal osteodystrophy include chronic metabolic acidosis resulting from dissolution of bone buffers and decalcification and the long-term administration of aluminum-containing antacids. No significant loss of vitamin D or calcium is associated with currently employed dialysis techniques, and the treatment of renal osteodystrophy often includes calcitriol.

**VIII-45.   The answer is A.**   *(Chap. 260)*   To offer optimal management to patients with acute renal failure, it is helpful to distinguish prerenal azotemia (generally managed with volume replacement or amelioration of cardiac dysfunction) from intrinsic renal dysfunction. Sodium reabsorption, which is quite avid in patients with prerenal azotemia, is impaired in those with intrinsic renal disease. However, creatinine is reabsorbed less efficiently than is sodium in both conditions. Therefore, the fractional excretion of sodium is very helpful in distinguishing between these two etiologies of renal failure. The fractional excretion of sodium is calculated by multiplying the urine sodium by the plasma creatinine, dividing this by the plasma sodium times the urine creatinine, and multiplying by 100. In this case the result is approximately 1.4, which suggests that impaired reabsorption of sodium is ongoing and that intrinsic renal failure is occurring. Only about 15% of patients receiving nephrotoxins such as aminoglycosides or radiocontrast agents have renal failure associated with a fractional excretion of sodium less than $<1\%$, and so an elevated value in this case points in the direction of nephrotoxic injury. The other causes of acute renal failure listed here are all associated with prerenal azotemia and therefore with a more avid reabsorption of sodium than that described.

**VIII-46.   The answer is B.**   *(Chap. 264)*   The characteristic pattern of focal (not all glomeruli) and segmental (not the entire glomerulus) glomerular scarring is shown. The history and laboratory features are also consistent with this lesion: some associated hypertension, diminution in creatinine clearance, and a relatively inactive urine sediment. The "nephropathy of obesity" may be associated with this lesion secondary to hyperfiltration; this condition may be more likely to occur in obese patients with hypoxemia, obstructive sleep apnea, and right-sided heart failure. Hypertensive nephrosclerosis exhibits more prominent vascular changes and patchy, ischemic, totally sclerosed glomeruli. In addition, nephrosclerosis seldom is associated with nephrotic-range proteinuria. Minimal-change disease usually is associated with symptomatic edema and normal-appearing glomeruli as demonstrated on light microscopy. This patient's presentation is consistent with that of membranous nephropathy, but the biopsy is not. With membranous glomerular nephritis all glomeruli are uniformly involved with subepithelial dense deposits. There are no features of crescentic glomerulonephritis present.

**VIII-47. The answer is E.** *(Chaps. 262 and 265)* The pathophysiology of nephrotoxic involvement by SLE is thought to be immune-complex deposition. Renal disease in SLE can range from mild abnormalities of the urinalysis to a fulminant inflammatory process that leads to progressive renal failure. Renal biopsy findings in patients with SLE who have worsening renal function can range from minimal glomerular lesions to diffuse proliferative lupus glomerulonephritis and membranous lupus glomerulonephritis. Patients with membranous lupus glomerulonephritis may be managed conservatively with therapy directed toward extrarenal manifestations. By contrast, those with more extensive or proliferative glomerular lesions require a more aggressive approach using glucocorticoids with or without another immunosuppressive agent, such as azathioprine or cyclophosphamide. However, little is gained by using immunosuppressant therapy in patients with advanced renal failure characterized by obliterative sclerosing lesions of the glomeruli. If such patients have other indications for dialysis, such as systemic symptoms and hyperkalemia, they are best managed with dialysis followed by renal transplantation. Measurement of serologic evidence of disease (e.g., double-strand DNA autoantibodies or a decrease in serum complement components) may be helpful. Patients with end-stage lupus nephritis can be managed successfully with hemodialysis. Moreover, patients with SLE who have undergone renal allografting rarely experience recurrence of disease in the new kidney.

**VIII-48. The answer is C.** *(Chaps. 41 and 265)* The evaluation of patients with hypokalemia should first include a consideration of redistribution of body potassium into cells such as that which occurs in alkalosis, $\beta_2$-agonist excess with refeeding syndrome and/or insulin therapy, vitamin $B_{12}$ therapy, pernicious anemia, and periodic paralysis. In periodic paralysis serum bicarbonate is normal. If the patient is hypertensive and plasma renin is elevated, renovascular hypertension or a renin-secreting tumor (including Wilms) must be considered and appropriate imaging studies must be carried out. If plasma renin levels are low, mineralocorticoid effect may be high as a result of either endogenous hormone (glucocorticoid overproduction or aldosterone overproduction as in Conn's syndrome) or exogenous agents (licorice or steroids). In a normotensive patient a high serum bicarbonate excludes renal tubular acidosis. High urine chloride excretion makes gastrointestinal losses less likely and implies primary renal potassium loss, as may be seen in diuretic abuse (ruled out by the urine screen) or Bartter's syndrome. In Bartter's syndrome, hyperplasia of the granular cells of the juxtaglomerular apparatus leads to high renin levels and secondary aldosterone elevations. Such hyperplasia appears to be secondary to chronic volume depletion caused by a hereditary (autosomal recessive) defect that interferes with salt reabsorption in the thick ascending loop of Henle. Chronic potassium depletion, which frequently presents initially in childhood, leads to polyuria and weakness.

**VIII-49. The answer is B.** *(Chap. 42; N Engl J Med 338:26–34, 1998.)* This represents a respiratory alkalosis with a combined metabolic acidosis. This is typical of salicylate toxicity. Salicylate intoxication can result in respiratory alkalosis, mixed respiratory alkalosis and metabolic acidosis, or, less commonly, a simple metabolic acidosis. Respiratory alkalosis is caused by direct stimulation of the respiratory center by salicylate. The accumulation of lactic acid and ketoacids leads to the concomitant metabolic acidosis. The severity of the neurologic manifestations largely depends on the concentration of salicylate in the central nervous system. Therapy is directed at limiting further drug absorption by administering activated charcoal and promoting the exit of salicylate from the CNS. This can be accomplished by alkalinizing the serum, typically by means of the addition of intravenous fluids with sodium bicarbonate, with the goal of raising the serum pH to between 7.45 and 7.50. Increasing the GFR will also enhance salicylate excretion. Hemodialysis is reserved for severe cases, especially those involving fulminant renal failure.

**VIII-50. The answer is D.** *(Chap. 260)* Cholesterol embolization (also known as atheroembolic renal disease) is characterized by pyuria, progressive renal failure (usually nonoliguric), and associated organ dysfunction (including bowel, pancreas, and CNS). Hypocomple-mentemia and eosinophiluria also may be seen. The urinalysis is not compatible with acute tubular necrosis because of the absence of granular casts.

**VIII-51.   The answer is B.**   *(Chap. 262; Rubin et al, JAMA 291:697–703, 2004.)*   Peritonitis is the most common serious complication of peritoneal dialysis. These patients typically present with abdominal pain, fever, and a cloudy peritoneal dialysate. Persistent or recur-rent peritonitis may require the removal of the catheter. Further complications include losses of amino acids as well as albumin, which may be as much as 5 to 15 g/d. In addition, patients can absorb glucose through the peritoneal dialysate, resulting in hyperglycemia, not hypoglycemia. The resulting hyperglycemia can cause a hypertriglyceridemia, espe-cially in patients with diabetes mellitus. Leakage of the dialysate fluid into the pleural space can also occur, more frequently on the right than on the left. It can be diagnosed by analysis of the pleural fluid, which typically has an elevated glucose concentration. Rapid fluid shifts are uncommon with peritoneal dialysis, and this approach may be favored for patients with congestive heart failure or unstable angina. A recent report suggested im-proved patient satisfaction with peritoneal dialysis compared with hemodialysis.

# IX. DISORDERS OF THE GASTROINTESTINAL SYSTEM

## QUESTIONS

**DIRECTIONS:** Each question below contains five suggested responses. Choose the **one best** response to each question.

**IX-1.** A 62-year-old male is evaluated in the emergency department for a complaint of vomiting and inability to tolerate oral intake. These symptoms have gradually progressed from occasional episodes of emesis after meals to an extent where the patient has not been able to tolerate solid foods for the last week. He notes no significant sensation of nausea before the emesis. Instead, the patient describes vomiting partially digested foods within a half hour of eating. The patient notes no abdominal pain. He has experienced an unintentional 30-lb weight loss over 6 months. The patient has a history of diabetes mellitus that is poorly controlled, with a glycosylated hemoglobin level of 8.9%. The patient underwent partial gastrectomy for peptic ulcer disease at age 52. His only medication is insulin therapy. On physical examination the patient is cachectic with a body mass index (BMI) of 17. He has temporal wasting. The abdominal examination reveals no masses and is nontender. The bowel sounds are normoactive, and the patient's stool is hemoccult-negative. An abdominal film shows an enlarged gastric bubble with decompressed small intestinal loops. What is the most likely diagnosis?

A. Small bowel obstruction
B. Gastroparesis
C. Esophageal stricture
D. Gastric outlet obstruction
E. Cholelithiasis

**IX-2.** The patient in Question IX-1 undergoes upper endoscopy for further evaluation, and a large mass is seen in the fundus of the stomach. Biopsy shows gastric adenocarcinoma. All the following are risk factors for the development of this disease *except*

A. atrophic gastritis
B. alcoholism
C. *Helicobacter pylori* infection
D. high consumption of salted and smoked food
E. juvenile hamartomatous polyps

**IX-3.** A 36-year-old male presents with fatigue and tea-colored urine for 5 days. Physical examination reveals

**IX-3.** *(Continued)*
jaundice and tender hepatomegaly but is otherwise unremarkable. Laboratories are remarkable for an aspartate aminotransferase (AST) of 2400 IU/L and an alanine aminotransferase (ALT) of 2640 IU/L. Alkaline phosphatase is 210 IU/L. Total bilirubin is 8.6 mg/dL. Which of the following is *least* likely to cause this clinical picture and these laboratory abnormalities?

A. Acute hepatitis A infection
B. Acute hepatitis B infection
C. Acute hepatitis C infection
D. Acetaminophen ingestion
E. Budd-Chiari syndrome

**IX-4.** A 34-year-old male reports "yellow eyes" for the last 2 days during a routine employment examination. He states that since his early twenties he has had similar episodes of yellow eyes lasting 2 to 4 days. He denies nausea, abdominal pain, dark urine, light-colored stools, pruritis, or weight loss. He has not sought prior medical attention because of finances, lack of symptoms, and the predictable resolution of the yellow eyes. He takes a multivitamin and some herbal medications. On examination he is mildly obese. He is icteric. There are no stigmata of chronic liver disease. The patient's abdomen is soft and nontender, and there is no organomegaly. Laboratory examinations are normal except for a total bilirubin of 3 mg/dL. Direct bilirubin is 0.2 mg/dL. AST, ALT, and alkaline phosphatase are normal. Hematocrit, lactate dehydrogenase (LDH), and haptoglobin are normal. Which of the following is the most likely diagnosis?

A. Crigler-Najjar syndrome type 1
B. Cholelithiasis
C. Dubin-Johnson syndrome
D. Gilbert's syndrome
E. Medication-induced hemolysis

**IX-5.** What is the appropriate next management step for this patient?

A. Genotype studies

**IX-5.** *(Continued)*
  B.   Peripheral blood smear
  C.   Prednisone
  D.   Reassurance
  E.   Right upper quadrant ultrasound

**IX-6.** A 34-year-old female presents to your clinic with 5 weeks of right upper quadrant pain. She denies nausea, changes in bowel habits, or weight loss. Her past medical history is unremarkable. Her only medications are a multivitamin and oral contraceptives. The examination is notable for a palpable liver mass 2 cm below the right costal margin. Serum $\alpha$ fetoprotein is normal. An abdominal CT scan shows two 3-cm hypervascular lesions in the right hepatic lobe that are suggestive of hepatocellular adenoma. What is the most appropriate next management step?

  A.   Observation
  B.   Discontinuation of oral contraceptives
  C.   Referral for surgical excision
  D.   Radiofrequency ablation (RFA)
  E.   CT-guided biopsy

**IX-7.** A 52-year-old male with chronic hepatitis C presents to your clinic with worsening right upper quadrant pain. Examination shows a palpable right upper quadrant mass. CT scan shows a large 5 × 5 cm mass in the right lobe of the liver. Serum $\alpha$ fetoprotein is elevated. A CT-guided liver biopsy confirms the suspected diagnosis of hepatocellular carcinoma. All the following are appropriate management steps *except*

  A.   referral for surgical resection
  B.   referral for radiofrequency ablation
  C.   referral for liver transplantation
  D.   systemic chemotherapy
  E.   chemoembolization

**IX-8.** All the following cancers commonly metastasize to the liver *except*

  A.   breast
  B.   colon
  C.   lung
  D.   melanoma
  E.   prostate

**IX-9.** All the following are risk factors for developing cholangiocarcinoma *except*

  A.   choledochal cyst
  B.   cholelithiasis
  C.   liver flukes
  D.   sclerosing cholangitis
  E.   working in the rubber industry

**IX-10.** All the following are associated with an increased risk for cholelithiasis *except*

**IX-10.** *(Continued)*
  A.   chronic hemolytic anemia
  B.   obesity
  C.   high-protein diet
  D.   pregnancy
  E.   female sex

**IX-11.** A 51-year-old male presents to the emergency room with fever, nausea, and right upper quadrant pain. Examination shows a tender right upper quadrant. There is a mild leukocytosis of 13,000 cells/mL. Bilirubin is 2.4 mg/dL. A poor-quality right upper quadrant ultrasound shows some mild intrahepatic ductal dilation and a thickened gallbladder but no obvious gallstones. You initiate broad-spectrum antibiotics. What is the most appropriate next management step?

  A.   Tc-HIDA scan
  B.   CT scan of the abdomen
  C.   Percutaneous cholecystostomy
  D.   Endoscopic retrograde cholangiopancreatography (ERCP)
  E.   Continued intravenous antibiotics and serial examinations

**IX-12.** A 41-year-old female presents to your clinic with a week of jaundice. She notes pruritis, icterus, and dark urine. She denies fever, abdominal pain, or weight loss. The examination is unremarkable except for yellow discoloration of the skin. Total bilirubin is 6.0 mg/dL, and direct bilirubin is 5.1 mg/dL. AST is 84 U/L, and ALT is 92 IU/L. Alkaline phosphatase is 662 IU/L. CT scan of the abdomen is unremarkable. Right upper quadrant ultrasound shows a normal gallbladder but does not visualize the common bile duct. What is the most appropriate next management step?

  A.   Antibiotics and observation
  B.   Endoscopic retrograde cholangiopancreaticography (ERCP)
  C.   Hepatitis serologies
  D.   HIDA scan
  E.   Serologies for antimitochondrial antibodies

**IX-13.** A 26-year-old female presents to the emergency room after ingesting "lots of pills." Her boyfriend discovered her crying on the floor of their bedroom, found numerous open bottles of acetaminophen scattered throughout the apartment, and called 911. He does not know when she first took the pills but had last seen her 4 h before finding her on the floor. She is nauseated and vomits once in the emergency room. Vital signs are stable. On examination she is alert and oriented. She has some epigastric tenderness to deep palpation. Otherwise the examination is unremarkable. Her acetaminophen level is 400 $\mu$g/mL. Liver function tests are normal. Which of the following statements regarding her clinical condition is not true?

**IX-13.** *(Continued)*

A. *N*-acetylcysteine is the treatment of choice for acetaminophen toxicity.

B. Alkalinization of the urine is not effective as a treatment for acetaminophen toxicity.

C. The patient should be admitted and observed for 48 to 72 h as her hepatic injury may manifest days after the initial ingestion.

D. Liver transplantation is the only option for patients who develop fulminant hepatic failure from acetaminophen.

E. Normal liver function tests at presentation make significant liver injury unlikely.

**IX-14.** The most common cause of upper gastrointestinal bleeding (UGIB) in the United States is

A. arteriovenous malformations
B. gastritis
C. Mallory-Weiss tears
D. neoplasia
E. peptic ulcer disease

**IX-15.** A 38-year-old male presents to the emergency room with coffee-ground emesis. He denies alcohol or nonsteroidal anti-inflammatory drug (NSAID) use. Heart rate is 92 beats/min, and blood pressure is 140/82 mmHg. Intravenous access is obtained, and he is stabilized hemodynamically. An endoscopy shows a duodenal ulcer. There is no active bleeding. However, there is a nonbleeding visible vessel in the ulcer base. All the following are appropriate management steps *except*

A. 24-h observation and discharge if the patient is stable hemodynamically
B. early surgical consultation
C. endoscopic injection with epinephrine
D. intravenous proton pump inhibitor
E. testing for *Helicobacter pylori*

**IX-16.** You are asked to see a 55-year-old male with chronic hepatitis C, cirrhosis, and a prior history of variceal bleeding. He presented to the hospital with upper gastrointestinal bleeding. He was intubated in the emergency room for airway protection and is now hemodynamically stable in the intensive care unit. The patient is encephalopathic and unable to communicate with you. The examination is notable for stable vital signs, icterus, multiple spider angiomata, ascites, and asterixis. The ammonia level is elevated. Hematocrit has dropped by 3% over the last 4 hours. All the following management recommendations are appropriate *except*

A. endoscopy with variceal banding
B. octreotide
C. propranolol
D. proton pump inhibitor

**IX-16.** *(Continued)*

E. transjugular intrahepatic portosystemic shunt (TIPS)

**IX-17.** A 51-year-old male with no significant past medical history comes to your clinic complaining of bright red blood per rectum. He denies nausea, weight loss, tenesmus, or diarrhea. He is constipated at times and often strains during a bowel movement. Over the last month he has noted blood streaking along the side of his stool. It is not mixed with the stool. There is also bright red blood on the toilet paper when he wipes himself. He has no family history of colon cancer and has never had a colonoscopy. The abdominal exam is soft and nontender. The digital rectal examination is guaiac-negative with a normal prostate. You perform anoscopy, which shows multiple nonbleeding internal hemorrhoids. What is the most appropriate next management step?

A. Colonoscopy
B. Fiber supplements
C. Observation
D. Referral for surgical banding
E. Glucocorticoid suppositories

**IX-18.** A 61-year-old male is admitted to your service for swelling of the abdomen. You detect ascites on clinical examination and perform a paracentesis. The results show a white blood cell count of 300 leukocytes/$\mu$L with 35% polymorphonuclear cells. The peritoneal albumin level is 1.2 g/dL, protein is 2.0 g/dL, and triglycerides are 320 mg/dL. Peritoneal cultures are pending. Serum albumin is 2.6 g/dL. Which of the following is the most likely diagnosis?

A. Congestive heart failure
B. Peritoneal tuberculosis
C. Peritoneal carcinomatosis
D. Chylous ascites
E. Bacterial peritonitis

**IX-19.** Which of the following statements about acute diarrhea is not true?

A. More than 90% of the cases are caused by infectious agents.
B. Most infectious diarrheas are transmitted via fecal-oral spread.
C. In hospitalized patients the most common etiology of infectious diarrhea is *Clostridium difficile* infection.
D. Traveler's diarrhea is commonly caused by gram-negative bacteria.
E. Viral causes of diarrhea such as Norwalk virus are usually mild and not contagious.

**IX-20.** All the following are causes of bloody diarrhea *except*

**IX-20.** *(Continued)*
A. *Campylobacter*
B. *Cryptosporidia*
C. *Escherichia coli*
D. *Entamoeba*
E. *Shigella*

**IX-21.** A 25-year-old female presents to walk-in clinic with diarrhea and crampy abdominal pain that has occurred for the last 2 days. It is watery, nonbloody, and voluminous. The patient denies fever, chills, or night sweats. She is nauseated and vomited twice in the morning but was able to tolerate her lunch. She has a 1-year-old son at home who she says has been "colicky" recently. She denies any recent travel. On examination her temperature is 38.2°C (100.5°F). Blood pressure is 112/72 mmHg, and heart rate is 82 beats/min. She is not orthostatic. Her mucus membranes are dry. The patient's abdomen is soft, nontender, and not distended. Her stool is heme-negative. What is the most appropriate next management step?

A. Admission for intravenous hydration
B. Flexible sigmoidoscopy
C. Observation
D. Oral ciprofloxacin for 5 days
E. Stool studies for fecal leukocytes and stool culture

**IX-22.** A 30-year-old canoe instructor comes to your clinic complaining of 4 weeks of crampy abdominal pain and diarrhea. He has low-grade fevers but denies bloody stool. He has lost 10 lb during that time. Your suspicion of *Giardia* infection is confirmed by a positive *Giardia* antigen stool study. What is the most appropriate next management step?

A. Flexible sigmoidoscopy
B. Oral ciprofloxacin
C. Oral metronidazole
D. CT scan of the abdomen to evaluate for extraintestinal giardiasis
E. Observation

**IX-23.** Which of the following statements about chronic diarrhea is not true?

A. Chronic pancreatitis is a common cause of malabsorption.
B. Iron deficiency and mucosal malabsorption are common in gluten-sensitive enteropathy.
C. Most of the causes of chronic diarrhea are noninfectious.
D. Osmotic diarrheas typically do not improve with fasting.
E. Secretory diarrheas are characterized clinically by large-volume watery fecal output.

**IX-24.** All the following are causes of diarrhea *except*

A. diabetes
B. hypercalcemia
C. hyperthyroidism
D. irritable bowel syndrome
E. metoclopramide

**IX-25.** A 55-year-old white male with a history of diabetes presents to your office with complaints of generalized weakness, weight loss, nonspecific diffuse abdominal pain, and erectile dysfunction. The examination is significant for hepatomegaly without tenderness, testicular atrophy, and gynecomastia. Skin examination shows a diffuse slate-gray hue slightly more pronounced on the face and neck. Joint examination shows mild swelling of the second and third metacarpophalangeal joints on the right hand. What is the recommended test for diagnosis?

A. Serum ferritin
B. Serum iron studies, including transferrin saturation
C. Urinary iron quantification in 24-h collection
D. Genetic screen for *HFE* gene mutation (C282Y and H63D)
E. Liver biopsy

**IX-26.** A 54-year-old male presents with 1 month of diarrhea. He states that he has 8 to 10 loose bowel movements a day. He has lost 8 lb during this time. Vital signs and physical examination are normal. Serum laboratory studies are normal. A 24-h stool collection reveals 500 g of stool with a measured stool osmolality of 200 mosmol/L and a calculated stool osmolarity of 210 mosmol/L. Based on these findings, what is the most likely cause of this patient's diarrhea?

A. Celiac sprue
B. Chronic pancreatitis
C. Lactase deficiency
D. Vasoactive intestinal peptide tumor
E. Whipple's disease

**IX-27.** A 25-year-old immigrant from Central America reports 2 years of crampy abdominal pain and diarrhea. She states that the diarrhea is loose and foul-smelling. She eats a normal diet but often eats irregularly because of finances. When she decreases her food intake, the pain and diarrhea lessen. She has lost 30 lb over the last 2 years. On physical examination she is thin with normal vital signs. The abdominal examination is soft with diffuse tenderness but normal bowel sounds, no rebound tenderness, and no masses. Stool is trace guaiac-positive. A 24-h stool collection while she is on a normal diet has an increased stool volume with elevated fat and bile acids. Which of the following is the most likely cause of the patient's diarrhea?

**IX-27.** *(Continued)*

A. Celiac sprue
B. Crohn's disease
C. Enterotoxigenic *Escherichia coli* infection
D. *Giardia* infection
E. Lactase deficiency

**IX-28.** A 17-year-old Asian student complains of abdominal bloating and diarrhea, particularly after eating ice cream and other milk products. Her parents have similar symptoms. The patient denies any weight loss or systemic symptoms. The physical examination is normal. Treatment with which of the following medications is most likely to reduce her symptoms?

A. Cholestyramine
B. Metoclopramide
C. Omeprazole
D. Viokase®
E. None of the above

**IX-29.** A 38-year-old male presents to his physician with 4 to 6 months of weight loss and joint complaints. He reports that his appetite is good, but he has had diarrhea with six to eight loose, foul-smelling stools each day. He has also had migratory pain in the knees and shoulders. Stool studies demonstrate steatorrhea. Which of the following diagnostic tests is most likely to be positive in this patient?

A. Serum IgA antiendomysial antibodies
B. Serum IgA antigliadin antibodies
C. Serum PCR for *Tropheryma whippelii*
D. Small bowel biopsy showing reduced villous height and crypt hyperplasia
E. Stool *Clostridium difficile* toxin

**IX-30.** A 70-year-old male with a history of cerebrovascular accidents is living at a nursing home, where he is noted to complain about mild diffuse abdominal pain for 3 days with associated anorexia. He is brought to the emergency department with altered mental status, where the examination is notable for a temperature of 38.1°C (100.6°F), pulse of 110/min, respiratory rate of 20/min, and blood pressure of 90/60 mmHg. The patient's lungs are clear, and cardiac examination, besides tachycardia, is normal. The abdomen had absent bowel sounds, diffuse tenderness with rebound, and guarding, most pronounced in the right lower quadrant. In addition to empirical antibiotics and fluid resuscitation, which of the following is the most appropriate next step?

A. Lumbar puncture
B. Nasogastric lavage
C. Mesenteric angiogram
D. Surgical consultation
E. CT of the abdomen without contrast

**IX-31.** Which of the following statements about this patient's condition is true?

A. Obstruction of the neck of the appendix can be identified in the majority of cases.
B. *Yersinia* complement fixation titers will be high in approximately 30% of cases.
C. The incidence of this disorder is higher in lower-socioeconomic-status groups.
D. This patient has a lower incidence of perforation than will a patient with a similar presentation who is 40 years old.
E. Colonoscopy probably will be normal.

**IX-32.** A 38-year-old male is seen in the urgent care center with several hours of severe abdominal pain. His symptoms began suddenly, but he reports several months of pain in the epigastrium after eating, with a resultant 10-lb weight loss. He takes no medications besides over-the-counter antacids and has no other medical problems or habits. On physical examination temperature is 38.0°C (100.4°F), pulse 130/min, respiratory rate 24/min, and blood pressure 110/50 mmHg. His abdomen has absent bowel sounds and is rigid with involuntary guarding diffusely. A plain film of the abdomen is obtained and shows free air under the diaphragm. Which of the following is most likely to be found in the operating room?

A. Necrotic bowel
B. Necrotic pancreas
C. Perforated duodenal ulcer
D. Perforated gallbladder
E. Perforated gastric ulcer

**IX-33.** Which of the following is the source of this patient's peritonitis?

A. Blood
B. Bile
C. Foreign body
D. Gastric contents
E. Pancreatic enzymes

**IX-34.** A 28-year-old male with HIV and a CD4 count of $4/\mu L$ is admitted to the hospital with several days of epigastric boring abdominal pain radiating to the back with associated nausea and bilious vomiting. He has a history of disseminated mycobacterial disease, cryptococcal pneumonia, and injection drug use. His current medications include fluconazole, trimethoprim-sulfamethoxazole, clarithromycin, ethambutol, and rifabutin. On physical examination he has normal vital signs, decreased bowel sounds, and tender epigastrium without rebound or guarding. Rectal exam is guaiac-negative. The remainder of the examination is normal. Amylase and lipase are elevated. The patient is treated conservatively with intravenous fluids and bowel rest, with resolution of symp-

**IX-34.**   *(Continued)*

toms. Right upper quadrant ultrasound is normal, and calcium and triglycerides are normal. Which of the following changes to his medical regimen should be recommended on discharge?

A.   Discontinue rifabutin.
B.   Substitute azithromycin for clarithromycin.
C.   Substitute dapsone for trimethoprim-sulfamethoxazole.
D.   Substitute amphotericin for fluconazole.
E.   Discontinue trimethoprim-sulfamethoxazole.

**IX-35.**   At presentation of acute pancreatitis, all the following predict a poor prognosis *except*

A.   hematocrit above 44%
B.   albumin <3.0 g/dL
C.   lactate dehydrogenase >500 U/dL
D.   lipase >600 U/L
E.   body mass index above 30

**IX-36.**   A 45-year-old male with a long history of alcohol dependence is admitted to the intensive care unit with acute onset of severe epigastric abdominal pain radiating to the back. He takes no medications and has no habits other than drinking two fifths of vodka per day. He has no other medical problems. Physical examination is notable for temperature of 38.3°C (100.9°F), pulse of 145/min, respiratory rate of 30/min, and blood pressure of 90/50. Oxygen saturation is 83% on room air but improves to 92% on an 80% oxygen face mask. The remainder of the examination is notable for tachycardia, diffuse inspiratory crackles with tachypnea, absent bowel sounds, and a diffusely tender abdomen. Cullen's sign is present. Laboratory tests show a white blood cell count of 20,000/mm$^3$ with a leftward shift, creatinine of 2.3 mg/dL, AST of 115 U/L, ALT of 50 IU/L, and total bilirubin of 2.1 mg/dL. Amylase is 400 IU/L, and lipase is 650 IU/L. A computed tomogram is obtained of the abdomen and is most likely to show which of the following findings?

A.   Cholelithiasis with obstruction of the cystic duct
B.   Necrotizing pancreatitis
C.   Pancreatitis without necrosis
D.   Mass in the head of the pancreas
E.   Pseudocyst

**IX-37.**   Which of the following medications has been proved to reduce mortality in the acute management of patients like this one?

A.   Calcitonin
B.   Ranitidine
C.   Imipenem
D.   Glucagon
E.   Methylprednisolone

**IX-38.**   The patient in Question IX-37 is admitted to the intensive care unit, where he requires intubation and mechanical ventilation for hypoxemic respiratory failure. His respiratory status stabilizes over the ensuing 3 days, but fevers persist. His medications are imipenem, omeprazole, subcutaneous minidose heparin, and acetaminophen. On the fifth hospital day his temperature is 39.5°C (103.1°F), heart rate is 130/min, and blood pressure is 80/38 mmHg; vasopressors are initiated. Blood and urine cultures are sterile, and chest radiography shows no new infiltrates. CT of the abdomen is repeated and shows extensive pancreatic necrosis with surrounding edema. CT-guided percutaneous needle aspiration of the necrotic area is obtained. On Gram stain there are many polymorphonuclear cells and heavy gram-negative rods. What is the most appropriate next management step?

A.   Percutaneous drain placement
B.   Discontinuation of imipenem and initiation of ceftazidime and vancomycin
C.   Initiation of amphotericin
D.   Endoscopic retrograde cholangiopancreatography
E.   Surgical consultation

**IX-39.**   A 25-year-old female with cystic fibrosis is diagnosed with chronic pancreatitis. She is at risk for all of the following complications *except*

A.   vitamin B$_{12}$ deficiency
B.   vitamin A deficiency
C.   pancreatic carcinoma
D.   niacin deficiency
E.   steatorrhea

**IX-40.**   A 55-year-old male with cirrhosis is seen in the clinic to follow up a recent hospitalization for spontaneous bacterial peritonitis. He is doing well and finishing his course of antibiotics. He is taking propranolol and lactulose; besides complications of end-stage liver disease, he has well-controlled diabetes mellitus and had a basal cell carcinoma resected 5 years ago. The cirrhosis is thought to be due to alcohol abuse, and his last drink of alcohol was 2 weeks ago. He and his wife ask if he is a liver transplant candidate. He can be counseled in which of the following ways?

A.   He is not a transplant candidate as he has a history of alcohol dependence.
B.   He is not a transplant candidate now, but may be after a sustained period of proven abstinence from alcohol.
C.   Because he has diabetes mellitus he is not a transplant candidate.
D.   Because he had a skin cancer he is not a transplant candidate.
E.   He is appropriate for liver transplantation and should be referred immediately.

**IX-41.** An 83-year-old male is brought urgently to the hospital with hematochezia and hypotension. He has no recent history of gastrointestinal symptoms. His past medical history is significant for hypertension and degenerative joint disease (DJD). His only medications are hydrochlorothiazide and ibuprofen. Physical examination is notable for a blood pressure of 85/60 mmHg with a heart rate of 125/min. Abdominal examination is normal. There is gross blood per rectum. After fluid resuscitation and stabilization upper and lower endoscopy is most likely to demonstrate

A. duodenal ulcer
B. fungating colonic mass
C. gastric ulcer
D. internal hemorrhoids
E. sigmoid diverticula

**IX-42.** A 67-year-old female is brought to the hospital with severe abdominal pain lasting 3 h. The pain came on suddenly while the patient was watching television. After the pain she had nausea and vomiting without hematemesis. Her last bowel movement was the night before admission and was normal. She has a past medical history of hypertension and atrial fibrillation. Her medications include hydrochlorothiazide, enalapril, and digoxin. Physical examination is notable for a blood pressure of 83/64 mmHg, an irregular heart rate of 115/min, a respiratory rate of 24/min, and a temperature of 38.6°C (101.5°F). Her abdomen has hypoactive sounds and is diffusely tender. Stool is heme occult-positive. Laboratory examination is notable for an anion-gap metabolic acidosis, elevated white blood cells with a left shift, normal serum amylase, and elevated serum lactate. CT scan of the abdomen demonstrates bowel wall edema and air in the area of the splenic flexure. What is the most likely source of this patient's abdominal findings?

A. Acute pancreatitis
B. Antibiotic-associated colitis
C. Colon cancer
D. Mesenteric ischemia
E. Perforated duodenal ulcer

**IX-43.** All the following increase the risk for the development of Crohn's disease *except*

A. cigarette smoking
B. female sex
C. history of appendectomy
D. Jewish ethnicity
E. oral contraceptive use

**IX-44.** Which of the following increases the risk of development of ulcerative colitis?

A. Appendectomy
B. Cigarette smoking

**IX-44.** *(Continued)*
C. Female sex
D. Jewish ethnicity
E. Oral contraceptive use

**IX-45.** A 50-year-old male with a history of alcohol dependence and chronic hepatitis C presents to your clinic with 3 months of fatigue, weakness, and weight loss. He has also noted some "yellowing of my eyes." You suspect cirrhosis. All the following are clinical signs of cirrhosis *except*

A. arthralgias
B. asterixis
C. Dupuytren's contracture
D. hemorrhoids
E. testicular atrophy

**IX-46.** Which of the following statements about alcoholic liver disease is not true?

A. Pathologically, alcoholic cirrhosis is often characterized by diffuse fine scarring with small regenerative nodules.
B. The ratio of AST to ALT is often higher than 2.
C. Serum aspartate aminotransferase levels are often greater than 1000 U/L.
D. Concomitant hepatitis C significantly accelerates the development of alcoholic cirrhosis.
E. Serum prothrombin times may be prolonged, but activated partial thromboplastin times are usually not affected.

**IX-47.** Which of the following statements regarding cirrhosis is true?

A. Hepatitis B is the most common viral cause of cirrhosis worldwide.
B. Fewer than 5% of patients with chronic hepatitis C will develop cirrhosis.
C. In the United States hepatitis B is transmitted primarily by fecal-oral spread.
D. Primary biliary cirrhosis is a common cause of cirrhosis in men in the fourth and fifth decades of life.
E. Cirrhosis secondary to hepatitis C most often has a micronodular appearance on gross pathology.

**IX-48.** You are asked to consult on a 62-year-old white female with pruritis for 4 months. She has noted progressive fatigue and a 5-lb weight loss. She has intermittent nausea but no vomiting and denies changes in her bowel habits. There is no history of prior alcohol use, blood transfusions, or illicit drug use. The patient is widowed and had two heterosexual partners in her lifetime. Her past medical history is significant only for hypothyroidism, for which she takes levothyroxine. Her family history is un-

**IX-48.** *(Continued)*

remarkable. On examination she is mildly icteric. She has spider angiomata on her torso. You palpate a nodular liver edge 2 cm below the right costal margin. The remainder of the examination is unremarkable. A right upper quadrant ultrasound confirms your suspicion of cirrhosis. You order a complete blood count and a comprehensive metabolic panel. What is the most appropriate next test?

A. 24-h urine copper
B. Antimitochondrial antibodies (AMA)
C. Endoscopic retrograde cholangiopancreatography (ERCP)
D. Hepatitis B serologies
E. Serum ferritin

**IX-49.** Which of the following statements about cardiac cirrhosis is true?

A. Prolonged passive congestion from right-sided heart failure results first in congestion and necrosis of portal triads, resulting in subsequent fibrosis.
B. AST and ALT levels may mimic the very high levels seen in acute hepatitis infection or acetaminophen toxicity.
C. Budd-Chiari syndrome cannot be distinguished clinically from cardiac cirrhosis.
D. Venoocclusive disease is a major cause of morbidity and mortality in patients undergoing liver transplantation.
E. Echocardiography is the gold standard for diagnosing constrictive pericarditis as a cause of cirrhosis.

**IX-50.** A 52-year-old male with alcoholic cirrhosis and ascites is admitted to the internal medicine service for increasing abdominal girth and peripheral edema. He has never had gastrointestinal bleeding or peritonitis. On examination he has the typical stigmata of chronic liver disease. He is alert and oriented and has a protuberant abdomen that is nontender. He has no asterixis. Hematocrit is stable at 33% on two values drawn 4 hours apart. Abdominal paracentesis shows a normal cell count. The serum ascites–albumin gradient is 1.4 g/dL. The peritoneal protein is 1.4 g/dL. Blood and peritoneal cultures are negative at 1 day. Serum sodium is 125 mEq/L. All the following are appropriate management steps at this time *except*

A. 2-g sodium diet
B. ciprofloxacin
C. furosemide
D. large-volume paracentesis
E. spironolactone

**IX-51.** A 22-year-old male complains of 4 months of worsening intermittent abdominal pain, bloating, diarrhea, and rectal bleeding. His past medical history is positive for

**IX-51.** *(Continued)*

genital herpes. The patient has normal vital signs and only diffuse abdominal pain on examination. Stool is positive for occult blood. Laboratory examination is remarkable only for a hematocrit of 34%. Flexible sigmoidoscopy reveals erythematous mucosa in the rectum, sigmoid, and distal descending colon. The mucosa has areas with a fine granular appearance with some focal hemorrhage and ulceration. Biopsies demonstrate abnormal crypt architecture, including crypt abcesses. There is acute and chronic inflammation localized to the mucosa and superficial submucosa. Which of the following is the most likely diagnosis?

A. Antibiotic-associated colitis
B. Celiac sprue
C. Crohn's disease
D. Herpes proctitis
E. Ulcerative colitis

**IX-52.** A 62-year-old female has a 3-month history of diffuse crampy abdominal pain and watery diarrhea and has lost 14 lb over this period. There is no prior history of abdominal or gynecologic disease. She is on no regular medications, is a nonsmoker, and does not consume alcohol. Colonoscopy reveals normal colonic mucosa. Biopsies of the colon reveal inflammation with extensive subepithelial collagen deposition and lymphocytic infiltration of the epithelium. Which of the following is the most likely diagnosis?

A. Collagenous colitis
B. Crohn's disease
C. Ischemic colitis
D. Lymphocytic colitis
E. Ulcerative colitis

**IX-53.** A 33-year-old male presents with a painful skin lesion on the leg. He reports that 3 days earlier he noticed a small hemorrhagic pustule on the anterior thigh that rapidly grew and ulcerated. The lesion is very painful. Past medical history is notable for ulcerative colitis for 8 years. He works as a landscaper and has kittens for pets. His only medication is sulfasalazine. Physical examination is notable for a temperature of 38.0°C (100.4°F) and the thigh lesion shown in Figure IX-53 (Color Atlas). Which of the following is the most appropriate therapy for the skin lesion?

A. Amphotericin B
B. Cefipime
C. Clarithromycin plus rifampin
D. Methylprednisolone
E. Vancomycin

**IX-54.** Which of the following extraintestinal manifestations of inflammatory bowel disease typically worsens with exacerbations of bowel activity?

**IX-54.** *(Continued)*

A. Ankylosing spondylitis
B. Arthritis
C. Nephrolithiasis
D. Primary sclerosing cholangitis
E. Uveitis

**IX-55.** All the following play a role in therapy for mild to fulminant ulcerative colitis *except*

A. 5-ASA
B. cyclosporine
C. glucocorticoid enema
D. infliximab
E. intravenous glucocorticoid
F. oral glucocorticoid

**IX-56.** All the following play a role in therapy for mild to severe Crohn's disease *except*

A. 5-ASA
B. bowel rest and total parenteral nutrition (TPN)
C. infliximab
D. intravenous glucocorticoid
E. oral glucocorticoid
F. oral vancomycin

**IX-57.** A 37-year-old female presents with a chief complaint of difficulty swallowing. She reports that she feels as if food gets stuck in her midchest. She notices no difference between liquids or solids but does note that the symptoms worsen when she eats hurriedly. She has had a 15-lb weight loss and reports regurgitation of undigested food after eating. The patient undergoes barium swallow. What is the most likely diagnosis?

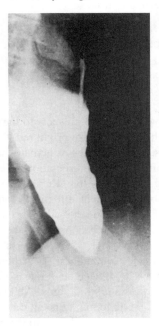

**IX-57.** *(Continued)*

A. Esophageal stricture
B. Esophageal spasm
C. Achalasia
D. Esophageal cancer
E. CREST syndrome

**IX-58.** A 42-year-old male presents for evaluation of recurrent sharp substernal chest pain that occurs primarily at rest and radiates to both arms and the sides of the chest. He notes that the pain is worse with eating and emotional stress. The pain lasts approximately 10 min before resolving entirely. He has undergone a full cardiac evaluation, including negative exercise echocardiography for inducible ischemia. You suspect diffuse esophageal spasm and order a barium swallow for further evaluation. Which of the following findings would best correlate with your suspected diagnosis?

A. Proximal esophageal dilatation with tapered beak-like appearance distally near the gastroesophageal junction
B. Uncoordinated distal esophageal contractions resulting in a corkscrew appearance of the esophagus
C. Dilation of the esophagus with loss of peristaltic contractions in the middle and distal portions of the esophagus
D. Reflux of barium back into the distal portion of the esophagus
E. A tapered narrowing in the distal esophagus with an apple core–like lesion

**IX-59.** All the following drugs can cause or exacerbate symptoms of gastroesophageal reflux disease *except*

A. sildenafil
B. atenolol
C. nifedipine
D. isosorbide mononitrate
E. donepezil

**IX-60.** A 68-year-old male presents with symptoms of heartburn, wheezing, and nocturnal cough. The symptoms have worsened recently after an inferior myocardial infarction as the patient notes a 20-lb weight gain related to decreased activity. In addition, the patient has had isosorbide mononitrate and metoprolol added to his medical regimen. He continues to smoke one pack of cigarettes daily. He reports that his largest meal of the day is dinner, which he normally eats at 8 P.M. You diagnose the patient with gastroesophageal reflux disease and initiate therapy with ranitidine 150 mg twice daily. In addition, all the following lifestyle modifications may help improve his symptoms *except*

A. elevating the head of the bed 6 in. with wooden blocks

**IX-60.** *(Continued)*
- B.   encouraging weight loss
- C.   avoiding meals within 2 to 4 h of lying down
- D.   encouraging smoking cessation
- E.   maintaining a low-sodium diet

**IX-61.** A 56-year-old patient with long-standing gastro-esophageal reflux disease seeks a second opinion regarding the recent finding of Barrett's esophagus on esophagogastroduodenoscopy (EGD). The patient originally was referred for EGD because of a recent diagnosis of iron-deficiency anemia with negative colonoscopy. On EGD he was found to have a 1.5-cm area of Barrett's esophagus with active reflux esophagitis. He is being maintained on esomeprazole 40 mg daily. He only occasionally has symptoms of heartburn but does have nocturnal cough. Which of the following statements regarding his disease process is false?

- A.   Acid suppression does not lead to regression of established metaplasia.
- B.   Up to 15 to 25% of the population will have evidence of short segment (less than 2 cm) Barrett's esophagus.
- C.   The patient's risk of developing adenocarcinoma of the esophagus is 0.5% per year.
- D.   The patient should be referred for photodynamic laser therapy for treatment to prevent the development of adenocarcinoma of the esophagus.
- E.   There are no recommendations for routine surveillance in patients with short-segment Barrett's esophagus.

**IX-62.** A 36-year-old female with AIDS and a CD4 count of 35/mm$^3$ presents with odynophagia and progressive dysphagia. The patient reports daily fevers and a 20-lb weight loss. The patient has been treated with clotrimazole troches without relief. On physical examination the patient is cachectic with a body mass index (BMI) of 16 and a weight of 86 lb. The patient has a temperature of 38.2°C (100.8°F). She is noted to be orthostatic by blood pressure and pulse. Examination of the oropharynx reveals no evidence of thrush. The patient undergoes EGD, which reveals serpinginous ulcers in the distal esophagus without vesicles. No yellow plaques are noted. Multiple biopsies are taken that show intranuclear and intracytoplasmic inclusions in large endothelial cells and fibroblasts. What is the best treatment for this patient's esophagitis?

- A.   Ganciclovir
- B.   Thalidomide
- C.   Glucocorticoids
- D.   Fluconazole
- E.   Foscarnet

**IX-63.** Which of the following medications is not associated with pill-induced esophagitis?

**IX-63.** *(Continued)*
- A.   Doxycycline
- B.   Ibuprofen
- C.   Cefuroxime
- D.   Alendronate
- E.   Ascorbic acid (vitamin C)

**IX-64.** A 42-year-old female presents with severe sharp chest pain after several days of nausea and vomiting. The patient reports that she believes that she contracted a viral gastroenteritis from the day-care center where she works. She has been ill for 4 days and feels that she was beginning to improve until late yesterday, when she experienced several episodes of retching without vomiting. Overnight the patient developed worsening chest pain. She has taken no fluids since yesterday because of the pain. This morning she felt as if she had swelling across the anterior portion of the neck. On physical examination the patient has a temperature of 38.4°C (101.1°F). Blood pressure is 110/62, and heart rate is 122 beats/min. Her mucous membranes are dry. She has crepitus with palpitation of the anterior neck. A mediastinal crunch is heard on inspiration. In addition, the patient has evidence of a left pleural effusion with dullness to percussion and decreased breath sounds throughout the lower one-half of the lung field. What test would you perform next to establish a diagnosis?

- A.   Chest radiogram
- B.   Swallow study with gastrograffin
- C.   Swallow study with thin barium
- D.   Thoracentesis
- E.   Esophagoscopy

**IX-65.** Which of the following increases the risk of bleeding with diverticular disease?

- A.   Hypertension
- B.   Low-fiber diet
- C.   Use of stimulant-containing laxatives
- D.   Constipation
- E.   History of diverticulitis

**IX-66.** A 68-year-old male presents to the emergency department with a complaint of bright red blood per rectum. He has had several episodes of hematochezia, beginning on the evening before presentation. He describes the bleeding as profuse and filling the toilet. On the morning of presentation the patient felt light-headed and almost passed out while sitting on the toilet. He has a past medical history of hypertension. He normally takes amlodipine for hypertension but did not take it because of these symptoms. On physical examination the patient appears pale. Blood pressure is 86/42, and heart rate is 134. He is unable to stand for orthostatic vital signs. Abdominal examination reveals slight abdominal distention with hyperactive bowel sounds. He has gross blood in the rectal vault. Ini-

**IX-66.** *(Continued)*

tially, the patient undergoes volume resuscitation with normal saline and receives 3 units of packed red blood cells. Blood pressure increases to 110/56 and heart rate decreases to 100 with these interventions. Initial hemoglobin is 7.2 mg/dL, and this rises to 9.8 mg /dL after transfusion. The patient is transferred to the medical intensive care unit, where he subsequently undergoes a radionucleotide localization scan that reveals a bleeding source in the right colon. What would be the most appropriate next step in this patient's management?

A. CT scan of the abdomen with intravenous contrast
B. Selective mesenteric angiogram with coiling
C. Colonoscopy
D. Total abdominal colectomy
E. Partial colectomy

**IX-67.** Despite appropriate intervention this patient continues to have bright red blood per rectum. Which of the following is an indication to proceed with surgical intervention?

A. Inability to localize the bleeding source
B. Transfusion of more than 6 units of packed red blood cells in 24 h
C. Rebleeding after initial therapy
D. Failure of bleeding to stop with vasopressin therapy
E. Right-sided site of bleeding

**IX-68.** A 26-year-old male presents with persistent perianal pain for 2 months that is worse with defecation. The patient notes that he occasionally sees small amounts of red blood on the toilet tissue. He never has had blood staining the toilet bowl. He reports persistent constipation but has not had any incontinence. He denies anal trauma. On physical examination there is a linear ulceration with raised edges with a skin tag at the distal end. Circular fibers of the hypertrophied internal sphincter are visible. What is the most appropriate treatment of this disease?

A. Sitz baths
B. Placement of a mechanical loop followed by surgical resection
C. Steroid enemas
D. Nitroglycerin ointment
E. Mesalamine enemas

**IX-69.** A 66-year-old female presents with an onset of abdominal pain that occurred acutely this afternoon. The pain rapidly progressed to the point where the patient sought evaluation within 1 h of its onset. The patient notes no association with food. She has had no fevers, chills, nausea, vomiting, or diarrhea. The patient has a history of coronary artery disease and atrial fibrillation. She currently takes aspirin, metoprolol, and warfarin. On physical

**IX-69.** *(Continued)*

examination the patient appears mildly uncomfortable. Blood pressure is 118/60, and heart rate is irregularly irregular at 122 beats/min. The cardiovascular exam is without murmurs or gallops. The abdomen is mildly distended with hypoactive bowel sounds. There is mild diffuse tenderness without rebound or guarding. Rectal examination shows no masses with hemoccult-negative brown stool in the vault. Initial laboratory examination reveals a lactic acid level of 3.2 mmol/L and a bicarbonate level of 17 meq/L. The patient is started on intravenous fluids, and a surgical consultation is called for. All the following findings are consistent with the suspected diagnosis of acute mesenteric arterial embolism causing ischemia *except*

A. pneumatosis intestinalis on plain radiography
B. thumbprinting on plain radiography
C. pale mucosa with ulcerations on endoscopy
D. filling defects of the mesenteric veins on CT imaging
E. diffuse bowel wall edema and portal vein gas

**IX-70.** All the following are indications for endoscopic retrograde cholangiopancreatography (ERCP) *except*

A. Unexplained jaundice
B. Acute pancreatitis without evidence of choledocholithiasis or cholangitis
C. Periampullary mass
D. Recurrent pancreatitis
E. Cholangitis with an impacted common bile duct stone

**IX-71.** Which of the following proteins does not cause secretion of gastric acid?

A. Acetylcholine
B. Caffeine
C. Gastrin
D. Histamine
E. Somatostatin

**IX-72.** A 36-year-old female presents with the chief complaint of burning epigastric pain. She notes that the pain is worse after she eats spicy or fatty food and occurs approximately 90 min after eating. Occasionally the patient awakens at night with the pain. Physical examination is unremarkable except for mild midepigastric tenderness with deep palpation. You suspect a duodenal ulcer. An EGD confirms this diagnosis, and biopsy specimens reveal *Helicobacter pylori*. Which of the following statements regarding the role of *H. pylori* in this disease is not correct?

A. *H. pylori* can be isolated in 95% or more of duodenal ulcers.

---

**IX-72.** *(Continued)*

B.  Among people infected with *H. pylori,* 15% will develop symptomatic ulcer disease.

C.  Urease production by *H. pylori* helps protect it from destruction by gastric acid and promotes colonization by *H. pylori.*

D.  Detection of *H. pylori* antibody in the serum is sufficient for a diagnosis of peptic ulcer disease.

E.  The 1-year relapse rate for peptic ulcer disease is less than 15% after eradication of *H. pylori.*

**IX-73.** All the following drugs for the treatment of peptic ulcer disease alter gastric acid pH *except*

A.  calcium carbonate
B.  cimetidine
C.  omeprazole
D.  pirenzepine
E.  sucralfate

**IX-74.** A 58-year-old female presents with epigastric pain that is worse after eating. The pain is so severe that the patient avoids eating and has lost 25 lb over 2 months. She describes the pain as burning in quality and somewhat relieved with antacid therapy. She has attempted to relieve the pain with ibuprofen but instead feels that the pain is worsening. What is the best test for diagnosis?

A.  Esophagogastroduodenoscopy
B.  Barium swallow
C.  Small bowel series
D.  CT scan of the abdomen
E.  Magnetic resonance angiogram of the mesenteric arteries

**IX-75.** A 48-year-old male seeks evaluation for diarrhea and malabsorptive symptoms. Approximately 5 years ago the patient underwent partial gastrectomy with gastrojejunostomy for a perforated duodenal ulcer. He had done well since that time until 5 months ago, when he developed abdominal pain and bloating after eating. In addition, the patient has had profound diarrhea that occurs after eating and is worse after he eats fatty foods. He notes that the diarrhea is foul-smelling and often leaves a greasy film in the toilet. On physical examination the patient is thin with a body mass index of 19. The examination is unremarkable. His stool is hemoccult-negative. Laboratory studies are remarkable except for an albumin of 3.1 g/dL. He is noted to have a hemoglobin of 9.6 mg/dL and a mean corpuscular volume (MCV) of 106. What is the most likely diagnosis?

A.  Dumping syndrome
B.  Bile reflux gastropathy
C.  Afferent loop syndrome
D.  Postvagotomy diarrhea
E.  Zollinger-Ellison syndrome

**IX-76.** A 42-year-old female presents to your office with complaints of right-sided abdominal pain for the last 3 months. She notes that the pain is episodic and characterizes it as crampy. She states that she has very loose stools but occasionally notes hard narrow-caliber stools and a feeling of incomplete evacuation. Symptoms worsen with stressful situations. She has found blood on the toilet tissue but no gross bleeding or melena. She denies weight loss. Her medications include ranitidine and a multivitamin. Examination of the abdomen and rectum is benign. What is your recommendation to this patient?

A.  Colonoscopy evaluation
B.  Initiation of an antidepressant
C.  Nutritional counseling and dietary modification
D.  Lomotil 5 mg every 6 h
E.  Tegaserod 2 mg before meals

**IX-77.** A 23-year-old Turkish female presents to the emergency department for evaluation of acute abdominal pain. She reports that she has had multiple episodes of severe abdominal pain since age 15. These episodes have been very severe, once prompting exploratory laparotomy at age 18 with removal of the appendix, which was histologically benign. She reports that the pain lasts approximately 2 or 3 days and then resolves entirely without intervention. There are no clear triggers for the pain. Past evaluation has included normal upper and lower endoscopy, normal small bowel series, and multiple CT scans that have shown only small amounts of free fluid in the abdominal cavity. In addition, the patient recently developed a migratory arthritis affecting her knees and ankles. The patient is currently on no medications. Multiple other family members have similar complaints. On physical examination the patient appears in moderate distress, lying very still. Temperature is 39.8°C (103.6°F). Heart rate is 130, and blood pressure is 112/66. She has evidence of a pleural effusion on the right with decreased breath sounds and dullness to percussion of half the lung field. She has a regular tachycardia without murmurs. Bowel sounds are hypoactive, and there is moderate diffuse abdominal tenderness. There is mild rebound tenderness diffusely throughout the abdomen without guarding. Her left knee is swollen and erythematous with an effusion. Laboratory studies show a white blood cell count of 15,300/mm³ (90% neutrophils). Erythrocyte sedimentation rate is 110 s. Arthrocentesis reveals a white blood cell count of 68,000 with 98% neutrophils. Culture is negative at 1 week. The patient's symptoms resolve over the course of 72 h. What is the best therapy for prevention of the patient's symptoms?

A.  Azathioprine
B.  Colchicine
C.  Hemin
D.  Indomethacin
E.  Prednisone

**IX-78.** A 54-year-old female comes to the hospital with 2 months of watery diarrhea and weight loss. She reports 8 to 10 loose watery stools per day that occur during the day or the night. They improve slightly but not completely with fasting. She has had no improvement with an empirical course of ciprofloxacin. Her past history is notable for hypertension and degenerative joint disease (DJD). Her medications include lisinopril, atenolol, hydrochlorothiazide, ibuprofen, and calcium carbonate. Colonoscopy reveals normal mucosa, but biopsies demonstrate a thickened subepithelial collagen band and epithelial lymphocytic infiltration. Which of the following medications is most likely to be responsible for her symptoms?

A. Atenolol
B. Calcium carbonate
C. Hydrochlorothiazide
D. Ibuprofen
E. Lisinopril

**IX-79.** A 24-year-old patient who is known to be infected with HIV-1 presents with a 2-week history of intermittent bloody diarrhea, urgency, abdominal pain, and malaise. Stool culture for enteropathogenic organisms is negative, and analysis for ova and parasites is similarly unrevealing. The patient is taking no medication. The diarrheal symptoms do not respond to a course of ciprofloxacin. Colonoscopic examination reveals multiple areas of ulceration and mucosal erosion. Biopsy reveals the presence of cells containing a large, densely staining nucleus and abundant intracytoplasmic inclusions. The most appropriate therapy for this patient is

A. acyclovir
B. clarithromycin
C. ganciclovir
D. pentamidine
E. pyrimethamine

**IX-80.** A 45-year-old male says that for the last year he occasionally has regurgitated particles from food eaten several days earlier. His wife complains that his breath has been foul-smelling. He has had occasional dysphagia for solid foods. The most likely diagnosis is

A. gastric outlet obstruction
B. scleroderma
C. achalasia
D. Zenker's diverticulum
E. diabetic gastroparesis

**IX-81.** Which of the following diagnostic studies for malabsorption is usually normal in persons who have bacterial overgrowth syndrome?

A. Fecal fat quantitation (24 h)
B. Stage II Schilling test (intrinsic factor given with vitamin B$_{12}$)

**IX-81.** *(Continued)*
C. D-Xylose absorption test
D. Lactulose breath test
E. Quantitative cultures of jejunal aspirates

**IX-82.** A 50-year-old male without a significant past medical history or recent exposure to alcohol presents with midepigastric abdominal pain, nausea, and vomiting. The physical examination is remarkable for the absence of jaundice and any other specific physical findings. Which of the following is the best strategy for screening for acute pancreatitis?

A. Measurement of serum amylase
B. Measurement of serum lipase
C. Measurement of both serum amylase and serum lipase
D. Isoamylase level analysis
E. Magnetic resonance imaging

**IX-83.** Which of the following could falsely depress the serum amylase level in a patient suspected of having acute pancreatitis?

A. Associated intestinal infarction
B. Associated pleural effusion
C. Hypercholesterolemia
D. Hypertriglyceridemia
E. Hypocalcemia

**IX-84.** A 35-year-old female complains of right upper quadrant pain that occurs after she eats a large meal. Occasionally the episodes are accompanied by nausea and vomiting. A plain x-ray of the abdomen discloses gallstones. Ultrasonography reveals gallstones and a normal-size common bile duct. The patient's blood chemistry and complete blood count (CBC) are normal. The most therapeutic maneuver at this time would be

A. observation
B. laparoscopic cholecystectomy
C. ursodeoxycholic acid
D. shock wave lithotripsy
E. ursodeoxycholic acid and shock wave lithotripsy

**IX-85.** One month ago a 21-year-old female was begun on daily isoniazid therapy because of a positive tuberculin skin test. She now feels well, and the physical examination is unremarkable. Routine laboratory data include the following: serum alanine aminotransferase (ALT) 2.5 $\mu$kat/L (150 Karmen units/mL), total bilirubin 17 $\mu$mol/L (1.0 mg/dL), and alkaline phosphatase 25 units. The most appropriate action by the patient's physician would be to order

A. another antituberculous drug
B. glucocorticoids
C. a liver biopsy

**IX-85.** *(Continued)*
   D. an ultrasound of the gallbladder
   E. continuation of isoniazid therapy

**IX-86.** Chronic active hepatitis is most reliably distinguished from chronic persistent hepatitis by the presence of

   A. extrahepatic manifestations
   B. hepatitis B surface antigen in the serum
   C. antibody to hepatitis B core antigen in the serum
   D. a significant titer of anti-smooth-muscle antibody
   E. characteristic liver histology

**IX-87.** A 35-year-old female with a history of acute lymphoblastic leukemia is seen 7 weeks after receiving an allogeneic bone marrow transplant. Routine prophylaxis for graft-versus-host disease with glucocorticoids and methotrexate is being administered. She complains of midsternal pain upon swallowing. Biopsy of one of the lesions noted on endoscopy would reveal (Fig. IX-87, Color Atlas)

   A. lymphoblasts on a Wright's-stained smear
   B. multinucleated giant cells on Wright's staining
   C. hyphal forms on silver staining
   D. small cysts on silver staining
   E. overgrowth of bacteria on Gram stain

**IX-88.** Chronic reflux esophagitis is *least* likely to result in the development of

   A. gastrointestinal bleeding
   B. an esophageal peptic stricture
   C. a lower esophageal ring
   D. Barrett's esophagus (esophagus lined by columnar epithelium)
   E. adenocarcinoma

**IX-89.** A 55-year-old male smoker presents with burning epigastric pain several hours after a meal that is relieved by antacids. Upper gastrointestinal endoscopy discloses an ulcer with a well-demarcated border at the duodenal bulb. Histologic examination of a biopsy specimen of the ulcer crater reveals eosinophilic necrosis with surrounding fibrosis without evidence of malignancy. Furthermore, analysis of a histologic section involving the gastric mucosa reveals invasion with a gram-negative rod. Which of the following is the most appropriate therapy?

   A. Metronidazole
   B. Ranitidine
   C. Omeprazole plus metronidazole
   D. Bismuth subsalicylate plus clarithromycin
   E. Omeprazole plus clarithromycin plus amoxicillin

**IX-90.** A 28-year-old female complains of chronic diarrhea. After a lengthy history and a negative physical examination, you suspect surreptitious laxative abuse.

**IX-90.** *(Continued)*
Which of the following tests would be most consistent with this hypothesis?

   A. Elevated stool osmotic gap
   B. Fecal leukocytes on stool examination
   C. Excess stool fat
   D. Charcot-Leyden crystals on stool examination
   E. Inflammatory cells on small bowel biopsy

**IX-91.** A 45-year-old male presents with a history of crushing nonradiating chest pain. Electrocardiography and exercise stress testing reveal no evidence of cardiac edema. A more detailed history is taken, and the patient states that he has had a sensation of sticking after swallowing. He notes this sensation equally whether he is eating solids or liquids. The diagnosis that is most likely to account for these symptoms is

   A. achalasia
   B. diffuse esophageal spasm
   C. lower esophageal (Schatzki) ring
   D. esophageal carcinoma
   E. Zenker's diverticulum

**IX-92.** Gastrointestinal complaints are common in clinical practice. Which of the following complaints is suggestive of a functional disorder?

   A. Diarrhea at night
   B. Acute abdominal pain
   C. Undigested meat in the stool
   D. Change in stool diameter
   E. Alternating periods of diarrhea and constipation

**IX-93.** The secretin-cholecystokinin test is useful in the evaluation of patients with suspected chronic pancreatitis. Which statement about this test is correct?

   A. Those with chronic pancreatitis usually have a high bicarbonate output after stimulation.
   B. Secretion of pancreatic enzymes may be measured.
   C. In patients with early chronic pancreatitis, enzyme output is relatively more deranged than failure to achieve an adequate bicarbonate concentration.
   D. Endocrine hormone output after stimulation is an end-point of the test.
   E. The test can distinguish between chronic pancreatitis and pancreatic carcinoma.

**IX-94.** A 57-year-old man with peptic ulcer disease experiences transient improvement with *Helicobacter pylori* eradication. However, 3 months later, symptoms recur despite acid-suppressing therapy. He does not take nonsteroidal anti-inflammatory agents. Stool analysis for *H. pylori* antigen is negative. Upper GI endoscopy reveals prominent gastric folds together with the persistent ulceration in the duodenal bulb previously detected and the

**IX-94.**  *(Continued)*

beginning of a new ulceration 4 cm proximal to the initial ulcer. Fasting gastrin levels are elevated and basal acid secretion is 15 meq/h. What is the best test to perform to make the diagnosis?

A.   No additional testing is necessary.

**IX-94.**  *(Continued)*

B.   Blood sampling for gastrin levels following a meal.

C.   Blood sampling for gastrin levels following secretin administration.

D.   Endoscopic ultrasonography of the pancreas.

E.   Genetic testing for mutations in the MEN1 gene.

# IX. DISORDERS OF THE GASTROINTESTINAL SYSTEM

## ANSWERS

**IX-1. The answer is D.** *(Chap. 34)* The patient's symptoms are most consistent with an obstructive process. The progressive and gradual nature of the process is evident in worsening tolerance for solid foods over the course of months. The patient's prior partial gastrectomy predisposes him to gastric outlet obstruction as a result of stricture at the previous anastomosis. In addition, gastric ulcers often undergo malignant transformation. Although the patient has no current symptoms of peptic ulcer disease, underlying malignancy with gastric outlet obstruction must be considered as gastric ulcers may develop into cancerous lesions if left untreated. Other factors that support the diagnosis of gastric outlet obstruction are the abdominal x-ray findings of dilated gastric bubble and the lack of air in the small bowel. Small bowel obstruction presents acutely with abdominal distention, pain, and vomiting. One would expect to find dilated small bowel loops with air-fluid levels. Gastroparesis is common in poorly controlled diabetic patients, symptomatically affecting approximately 10% of those patients. Frequent vomiting of poorly digested food is reported, as in this patient. However, no abnormal findings are associated on standard radiography. Finally, cholelithiasis is most often asymptomatic but can present as biliary colic. There should be associated pain in the right upper quadrant and epigastrium with eating. Again, the abdominal radiogram is normal in this condition with the possible exception of stones seen within the gallbladder.

**IX-2. The answer is E.** *(Chap. 34)* Juvenile hamartomatous polyps are lesions that consist of lamina propria and dilated cystic glands. They are at increased risk of bleeding, but not malignant transformation. Other polyposis syndromes including familial adenomatous polyposis, Peutz-Jeghers syndrome, and Gardner's syndrome confer increased malignant potential throughout the GI tract. Gastric adenocarcinoma remains a prevalent malignancy worldwide despite significant decline in incidence over the last 50 years. The highest incidence of gastric cancer occurs in Japan. A major pathophysiologic risk appears to be related to bacterial conversion of ingested nitrites into carcinogens in the stomach. Risk factors for the development of gastric cancer include long-term ingestion of foods with high concentrations of nitrite (dried, smoked, salted foods) and conditions that promote bacterial colonization/infection in the stomach, such as helicobacter infection, chronic gastritis, and achlorhydria. Duodenal ulcers are not a risk factor for gastric carcinoma.

**IX-3. The answer is C.** *(Chaps. 285 and 287)* Causes of extreme elevations in serum transaminases generally fall into a few major categories, including viral infections, toxic ingestions, and vascular/hemodynamic causes. Both acute hepatitis A and hepatitis B infections may be characterized by high transaminases. Fulminant hepatic failure may occur, particularly in situations in which acute hepatitis A occurs on top of chronic hepatitis C infection or if hepatitis B and hepatitis D are cotransmitted. Most cases of acute hepatitis A or B infection in adults are self-limited. Hepatitis C is an RNA virus that does not typically cause acute hepatitis. However, it is associated with a high probability of chronic infection. Therefore, progression to cirrhosis and hepatoma is increased in patients with chronic hepatitis C infection. Extreme transaminitis is highly unlikely with acute hepatitis C infection. Acetaminophen remains one of the major causes of fulminant hepatic failure and is managed by prompt administration of *N*-acetylcysteine. Budd-Chiari syndrome is characterized by posthepatic thrombus formation. It often presents with jaundice, painful hepatomegaly, ascites, and elevated transaminases.

**IX-4 and IX-5.   The answers are D and D.**   *(Chap. 284)*   Gilbert's syndrome is characterized by a mild unconjugated hyperbilirubinemia. UGT1A1 activity is typically reduced to 10 to 35% of normal, resulting in impaired conjugation. Diagnosis occurs during young adulthood. Exacerbations occur during times of stress, fatigue, alcohol use, or decreased caloric intake. Episodes are self-limited and benign. No treatment is required, and patient reassurance is recommended. Crigler-Najjar syndrome type 1 is a congenital disease characterized by more dramatic elevations in bilirubin that occur first in the neonatal period. Dubin-Johnson syndrome is another congenital hyperbilirubinemia. However, it is a predominantly conjugated hyperbilirubinemia. Medications and toxins may produce jaundice in the setting of cholestasis or hepatocellular injury. Similarly, medications may induce hemolysis; however, the normal hematocrit, LDH, and haptoglobin eliminate hemolysis as a possibility. Obstructive cholelithiasis is characterized by right upper quadrant pain that is often exacerbated by fatty meals. The absence of symptoms or elevation in other liver function tests also makes this diagnosis unlikely.

**IX-6.   The answer is B.**   *(Chaps. 78 and 282)*   Hepatic adenomas are benign tumors of the liver found in women in the third and fourth decades. Hormones are thought to play an essential pathophysiologic role. The risk of adenomas is increased among those taking oral contraceptives, anabolic steroids, and exogenous androgens. These adenomas typically occur in the right lobe and are often asymptomatic and are discovered incidentally. Clinical features may include pain or a palpable mass. Diagnosis is usually made by a combination of modalities, including ultrasound, CT, MRI, and nuclear medicine. The risk of malignant transformation is low. Surveillance is recommended for asymptomatic small lesions. However, since this patient has significant pain, an intervention is necessary. In light of the relationship with hormones and the low risk of malignant transformation, the first option would be discontinuation of oral contraceptive therapy and follow-up in 4 to 6 weeks. Tumors that do not shrink after discontinuation of oral contraceptives may require surgical excision. RFA has no established role, and biopsy is not indicated as the clinical picture is highly suggestive of a benign lesion. Advice should be given to patients with large adenomas that pregnancy may exacerbate symptoms and promote hemorrhage.

**IX-7.   The answer is D.**   *(Chaps. 78 and 287)*   Hepatocelluar carcinoma (HCC) is one of the most common tumors in the world. Its high prevalence in Asia and sub-Saharan Africa is related to the prevalence of chronic hepatitis B infection in those areas. The rising incidence in the United States is related to the presence of chronic hepatitis C. It is more common in men than in women and usually arises from a cirrhotic liver. The incidence peaks in the fifth and sixth decades of life in Western countries but one to two decades earlier in regions of Asia and Africa. Chronic liver disease with other etiologies, such as hemochromatosis, primary biliary cirrhosis, and alcoholic cirrhosis, also carries an increased risk of HCC. Patients often present with an enlarging abdomen in the setting of chronic liver failure. $\alpha$ Fetoprotein levels may be elevated. The primary treatment modality is surgery. Surgical resection offers the best hope for a cure. In cases in which there are multiple lesions or resection is technically not feasible, other options, such as radiofrequency ablation, may be tried. Liver transplantation in selected patients offers a survival that is the same as the survival after transplantation for nonmalignant liver disease. Chemoembolization may confer a survival benefit in patients with nonresectable disease. Systemic chemotherapy is generally not effective and is reserved for palliation when other, more local strategies have been tried.

**IX-8.   The answer is E.**   *(Chaps. 78 and 282)*   The liver is particularly vulnerable to invasion by tumor cells because of its dual blood supply by the portal vein and the hepatic arteries. Most patients with liver metastases present with symptoms from the primary tumor. Sometimes hepatic involvement is suggested by features of active hepatic disease, including abdominal pain, hepatomegaly, and ascites. Liver biochemical tests are often the first clue to metastatic disease, but the elevations are often mild and nonspecific. Typically, alkaline phosphatase is the most sensitive indicator of metastatic disease. Lung, breast, and colon cancer are the most common tumors that metastasize to the liver. Melanoma, particularly ocular melanoma, also commonly seeds the hepatic circulation. Prostate cancer is a much less common cause of hepatic metastases.

**IX-9. The answer is B.** *(Chaps. 78 and 292)* Cholangiocarcinoma occurs most commonly in the sixth and seventh decades of life. Patients often present with symptoms and signs of biliary obstruction, including right upper quadrant pain, jaundice, and cholangitis. Unfortunately, most patients present with unresectable disease, and 5-year survival is dismal. Diagnosis is often made by cholangiography. Chronic infection with the liver flukes *Opisthorchis* and *Clonorchis* confers an added risk of cholangiocarcinoma. Similarly, exposure to toxic dyes in the automobile and rubber industries, primary sclerosing cholangitis, and congenital malformations of the biliary tree such as choledochal cysts and Caroli disease predispose to the development of cholangiocarcinoma. Cholelithiasis is not clearly a predisposing factor.

**IX-10. The answer is C.** *(Chap. 292)* Gallstones are very common, particularly in Western countries. Cholesterol stones are responsible for 80% of cases of cholelithiasis; pigment stones account for the remaining 20%. Cholesterol is essentially water-insoluble. Stone formation occurs in the setting of factors that upset cholesterol balance. Obesity, cholesterol-rich diets, high-calorie diets, and certain medications affect biliary secretion of cholesterol. Intrinsic genetic mutations in certain populations may affect the processing and secretion of cholesterol in the liver. Pregnancy results in both an increase in cholesterol saturation during the third trimester and changes in gallbladder contractility. Pigment stones are increased in patients with chronic hemolysis, cirrhosis, Gilbert's syndrome, and disruptions in the enterohepatic circulation. Although rapid weight loss and low-calorie diets are associated with gallstones, there is no evidence that a high-protein diet confers an added risk of cholelithiasis.

**IX-11. The answer is A.** *(Chap. 292)* The patient has a clinical presentation suggestive of acute cholecystitis. The gallbladder was not visualized adequately. The most appropriate next step is to confirm patency of the cystic duct. Technetium-labeled hepatic iminodiacetic acid (HIDA) is injected intravenously and taken up by hepatocytes and excreted in bile. If the cystic duct is patent, the gallbladder will be visualized on nuclear imaging. In patients with cholecystitis, either calculous or acalculous, the cystic duct will not be patent and the gallbladder will not be visualized. CT scan of the abdomen will not help in the diagnosis of cholecystitis. There is no evidence of choledocholithiasis, and so ERCP is not indicated. Similarly, until the diagnosis of cholecystitis is confirmed, procedural intervention with a cholecystostomy is not warranted. Observation is insufficient. Attempts to establish a definitive diagnosis are important in guiding medical and surgical therapy.

**IX-12. The answer is B.** *(Chap. 292)* The clinical presentation is consistent with a cholestatic picture. Painless jaundice always requires an extensive workup, as many of the underlying pathologies are ominous and early detection and intervention often offers the only hope for a good outcome. The gallbladder showed no evidence of stones and the patient shows no evidence of clinical cholecystitis, and so a HIDA scan is not indicated. Similarly, antibiotics are not necessary at this point. The cholestatic picture without significant elevation of the transaminases on the liver function tests makes acute hepatitis unlikely. Antimitochondrial antibodies are elevated in cases of primary biliary cirrhosis (PBC), which may present in a similar fashion. However, PBC is far more common in women than in men, and the average age of onset is the fifth or sixth decade. The lack of an obvious lesion on CT scan does not rule out a source of the cholestasis in the biliary tree. Malignant causes such as cholangiocarcinoma and tumor of the ampulla of Vater and nonmalignant causes such as sclerosing cholangitis and Caroli's disease may be detected only by direct visualization with ERCP. ERCP is useful both diagnostically and therapeutically as stenting procedures may be done to alleviate the obstruction.

**IX-13.** **The answer is E.** *(Chaps. 286 and 377)* Drug-induced liver injury is common. Acetaminophen is one of the most common causes of drug-induced injury. It is often ingested in suicide attempts or accidentally by children. Acetaminophen is metabolized by a phase II reaction to innocuous sulfate and glucuronide metabolites. However, a small proportion of acetaminophen is metabolized by a phase I reaction to a hepatoxic metabolite, *N*-acetyl-benzoquinone-imide (NAPQI). When excessive amounts of NAPQI are formed, glutathione levels are depleted and covalent binding of NAPQI is thought to occur, with hepatocyte macromolecules leading to hepatic injury. Patients often present with confusion, abdominal pain, and sometimes shock. Treatment includes gastric lavage, activated charcoal, and supportive measures. The risk of toxicity is derived from a nomogram plot where acetaminophen plasma levels are plotted against time after ingestion. In this patient the level was above 200 μg/mL at 4 h, indicating a risk of toxicity. Therefore, *N*-acetylcysteine, a sulfhydryl compound, is administered as a reservoir of sulfhydryl groups to support the reserves of glutathione. Normal liver function tests at the time of presentation do not indicate a benign course. Rather, patients must be observed for a period of days as the hepatic toxicity and transaminitis may manifest 4 to 6 days after the initial ingestion. Alkalinization plays no role. However, in patients who develop signs of hepatic failure (e.g., progressive jaundice, coagulopathy, confusion), liver transplantation is the only established option.

**IX-14.** **The answer is E.** *(Chaps. 37 and 272)* The annual incidence of hospital admissions for UGIB in the United States and Europe is approximately 0.1%, with a mortality rate of 5 to 10%. Patients die more frequently as a result of decompensation of the underlying illness than from exsanguinations. Age, comorbidities, and hemodynamic compromise predict an adverse outcome. Peptic ulcer disease accounts for approximately 50% of the cases. Mallory-Weiss tears, esophageal varices, and nonerosive gastritis account for the vast majority of the remaining cases. Arteriovenous malformation (AVMs), neoplasia, and Dieulafoy lesions are more rare cause of UGIB.

**IX-15.** **The answer is A.** *(Chaps. 37 and 274)* In addition to clinical features, characteristics of an ulcer at the time of endoscopy provide important prognostic information. One-third of patients with either active bleeding or a nonbleeding visible vessel will have further bleeding if they are treated only medically. This contrasts with the virtually nonexistent risk of rebleeding if the ulcer has a clean base. In this case, although the patient is hemodynamically stable and shows no active bleeding, endoscopy shows a visible vessel that is at significant risk of rebleeding. Therefore, intervention with electrocoagulation, heater probe, or injection therapy is appropriate. Treatment with proton pump inhibition and eradication of *H. pylori* if present clearly lowers the risk of recurrent bleeding episodes. Early consultation with surgery or interventional radiology is reasonable in patients with risk factors for rebleeding. Although patients with clean-based ulcers may be discharged after endoscopy, patients with ulcers that are not clean-based should be observed for 3 days as the vast majority of recurrent bleeding episodes occur within 72 h.

**IX-16.** **The answer is E.** *(Chaps. 37 and 289)* Patients with variceal bleeding have poorer outcomes than do patients with other sources of UGIB. Endoscopic therapy significantly reduces rebleeding and mortality. Ligation therapy (e.g., banding) is the treatment of choice, resulting in fewer complications than sclerotherapy. Octreotide, a somatostatin analogue, given as an intravenous infusion may help control acute bleeding. Similarly, if blood pressure permits, treatment with nonselective beta blockers decreases significantly recurrent bleeding from esophageal varices. Proton pump inhibition in patients admitted to the intensive care unit (ICU) with UGIB is reasonable and may ameliorate complications from gastritis, although most of the data are with the use of $H_2$ blockers. For patients with severe varices and decompensated cirrhosis TIPS may be an option to improve rates of rebleeding. However, one of the primary complications is worsening hepatic encephalopathy. In this patient with encephalopathy TIPS cannot be recommended. If the patient improved clinically, elective TIPS might be considered.

**IX-17.** **The answer is A.** *(Chap. 37)* Lower gastrointestinal bleeding (LGIB) results in far fewer hospitalizations than does upper GI bleeding. Hemorrhoids are probably the most common cause of LGIB. Anal fissures are also causes of minor bleeding and pain. If these local causes are excluded, diverticula, vascular ectasias, neoplasms, and colitis account for the majority of the remaining cases. Acute LGIB with hemodynamic instability requires urgent hospitalization and colonoscopy. In younger patients (under 40 years of age) with apparent risk factors for malignancy (constitutional symptoms, weight loss, family history) the identification of hemorrhoids combined with the appropriate history makes further diagnostic testing less necessary. In this group the risk of malignancy is exceedingly low. In patients older than 50 years, the presence of hemorrhoids does not eliminate other diagnoses from the potential causes of LGIB. Therefore, despite the presence of internal hemorrhoids, in light of the potential for other pathologies in this 51-year-old male, further endoscopy is advised. He is eligible for age-appropriate colonoscopy at age 50 and therefore should undergo this procedure. Fiber supplements, increased oral hydration, and suppositories all may aid in the treatment of hemorroids. In more refractory cases surgical banding or hemorroidectomy may be indicated.

**IX-18.** **The answer is A.** *(Chaps. 39 and 283)* Diagnostic paracentesis is part of the routine evaluation in a patient with ascites. Fluid should be examined for its gross appearance, protein content, cell count and differential, and albumin. Cytologic and culture studies should be performed when one suspects infection or malignancy. The serum-ascites albumin gradient (SAG) offers the best correlation with portal pressure. A high gradient (>1.1 g/dL) is characteristic of uncomplicated cirrhotic ascites and differentiates ascites caused by portal hypertension from ascites not caused by portal hypertension in more than 95% of cases. Conditions that cause a low gradient include more "exudative" processes such as infection, malignancy, and inflammatory processes. Similarly, congestive heart failure and nephrotic syndrome cause high gradients. In this patient the SAG is 1.5 g/dL, indicating a high gradient. The low number of leukocytes and polymorphonuclear cells makes bacterial or tubercular infection unlikely. Chylous ascites often is characterized by an opaque milky fluid with a triglyceride level greater than 1000 mg/dL in addition to a low SAG.

**IX-19.** **The answer is E.** *(Chap. 35)* Acute diarrhea is an extremely common condition. Most cases of acute diarrhea are caused by infectious agents. The remainder are caused by medications, toxic ingestions, ischemia, and presentations of more chronic conditions. Fecal-oral transmission via direct personal contact or ingestion of contaminated food or water is the usual route of spread. Viral causes such as rotavirus and Norwalk virus account for most cases of pediatric acute diarrhea. Bacterial pathogens are more common in adults. Hospitalized patients may be affected by a variety of pathogens, but *C. difficile* accounts for the majority of cases. Travelers to some regions of Latin America, Africa, and Asia are at risk for a variety of pathogens, with enterotoxigenic *Escherichia coli* and other aerobic gram-negative bacilli being common pathogens. Campers, backpackers, and swimmers in wilderness areas are at risk for *Giardia* infection. Norwalk and Norwalk-like viruses are extremely contagious pathogens. Infection with these agents often results in dramatic symptoms of nausea, vomiting, abdominal pain, and profuse watery diarrhea. The infection may be highly contagious as patients may shed virus for many days after the resolution of symptoms. The viruses are the etiology of a number of well-publicized outbreaks of diarrhea on cruise ships and in close environments.

**IX-20.** **The answer is B.** *(Chap. 35)* *Campylobacter* and *Shigella* are associated with bloody diarrhea. Fecal-oral transmission and exposure to undercooked poultry products are routes of transmission. Although bloody diarrhea is a common occurrence in amebic dysentery, patients may develop extraintestinal manifestations in the liver, lungs, heart, and brain. Enterotoxigenic *E. coli* causes a watery diarrhea, but enterohemorrhagic *E. coli* O157:H7 (often from undercooked hamburger) may cause a severe dysentery and the development of hemolytic-uremic syndrome. Cryptosporidiosis is a common cause of diarrhea in immunodeficient individuals. It causes a profuse watery diarrhea with mucus, but blood and fecal leukocytes are extremely rare.

**IX-21.  The answer is C.**  *(Chap. 35)*  The decision to evaluate and presumptively treat acute diarrhea depends on the severity and duration of symptoms and host factors. The majority of episodes of acute diarrhea are self-limited and require no evaluation or treatment. Indications for evaluation include profuse diarrhea with dehydration, grossly bloody stools, fever above 38.5°C (101.3°F), prolonged-duration severe abdominal pain, and extensive comorbidities. This patient is able to tolerate oral fluids and therefore does not require admission to the hospital. Most likely she has a self-limited form of diarrhea, possibly related to her child's recent illness. Empirical antibiotics may be a cost-effective alternative to extensive evaluation in patients with symptoms and signs suggestive of bacterial diarrhea but are not indicated in this case. Similarly, stool studies and endoscopy should be reserved for patients with more worrisome clinical features.

**IX-22.  The answer is C.**  *(Chap. 35)*  The presence of prolonged diarrhea in an individual with possible wilderness exposure should raise the possibility of a diagnosis of giardiasis. *Giardia* is a protozoon that is a common cause of prolonged diarrhea in campers and hikers. Although quinolones are standard therapy for many bacterial causes of diarrhea, they are ineffective in patients with protozoal causes. This type of diarrhea is highly treatable with oral metronidazole. Observation is inappropriate as this patient shows no sign of resolution of symptoms and is symptomatic. Extraintestinal manifestations are not seen in *Giardia* infections. Sigmoidoscopy does not contribute further information and is not cost-effective.

**IX-23.  The answer is D.**  *(Chaps. 35 and 275)*  Diarrhea lasting more than 4 weeks should raise the possibility of chronic diarrhea. As opposed to acute diarrhea, noninfectious etiologies are the cause in the majority of cases of chronic diarrhea. Chronic diarrhea may be divided into different categories: secretory, osmotic, malabsorptive, inflammatory, and miscellaneous causes. The classic examples of secretory diarrhea are those mediated by hormones. Metastatic carcinoid tumors or neuroendocrine tumors such as gastrinoma, VIPoma, and somatostatinoma all may present with chronic diarrhea. Secretory diarrheas are characterized classically by painless, high-volume watery diarrhea. Malabsorptive diarrhea may result from improper excretion of pancreatic enzymes, as in the case of chronic pancreatitis, or from problems at the brush border. Celiac sprue, or gluten enteropathy, causes villous atrophy and crypt hyperplasia in the proximal small bowel and may result in inadequate iron absorption as well as various nutritional deficiencies. Osmotic diarrhea is caused by ingested, poorly absorbable, osmotically active solutes that draw fluid into the luminal space. Examples include osmotic laxatives and carbohydrate malabsorption secondary to lactase deficiency. Fasting often removes the osmotically active solute and causes resolution of the diarrhea.

**IX-24.  The answer is B.**  *(Chap. 35)*  Rapid transit may accompany many diarrheas as a secondary or contributing process, but primary dysmotility is an unusual cause of diarrhea. Hormonal and metabolic processes may result in increased motility. Hyperthyroidism is often clinically accompanied by complaints of diarrhea. Medications are a common cause of diarrhea either as a primary cause of motility as in the case of "prokinetic" agents such as metoclopramide and erythromycin or as a side effect of bacterial overgrowth as in the case of prolonged antibiotic administration. Diabetes results in microvascular complications of peripheral and autonomic neuropathies and may result in gastroparesis and intestinal dysmotility. Irritable bowel syndrome is extremely common. It is characterized by disturbed intestinal and colonic motor and sensory responses to various stimuli. Clinically, it is characterized by episodes of constipation and diarrhea. Although disturbances in electrolytes may cause changes in intestinal motility, hypercalcemia is typically associated with constipation, not diarrhea.

**IX-25. The answer is D.** *(Chap. 336)* Hemochromatosis is a common disorder of iron storage in which inappropriate increases in intestinal iron absorption result in excessive deposition in multiple organs but predominantly in the liver. There are two forms: hereditary hemochromatosis, in which the majority of cases are associated with mutations of the *HFE* gene, and secondary iron overload, which usually is associated with iron-loading anemias such as thalassemia and sideroblastic anemia. Serum ferritin testing and plasma iron studies can be very suggestive of the diagnosis, with the ferritin often >500 $\mu$g/L and transferrin saturation of 50 to 100%. However, these tests are not conclusive, and further testing is still required for the diagnosis. Although liver biopsy and evaluation for iron deposition or a hepatic iron index ($\mu$g/g dry weight)/56 $\times$ age > 2 is the definitive diagnosis, genetic testing is widely available today, and because of the high prevalence of *HFE* gene mutations associated with hereditary hemochromatosis, it is recommended for diagnostic evaluation. If the genetic testing is inconclusive, the invasive liver biopsy evaluation may be indicated.

**IX-26. The answer is D.** *(Chap. 275)* This patient has a stool osmolality gap (measured stool osmolality – calculated stool osmolality) of <50 mosmol/L, suggesting a secretory rather than an osmotic cause for diarrhea. Secretory causes of diarrhea include toxin-mediated diarrhea (cholera, enterotoxigenic *Escherichia coli*) and intestinal peptide–mediated diarrhea in which the major pathophysiology is a luminal or circulating secretagogue. The distinction between secretory diarrhea and osmotic diarrhea aids in forming a differential diagnosis. Secretory diarrhea will not decrease substantially during a fast and has a low osmolality gap. Osmotic diarrhea will generally decrease during a fast and has a high (>50 mosmol/L) osmolality gap. Celiac sprue, chronic pancreatitis, lactase deficiency, and Whipple's disease all cause an osmotic diarrhea.

**IX-27. The answer is B.** *(Chap. 275)* This patient's presentation with steatorrhea that decreases during a fast is consistent with an osmotic diarrhea such as that with Crohn's disease, *Giardia* infection, lactase deficiency, or Whipple's disease. Enterotoxigenic *E. coli* causes secretory diarrhea. Bile salts are reabsorbed in the ileum, and elevation of bile salts in the stool suggests extensive ileal pathology such as that seen in Crohn's disease. The presence of steatorrhea is determined in these cases by the degree of ileal disease. Patients with mild disease will have diarrhea resulting from bile salt irritation of the colon (bile acid diarrhea) but not steatorrhea resulting from increased hepatic synthesis of bile acids. In cases of severe ileal disease, hepatic bile acid synthesis cannot increase sufficiently to maintain micelle formation and normal fat absorption, resulting in steatorrhea. Similar symptoms develop in patients with surgical ileal resection, depending on the extent of the residual ileum. Treatment of diarrhea with cholestyramine is effective in improving bile acid diarrhea when ileal disease is mild but is usually not effective in treating extensive ileal disease with steatorrhea.

**IX-28. The answer is E.** *(Chap. 275)* This patient most likely has primary lactase deficiency. Carbohydrates in the diet are composed of starches, disaccharides (lactose, sucrose), and glucose. Only monosaccharides (glucose, galactose) are absorbed in the small intestine so that starches and disaccharides must be digested before absorption. Starches are digested by amylase (pancreatic > salivary). Lactose, the disaccharide present in milk, requires digestion by brush border lactase into glucose and galactose. Lactase is present in the intestinal brush border in all species during the postnatal period but disappears except in humans. There are marked racial differences in the persistence of lactase, with Asians having among the highest prevalence of lactase deficiency and Northern Europeans having the lowest prevalence. In primary lactase deficiency other aspects of intestinal nutrient absorption and brush border function are normal. Symptoms usually arise in adolescence or adulthood and consist of diarrhea, abdominal pain, cramps, bloating, and flatus after the consumption of milk products. The differential diagnosis includes irritable bowel syndrome. Treatment involves avoidance of foods with a high lactose content (milk, ice cream)

| Primary Lactase Deficiency in Different Adult Ethnic Groups | |
| --- | --- |
| Ethnic Group | Prevalence of Lactase Deficiency, % |
| Northern European | 5–15 |
| Mediterranean | 60–85 |
| African black | 85–100 |
| American black | 45–80 |
| American Caucasian | 10–25 |
| Native American | 50–95 |
| Mexican American | 40–75 |
| Asian | 90–100 |

*Source*: From FJ Simons: Am J Dig Dis 23:963, 1978.

and use of oral galactosidase ("lactase") enzyme replacement. The efficacy of the enzyme replacement treatments varies with the product, the food, and the individual. Cholestyramine is useful in cases of bile acid diarrhea. Viokase is used in patients with chronic pancreatic insufficiency (chronic pancreatitis, resection, cystic fibrosis) and contains amylase, protease, and lipase. Metoclopramide is a promotility agent and will not help symptoms of lactase deficiency. Omeprazole is a proton pump inhibitor and will decrease gastric acid secretion.

**IX-29.   The answer is C.**   *(Chap. 275)*   The combination of steatorrhea, weight loss, and migratory large joint arthralgias is consistent with the diagnosis of Whipple's disease. Whipple's disease may also cause cardiac and central nervous system (CNS) disease, including dementia. It is caused by chronic infection with *T. whippelii*. The disease occurs predominantly in middle-aged white men. Whipple's disease may also be diagnosed by a small bowel (or other involved organ) showing macrophages staining positive for PAS and containing the small Whipple's bacillus. Treatment for Whipple's disease requires prolonged (1 year) therapy with trimethoprim-sulfamethoxazole or chloramphenicol. Antiendomysial antibodies, antigliadin IgA antibodies, and the small bowel biopsy findings described above are characteristic of celiac sprue. Antibiotic-associated colitis caused by *C. difficile* does not cause steatorrhea.

**IX-30 and IX-31.   The answers are D and B.**   *(Chap. 281)*   The patient presents with acute appendicitis, with initially diffuse abdominal pain and later localized pain, in this case on physical examination, to the right lower quadrant. Interestingly, the incidence of acute appendicitis is decreasing in the United States and Europe. Furthermore, acute appendicitis has a lower incidence among lower-socioeconomic-status groups and in underdeveloped countries. Pathologically, obstruction of the appendix is found in a minority of cases: 30 to 40%. *Yersinia* complement-fixing antibody titers are found in approximately 30% of cases of appendicitis. In addition to the classic diffuse abdominal pain that progresses over several hours to right lower quadrant pain, anorexia is a common complaint, with the majority of patients having associated nausea and vomiting. Depending on the location of the appendix and its potential juxtaposition to other intraabdominal structures, urinary symptoms or diarrhea may be present or absent. It is important to note that atypical presentations of acute appendicitis may occur, particularly in the extremes of age and pregnancy. Elderly patients often have milder symptoms and have a 30% incidence of perforation. Often they present with a palpable mass resulting from abscess formation after perforation. In pregnancy the appendix is displaced generally to the right upper quadrant, and this leads to confusion in making the diagnosis, resulting in higher mortality. After it has been ascertained that the patient has an acute abdomen manifest by peritoneal signs with a high index of suspicion for appendicitis, surgical consultation is indicated. The patient's altered mental status most likely is due to his intra-abdominal process, not bacterial meningitis. Nasogastric lavage may be indicated if the patient has grossly bloody stool on rectal examination or has an unexplained anemia, but a gastrointestinal hemorrhage is unlikely to present with right lower quadrant pain. Abdominal CT without contrast will visualize nephrolitiasis well but is unlikely to show appendicitis.

**IX-32 and IX-33.   The answers are C and D.**   *(Chap. 281)*   The patient presents with several months of epigastric abdominal pain that is worse after eating. His symptoms are highly suggestive of peptic ulcer disease, with the worsening pain after eating suggesting a duodenal ulcer. The current presentation with acute abdomen and free air under the diaphragm diagnoses perforated viscus. Perforated gallbladder is less likely in light of the duration of symptoms and the absence of the significant systemic symptoms that often accompany this condition. As the patient is relatively young with no risk factors for mesenteric ischemia, necrotic bowel from an infarction is highly unlikely. Pancreatitis can have a similar presentation, but a pancreas cannot perforate and liberate free air. Peritonitis is most commonly associated with bacterial infection, but it can be caused by the abnormal presence of physiologic fluids, for example, gastric contents, bile, pancreatic enzymes, blood, or urine, or by foreign bodies. In this case peritonitis most likely is due to the presence of gastric juice in the peritoneal cavity after perforation of a duodenal ulcer has allowed these juices to leave the gut lumen.

**IX-34. The answer is C.** *(Chap. 294)*   A diagnosis of pancreatitis is made in an appropriate clinical setting with abdominal pain radiating to the back and elevated amylase and lipase. Although there are many causes of acute pancreatitis, among the most common are medications, alcohol, and gallstones. This patient does not drink alcohol and right upper quadrant ultrasound does not show cholelithiasis, leaving medications as the likely etiology. Commonly associated drugs are sulfonamides, estrogens, 6-mercaptopurine, azathiaprine, anti-HIV medications, and valproic acid. The patient was taking sulfamethoxazole, which is a sulfonamide. He should be advised to discontinue this medication, and different *Pneumocystis carinii* pneumonia prophylaxis should be prescribed. Alternative regimens include dapsone, aerosolized pentamidine, and atovaquone. Discontinuation of all *Pneumocystis* pneumonia prophylaxis with his degree of immune suppression is unadvisable.

**IX-35. The answer is D.** *(Chap. 294)* In acute pancreatitis there are many scoring systems to predict the severity of illness and/or likelihood of mortality; however, they are difficult to use and are not uniformly applied. However, there are certain key features of a severe attack, including age over 70, body mass index over 30, hematocrit over 44% indicating dehydration with hemoconcentration, markedly elevated lactate dehydrogenase, hypoalbuminemia, and organ failure, among others. It is important to note that the degree of elevation of amylase and lipase has never been correlated with the severity of disease.

Risk Factors That Adversely Affect Survival in Acute Pancreatitis

1. Organ failure[a]
   a. Cardiovascular: hypotension (systolic blood pressure < 90 mmHg) or tachycardia > 130 beats/min
   b. Pulmonary: $P_{O_2}$ < 60 mmHg
   c. Renal: oliguria (<50 mL/h) or increasing BUN or creatinine
   d. Gastrointestinal bleeding
2. Pancreatic necrosis[a] (see Table 294-4)
3. Obesity[a] (BMI > 29); age > 70
4. Hemoconcentration[a] (hematocrit > 44%)
5. C-Reactive protein > 150 mg/L
6. Trypsinogen activation peptide
   a. >3 Ranson criteria (not fully utilizable until 48 h)[b]
   b. Apache II score > 8 (cumbersome)[b]

[a] Most useful.
[b] Often cited, but less useful.
*Note*: BUN, blood urea nitrogen; BMI, body mass index.

**IX-36 and IX-37. The answers are B and C.** *(Chap. 294)*   This patient presents with a clinical diagnosis of pancreatitis with classic location of epigastric pain radiating to the back with nausea and vomiting and the risk factor of alcohol abuse. This suspicion is confirmed by elevated amylase and lipase. On physical examination Cullen's sign, or periumbilical ecchymosis, is noted. This finding, which occurs when there is retroperitoneal hemorrhage tracking up the umbilical ligaments and surrounding the umbilicus, is a marker of necrotizing pancreatitis. CT is likely to comfirm this clinical suspicion. The cystic duct is not in communication with the pancreatic duct; therefore, its obstruction should not lead to pancreatitis. Pseudocyst is generally a late complication of pancreatitis and therefore is unlikely to be found this early in the presentation. Finally, there is little clinical evidence to suggest a more chronic process such as pancreatic cancer. In acute pancreatitis with significant swelling at the head of the pancreas there can be mild obstruction of the common bile duct, leading to transient elevation of transaminases and bilurubin. In severe necrotizing pancreatitis a number of therapies have been attempted to improve outcomes, including glucocorticoids, nonsteroidal anti-inflammatory drugs, calcitonin, octreotide, somatostatin, and antibiotics. Early implementation of prophylactic antibiotics in these patients has been shown to result in a decreased incidence of sepsis and decreased mortality. Both somatostatin and octreotide have been shown in a meta-analysis to lead to decreased mortality but no change in complications. The other drugs mentioned have no proven benefit.

**IX-38.** **The answer is E.** *(Chap. 294)* Ongoing fevers with no clear source in a patient with necrotizing pancreatitis should prompt imaging of the pancreas for fluid collections, abscess formation, or other complications. The patient in this case was appropriately referred for CT-guided percutaneous aspiration to determine if the necrosis was infected, which occurs in 40 to 60% of cases. The most commonly found organisms are gram-negative rods of enteric origin. The diagnosis of infected pancreatic necrosis warrants prompt surgical debridement as the solid portion of the pancreas is not amenable to percutaneous drainage. In contrast, infected pseudocysts and pancreatic abscesses that have defined areas of infection can be managed with percutaneous drains in selected patients.

**IX-39.** **The answer is D.** *(Chap. 294)* Chronic pancreatitis is a common disorder in any patient population with relapsing acute pancreatitis, especially patients with alcohol dependence, pancreas divisum, and cystic fibrosis. The disorder is notable for both endocrine and exocrine dysfunction of the pancreas. Often diabetes ensues as a result of loss of islet cell function; though insulin-dependent, it is generally not as prone to diabetic ketoacidosis or coma as are other forms of diabetes mellitus. As pancreatic enzymes are essential to fat digestion, their absence leads to fat malabsorption and steatorrhea. In addition, the fat-soluble vitamins, A, D, E, and K, are not absorbed. Vitamin A deficiency can lead to neuropathy. Vitamin $B_{12}$, or cobalamin, is often deficient. This deficiency is hypothesized to be due to excessive binding of cobalamin by cobalamin-binding proteins other than intrinsic factor that are normally digested by pancreatic enzymes. Replacement of pancreatic enzymes orally with meals will correct the vitamin deficiencies and steatorrhea. The incidence of pancreatic adenocarcinoma is increased in patients with chronic pancreatitis, with a 20-year cumulative incidence of 4%. Chronic abdominal pain is nearly ubiquitous in this disorder, and narcotic dependence is common. Niacin is a water-soluble vitamin, and absorption is not affected by pancreatic exocrine dysfunction.

**IX-40.** **The answer is B.** *(Chap. 291)* The patient has advanced cirrhosis with a high risk of mortality as evidenced by his episode of spontaneous bacterial peritonitis. His diabetes and remote skin cancers are not absolute contraindications for liver transplantation, but active alcohol abuse is. The other absolute contraindications to transplantation are life-threatening systemic disease, uncontrolled infections, preexisting advanced cardiac or pulmonary disease, metastatic malignancy, and life-threatening congenital malignancies. Ongoing drug or alcohol abuse is an absolute contraindication, and patients who would otherwise be suitable candidates should immediately be referred to appropriate counseling centers to achieve abstinence. Once that is achieved for an acceptable period of time, transplantation can be considered. Indeed, alcoholic cirrhosis accounts for a substantial portion of the patients who undergo liver transplantation.

**IX-41.** **The answer is E.** *(Chap. 279)* Diverticulosis is extremely common in Western countries, affecting over 50% of people over age 60 years. Diverticulosis typically involves the sigmoid colon, probably as a result of the relatively high-pressure zone in the sigmoid. Hemorrhage from colonic diverticula is the most common cause of significant hematochezia in a patient over 60 years old. Hypertension, atherosclerosis, and nonsteroidal anti-inflammatory medications increase the risk of bleeding in patients with diverticulosis.

Colonoscopy may be diagnostic and therapeutic. For ongoing significant bleeding, angiography may localize the site of bleeding and allow treatment with coil embolization. Patients requiring emergent surgery should undergo total colectomy because of the frequency of lesions in the right colon. Colonic carcinoma and internal hemorrhoids seldom present with hemodynamically significant hematochezia. Duodenal and gastric ulcers that are bleeding profusely may present with hematochezia; however, this patient's age and presentation make diverticulosis more likely.

**IX-42. The answer is D.** *(Chap. 279)* This presentation is classic for mesenteric ischemia caused by an arterial thromboembolus, probably at Sudek's point (the watershed area at the confluence of collateral vessels at the splenic flexure of the colon). In this case the history of atrial fibrillation increased the risk of an embolic event. Emboli originate from the heart in more than 75% of cases. Atherosclerosis is a risk factor for thrombotic disease. The CT in this case is classic for mesenteric ischemia, demonstrating bowel wall edema ("thumbprinting") and pneumatosis intestinalis. Surgical exploration with bowel resection and restoration of blood supply is the appropriate therapy for patients with acute mesenteric ischemia. Acute pancreatitis is not likely in this case because of the negative amylase and CT findings. Antibiotic-associated colitis may present with an acute abdomen and hemodynamic collapse, but with the acute presentation, with the atrial fibrillation, and in the absence of antibiotics or hospitalization this is less likely. A perforated duodenal ulcer will show free intraperitoneal air, not air in the bowel wall. Colon cancer seldom presents with an acute abdomen and critical illness.

**IX-43 and IX-44. The answers are C and D.** *(Chap. 276)* There are similarities and differences in the epidemiology of Crohn's disease (CD) and that of ulcerative colitis (UC). Both diseases have peaks of onset at ages 15 to 30 and 60 to 80 years, and people of Jewish descent are at greatest risk. Asians and Hispanics have the lowest prevalence of these diseases. Both diseases also

Epidemiology of IBD

|  | Ulcerative Colitis | Crohn's Disease |
|---|---|---|
| Incidence (U.S.) | 11/100,000 | 7/100,000 |
| Age of onset | 15–30 & 60–80 | 15–30 & 60–80 |
| Ethnicity | Jewish > Non-Jewish Caucasian > African American > Hispanic > Asian | |
| Male:female ratio | 1:1 | 1.1–1.8:1 |
| Smoking | May prevent disease | May cause disease |
| Oral contraceptives | No increased risk | Relative risk 1.9 |
| Appendectomy | Protective | Not protective |
| Monozygotic twins | 20% concordance | 67% concordance |
| Dizygotic twins | 0% concordance | 8% concordance |

increase the risk of colon cancer, although the magnitude of risk is greater in UC. Interestingly, cigarette smoking seems to decrease the risk of UC and increase the risk of CD. Oral contraceptives increase the risk of CD but not that of UC. A history of appendectomy decreases the risk of UC. CD is approximately 50% more common in women, but there is no sex predominance for UC. CD also has a substantially higher concordance in monozygotic and dizygotic twins than does UC. All these epidemiologic associations may provide insight into the pathogenesis of the inflammatory bowel diseases. A consensus view is that in a genetically predisposed individual a combination of exogenous and host factors causes dysregulated mucosal immune function.

**IX-45. The answer is A.** *(Chap. 289)* Cirrhosis is a pathologically defined entity that is associated with a spectrum of characteristic clinical manifestations. Pathologic features reflect irreversible injury to hepatic parenchyma with extensive fibrosis and formation of regenerative nodules. Clinical symptoms and signs result from both reduced "synthetic" function of the liver and increased portal systemic pressure. Loss of functioning hepatocellular mass results in hyperbilirubinemia with subsequent scleral icterus and jaundice. Pruritis may be a common symptom of bilirubin deposition in the skin. Decreased synthesis of proteins such as albumin results in decreased oncotic pressure and subsequent edema.

Bleeding and easy bruisability may result from decreased production of coagulation factors and thrombocytopenia secondary to splenomegaly. Hormonal imbalance from decreased liver clearance of circulating androstenedione may result in gynecomastia, decreased body hair, palmar erythema, and testicular atrophy. Portal hypertension manifests with esophageal and gastric varices, splenomegaly, and hemorrhoids. Other common signs include asterixis, encephalopathy, parotid and lacrimal gland hypertrophy, spider angiomata, caput medusa, and Dupuytren's contractures. The liver is nodular in texture. Although the common conception is that it is small, it may be normal or enlarged. Arthralgias are not a common feature of cirrhosis.

**IX-46.    The answer is C.**    *(Chap. 289)*    Alcoholic cirrhosis is the most common type of cirrhosis encountered in North America. Unlike some other causes of cirrhosis, pathologically it is characterized by small, fine scarring and small regenerative nodules. Therefore, it sometimes is referred to as micronodular cirrhosis. There is clear evidence that excessive alcohol use in the setting of chronic hepatitis C strongly increases the risk of development of cirrhosis; therefore, screening and appropriate counseling are essential. Ethanol results in proportionally greater inhibition of ALT synthesis than AST synthesis. Therefore, serum AST is usually disproportionately elevated relative to ALT, resulting in a ratio greater than 2. The liver is the site of vitamin K–dependent carboxylation of coagulation factors II, VII, IX, and X. Therefore, with progressive deterioration in liver function, elevations in serum prothrombin time result, as the extrinsic pathway of coagulation is primarily dependent on tissue factor and factor II. The intrinsic pathway contains many other unaffected factors, and the activated partial thromboplastin time is often normal. Unlike the case in acute viral hepatitis, acetaminophen toxicity, and vascular congestion, alcoholic injury to the liver rarely elevates the transaminases above levels in the hundreds. Elevations in the AST above 500 to 600 U/L should prompt a search for alternative or coincident diagnoses.

**IX-47.    The answer is A.**    *(Chap. 289)*    Unlike cirrhosis secondary to alcohol use, posthepatitic cirrhosis typically has a coarsely nodular appearance. Hepatitis B (HBV) is the most common cause of cirrhosis worldwide. Infection is typically perinatal or occurs in early childhood. The HBV vaccine has had a significant impact on the incidence of HBV infection and subsequent cirrhosis and hepatoma. In the United States, HBV infection is much less prevalent. However, certain high-risk behavioral groups (e.g., those with multiple sexual partners, injection drug users, men who have sex with men) are at increased risk for infection. Hepatitis A, not hepatitis B or C, is spread via the fecal-oral route. Hepatitis C accounts for many cases of cirrhosis after blood transfusions and is a major cause of morbidity in injection drug users. Unlike HBV infection, HCV infection in adulthood carries a high risk of transformation to chronic hepatitis. These individuals develop cirrhosis more than 20% of the time. Primary biliary cirrhosis is a rare cause of cirrhosis. It most frequently affects women in the fourth through sixth decades. It is associated with autoimmune phenomena and antimitochondrial antibodies.

**IX-48.    The answer is B.**    *(Chap. 289)*    The presence of cirrhosis in an elderly woman with no prior risk factors for viral or alcoholic cirrhosis should raise the possibility of primary biliary cirrhosis (PBC). It is characterized by chronic inflammation and fibrous obliteration of intrahepatic ductules. The cause is unknown, but autoimmunity is assumed as there is an association with other autoimmune disorders, such as autoimmune thyroiditis, CREST syndrome, and the sicca syndrome. The vast majority of patients with symptomatic disease are women. AMA is positive in over 90% of patients with PBC and only rarely is positive in other conditions. This makes it the most useful initial test in the diagnosis of PBC. Since there are false-positives, if AMA is positive, a liver biopsy is performed to confirm the diagnosis. The 24-h urine copper collection is useful in the diagnosis of Wilson's disease. Hepatic failure from Wilson's disease typically occurs before age 50 years. Hemochromatosis may result in cirrhosis. It is associated with lethargy, fatigue, loss of libido, discoloration of the skin, arthralgias, diabetes, and cardiomyopathy. Ferritin levels are usually increased, and the most suggestive laboratory abnormality is an elevated transferrin saturation percentage. Although hemochromatosis is a possible diagnosis in this case, PBC is more likely in light of the clinical scenario. Although chronic hepatitis B and hepatitis C are certainly in the differential diagnosis and must be ruled out, they are unlikely because of the patient's history and lack of risk factors.

IX-49.  **The answer is B.**  *(Chap. 289)*  Severe right-sided heart failure may lead to chronic liver injury and cardiac cirrhosis. Elevated venous pressure leads to congestion of the hepatic sinusoids and of the central vein and centrilobular hepatocytes. Centrilobular fibrosis develops, and fibrosis extends outward from the central vein, not the portal triads. Gross examination of the liver shows a pattern of "nutmeg liver." Although transaminases are typically mildly elevated, severe congestion, particularly associated with hypotension, may result in dramatic elevation of AST and ALT 50- to 100-fold above normal. Budd-Chiari syndrome, or occlusion of the hepatic veins or inferior vena cava, may be confused with congestive hepatopathy. However, the signs and symptoms of congestive heart failure are absent in patients with Budd-Chiari syndrome, and these patients can be easily distinguished clinically from those with heart failure. Venoocclusive disease may result from hepatic irradiation and high-dose chemotherapy in preparation for hematopoietic stem cell transplantation. It is not a typical complication of liver transplantation. Although echocardiography is a useful tool for assessing left and right ventricular function, findings may be unimpressive in patients with constrictive pericarditis. A high index of suspicion for constrictive pericarditis (e.g., prior episodes of pericarditis, mediastinal irradiation) should lead to a right-sided heart catheterization with demonstration of "square root sign," limitation of right heart filling pressure in diastole that is suggestive of restrictive cardiomyopathy. Cardiac magnetic resonance imaging may also be helpful in determining which patients should proceed to cardiac surgery.

IX-50.  **The answer is B.**  *(Chap. 289)*  Ascites is the accumulation of excess fluid in the peritoneal cavity. It may be "transudative" as a result of hydrostatic and oncotic forces. It may also be "exudative" as a result of inflammatory, infectious, or malignant processes. Portal hypertension plays an important role in the formation of ascites by raising hydrostatic pressure within the splanchnic capillary bed. Increased sympathetic output results in diminished natriuresis through activation of the renin-angiotensin system. Reduced oncotic pressure from hypoalbuminemia also favors extravasation of fluid into the peritoneal cavity. Cirrhotic patients with ascites also have an impaired ability to excrete a water load from the kidney in a normal fashion. Renal vasoconstriction may also contribute to sodium retention. The presence of ascites in a patient with cirrhosis necessitates evaluation with paracentesis. Once infectious or other exudative processes have been eliminated, the focus shifts toward improvement of salt balance. Critical measures include limitation of sodium intake through salt-restricted diets. Fluid restriction does little to help diuresis but may be necessary to improve hyponatremia. Diuretics favor increased sodium excretion. Care must be made not to "overdiurese" patients and reduce renal perfusion too quickly and precipitate renal impairment. Inhibition of the renin-angiotensin system with spironolactone has been shown to improve salt balance. Hyperkalemia must be monitored closely. Patients with pronounced ascites requiring hospitalization benefit from large-volume paracentesis. Although patients with ascites are at high risk for spontaneous bacterial peritonitis, especially those with a prior history of variceal bleeding or a low peritoneal protein level, prophylactic antibiotics in non-high-risk patients such as this one have not shown any survival benefit, and this regimen may promote bacterial resistance.

IX-51.  **The answer is E.**  *(Chap. 276)*  The clinical presentation is consistent with inflammatory bowel disease, antibiotic-associated colitis, or herpes proctitis. Celiac sprue is a disease of the small intestine that presents with malabsorption. The macroscopic and microscopic finding described are classic for ulcerative colitis (UC). With mild inflammation the mucosa appears granular ("sandpaper"), and with increasing severity it develops ulcers and focal hemorrhage. In long-standing disease areas of mucosal regeneration may appear as "pseudopolyps." Microscopically, it is important to note that UC typically causes superficial inflammation whereas Crohn's disease involves all layers of the bowel from the mucosa to the serosa with normal areas interspersed with involved regions ("skip lesions"). In this case the limitation to the superficial submucosa with crypt abscesses confirms the diagnosis of UC. Antibiotic-associated colitis typically presents with pseudomembranes. Herpes proctitis may mimic inflammatory bowel disease in immunocompromised and immune-competent patients macroscopically but is limited to the anorectum.

**IX-52. The answer is A.** *[Chap. 276; Am J Gastroenterol 98(12 Suppl):S31–S36, 2003.]* Collagenous colitis is one of the two atypical (microscopic) colitides that should be included in the differential diagnosis of inflammatory bowel disease. The other atypical colitis is lymphocytic colitis. These diseases present typically with watery diarrhea in 50- to 60-year-old patients. Collagenous colitis is markedly more common in women, whereas lymphocytic colitis has an equal sex distribution. Both have normal endoscopic appearances and require biopsy for diagnosis. Collagenous colitis features increased subepithelial collagen deposition and inflammation with increased intraepithelial lymphocytes. In lymphocytic colitis, there is no collagen deposition and there are greater numbers of intraepithelial lymphocytes than is the case in collagenous colitis. Treatment for collagenous colitis ranges from sulfasalazine or mesalamine to glucocorticoids, depending on severity. Lymphocytic colitis is usually treated with 5-ASA or prednisone.

**IX-53. The answer is D.** *(Chap. 276)* The lesion shown is pyoderma gangrenosum (PG). PG occurs in approximately 10% of cases of UC, and less commonly in cases of Crohn's disease. It is usually associated with severe disease. PG usually begins as a pustule that spreads rapidly in a concentric fashion and eventually ulcerates. The lesions are tender with necrotic tissue and exudate. They are most commonly found on the dorsal surfaces of the feet and legs but may involve the arms, torso, or face. Intravenous glucocorticoids are the usual therapy, but antibiotics may be administered if secondary infection is suspected. The differential diagnosis includes deep fungal infections (treated with amphotericin B), ecthyma gangrenosum (which is typically painless) as a result of disseminated *Pseudomonas* infection, sporotrichosis, and *Mycobacterium marinum* (treated with clarithromycin plus rifampin). Other extracolonic dermatologic manifestations of inflammatory bowel disease include erythema nodosum and neutrophilic dermatosis (Sweet's syndrome).

**IX-54. The answer is B.** *(Chap. 276)* Arthritis, typically involving the large joints of the upper and lower extremities, develops in 15 to 20 % of patients with inflammatory bowel disease (IBD). It is more common in Crohn's disease (CD) than in ulcerative colitis (UC) and flares with disease activity. Treatment is focused on controlling bowel inflammation. Erythema nodosum and venous thromboembolism also generally correlate with intestinal disease activity. In contrast, the other extraintestinal manifestations of IBD listed above typically do not correlate with disease activity. Ankylosing spondylitis is more common in CD than in UC and may occur in up to 10% of these patients. The course is often progressive and debilitating. Nephrolithiasis occurs more frequently in CD with ileal disease resulting from calcium oxalate stones. Primary sclerosing cholangitis (PSC) occurs in 1 to 5% of patients with IBD. Most patients with PSC have IBD. PSC may be detected before active bowel disease and may even occur years after proctocolectomy in patients with UC. Ten percent of patients with PSC will develop cholangiocarcinoma. Uveitis is associated with UC and CD and may occur during remission or after bowel resection. Without timely treatment with corticosteroids, vision loss may ensue.

**IX-55 and IX-56. The answers are D and F.** *(Chap. 276)* Therapy for ulcerative colitis (UC) and Crohn's disease (CD) is similar in most respects with a few differences. The mainstay of therapy is 5-ASA or its derivatives. Since UC typically involves the colon with little small bowel involvement, enemas may be used in mild to severe disease. The tumor necrosis factor (TNF) antibody infliximab is extremely effective in therapy for Crohn's disease, with efficacy in patients who are refractory to glucocorticoids and patients with perianal or enterocutaneous fistulas. The effects of infliximab last an average of 3 months. Patients may develop antibodies to infliximab or may develop a lupus-like syndrome, and there is a possible association with the development of lymphoma. Infliximab has not consistently been shown to be beneficial in patients with UC. Bowel rest plus TPN or an elemental diet can induce remission in Crohn's disease but not in UC. Metronidazole and ciprofloxacin are effective in active inflammatory, fistulous, and perianal CD. Antibiotics have no role in therapy for active or quiescent UC. Oral vancomycin is effective in the treatment of antibiotic-associated colitis but not CD.

**Medical Management of IBD**

**Ulcerative Colitis: Active Disease**

|  | Mild | Moderate | Severe | Fulminant |
|---|---|---|---|---|
| Distal | 5-ASA oral and/or enema | 5-ASA oral and/or enema<br>Glucocorticoid enema<br>Oral glucocorticoid | 5-ASA oral and/or enema<br>Glucocorticoid enema<br>Oral or IV glucocorticoid | Intravenous glucocorticoid<br>Intravenous CSA |
| Extensive | 5-ASA oral and/or enema | 5-ASA oral and/or enema<br>Glucocorticoid enema<br>Oral glucocorticoid | 5-ASA oral and/or enema<br>Glucocorticoid enema<br>Oral or IV glucocorticoid | Intravenous glucocorticoid<br>Intravenous CSA |

**Ulcerative Colitis: Maintenance Therapy**

| Distal | 5-ASA oral and/or enema<br>6-MP or azathioprine |
|---|---|
| Extensive | 5-ASA oral and/or enema<br>6-MP or azathioprine |

**Crohn's Disease: Active Disease**

| Mild–Moderate | Severe | Perianal or Fistulizing Disease |
|---|---|---|
| 5-ASA oral and/or enema<br>Metronidazole and/or ciprofloxacin<br>Oral glucocorticoids<br>Infliximab<br>Budesonide | 5-ASA oral and/or enema<br>Metronidazole and/or ciprofloxacin<br>Oral or IV glucocorticoids<br>Infliximab<br>TPN or elemental diet | Metronidazole and/or ciprofloxacin<br>Azathioprine or 6-MP<br>Infliximab<br>Intravenous CSA |

**Crohn's Disease: Maintenance Therapy**

| Inflammatory | Perianal or Fistulizing Disease |
|---|---|
| 5-ASA oral and/or enema<br>Azathioprine or 6-MP<br>Infliximab | Metronidazole and/or ciprofloxacin<br>Azathioprine or 6-MP<br>Infliximab |

*Note*: CSA, cyclosporine; 6-MP, 6-mercaptopurine; TPN, total parenteral nutrition.

**IX-57.   The answer is C.**   *(Chap. 273)*   The patient has typical symptoms of and barium findings for achalasia, an esophageal disease marked by abnormal motility and failure of the lower esophageal sphincter to relax normally with swallowing. The underlying abnormality is loss of the intramural neurons that control the inhibitory neurotransmitters. Other diseases that can cause secondary achalasia through destruction of these neurons include Chagas' disease, malignancy, and viral infections. Typical clinical symptoms of achalasia include dysphagia with both solids and liquids equally and worsening of symptoms with emotional stressors and rapid eating. Aspiration and regurgitation of undigested food are also common. The presence of esophageal reflux symptoms is inconsistent with the diagnosis of achalasia. The course is usually progressive, with weight loss occurring over several months. Diagnosis can be made from the classic appearance on barium swallow of esophageal dilatation with a beaklike appearance of the lower esophagus representing the failure of the lower esophageal sphincter (LES) to relax. Other diagnostic maneuvers include manometry demonstrating increased LES tone, and endoscopy should be performed to exclude coincident carcinoma. Treatment is often difficult. Nitrates and calcium channel blockers offer short-term benefits for relief of symptoms but lose efficacy over time. Endoscopic injections of botulinum toxin are also effective for short periods but may lead to fibrosis with repeated injections. Balloon dilatation is effective in approximately 85% of patients with the side effect of perforation or bleeding. Finally, some patients ultimately require surgical intervention with myotomy, which has equal success compared to balloon dilatation.

**IX-58.** **The answer is B.** *(Chap. 273)* Diffuse esophageal spasm is a disorder of esophageal motility marked by disorganized nonperistaltic contractions. The contractions are due to dysfunction of the inhibitory nerves, with pain correlating with contractions of long duration and large amplitude. Clinically, patients present with sharp substernal chest pain that may mimic cardiac disease with radiation to the arms, chest, and jaw. Symptoms last for a few seconds to minutes and may be related to swallowing or emotional stress. Dysphagia with or without pain often coexists. The presence of cardiac disease needs to be evaluated before consideration of a noncardiac cause of chest pain. The diagnostic procedure of choice is barium swallow, which shows loss of normal peristaltic contractions below the level of the aortic arch. Instead, there are numerous uncoordinated simultaneous contractions that produce multiple ripples in the esophageal wall with sacculation and pseudodiverticula. This creates the characteristic appearance of a "corkscrew" esophagus. Treatment is aimed primarily at preventing these contractions with medications that cause smooth muscle relaxation, such as nitrates and calcium channel blockers.

The other options listed describe other diseases of the esophagus. A beaklike appearance of the distal esophagus is characteristic of achalasia. Scleroderma causes atrophy of the smooth muscle within the lower two-thirds of the esophagus and is represented on barium swallow as dilation of the distal esophagus with loss of peristaltic contractions. Gastroesophageal reflux disease is a common disorder that affects 15% of persons at least once per week and is marked by loss of lower esophageal sphincter tone with reflux of barium back into the distal esophagus. Esophageal narrowing with apple-core lesions is typical of esophageal cancer.

**IX-59.** **The answer is E.** *(Chap. 273)* Many different classes of drugs cause decreases in lower esophageal sphincter tone. They include calcium channel blockers, nitrates, beta blockers, phophodiesterase inhibitors including sildenafil, and anticholinergic agents such as scolpalamine. Donepezil is an acetylcholinesterase inhibitor that increases cholinergic activity. It is used for the treatment of Alzheimer's dementia and is associated with increased GI motility as a side effect.

**IX-60.** **The answer is E.** *(Chap. 273)* Mild cases of gastroesophageal reflux disease (GERD) can often be managed with lifestyle modifications alone. These interventions include weight loss, avoidance of tightly fitting clothing, and elevation of the head of the bed with wooden blocks by 6 in. Simply using more pillows to raise one's head higher off the bed often creates more reflux as it causes increased intra-abdominal pressure and thus should be discouraged. Other factors that have been shown to cause increased GERD symptoms include smoking and eating large meals before lying down, especially meals taken with large quantities of fluid. Finally, certain foods and drugs often increase GERD symptoms, including chocolate, alcohol, mint, coffee, fatty foods, orange juice, beta blockers, nitrates, and anticholinergics. High sodium intake is not associated with an increased incidence of GERD.

**IX-61.** **The answer is D.** *(Chap. 273)* Barrett's esophagus is a condition of metaplasia of the squamous epithelium of the distal esophagus to columnar epithelium. This occurs after severe reflux esophagitis and is the strongest risk factor for the development of adenocarcinoma of the esophagus. The risk of development to adenocarcinoma increases with increasing size of the lesion, and once Barrett's esophagus develops, treatment with acid suppression does not cause regression of metaplasia. Barrett's esophagus is divided into long segment (more than 2 to 3 cm) and short segment (less than 2 to 3 cm). Long-segment disease is present in 0.5% of the population, and short-segment disease may be found in up to 15 to 25%. The risk of adenocarcinoma is 0.5% per year. Barrett's esophagus develops more commonly in white men, and the incidence increases with age. Recommendations for surveillance for metaplasia are not firmly established. A one-time esophagoscopy is recommended after age 50 in patients with persistent GERD symptoms. Patients with short-segment disease are not routinely followed with repeated esophagoscopy, whereas those with long-segment disease require surveillance at 1-year intervals for the first 2 years. If no progression is detected, surveillance can be done every 2 to 3 years. The treatment of choice for high-grade dysplasia is esophagectomy of the diseased segment. Photodynamic laser therapy and thermocoagulation are being developed as alternatives to esophagectomy in patients with established high-grade dysplasia.

**IX-62.   The answer is A.**   *(Chap. 273)*   This patient has symptoms of esophagitis. In patients with HIV various infections can cause this disease, including herpes simplex virus (HSV), cytomegalovirus (CMV), varicella zoster virus (VZV), *Candida,* and HIV itself. The lack of thrush does not rule out *Candida* as a cause of esophagitis, and EGD is necessary for diagnosis. CMV classically causes serpiginous ulcers in the distal esophagus that may coalesce to form large giant ulcers. Brushings alone are insufficient for diagnosis, and biopsies must be performed. Biopsies reveal intranuclear and intracytoplasmic inclusions with enlarged nuclei in large fibroblasts and endothelial cells. Ganciclovir intravenously is the treatment of choice, and valganciclovir is an oral preparation that has been introduced recently. Foscarnet is useful in treating ganciclovir-resistant CMV.

Herpes simplex virus manifests as vesicles and punched-out lesions in the esophagus with the characteristic finding on biopsy of ballooning degeneration with ground-glass changes in the nuclei. It can be treated with acyclovir or foscarnet in resistant cases. *Candida* esophagitis has the appearance of yellow nodular plaques with surrounding erythema. Treatment usually requires fluconazole therapy. Finally, HIV alone can cause esophagitis that can be quite resistant to therapy. On EGD these ulcers appear deep and linear. Treatment with thalidomide or oral glucocorticoids is employed, and highly active antiretroviral therapy should be considered.

**IX-63.   The answer is C.**   *(Chap. 273)*   The most common medications causing pill-induced esophagitis are antibiotics, especially tetracyclines, penicillin, and clindamycin. Other medications include nonsteroidal anti-inflammatory drugs and bisphosphonates. Over-the-counter medications and vitamins may also be implicated. The most common offenders are vitamin C and ferrous sulfate.

**IX-64.   The answer is B.**   *(Chap. 273)*   The patient has symptoms of and a physical examination indicating esophageal rupture, also known as Boerhaave's syndrome. This may follow forceful vomiting or retching with increased intraesophageal pressure. Esophageal perforation usually causes severe retrosternal chest pain, although the symptoms may be mild in the elderly. Free air enters the mediastinum and may track upward, causing subcutaneous emphysema in the neck and chest wall. The clinical manifestations of this are palpable crepitus and a mediastinal crunch with inspiration. A left pleural effusion with high amylase levels may also be seen. A chest radiogram may show mediastinal air. The diagnosis is established by demonstration of leaking of contrast material into the mediastinum. The contrast of choice is water-soluble gastrograffin. If this fails to yield a diagnosis, thin barium may be used. Treatment includes broad-spectrum antibiotics and surgical repair of the laceration.

**IX-65.   The answer is A.**   *(Chap. 279)*   Hemorrhage from diverticular disease is the most common cause of lower gastrointestinal bleeding in older adults. Although one-half of adults older than 60 years will have evidence of diverticular disease, only 20% will have an episode of bleeding. Once a person has an episode of bleeding, there is a 25% chance of rebleeding. Risk factors for bleeding include hypertension, athersclerosis, and use of non-steroidal anti-inflammatory medications. Constipation, a low-fiber diet, laxatives, and diverticulitis are not risk factors for bleeding.

**IX-66 and IX-67. The answers are B and B.** *(Chap. 279)* The patient is presenting with a large-volume lower GI bleed that most likely is due to diverticular disease in light of his age and history of hypertension. Other common causes of lower GI bleeding include arteriovenous malformations and colon cancer. The patient received appropriate initial management with volume resuscitation and blood transfusion therapy. The other initial step in management is localization of the bleeding source. Modalities to localize the bleeding site include radionucleotide-tagged red blood cell scan and colonoscopy. This patient has undergone a tagged red blood cell scan that localized the bleeding source to the right side of the colon. Thus, colonoscopy would not aid in localization and would only delay the procedure of choice: mesenteric angiography with selective embolization or coiling of the culprit artery. The complication rate of this procedure is low, with fewer than 10% of patients developing colonic ischemia. There is an approximately 25% risk of acute rebleeding. Indications to proceed with surgical intervention include unstable vital signs or a requirement of more than 6 units of packed red blood cells in 24 h. Vasopressin therapy was used in the past for acute treatment of diverticular bleeding but has fallen out of favor because of a high complication rate and a high rebleeding rate. Myocardial infarction or intestinal ischemia occurs in over 40% of patients, with rebleeding occurring in 50% after discontinuation of the drug.

**IX-68. The answer is D.** *(Chap. 279)* The patient has a chronic anal fissure. Anal fissures are often diagnosed by history alone, with severe anal pain made worse with defecation. There is often mild associated bleeding, but less than that seen with hemorrhoidal bleeding. The blood is usually described as staining the toilet paper or coating the stool. Associated conditions include constipation, trauma, Crohn's disease, and infections, including tuberculosis and syphilis. Acute anal fissures appear like a linear laceration, whereas chronic fissures show evidence of hypertrophied anal papillae at the proximal end with a skin tag at the distal end. Often the circular fibers of the internal anal sphincter can be seen at the base of the fissure. Acute anal fissures are treated conservatively with increased dietary fiber intake, topical anesthetics or glucocorticoids, and sitz baths. Treatment for chronic anal fissures is aimed at finding methods to decrease anal sphincter tone. Topical nitroglycerin or botulinum toxin injections may be used. In some cases surgical therapy becomes necessary with lateral internal sphincterotomy and dilatation.

**IX-69. The answer is D.** *(Chap. 279)* This patient presents with acute abdominal pain out of proportion to the examination. With her history of atrial fibrillation, the most likely diagnosis is arterial mesenteric embolism. A high index of suspicion must be maintained as patients often present early in the course of ischemia with only minimal signs of illness. However, the mortality rate is more than 50%. The most significant predictor of mortality is timeliness of diagnosis and treatment. In this patient there is a slight elevation in the lactic acid level, and this should prompt further evaluation. Abdominal plain radiograms are frequently normal but may show thumbprinting or pneumatosis intestinalis. Thumbprinting refers to the appearance of bowel wall edema on plain radiograms, whereas pneumatosis intestinalis describes the presence of air within the abdominal wall. Dynamic CT imaging with oral and intravenous contrast also can show pneumatosis intestinalis, bowel wall edema, and portal vein gas. In patients with arterial ischemia, lack of enhancement on arterial imaging can be seen. Filling defects of mesenteric veins are indicative of mesenteric venous ischemia, which can be associated with acute clots. Hypercoagulable disorders such as protein C deficiency are associated with mesenteric vein clots. Finally, endoscopy can be performed to show intestinal ischemia. Mild ischemia shows minimal mucosal erythema only, whereas moderate ischemia demonstrates pale mucosa with evidence of extension to the muscular layer of the bowel. More severe ischemia is marked by black or green discoloration of the mucosa and is associated with full-thickness necrosis of the intestines.

**IX-70. The answer is B.** *(Chap. 272)* Endoscopic retrograde cholangiopancreatography has become a commonly used modality to diagnose and treat disorders of the pancreas and biliary tree. In 2002 the National Institutes of Health released a consensus statement on the use of ERCP as a diagnostic and therapeutic tool (*http://consensus.nih.gov/ta/020/020sos_intro.htm*). Accepted indications for ERCP include a diagnosis of unexplained jaundice and for the evaluation of periampullary masses. Additionally, ERCP can be used with sphincter of Oddi manometry to aid in the diagnosis of unexplained recurrent pancreatitis. Therapeutically, ERCP is used to retrieve impacted common bile stones and relieve strictures, both pancreatic and biliary. This can be especially useful in relieving pseudocysts when there is a pancreatic duct stricture preventing adequate drainage. However, there is no role for ERCP in acute pancreatitis if there is no evidence of a complicating common bile duct stone. In fact, ERCP is likely to worsen acute pancreatitis.

**IX-71. The answer is E.** *(Chap. 274)* Gastric parietal cells create hydrochloric acid through a process of oxidative phosphorylation involving the $H^+$-$K^+$-ATPase pump. For each molecule of hydrochloric acid produced, a bicarbonate ion is released into the gastric venous circulation, creating the "bicarbonate tide." Control of gastric acid secretion is primarily under the control of the parasympathetic system. Postganglionic vagal fibers stimulate muscarinic receptors on parietal cells to increase acid secretion. In addition, cholinergic stimulation increases gastrin release from antral G cells as well as increasing the sensitivity of parietal cells to circulating gastrin. Gastrin is the most potent stimulus of gastric acid secretion and is released from antral G cells in response to cholinergic stimuli. Histamine is also a potent stimulus for gastric acid secretion. It is stored in enterochromaffin-like cells in the oxyntic glands of the stomach. Stimuli for histamine release include gastrin and acetylcholine. Finally, caffeine stimulates gastrin release and thus increases acid secretion.

The most important protein produced in the stomach for inhibition of acid secretion is somatostatin. It is produced in the D cells of the antrum, and its release is stimulated by a fall in the gastric pH to less than 3.0. Further inhibition of gastric acid secretion is mediated by intestinal peptides secreted from the duodenum in response to acid pH. These peptides include gastric inhibitory peptide and vasoactive intestinal peptide. Finally, hyperglycemia and hypertonic fluids in the duodenum also inhibit gastric acid secretion through mechanisms that are unknown.

**IX-72. The answer is D.** *(Chap. 274)* *Helicobacter pylori* is a spiral-shaped, microaerophilic gram-negative rod that is found in 95% of duodenal ulcers and 75 to 85% of gastric ulcers. However, only 15% of infected individuals with documented *H. pylori* infections develop peptic ulcer disease over the course of their lifetimes. *H. pylori* colonization of the gastric mucosa is promoted by the organism's production of urease, which hydrolyzes urea to ammonium ion and carbon dioxide. This increases the gastric pH and helps the organism avoid the harmful effects of gastric acid. *H. pylori* further promotes inflammation in the gastric mucosa by means of the generation of inflammatory cytokines and increased generation of hydrogen ions created by the breakdown of ammonium ion. Furthermore, the organism produces proteases and phospholipases that cause degradation of the mucus gel layer that protects the gastric mucosa from the stomach acid. The reason for *H. pylori*–mediated duodenal ulcer is unclear. One possibility is that *H. pylori* infection causes gastric metaplasia in the duodenum and thus creates an environment for infection. Another possibility is that *H. pylori* infection in the stomach increases acid secretion and decreases duodenal pH, causing duodenal ulceration. Detection of *H. pylori* antibody in the serum of someone suspected of having a duodenal or gastric ulcer is insufficient for the diagnosis as this only signifies prior infection. Demonstration of organisms on biopsy, detection by the urease breath test, or detection of *H. pylori* in the stool is needed for the diagnosis. Treatment of *H. pylori* requires triple-drug therapy, with a variety of regimens available.

All include some form of acid suppression in the form of bismuth sulfate or proton pump inhibitors. The 1-year relapse rate of duodenal ulcers after eradication of *H. pylori* is less than 15%.

**IX-73. The answer is E.** *(Chap. 274)* Sucralfate is a complex polyaluminum hydroxide salt of sucrose sulfate. It acts neither to neutralize acid nor to alter gastric acid secretion. Instead, sucralfate binds tightly to the ulcer bed at acid pH to promote healing. It also protects the ulcer bed from diffusion of hydrogen ion to the base of the ulcer and binds bile salts and pepsins, further preventing the ulcer from causing further damage. The other options listed above include the neutralizing antacid calcium carbonate and multiple medications that alter gastric acid secretion. Omeprazole is a proton pump inhibitor that irreversibly inactivates the $H^+$-$K^+$-ATPase pump. Cimetidine was the first $H_2$ receptor blocker to be developed, and pirenzepine is a selective anticholinergic agent for the treatment of peptic ulcer disease.

**IX-74. The answer is A.** *(Chap. 274)* The patient describes symptoms consistent with the diagnosis of a gastric ulcer. Gastric ulcers most frequently have an onset in the sixth decade of life. The symptoms associated with gastric ulcers are less characteristic than those associated with duodenal ulcers. Many patients complain of pain with eating and may have food aversion with weight loss. This patient's symptoms have been worsened by the use of nonsteroidal anti-inflammatory drugs. *Helicobacter pylori* can be identified in up to 85% of gastric ulcers. The diagnosis should be made by esophagogastroduodenoscopy as there is an increased risk of gastric adenocarcinoma in patients with gastric ulcers. In light of the patient's symptoms of weight loss and anorexia, care should be taken to ensure that no concurrent malignancy exists.

**IX-75. The answer is C.** *(Chap. 275)* The patient's symptoms are consistent with bacterial overgrowth in the afferent loop. These patients complain of abdominal bloating and pain 20 min to 1 h after eating. There may be associated vomiting. In addition, malabsorptive diarrhea is common and ceases with fasting. The report of foul-smelling diarrhea that floats should prompt an evaluation for fat malabsorption. This patient also has a macrocytic anemia, which can result from vitamin $B_{12}$ deficiency.

Many other complications have been noted after surgery for peptic ulcer disease. Dumping syndrome refers to a spectrum of vasomotor symptoms that occur after peptic ulcer surgery, including tachycardia, light-headedness, and diaphoresis. It can occur within 30 min of eating and is related to rapid delivery of hyperosmolar contents to the proximal small intestine, resulting in large fluid shifts. A late dumping syndrome can also occur, with similar symptoms developing 90 min to 3 h after eating. It is related to meals containing large amounts of simple carbohydrates and thus causes insulin surges and hypoglycemia. Bile reflux gastropathy presents after partial gastrectomy with abdominal pain, early satiety, and vomiting. Histologic examination reveals minimal inflammation but extensive epithelial injury. Treatment consists of prokinetic agents and bile acid sequestrants. Finally, postvagotomy diarrhea occurs in 10% of patients after peptic ulcer surgery. These patients usually complain of severe diarrhea that occurs 1 to 2 h after meals. Abdominal bloating and malabsorption are not usually part of this syndrome.

**IX-76. The answer is A.** *(Chap. 277)* Although it is likely that this patient has a diagnosis of irritable bowel syndrome (IBS), this is a diagnosis of exclusion. The American Gastroenterological Association recommends that any patient with IBS symptoms who is over the age of 40 or has associated abnormalities such as weight loss, iron deficiency anemia, elevated erythrocyte sedimentation rate, leuckocytes or blood in the stool, and stool volume >200 mL/d should be evaluated for other possible etiologies. The Rome II Criteria for the diagnosis of IBS are that the symptoms must be present for at least 12 weeks, must not necessarily be consecutive, must occur within the preceding 12 months, and must include two of the following features: (1) relieved by defecation, (2) onset associated with changes in stool frequency, (3) onset associated with changes in stool form. Patients may have pain associated with alternating bowel habits or, less commonly, associated with painless diarrhea. Women are more two or three times as likely to be affected, and 80% of severe IBS patients are women. A multidimensional approach to therapy includes nutritional counseling with a trial of dietary modification, stool-bulking agents (bran), antispasmodics, antidiarrheal agents, antidepressants, and more recently serotonin receptor agonists and antagonists. The serotonin receptor antagonists, such as alosetron, are used in diarrhea-predominant IBS with monitoring for hepatic toxicity. In constipation-predominant IBS serotonin receptor agonists such as tegaserod may be initiated.

**IX-77. The answer is B.** *(Chap. 278)*   This is a classic presentation of familial Mediterranean fever, an inherited disease most common in Armenians, Arabs, Turks, and non-Ashkenazi Jews. Febrile episodes begin in early childhood, with more than 90% of patients experiencing the first attack by age 20. Fever is invariably a feature of an acute attack. Other common features include severe serositis presenting most frequently as peritonitis or pleuritis. The pain is often so severe that exploratory laparotomy may be performed to search for a source of peritonitis. CT imaging shows only small amounts of free fluid in the abdomen or pleural space. On laboratory testing this fluid represents sterile neutrophilia in response to the intense serosal inflammation. Other manifestations of the disease include acute monoarthritis with large sterile, neutrophilic effusions and a rash that resembles erysipelas on the lower extremity. The attacks are self-limited and resolve within 72 h, although the joint symptoms may persist. Amyloidosis as a result of chronic inflammation is a common manifestation late in the disease. Laboratory studies are nonspecific, showing changes expected with acute inflammation. Diagnosis usually can be made with clinical criteria alone, although there is gene testing available for the most common mutations that cause the disease. Treatment is targeted at preventing attacks with colchicine, a drug that inhibits microtubule formation and has been demonstrated to decrease the frequency and intensity of the attacks. In addition, it can prevent the development of amyloidosis. There are no alternative therapies available, although investigations into the use of interferon and tumor necrosis factor inhibitors are ongoing.

**IX-78. The answer is D.** *[Chap. 276; Am J Gastroenterol 98(12 Supp):S31–S36, 2003.]* Nonsteroidal anti-inflammatory drugs (NSAIDs) may cause atypical (microscopic) colitis, as in this case of collagenous colitis. Collagenous colitis typically presents in woman age 50 to 60 with persistent watery diarrhea. The mucosa appears normal by endoscopy but shows acute and chronic inflammation on histology. The subepithelial collagen band distinguishes collagenous colitis from lymphocytic colitis. NSAIDs may also cause acute colitis and present with diarrhea, abdominal pain, and bleeding. Complications of NSAID colitis may include stricture, obstruction, perforation, and fistulization. The other medications listed do not cause atypical or acute colitis.

**IX-79. The answer is C.** *(Chaps. 35, 173, and 271)*   Diarrhea in patients with AIDS may be due to many microbiologic agents. Patients infected with HIV-1 are at risk of infection with nonopportunistic pathogens such as *Salmonella, Shigella, Campylobacter, Entamoeba, Chlamydia, Neisseria gonorrhoeae, Treponema pallidum,* and *Giardia lamblia* and are also at risk for infections that occur in the presence of immunodeficiency. Infectious agents in the latter category include protozoa such as *Cryptosporidium, Isospora belli,* and *Blastocystis*; bacteria such as *Mycobacterium avium-intracellulare*; and viral pathogens such as cytomegalovirus (CMV), herpes simplex virus, adenovirus, and HIV itself. CMV infection of the gastrointestinal tract may present with upper GI symptoms, nausea, vomiting, abdominal pain, or symptoms of ulcerative colitis such as bloody diarrhea. A diagnosis of CMV infection, which almost certainly represents reinfection or reactivation since affected persons virtually always previously were exposed to CMV, can be made by finding typical cytomegalic cells on histopathologic analysis. Such cells, which provide evidence of the CMV-mediated cytopathic effect, are characterized by being large (25 to 35 μm) with a basophilic intranuclear inclusion (sometimes surrounded by a clear halo: the "owl's eye" effect) and frequently are associated with clusters of intracytoplasmic inclusions.

Serious CMV-mediated gastroenteritis should be treated with ganciclovir, which may result in weight gain and an improved quality of life. Foscarnet, an inhibitor of viral DNA polymerase, may be useful in cases of ganciclovir failure or intolerance. Antibacterial antibiotics, antifungal agents, antituberculous drugs, and acyclovir play no role in treating histologically proven CMV colitis.

**IX-80. The answer is D.** *(Chaps. 34 and 273)* A Zenker's diverticulum typically causes halitosis and regurgitation of saliva and particles of food consumed several days earlier. When a Zenker's diverticulum fills with food, it may produce dysphagia by compressing the esophagus. Gastric outlet obstruction can cause bloating and regurgitation of newly ingested food. Gastrointestinal disorders associated with scleroderma include esophageal reflux, the development of wide-mouthed colonic diverticula, and stasis with bacterial overgrowth. Achalasia typically presents with dysphagia for both solids and liquids. Gastric retention caused by the autonomic neuropathy of diabetes mellitus usually results in postprandial epigastric discomfort and bloating.

**IX-81. The answer is C.** *(Chap. 275)* Malabsorption caused by bacterial overgrowth results from bacterial utilization of ingested vitamins and the deconjugation of bile salts by bacteria in the proximal jejunum. Deconjugated bile salts do not form micelles in the jejunum, and long-chain fatty acids cannot be absorbed. The bacteria also separate ingested vitamin $B_{12}$ from intrinsic factor, thus interfering with its absorption from the ileum. The absorption of simple carbohydrates generally is not impaired, though complex carbohydrates may be metabolized by bacteria. Thus, persons with bacterial overgrowth have steatorrhea, an abnormal Schilling test (even with the administration of intrinsic factor), increased metabolism of nonabsorbable carbohydrates (e.g., lactulose), and increased bacterial concentrations in jejunal aspirates. Absorption of D-xylose, a simple carbohydrate, is often normal.

**IX-82. The answer is C.** *(Chap. 294)* Though it is widely used as a screening test to rule out acute pancreatitis in a patient with acute abdominal or back pain, only about 85% of patients with acute pancreatitis have an elevated serum amylase level. Confounding issues include delay between symptoms and the obtaining of blood samples, the presence of chronic pancreatitis, and hypertriglyceridemia, which can falsely lower levels of both amylase and lipase. Because the serum amylase level may be elevated in other conditions, such as renal insufficiency, salivary gland lesions, tumors, burns, and diabetic ketoacidosis, as well as in other abdominal diseases, such as intestinal obstruction and peritonitis, amylase isoenzyme levels have been used to distinguish among these possibilities. Therefore, the pancreatic isoenzyme level can be used to diagnose acute pancreatitis more specifically in the setting of a confounding condition. The serum lipase assay is less subject to confounding variables. However, the sensitivity of the serum lipase level for acute pancreatitis may be as low as 70%. Therefore, the recommended screening test for acute pancreatitis is both serum amylase and serum lipase activities.

**IX-83. The answer is D.** *(Chaps. 293 and 294)* Serum amylase is a sensitive screening test for acute pancreatitis. Levels >300 U/dL make the diagnosis extremely likely, especially if intestinal perforation and infarction are excluded (both conditions can raise serum amylase). In all but 15% of patients with acute pancreatitis, the serum amylase level is elevated within 24 h and begins to decline by 3 to 5 days in the absence of extensive pancreatic necrosis, partial infarction, or pseudocyst formation. Reasons for normal values could be a delay in obtaining the blood test, the presence of chronic rather than acute pancreatitis, and the presence of hypertriglyceridemia. Both serum amylase and lipase (perhaps the best enzyme to diagnose acute pancreatitis) will be falsely low in patients with hypertriglyceridemia. Serum trypsinogen may have theoretical advantages over amylase and lipase insofar as the pancreas is the only source of this enzyme.

**IX-84. The answer is B.** *(Chap. 292)* Though the presence of asymptomatic gallstones in a patient without a comorbid disease such as diabetes requires prophylactic cholecystectomy, those with symptomatic biliary stone disease are more likely to have complications and probably should also receive definitive therapy. Complications from gallbladder surgery are low, especially with laparoscopic cholecystectomy; surgical treatment is probably the best approach. This patient's symptoms are beginning to interfere with her general routine, and an operation is indicated. Selected patients may be candidates for gallstone dissolution therapy with ursodeoxycholic acid with or without shock wave lithotripsy. Patients most appropriate for the approach of gallstone dissolution include those with a radiolucent, solitary stone less than 2 cm in diameter in a well-contracted gallbladder. In this patient's case the stone is radiopaque. Moreover, gallstones will recur in about 30% of patients treated with a nonsurgical therapy.

**IX-85.    The answer is E.**    *(Chap. 286)*    About 10% of persons treated with isoniazid develop mild elevations of serum aminotransferase levels during the first few weeks of therapy. These levels usually return to normal despite continued use of isoniazid. About 1% of persons with elevated aminotransferase levels develop symptoms of hepatitis and are at high risk for developing fatal hepatic failure. The older the patient, the higher the risk of isoniazid hepatitis; thus, because this patient is young and asymptomatic, isoniazid can safely be continued as long as she is watched for symptoms of hepatitis. A liver biopsy would not be indicated at this time.

**IX-86.    The answer is E.**    *(Chap. 287)*    Although chronic active hepatitis may be associated with extraintestinal manifestations (e.g., arthritis) and the presence in the serum of auto-antibodies (e.g., anti-smooth-muscle antibody), these factors are not invariably present. The distinction between chronic active hepatitis and chronic persistent hepatitis can be established only by doing a liver biopsy. In chronic active hepatitis there is piecemeal necrosis (erosion of the limiting plate of hepatocytes surrounding the portal triads), hepatocellular regeneration, and extension of inflammation into the liver lobule; these features are not seen in chronic persistent hepatitis. Both diseases may be associated with serologic evidence of hepatitis B infection.

**IX-87.    The answer is C.**    *(Chaps. 272 and 273)*    Though candidal infection is a common cause of esophagitis, typically manifested by dysphagia, it may be seen with immunodeficiency states such as AIDS, with the use of immunosuppressive agents including glucocorticoids, and with the use of broad-spectrum antibiotics. Esophagitis also may be seen in diabetic patients, patients with systemic lupus erythematosus, and those who have experienced a corrosive esophageal injury. Oral thrush is a helpful but not invariant coexisting finding. Candidal esophagitis may be complicated by bleeding, perforation, stricture, or systemic invasion. Upper gastrointestinal radiography may reveal multiple nodular filling defects. Endoscopic evaluation typically reveals a whitish exudate in the setting of underlying erythematous mucosa. The definitive diagnosis would require the demonstration of yeast or hyphal forms on Gram stain, PAS, or silver stain. Uncomplicated cases of candidal esophagitis respond well to fluconazole, which is preferred to ketoconazole because of reduced bioavailability of ketoconazole at increased gastric pH.

**IX-88.    The answer is C.**    *(Chap. 273)*    Chronic acid-induced (reflux) esophagitis may cause bleeding from diffuse erosions or discrete ulcerations. Peptic damage to the submucosa can result in fibrosis and subsequent stricture. Barrett's esophagus is formed as destroyed squamous epithelium is replaced by columnar epithelium, usually similar to that of the adjacent gastric mucosa. Adenocarcinoma may develop in 2 to 5% of persons with a Barrett's esophagus. A lower esophageal ring is a structural lesion that is not related to reflux esophagitis.

**IX-89.    The answer is E.**    *(Chap. 274)*    This patient has the classic clinical symptoms and endoscopic findings of a duodenal ulcer. The incidence of duodenal ulcers is about 10% of the population in industrialized countries. The pathophysiology of duodenal ulcers includes excess gastric acid secretion; however, *Helicobacter pylori* infection, as documented in this patient, may play a critical role. The mechanism by which gastric infection with *H. pylori* causes duodenal ulcers is not clear. However, *H. pylori* gastric infection might induce increased acid secretion through both direct actions of the bacterium and indirect stimulation of proinflammatory cytokines such as interleukin 8 (IL-8), tumor necrosis factor (TNF), and IL-11. Regardless of the mechanism, there is now a consensus recommendation that *H. pylori* infection be eradicated in patients with documented peptic ulcer disease. No single- or double-agent regimen has been reliably effective in eradicating the organism. In general, a combination of two antibiotics plus a proton pump inhibitor (omeprazole or lansoprazole) is required to achieve a high likelihood (over 85%) of eradication. Therefore, recommended regimens include bismuth plus metronidazole and tetracycline, rantidine plus a tetracycline and clarithromycin or metronidazole, and omeprazole plus clarithromycin and metronidazole or amoxicillin. This triple therapy is effective in eradicating the organism in approximately 90% of cases; drawbacks include poor patient compliance and side effects. Because of the emergence of resistant strains, metronidazole should be used in penicillin-allergic patients as a substitute for amoxicillin. U.S. Food and Drug Administration (FDA)-approved regimens utilizing two agents (proton pump inhibitor plus one antibiotic) have lower eradication rates (65 to 80%) than the triple regimen.

**IX-90.** **The answer is A.** *(Chaps. 35 and 275; Fine, Schiller, Gastroenterology 116:1464–1486, 1999.)* Chronic diarrhea (lasting more than 4 weeks) may be due to a host of causes, including medications [especially habitual use of laxatives, which may be stimulant (senna, castor oil) or osmotic (e.g., Mg-containing) in nature], enterocolic fistulas, hormones (from certain endocrine tumors, such as carcinoid, VIPoma, and medullary carcinoma of the thyroid), carbohydrate malabsorption (e.g., lactase deficiency, which leads to a low stool pH), fat malabsorption, pancreatic exocrine insufficiency, mucosal malabsorption (e.g., celiac sprue, seen on small-bowel biopsy), or IBD. Diarrhea can result from invasion of the small bowel with lymphoma cells or eosinophils in which the Charcot-Leyden crystals from extruded eosinophils may be seen. If inflammation or infection is the cause, fecal leukocytes will usually be found. Laxative use is consistent with an osmotic gap: 2([Na] + [K]) <290 mosmol/kg. However, certain anionic laxatives containing sulfates or phosphates produce diarrhea without an osmotic gap, since sodium secretion occurs in response. In these cases direct measurement of the laxative in the stool is required to confirm the suspicion of laxative abuse.

**IX-91.** **The answer is B.** *(Chaps. 33 and 273)* "Sticking" during the passage of food through the mouth, pharynx, or esophagus is almost always associated with a significant pathologic problem. The history can provide the correct diagnosis in over three-fourths of patients with dysphagia. Motor dysphagias such as those caused by achalasia and diffuse esophageal spasm are equally affected by solids and liquids from the onset. Patients with an esophageal carcinoma typically initially have problems swallowing solid food, but with progression of the cancer, difficulty with liquids also is encountered. Since this patient has dysphagia with both solids and liquids and has severe chest pain, diffuse esophageal spasm is the likely diagnosis. Diagnostic studies would include both barium swallow esophagastroscopy and upper endoscopy to exclude an associated structural abnormality.

**IX-92.** **The answer is E.** *(Chap. 271)* As in most aspects of internal medicine, a thorough clinical history is likely to yield important, if not essential, clues to the primary pathologic abnormality. Complaints of abdominal pain, distention, and stool frequency and type are very common. Abdominal pain is likely to be more serious if it is acute rather than chronic. The character of the pain, its location, and the exacerbating factors (especially those related to eating) must be elicited carefully. If a patient complains of diarrhea only during the day, it is much more likely to be functional than it would be if the diarrhea occurred at night or during both the day and the night. Blood loss is almost always suggestive of an organic cause, as is fever or weight loss. Crampy abdominal pain is relieved by defecation; it may well be due to a functional bowel syndrome. Either pelletlike stools or alternation of diarrhea and constipation is similarly compatible with functional bowel syndrome. However, a definite change in stool diameter suggests a colonic neoplasm. Stool characteristics also may be helpful historic features. For example, a pungent stool odor with the presence of undigested meat in the stool may be suggestive of pancreatic insufficiency. White-colored stool signifies cholestasis or steatorrhea. Mucus mixed in with the stool is also suggestive of functional bowel syndromes, whereas pus is more likely to be found in association with an infection or inflammation.

**IX-93.   The answer is B.**   *(Chap. 293)*   The secretin test may be used to detect diffuse pancreatic disease. The secretin response of the pancreas is directly related to the functional mass of pancreatic tissue; therefore, failure to secrete adequate amounts of bicarbonate-containing fluid and/or pancreatic enzymes indicates some degree of pancreatic insufficiency. In patients with early chronic pancreatitis the bicarbonate output is usually low, without a concomitant severe drop in enzyme levels. The test involves the administration of secretin and cholecystokinin, followed by the collection and measurement of duodenal contents. The contents are assayed for the volume of output and bicarbonate content as well as for pancreatic amylase, lipase, trypsin, and chymotrypsin. The pancreas has a great reserve of enzyme secretion ability; intraluminal lipolytic and other digestive functions require only small amounts of enzymes. Consequently, patients with chronic pancreatitis often have low outputs of bicarbonate after secretin but still have normal fecal fat excretion. Steatorrhea occurs only in the setting of markedly low intraluminal levels of pancreatic lipase. Since the normal secretin-CCK test permits only the identification of chronic pancreatic damage, it cannot distinguish between chronic pancreatitis and pancreatic carcinoma, which usually does not produce a major loss of exocrine pancreatic function.

**IX-94.   The answer is C.**   *(Chap. 274)*   Fasting gastrin levels can be elevated in a variety of conditions including atrophic gastritis with or without pernicious anemia, G-cell hyperplasia, and acid suppressive therapy (gastrin levels increase as a consequence of loss of negative feedback). The diagnostic concern in a patient with persistent ulcers following optimal therapy is Zollinger-Ellison syndrome (ZES). The result is not sufficient to make a diagnosis because gastrin levels may be elevated in a variety of conditions. Elevated basal acid secretion also is consistent with ZES, but up to 12% of patients with peptic ulcer disease may have basal acid secretion as high as 15 meq/h. Thus, additional testing is necessary. Gastrin levels may go up with a meal ($>$200%) but this test does not distinguish G-cell hyperfunction from ZES. The best test in this setting is the secretin stimulation test. An increase in gastrin levels $>$200 pg within 15 min of administering 2 $\mu$g/kg of secretin by intravenous bolus has a sensitivity and specificity of $>$90% for ZES. Endoscopic ultrasonography is useful in locating the gastrin-secreting tumor once the positive secretin test is obtained. Genetic testing for mutations in the gene that encodes the menin protein can detect the fraction of patients with gastrinomas that are a manifestation of Multiple Endocrine Neoplasia type I (Wermer's syndrome). Gastrinoma is the second most common tumor in this syndrome behind parathyroid adenoma, but its peak incidence is generally in the third decade.

# X. RHEUMATOLOGY AND IMMUNOLOGY

## QUESTIONS

**DIRECTIONS:** Each question below contains four or five suggested responses. Choose the **one best** response to each question.

**X-1.** A 63-year-old white female is admitted to the hospital complaining of hemoptysis and shortness of breath. She had been well until 3 months ago, when she noted vague symptoms of fatigue and a 10-lb unintentional weight loss. Past medical history is notable only for osteoporosis. Her current symptoms began on the day of presentation with the expectoration of >200 mL of red blood in the emergency department. On physical examination, the patient is in marked respiratory distress with a respiratory rate of 44 breaths per minute. Oxygen saturation is 78% on room air and 88% on nonrebreather mask. Pulse is 120 beats/min, with a blood pressure of 170/110. There are diffuse crackles throughout both lung fields, and the cardiac examination is significant only for a regular tachycardia. There are no rashes or joint swellings. Laboratory studies reveal a hemoglobin of 10.2 mg/dL with a mean corpuscular volume (MCV) of 88 $\mu m^3$ (fL). The white blood cell count is 9760/$mm^3$. Blood urea nitrogen (BUN) is 78 mg/dL, and creatinine is 3.2 mg/dL. The urinalysis shows 1+ proteinuria, moderate hemoglobin, 25 to 35 red blood cells (RBC) per high-power field, and occasional RBC casts. Chest computed tomography (CT) shows diffuse alveolar infiltrates consistent with alveolar hemorrhage. The antimyeloperoxidase titer is positive at 126 U/mL (normal <1.4 U/mL). What is the most likely diagnosis?

A. Goodpasture's disease
B. Wegener's granulomatosis
C. Microscopic polyangiitis
D. Polyarteritis nodosa
E. Cryoglobulinemia

**X-2.** A 43-year-old male presents to your office complaining of weakness in the right hand for 2 days. He reports that he had been in excellent health until 2 months ago, when he was diagnosed with hypertension. Since that diagnosis, he has lost 20 lb unintentionally and complains of frequent headaches and abdominal pain that is worse after eating. He previously was an injection drug user but now is maintained on methadone. His only medications

**X-2.** *(Continued)*
are hydrochlorothiazide 25 mg/d, methadone 70 mg/d, and lisinopril 5 mg/d. On physical examination, the patient appears well developed and without distress. Blood pressure is 148/94. He is not tachycardic. The examination is otherwise notable only for the inability to extend the right wrist and fingers against gravity. Laboratory studies show an erythrocyte sedimentation rate (ESR) of 88 mm/h, an aspartate aminotransferase (AST) of 154 IU/L, and an alanine aminotransferase (ALT) of 176 IU/L. Which of the following tests is most useful in establishing a diagnosis?

A. Hepatitis B surface antigen
B. Hepatitis C viral load
C. Anticytoplasmic neutrophil antibodies
D. Mesenteric angiography
E. Radial nerve biopsy

**X-3.** A 64-year-old male presents to your clinic with a complaint of worsening sinusitis over the last several months and hemoptysis for several days. On urinalysis, RBC casts and dysmorphic red blood cells are noted. Creatinine is 1.3 mg/dL. You diagnose Wegener's granulomatosis based on clinical symptoms and an elevated antiproteinase-3 titer. What is the initial choice of therapy?

A. Prednisone 1 mg/kg orally per day
B. Methylprednisolone 1000 mg intravenously per day
C. Prednisone 1 mg/kg orally per day plus cyclophosphamide 2 mg/kg orally per day
D. Cyclophosphamide 2 mg/kg orally per day
E. Methylprednisolone 1000 mg intravenously per day plus methotrexate 0.3 mg/kg subcutaneously each week

**X-4.** A 62-year-old white male presents with a chief complaint of right knee pain and swelling. Past medical history is significant for obesity with a body mass index (BMI) of 34 kg/$m^2$, diet-controlled type 2 diabetes mellitus, and

**X-4.** *(Continued)*

hypertension. His medications include hydrochlorothiazide and acetaminophen as needed for pain. Physical examination is remarkable for a moderate-size effusion of the right knee, with range of motion limited to 90° of flexion and 160° of extension. There is minimal warmth and no redness. He has crepitus with range of motion. With weight bearing, he has outward bowing of the legs bilaterally. A radiogram of the right knee shows osteophytes and joint space narrowing. Which of the following is the most likely finding on joint fluid examination?

A.  A Gram stain showing gram-positive cocci in clusters
B.  A white blood cell count of $1110/mm^3$
C.  A white blood cell count of $22,000/mm^3$
D.  Positively birefringent crystals on polarizing light microscopy
E.  Negatively birefringent crystals on polarizing light microscopy

**X-5.** A 41-year-old female presents to your clinic with 3 weeks of weakness, lethargy. and depressed mood. She notes increasing difficulty with climbing steps, rising from a chair, and combing her hair. She has no difficulty buttoning her blouse or writing. The patient also notes some dyspnea on exertion and orthopnea. She denies rash, joint aches, or constitutional symptoms. She is on no medications, and the past medical history is otherwise uninformative. The family history is notable only for coronary artery disease. The physical examination is notable for an elevated jugular venous pressure, an $S_3$, and some bibasilar crackles. The neurologic examination shows some marked proximal muscle weakness in the deltoids and biceps and the hip flexors. Distal muscle strength is normal. Sensory examination and reflexes are normal. Laboratories are unremarkable except for a negative antinuclear antibody screen and a creatinine kinase of 3200 IU/L. You suspect a diagnosis of polymyositis. All the following clinical conditions may occur in polymyositis *except*

A.  an increased incidence of malignancy
B.  interstitial lung disease
C.  dilated cardiomyopathy
D.  dysphagia
E.  Raynaud's phenomenon

**X-6.** A 62-year-old female complains of aching joints. She notes intermittent stiffness and pain in the knees, hips, wrists, and hands. She also describes easy fatigability, dyspepsia, a dry cough, and itchy red eyes and also has trouble keeping her dentures in place. There is a history of diabetes but no other significant history. Medications include insulin and naproxen. She has no HIV risk factors.

**X-6.** *(Continued)*

Examination is significant for dry mucous membranes in the oropharynx. There is no evidence of joint destruction or active inflammation. Laboratory studies show a negative antinucleolar antibody but a positive Ro/SSA autoantigen. What is the most likely diagnosis?

A.  Sarcoidosis
B.  Sjögren's syndrome
C.  Rheumatoid arthritis
D.  Psychogenic illness
E.  Vitamin A deficiency

**X-7.** A patient with primary Sjögren's syndrome that was diagnosed 6 years ago and treated with tear replacement for symptomatic relief notes continued parotid swelling for the last 3 months. She has also noted enlarging posterior cervical lymph nodes. Evaluation shows leukopenia and low C4 complement levels. What is the most likely diagnosis?

A.  Chronic pancreatitis
B.  Secondary Sjögren's syndrome
C.  HIV infection
D.  Lymphoma
E.  Amyloidosis

**X-8.** A 51-year-old male presents to your office complaining of lower back pain. When he exerts himself or lifts items, he describes worsening of the pain and also pain in the left buttock that radiates down the posterior left thigh. The patient denies pain at rest and any history of trauma. You examine his lower back. Which examination maneuver is the most specific for lumbar disk herniation?

A.  Right straight leg raise
B.  Left straight leg raise
C.  Right crossed straight leg raise
D.  Left crossed straight leg raise
E.  Reverse straight leg raise

**X-9.** A 45-year-old male comes to the physician complaining of a red, tender ear for the last 4 days. He also reports a painful left knee and nose pain of about the same duration. Eight months ago the patient had a similar episode of pain in the other ear that healed spontaneously over approximately 1 week. Past medical history is unremarkable. The patient works as a construction worker and takes no medications. He uses alcohol socially and does not smoke. Physical examination is notable for a temperature of 38.1°C (100.6°F), the bridge of the nose is tender to palpation, and there is redness, pain, and decreased mobility of the left knee with a small effusion. His ear is shown below. Without treatment, this patient may develop all the following complications of his disease *except*

**X-9.** *(Continued)*

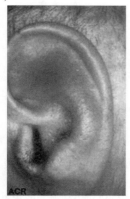

A.  aortic regurgitation
B.  diabetes mellitus
C.  glomerulonephritis
D.  respiratory failure
E.  stroke

**X-10.** In this patient, which of the following would be the most appropriate therapy?

A.  Amphotericin
B.  Cyclophosphamide
C.  Etanercept
D.  Plasmapheresis
E.  Prednisone

**X-11.** During a routine health examination, a 22-year-old female inquires about her risk of developing diabetes mellitus. Her identical twin sister was recently diagnosed with type 1 diabetes mellitus after developing ketoacidosis. This patient is asymptomatic, and a fasting blood sugar is normal. Her risk for developing type 1 diabetes is approximately

A.  5%
B.  25%
C.  50%
D.  75%
E.  100%

**X-12.** The patient shown in Figure X-12 (Color Atlas) is most likely to have

A.  diabetes mellitus
B.  glomerulonephritis
C.  hypothyroidism
D.  muscle weakness
E.  seizures

**X-13.** A 42-year-old female presents to the physician with 3 months of worsening dyspnea on exertion, malaise, and weakness. She reports that the symptoms have worsened

**X-13.** *(Continued)*

gradually and are associated with low-grade fever, anorexia, and an 8-lb weight loss. She has trouble climbing stairs because of leg weakness and shortness of breath. Recently she has noticed that her arms tire while she is brushing her teeth or combing her hair. Her mother also commented that the patient seems to have difficulty rising from the couch. Her writing is normal, and she has no sensory symptoms. Physical examination is notable for a temperature of 37.8°C (100°F), bilateral lung crackles, and diminished strength in the deltoids, quadriceps, and psoas muscles. Laboratory studies are notable for an elevated creatine kinase. Chest radiography shows bilateral interstitial infiltrates, and lung volumes are reduced to 70% of the predicted values. Which of the following autoantibodies is most likely to be present in this patient?

A.  Antiglomerular basement membrane antibody
B.  Antihistone antibody
C.  Anti-Jo-1 antibody
D.  Antimicrosomal antibody
E.  Antineutrophil cytoplasmic antibody (ANCA)

**X-14.** A patient presents with 3 weeks of pain in the lower back. All the following are risk factors for serious causes of spine pathology *except*

A.  Age more than 50 years
B.  Urinary incontinence
C.  Duration of pain more than 2 weeks
D.  Bed rest without relief
E.  History of intravenous drug use

**X-15.** A 42-year-old obese male presents to your office with complaints of paresthesias in the right hand that are worst in the fourth and fifth fingers. Symptoms have been present intermittently for the last 4 months. He has no other past medical history and takes no medications. The examination is significant for an intact neurologic examination of the right upper extremity but mild wasting of the intrinsic muscles on inspection of the right hand. Laboratories show a normal white blood cell count, hemoglobin, and sedimentation rate. Electrolytes and creatinine and liver function tests are normal except for a serum glucose of 148 mg/dL. What is the most likely etiology of this patient's symptoms?

A.  Diabetes mellitus
B.  Cholesterol emboli
C.  Churg-Strauss disease
D.  Cervical spondylosis
E.  Neurogenic thoracic outlet syndrome

**X-16.** A 25-year-old female presents with a complaint of painful mouth ulcerations. She describes these lesions as shallow ulcers that last for 1 or 2 weeks. The ulcers have

**X-16.** *(Continued)*

been appearing for the last 6 months. For the last 2 days, the patient has had a painful red eye. She has had no genital ulcerations, arthritis, skin rashes, or photosensitivity. On physical examination, the patient appears well developed and in no distress. She has a temperature of 37.6°C (99.7°F), heart rate of 86, blood pressure of 126/72, and respiratory rate of 16. Examination of the oral mucosa reveals two shallow ulcers with a yellow base on the buccal mucosa. The ophthalomologic examination is consistent with anterior uveitis. The cardiopulmonary examination is normal. She has no arthritis, but medially on the right thigh there is a palpable cord in the saphenous vein. Laboratory studies reveal an erythrocyte sedimentation rate of 68 s. White blood cell count is 10,230/mm³ with a differential of 68% polymorphonuclear cells, 28% lymphocytes, and 4% monocytes. The antinuclear antibody and anti-dsDNA antibody are negative. C3 is 89

**X-16.** *(Continued)*

mg/dL, and C4 is 24 mg/dL. What is the most likely diagnosis?

   A.   Behçet's syndrome
   B.   Systemic lupus erythematosus
   C.   Discoid lupus erythematosus
   D.   Sjögren's syndrome
   E.   Cicatricial pemphigoid

**X-17.** What is the best initial treatment for this patient?

   A.   Topical glucocorticoids including ophthalmic prednisolone
   B.   Systemic glucocorticoids and azathioprine
   C.   Thalidomide
   D.   Colchicine
   E.   Intralesional interferon $\alpha$

**X-18.** A 24-year-old female presents with symptoms of low back pain and stiffness. She reports that the pain is greatest on awakening in the morning and gradually improves throughout the day. These symptoms have been present for 5 months and are worsening. She initially attributed the pain to starting a cardiovascular exercise program and stopped the workout for 6 weeks. During that time there was no change in the pain. She has tried intermittent use of naproxen 500 mg daily without relief. There is no radiation of the pain down the legs or any weakness. On physical examination, the patient appears her stated age and is in no distress. Vital signs are normal for age. She is noted to have a chest expansion of 4 cm as measured by the distance between maximal inspiration and maximal forced expiration. With bending forward, lumbar spine flexion is noted to be 4 cm as well. Laboratory studies reveal the presence of HLA-B27. Erythrocyte sedimentation rate is 37 s by the Westergren method. An MRI of the pelvis is shown below. Which of the following statements about this patient's disease is true?

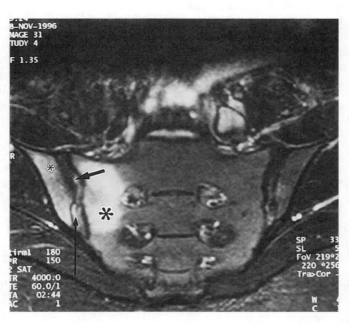

   A.   Decreased bone mineral density is a common feature but is seen only after the onset of limited mobility.

   B.   More than 90% of individuals with this patient's diagnosis are HLA-B27-positive.

**X-18.** *(Continued)*

C. If a person with no family history of inflammatory arthritis is HLA-B27-positive, that person has a lifetime incidence of 15% for the development of disease.

D. Males and females are equally affected.

E. The median age of onset of symptoms is 30 years.

**X-19.** Which of the following tests is not used as a diagnostic criterion for the diagnosis of the disease in Question 18?

A. History of inflammatory back pain described as pain worse in the morning and improving with exercise, lasting more than 3 months, and of insidious onset

B. HLA-B27 positivity

C. Limitation of motion of the lumbar spine in the frontal and sagittal planes

D. Limitation of chest expansion

E. Presence of sacroiliitis on pelvic radiography

**X-20.** What is the most common extraarticular manifestation of ankylosing spondylitis?

A. Anterior uveitis

B. Aortic regurgitation

C. Cataracts

D. Inflammatory bowel disease

E. Third-degree heart block

**X-21.** A 48-year-old male has a long-standing history of ankylosing spondylitis. His most recent spinal film shows straightening of the lumbar spine, loss of lordosis, and "squaring" of the vertebral bodies. He currently is limited by pain with ambulation that is not improved with nonsteroidal anti-inflammatory medications. Which of the following treatments has been shown to improve symptoms the best at this stage of the illness?

A. Celecoxib

B. Etanercept

C. Prednisone

D. Sulfasalazine

E. Thalidomide

**X-22.** A 54-year-old female with rheumatoid arthritis is treated with infliximab for refractory disease. All the following are potential side effects of this treatment *except*

A. Demyelinating disorders

B. Disseminated tuberculosis

C. Exacerbation of congestive heart failure

D. Pancytopenia

E. Pulmonary fibrosis

**X-23.** All the following organisms have been implicated in reactive arthritis *except*

A. *Chlamydia trachomatis*

B. *Neisseria gonorrhoeae*

C. *Salmonella enteritidis*

D. *Shigella dysenteriae*

E. *Yersinia enterocolitica*

**X-24.** Which of the following definitions best fits the term *enthesitis*?

A. Alteration of joint alignment so that articulating surfaces incompletely approximate each other

B. Inflammation at the site of tendinous or ligamentous insertion into bone

C. Inflammation of the periarticular membrane lining the joint capsule

D. Inflammation of a saclike cavity near a joint that decreases friction

E. A palpable vibratory or crackling sensation elicited with joint motion

**X-25.** A 44-year-old female is seen in consultation for renal failure. The past history is notable for episodes of severe pleuritic chest pain and abdominal pain that are unexplained. These symptoms are usually accompanied by fevers to 38.9°C (102°F). Occasionally, the patient describes swelling and pain in the knees. In the past, the patient was given the diagnosis of systemic lupus erythematosus and empirically treated with steroids. However, her symptoms did not improve. Notably, the patient has never had a positive test for antinuclear antibodies, antibodies to double-strand DNA, or low complements. On presentation, the patient has no rashes or joint inflammation. Blood pressure is 142/90. She has pitting edema in bilateral lower extremities. A 24-h urine collection shows 4.2 g of protein. BUN is 68 mg/dL, and creatinine is 3.4 mg/dL. A renal biopsy is performed; it reveals glomerular deposits of dense eosinophilic amorphous material. On Congo red stain, an apple-green birefringence is seen under polarized light microscopy. What medication could have been prescribed to prevent this complication from occurring?

A. Colchicine

B. Cyclophosphamide

C. Etanercept

D. Methotrexate

E. Prednisone

**X-26.** A 64-year-old African-American male is evaluated in the hospital for congestive heart failure, renal failure, and polyneuropathy. Physical examination on admission was notable for these findings and raised waxy papules in the axilla and inguinal region. Admission laboratories

**X-26.** *(Continued)*

showed a BUN of 90 mg/dL and a creatinine of 6.3 mg/dL. Total protein was 9.0 g/dL, with an albumin of 3.2 g/dL. Hematocrit was 24%, and white blood cell and platelet counts were normal. Urinalysis was remarkable for 3+ proteinuria but no cellular casts. Further evaluation included an echocardiogram with a thickened left ventricle and preserved systolic function. Which of the following tests is most likely to diagnose the underlying condition?

A. Bone marrow biopsy
B. Electromyogram (EMG) with nerve conduction studies
C. Fat pad biopsy
D. Right heart catheterization
E. Renal ultrasound

**X-27.** A 38-year-old female presents to the clinic with symptoms of malaise and fatigue for the last 5 months after what she believes was a viral upper respiratory tract illness. In addition to these symptoms, she reports impaired concentration, unrefreshing sleep, headaches, sore throat, and swollen red joints. Physical examination is notable for shoddy, tender cervical adenopathy. Which of the following symptoms is not consistent with a diagnosis of chronic fatigue syndrome according to the Centers for Disease Control and Prevention (CDC) criteria?

A. Unrefreshing sleep
B. Headaches
C. Sore throat
D. Swollen red joints
E. Tender cervical adenopathy

**X-28.** Which of the following therapies is indicated for patients with chronic fatigue syndrome?

A. Acyclovir
B. Cognitive-behavioral therapy
C. Immunoglobulin
D. A and C
E. A, B, and C

**X-29.** A 45-year-old male has been hospitalized for several weeks in the intensive care unit for postsurgical complications after gastrojejunal bypass surgery. He is noted to have persistent fevers and on examination is found to have erythema, fluctuance, and tenderness over the posterior surface of the left elbow. Initial management of this disorder should include all the following *except*

A. incision and drainage
B. empirical antibiotics for gram-positive organisms
C. aspiration of the collection for Gram stain and culture
D. microscopic evaluation of aspirate for crystals
E. pressure-relieving devices

**X-30.** A 26-year-old female presents complaining of joint pain involving the right knee, both ankles, the left elbow, and the right third toe. The pain began acutely in the right knee 7 days ago, with other joints becoming affected in an additive process. She also has had fatigue and fevers to 38.3°C (101°F). She had a painful red eye last week that spontaneously resolved. She did not seek evaluation. The patient denies any rash, weight loss, or lymph node swelling. She has not had diarrhea, nausea, vomiting, dysuria, or vaginal discharge. The patient does report a new sexual partner approximately 1 month ago. She has no past medical history and takes only oral contraceptive pills. On physical examination, the patient appears fatigued. Vital signs are heart rate 112 beats/min, blood pressure 126/78 mmHg, respiratory rate 16/min, and temperature 38.2°C (100.8°F). The patient's right knee is warm to touch with a large effusion. The left elbow shows tenderness and warmth at the insertion sites of the wrist extensors, and the ankles are swollen and warm. There is pain with dorsiflexion and with palpation of the insertion site of the Achilles tendons. The right third toe shows diffuse swelling. Laboratory examination shows a white blood cell count of 9890/mm³ with 56% polymorphonuclear cells, 30% lymphocytes, 9% monocytes, 4% eosinophils, and 1% basophils. Hematocrit is 34.6%. MCV is 84. ESR is 36 s by the Westergren method. DNA probes for *N. gonorrhoeae* and *C. trachomatis* are negative. What is the most likely diagnosis?

A. Disseminated gonococcal infection
B. Epstein-Barr virus infection
C. HIV seroconversion
D. Reactive arthritis
E. Rheumatoid arthritis

**X-31.** A 45-year-old male develops reactive arthritis after an episode of *Yersinia enterocolitica* diarrhea. He is improving after 3 days of indomethacin 50 mg tid. He is asking about the long-term prognosis because he has been quite disabled since his illness. He is currently ambulating with crutches owing to severe right knee and ankle pain. In addition, he has had significant low back pain and dactylitis in the hands and feet. He had an episode of uveitis that has resolved. He is known to be HLA-B27-negative. What information do you give the patient in regard to the prognosis?

A. The likelihood of recurrence is less than 10% because this is a self-limited process after an acute infection.
B. As he is HLA-B27-negative, he has a higher chance of recurrence compared with persons who are HLA-B27-positive.
C. Persons who develop reactive arthritis after *Yersinia* infection have less chronic disease compared with those who have had *Shigella* infection.

**X-31.** *(Continued)*

D.  Joint symptoms persist in more than 80% of patients with reactive arthritis.

E.  The patient should expect to be disabled as a result of his episode of reactive arthritis as 50% of per-

**X-31.** *(Continued)*

sons are unable to work after the onset of this disease.

**X-32.** A 42-year-old male presents with complaints of a rash and joint pain. He first noticed the rash 6 months ago. It is primarily on the hands, the extensor surfaces of the elbows, and the knees, low back, and scalp. Although he complains of the appearance of these lesions, they do not itch or hurt. The patient has not been previously evaluated for them and has recently noticed changes in the nail beds. For the last 2 weeks, the patient has had increasingly severe pain in the distal joints of the hands and feet. His hands are so painful that he is having trouble writing and holding utensils. The patient denies fevers, weight loss, fatigue, cough, shortness of breath, or changes in bowel or bladder habits. Which of the following is the most likely diagnosis?

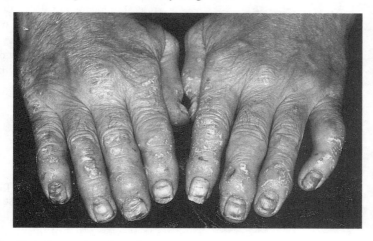

A.  Arthritis associated with inflammatory bowel disease

B.  Gout

C.  Osteoarthritis

D.  Psoriatic arthritis

E.  Rheumatoid arthritis

**X-33.** Which of the following does not cause small-vessel vasculitis?

A.  Churg-Strauss syndrome

B.  Essential mixed cryoglobulinemia

C.  Henoch-Schönlein purpura

D.  Kawasaki disease

E.  Microscopic polyangiitis

**X-34.** All but which of the following statements regarding the pathogenesis of vasculitis are true?

A.  Deposition of immune complexes in vessel walls activates complement that further perpetuates damage by attracting neutrophils to the diseased vessel.

B.  A multitude of protein targets have been described as causative of vasculitis when associated with a perinuclear pattern of staining in antineutrophil cytoplasmic antibodies.

C.  The primary protein target of antineutrophil cytoplasmic antibodies in a cytoplasmic pattern is proteinase-3.

D.  When neutrophils are under the influence of TNF-$\alpha$ and interleukin 1 (IL-1), proteinase-3 and myeloperoxidase are translocated to the neutrophil surface and thus supply a target for antibody binding and stimulation of an inflammatory reaction.

**X-35.** A 48-year-old female presents in May with a complaint of worsening sinusitis. Since adolescence, the patient has had seasonal allergies in the late summer and early fall. However, the patient now reports that she has had significant sinus congestion and pain since January. She recently developed severe tinnitus that disrupts her sleep as well as recurrent epistaxis. On physical examination, the patient appears comfortable. A head, eyes, ears, nose, and throat (HEENT) examination reveals a na-

**X-35.** *(Continued)*

sal septal perforation with sinus pain with palpation and bloody drainage. There are coarse rhonchi in the right upper lung. The neurologic examination demonstrates decreased sensorineural hearing in the left ear. A chest radiogram is shown below. Urinalysis demonstrates multiple dysmorphic red blood cells and a few red blood cell casts with 2+ proteinuria. Creatinine is 1.9 mg/dL. What is the best way to establish the diagnosis definitively?

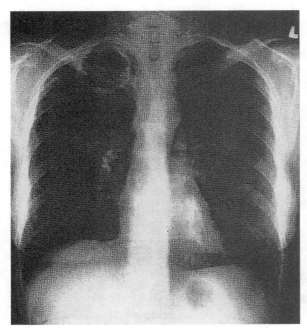

A. Assess for the presence of Epstein-Barr virus.
B. Demonstrate the presence of cytoplasmic antineutrophil cytoplasmic antibodies.
C. Demonstrate the presence of perinuclear antineutrophil cytoplasmic antibodies.
D. Perform a lung biopsy.
E. Perform a biopsy of the upper airway.

**X-36.** What do you tell the patient about the prognosis?

A. Before the introduction of cyclophosphamide, the disease was uniformly fatal, with a mean survival of 2 years.
B. More than 75% of these patients have a complete remission.
C. Among patients who go into remission, 50% will have a relapse.
D. The current 5-year survival rate for patients with this diagnosis is more than 90%.
E. All of the above.

**X-37.** Which of the following autoantibodies is most commonly seen in patients with Churg-Strauss vasculitis?

A. Antimyeloperoxidase antineutrophil cytoplasmic antibody

**X-37.** *(Continued)*

B. Antinuclear antibody
C. Anti-Smith antibody
D. Anti–tRNA synthetase antibody
E. Antihistone antibody

**X-38.** A 58-year-old female presents complaining of right shoulder pain. She does not recall any prior injury but notes that she feels that the shoulder has been getting progressively more stiff over the last several months. She previously had several episodes of bursitis of the right shoulder that were treated successfully with NSAIDs and steroid injections. The patient's past medical history is also significant for diabetes mellitus, for which she takes proglitazone and glyburide. On physical examination, the right shoulder is not warm or red but is tender to touch. Passive and active range of motion is limited in flexion, extension, and abduction. A right shoulder radiogram shows osteopenia without evidence of joint erosion or osteophytes. What is the most likely diagnosis?

A. Adhesive capsulitis
B. Avascular necrosis
C. Bicipital tendinitis
D. Osteoarthritis
E. Rotator cuff tear

**X-39.** A 35-year-old female presents to her primary care doctor complaining of diffuse body and joint pain. When asked to describe which of her joints are most affected, she answers, "All of them." There is no associated stiffness, redness, or swelling of the joints. No Raynaud's phenomenon has been appreciated. Occasionally she notes numbness in the fingers and toes. The patient complains of chronic pain and poor sleep quality that she feels is due to her pain. She previously was seen in the clinic for chronic headaches that were felt to be tension-related. She has tried taking over-the-counter Motrin twice daily without relief of pain. She has no other medical problems. On physical examination, the patient appears comfortable. Her joints exhibit full range of motion without evidence of inflammatory arthritis. She does have pain with palpation at bilateral suboccipital muscle insertions, at C5, at the lateral epicondyle, in the upper outer quadrant of the buttock, at the medial fat pad of the knee proximal to the joint line, and unilaterally on the second right rib. The erythrocyte sedimentation rate is 12 s. Antinuclear antibodies are positive at a titer of 1:40 in a speckled pattern. The patient is HLA-B27-positive. Rheumatoid factor is negative. Radiograms of the cervical spine, hips, and elbows are normal. What is the most likely diagnosis?

A. Ankylosing spondylitis
B. Disseminated gonococcal infection
C. Fibromyalgia
D. Rheumatoid arthritis
E. Systemic lupus erythematosus

**X-40.** All the following are treatments for fibromyalgia *except*

A. Aerobic and stretching exercises
B. Cyclobenzaprine
C. Methylprednisolone
D. Tricyclic antidepressants
E. Zolpidem

**X-41.** A 68-year-old male with a past history of type 2 diabetes mellitus presents complaining of right foot pain. He attributes the pain to twisting his ankle a week ago, when he stepped off a curb. The patient has been able to bear his weight and denies fevers and redness. He does feel that the right foot is slightly more swollen than the left. He has had diabetes mellitus for the last 20 years, and this has been complicated by retinopathy requiring laser photocoagulation and nephropathy with nephritic range proteinuria. Baseline creatinine is 2.0 mg/dL. The patient's last hemoglobin $A_{1C}$ was 9.4%. On physical examination, the patient is noted to have bilateral sensory neuropathy in a stocking-glove distribution. The loss of sensation is greatest in the feet. The pulses are diminished in the left dorsalis pedis but otherwise are full and strong. There is no delay in capillary refill. The right foot is slightly swollen compared with the left. Large bony lesions are present on the top of the right foot. The ankle joint appears enlarged, and loose bodies are palpable. There is little pain. What is the diagnosis?

A. Ankle dislocation
B. Charcot joint
C. Gout
D. Hypertrophic osteoarthropathy
E. Torn deltoid ligament of the ankle

**X-42.** In a patient with acute bacterial arthritis, all the following are portals of entry for bacteria into the joint *except*

A. Direct inoculation during surgery
B. Lymphangitic spread
C. Inoculation from the bloodstream
D. Contiguous infection from bone or soft tissue
E. Traumatic injury

**X-43.** You are working in an urgent care clinic. A female patient presents to you with complaints of left knee pain. Temperature is 38.3°C (101°F), and her left knee is swollen, with warmth and overlying erythema. Which of the following associated medical conditions puts this patient at highest risk of developing nongonococcal bacterial arthritis?

A. Hypertension
B. End-stage renal disease
C. Diabetes mellitus
D. Rheumatoid arthritis
E. Osteoarthritis

**X-44.** A 38-year-old female presents to her primary care doctor with the complaint of pain in both hands and the wrists, knees, and feet that has worsened over 2 months. In addition, the patient has experienced fatigue, anorexia, and a 10-lb weight loss over the last 6 months. She reports that the joint symptoms began in the hands and now involve progressively more of her joints. The pain is worse in the morning to such an extent that she feels unable to perform her usual household tasks for approximately 90 min after waking. She has taken ibuprofen 400 mg every 6 h, and this occasionally helps. In fact, she states that she would be unable to move at all without the anti-inflammatory medication. There is a past medical history of peptic ulcer disease, and she was treated for *Helicobacter pylori*. With NSAID use, the symptoms of epigastric pain with eating have begun to recur. The patient occasionally has loose bowel movements without blood or mucus. She currently takes only over-the-counter ibuprofen. On physical examination the patient appears uncomfortable with any movement. Temperature is 37.8°C (100°F). She has a heart rate of 89, a blood pressure of 112/68, and a respiratory rate of 12. Heart, lung, and abdominal examinations are normal. The neurologic examination is limited by pain. On joint examination, the patient has diffuse periarticular swelling with boggy inflamed synovium of the wrists, metacarpal-phalangeal joints, and distal interphalangeal joints. There is no clear joint effusion or redness, although the joints are mildly warm to touch. The left knee has a large effusion with a limited range of motion but without redness. The right knee is moderately swollen as well but without effusion. The feet are also swollen and tender to touch. Which of the following tests is most likely to yield a definitive diagnosis?

A. Arthrocentesis with examination for crystals
B. Colonoscopy with biopsy
C. Erythrocyte sedimentation rate
D. Radiograms of the hands and feet
E. Serum rheumatoid factor testing

**X-45.** Which of the following statements regarding rheumatoid arthritis is true?

A. There is an association with the class II major histocompatibility complex allele HLA-B27.
B. The earliest lesion in rheumatoid arthritis is an increase in the number of synovial lining cells with microvascular injury.
C. Females are affected three times more often than are males, and this difference is maintained throughout life.
D. Africans and African Americans most commonly have the class II major histocomatibility complex allele HLA-DR4.
E. Titers of rheumatoid factor are not predictive of the severity of rheumatoid arthritis or its extraarticular manifestations.

**X-46.** A 62-year-old male has had rheumatoid arthritis for 12 years. During that time, his disease has primarily been manifested as wrist, hand, and ankle arthritis. Early in the disease course he was treated with NSAIDs and prednisone. Methotrexate was added by weekly injection 6 years ago. The joint symptoms are moderately well controlled. He has morning pain and stiffness that lasts approximately 15 min upon awakening. He continues to work as a bank manager. The patient has had no difficulties with joint destruction. However, recently the patient has noted dyspnea on exertion at one city block. He no longer can climb from the basement of his home to the second floor without stopping twice. On physical examination, the patient is comfortable at rest but quickly gets out of breath with rapid walking. Respiratory rate is 22 breaths/min. Oxygen saturation is 94% on room air at rest and 91% with ambulation. On lung examination the patient has normal percussion and fremitus. Velcro-like crackles are heard throughout the lower third of the bilateral lung fields. A cardiovascular examination is normal. There are no rheumatoid nodules. The synovium of his wrists and metacarpal-phalangeal joints shows mild thickening. There is no warmth, effusions, or joint deviation. Rheumatoid factor is 22. The last measurement was 1 year ago and showed a level of 25. A high-resolution CT scan of the chest shows fibrosis with ground-glass infiltrates at the lung bases. What is the most likely diagnosis?

A. Caplan's syndrome
B. Cytomegalovirus infection
C. Idiopathic pulmonary fibrosis
D. Idiosyncratic reaction to methotrexate
E. *Pneumocystis carinii* infection

**X-47.** A 52-year-old female has poorly controlled rheumatoid arthritis on prednisone 5 mg daily and etanercept 50 mg weekly by subcutaneous injection. Despite this, she has ongoing symptoms with severe pain in the wrists, hands, feet, and ankles. She also has destructive arthritis causing swan-neck and boutonnière deformities in the hands as well as plantar subluxation of the metatarsal heads that prevents ambulation. She has subcutaneous nodules on the extensor surfaces of the arms. She presents to the emergency room complaining of fevers and dysuria. On physical examination temperature is 39.1°C (102.3°F). Heart rate is 112, and blood pressure is 122/76. The examination is unremarkable except for right costovertebral angle tenderness and splenomegaly. Laboratory studies at the time of presentation reveal a white blood cell count of 2300/mm³ with 15% polymorphonuclear cells, 75% lymphocytes, 8% monocytes, and 2% eosinophils. She is also anemic with a hemoglobin of 9.2 mg/dL and a hematocrit of 28.7%. The mean corpuscular volume is 88 fL. The platelet count is 132,000/mm³. A peripheral blood smear shows normocytic anemia without anisocytosis or poikilocytosis. She is found to have *Escherichia coli* bacteremia

**X-47.** *(Continued)*
related to a urinary tract infection. She is treated with ceftriaxone and does well. However, she remains anemic and neutropenic. The patient undergoes a bone marrow biopsy that shows hypercellularity with a lack of mature neutrophils. What is the most likely diagnosis?

A. Acute myelogenous leukemia
B. B cell lymphoma
C. Disseminated *Mycobacterium tuberculosis* infection
D. Felty's syndrome
E. Idiosyncratic reaction to etanercept

**X-48.** Which of the following statements best describes the course of disease with rheumatoid arthritis?

A. At 10 years, more than 40% of patients have no evidence of joint destruction or disability.
B. At 10 years, approximately 50% of patients have work disability.
C. Progression of disease does not correlate with titers of rheumatoid factor or an elevated erythrocyte sedimentation rate.
D. White males have more persistent synovitis and more progressively destructive disease than do white females.
E. The median life expectancy of patients with rheumatoid arthritis is not shortened compared with their peers.

**X-49.** A 48-year-old female is diagnosed with rheumatoid arthritis after 9 months of symptoms. Current symptoms involve pain and stiffness in the bilateral proximal interphalangeal joints, metacarpal-phalangeal joints, right wrist, left knee, and bilateral ankles. The patient has morning stiffness for 1 h daily. She has not been able to work in her job as a computer operator for the last month. Past medical history is significant for chronic active hepatitis B. She is currently receiving therapy with lamivudine. Rheumatoid factor is 132. The erythrocyte sedimentation rate is 108 s. She has a hemoglobin of 10.2 mg/dL and a hematocrit of 32.4%. AST is 132 IU/L, ALT is 116 IU/L, total bilirubin is 1.4 mg/dL, and alkaline phosphatase is 112 IU/L. Radiograms show no evidence of erosions in the hands, wrists, or ankles. What is the best initial treatment?

A. Indomethacin 50 mg orally three times daily
B. Infliximab 3 mg/kg intravenously monthly
C. Methotrexate 15 mg subcutaneously once weekly
D. Physical therapy
E. Prednisone 60 mg orally once daily

**X-50.** A 58-year-old male presents to his primary care physician complaining of recent onset of blisters on the skin. The initial lesion was on the patient's buccal mucosa but

**X-50.** *(Continued)*

rapidly progressed to include the scalp and trunk. He reports that the lesions seem to appear in any areas of trauma or pressure. When the blisters rupture, there is significant pain, but they heal without scarring. The patient's chest is shown in Figure X-50 (Color Atlas). The patient has a past medical history of hypertension and diabetes mellitus. He currently takes hydrochlorothiazide 25 mg/d, ramipril 5 mg/d, and glyburide 5 mg/d. What is the diagnosis?

A. Bullous pemphigoid
B. Dermatitis herpetiformis
C. Discoid lupus erythematosus
D. Pemphigus vulgaris
E. Toxic epidermal necrolysis

**X-51.** A 36-year-old female presents to the emergency department for evaluation of a pruritic rash on the back, knees, buttocks, and elbows. She has noticed the rash for the last 2 weeks, and in addition to the pruritus, she has noted a severe burning quality to the rash. It has progressed despite the application of 1% hydrocortisone cream. The patient also has had a long history of mild diarrhea that previously was diagnosed as most likely being diarrhea-predominant irritable bowel syndrome. She has lost 10 lb despite having a good appetite. She has also had bouts of an unexplained arthritis affecting the knees. She currently takes no medications. On physical examination, there are multiple excoriations and a papulovesicular rash on the back and buttocks. Similar lesions are present on the elbows and knees with plaquelike lesions. A biopsy of one of the lesions shows granular deposits of IgA in the papillary dermis and along the epidermal basement membrane zone. The patient is started on therapy with dapsone 100 mg daily. What adjunctive treatment is likely to control the skin disease?

A. Azathioprine 100 mg/d
B. Cyclophosphamide 50 mg/d
C. Initiation of a gluten-free diet
D. Initiation of psoralen plus ultraviolet light (PUVA) therapy
E. Triamcinolone 0.5% cream

**X-52.** A 29-year-old male with episodic abdominal pain and stress-induced edema of the lips, the tongue, and occasionally the larynx is likely to have low functional or absolute levels of which of the following proteins?

A. C5A (complement cascade)
B. IgE
C. T cell receptor, α chain
D. Cyclooxygenase
E. C1 esterase inhibitor

**X-53.** A 35-year-old female comes to the local health clinic because for the last 6 months she has had recurrent

**X-53.** *(Continued)*

urticarial lesions, which occasionally leave a residual discoloration. She also has had arthralgias. The sedimentation rate now is 85 mm/h. The procedure most likely to yield the correct diagnosis in this case would be

A. a battery of wheal-and-flare allergy skin tests
B. measurement of total serum IgE concentration
C. measurement of C1 esterase inhibitor activity
D. skin biopsy
E. patch testing

**X-54.** A 23-year-old male seeks medical attention for perennial nasal congestion and postnasal discharge. He states that he does not have asthma, eczema, conjunctivitis, or a family history of allergic disease. Nasal secretions are rich in eosinophils. The test most likely to yield a specific diagnosis in this setting is

A. serum IgE level (competitive radioimmunosorbent technique)
B. serum IgE level (radiodiffusion technique)
C. elimination diet test
D. skin testing
E. sinus x-rays

**X-55.** Which of the following statements regarding the renal involvement associated with systemic lupus erythematosus (SLE) is true?

A. Clinically apparent renal disease occurs in 90% of affected persons.
B. Interstitial nephritis is a rare finding on renal biopsy.
C. Renal biopsy is not initially necessary in patients with deteriorating renal function and active urine sediment.
D. Renal disease is uncommon in patients with high-titer anti-double-strand DNA antibodies.
E. Urinalysis in affected persons usually reveals proteinuria but little sediment and no red blood cells.

**X-56.** A 25-year-old female presents with a history of recurrent expectoration of foul-smelling sputum and intermittent fevers. Chest x-ray discloses characteristic "tram-tracking" bronchial thickening. Physical examination reveals coarse rhonchi in the right chest and splenomegaly. Blood test results are normal except for low levels of serum IgG and IgA. The past medical history is remarkable for frequent upper respiratory infections and for a history of diarrhea 3 years ago resulting from *Giardia lamblia* infection. The most appropriate therapy would be

A. glucocorticoids
B. glucocorticoids and an alkylating agent
C. monthly intravenous immunoglobulin
D. splenectomy
E. bone marrow transplantation

**X-57.** A 30-year-old Turkish sailor reports several occurrences of painful oral ulcers in the tongue and the inner aspect of the cheek over the last year. He currently presents with several painful skin lesions, including an ulcer on the left side of the scrotum and painful red nodules on both shins. He also reports occasional bilateral knee and wrist pain. Which of the following tests would be compatible with the patient's diagnosis?

A. Elevated level of serum IgE levels
B. Biopsy of the skin lesion showing infiltration with neutrophils
C. Positive syphilis fluorescent antibody test from material obtained from the scrotal lesion
D. The formation of a red nodule 2 days after a sterile needle is pricked into the forearm
E. Positive herpes simplex virus culture from the genital lesion

**X-58.** A 70-year-old female presents with blurring of vision in the left eye since waking earlier in the morning. She reports 2 months of fevers, sweats, anorexia, and a 4.5-kg (10-lb) weight loss. She also reports increasingly severe left temporal headaches over the same period. Physical examination reveals scalp tenderness over the left temporal region. Laboratories reveal a normochromic, normocytic anemia, mildly elevated alkaline phosphatase, and an erythrocyte sedimentation rate of 92. Appropriate action includes

A. obtaining an emergent MRI/magnetic resonance angiogram (MRA) of the head
B. referring the patient for a biopsy of the temporal artery but abstaining from initiating therapy until the biopsy results are available
C. initiating high-dose glucocorticoid therapy and referring the patient for a temporal artery biopsy
D. obtaining a head CT to rule out metastatic disease and scheduling a colonoscopy
E. performing a lumbar puncture to rule out meningitis

**X-59.** Within minutes after the injection of radiocontrast at the time of abdominal CT, a patient develops urticaria, flushing, and congestion of the tongue and larynx. Respiratory stridor develops, and intubation is emergently required. The mechanism of this event is

A. direct activation of mediator release from mast cells, basophils, or both
B. IgE-mediated reaction against protein-hapten conjugates
C. IgE-mediated reaction against native proteins
D. deficiency of C1 esterase inhibitor
E. inherited inability to catabolize the radiocontrast agent normally

**X-60.** A 30-year-old female presents complaining of frequent upper respiratory infections characterized by heavy sputum production. She has a history of eczema, wheezing, and intermittent diarrhea. She has never been hospitalized for any of her infections but is concerned about their recurrent nature. At this time she feels well, and the physical examination is unremarkable. Routine laboratory studies are unremarkable; however, quantitative immunoglobulin levels show that she has normal levels of serum IgM and IgG but depressed levels of serum IgA. The most important thing to tell this patient is that

A. she will require lifelong infusions of intravenous immunoglobulin
B. she will require immunoglobulin infusions at times when she develops a bacterial infection
C. she is likely to develop systemic lupus erythematosus
D. blood transfusions could have grave consequences
E. prophylactic therapy with trimethoprim-sulfamethoxazole should be initiated at this time

**X-61.** A 26-year-old female with SLE is noted to have a prolonged partial thromboplastin time. This abnormality is associated with

A. leukopenia
B. drug-induced lupus
C. central nervous system vasculitis
D. central nervous system hemorrhage
E. deep venous thrombosis

**X-62.** A patient with diffuse cutaneous scleroderma (systemic sclerosis) who had been stable for several years is noted to have hypertension. This patient is at significant risk of dying from

A. thrombotic stroke
B. central nervous system hemorrhage
C. renal failure
D. pulmonary hypertension
E. pulmonary fibrosis

**X-63.** A 37-year-old female with Raynaud's phenomenon complains of progressive weakness with inability to arise from a sitting position without assistance. On examination, the patient has swollen "sausage-like" fingers, alopecia, erythematous patches on the knuckles, facial telangiectasias, and proximal muscle weakness. Laboratory evaluation includes a normal complete blood count (CBC) and serum chemistries except for creatine phosphokinase 4.5 μkat/L (270 U/L) and aldolase 500 nkat/L (30 U/L). The following serologic profile is found: rheumatoid factor is positive at 1:1600; ANA is also positive at 1:1600 with a speckled pattern and very high titers of antibodies against the ribonuclease-sensitive ribonucleoprotein component of extractable nuclear antigen. This patient probably has

**X-63.** *(Continued)*
A. early rheumatoid arthritis
B. systemic sclerosis
C. systemic lupus erythematosus
D. dermatomyositis
E. mixed connective tissue disease (MCTD)

**X-64.** A 70-year-old male with a history of hypertension, peptic ulcer disease, chronic renal insufficiency, and diabetes presents with an acutely swollen and painful left knee. Vital signs and general physical examination are unremarkable, but the left knee has an obvious effusion and is warm, swollen, and red. Arthrocentesis reveals a white blood cell count of 50,000/$\mu$L, a negative Gram stain, and strongly birefringent needle-shaped intracellular crystals. Which of the following statements concerning this situation is correct?

A. The serum uric acid level will be elevated.
B. Intraarticular glucocorticoid may be given now.
C. Antibiotics are required.
D. A 24-h urine collection will reveal a high level of uric acid.
E. Allopurinol should be given now.

**X-65.** A 50-year-old female has had Raynaud's phenomenon of the hands for 15 years. The condition has become worse during the last year, and she has developed arthralgias and arthritis involving the hands and wrists as well as mild sclerodactyly and difficulty swallowing solid foods. Laboratory studies reveal a positive serum antinuclear antibody assay at a dilution of 1:160. Anticentromere antibodies are present in high titers; antiribonucleoprotein antibodies are not detectable. The most likely diagnosis of this female's disorder is

A. systemic sclerosis
B. mixed connective tissue disease
C. overlap syndrome
D. dermatomyositis
E. systemic lupus erythematosus

**X-66.** A 27-year-old female with SLE is in remission; current treatment consists of azathioprine 75 mg/d and prednisone 5 mg/d. Last year she had a life-threatening exacerbation of her disease. She now strongly desires to become pregnant. Which of the following is the least appropriate action to take?

A. Advise her that the risk of spontaneous abortion is high.

**X-66.** *(Continued)*
B. Warn her that exacerbations can occur in the first trimester and in the postpartum period.
C. Tell her it is unlikely that a newborn will have lupus.
D. Advise her that fetal loss rates are higher if anti-cardiolipin antibodies are detected in her serum.
E. Stop the prednisone just before she attempts to become pregnant.

**X-67.** Which of the following is least likely to be seen in patients with Sjögren's syndrome?

A. Dental caries
B. Corneal ulceration
C. Renal tubular acidosis
D. Lymphoma
E. Cardiac fibrosis

**X-68.** Acute sarcoidosis is characterized by which of the following syndromes?

A. Cough, hemoptysis, and interstitial pulmonary involvement
B. Myopathy, keratotic skin lesions on the palms and soles, and arthralgias
C. Fever, pulmonary stenotic murmur, and nail bed lesions
D. Erythema nodosum, arthralgias, and pulmonary nodules
E. Fever, parotid enlargement, uveitis, and facial nerve palsy

**X-69.** Which of the following findings on joint aspiration is most likely to be associated with calcium pyrophosphate deposition disease (pseudogout)?

A. Fluid, clear and viscous; white blood cell count, 400/$\mu$L; crystals, rhomboidal and weakly positively birefringent
B. Fluid, cloudy and watery; white blood cell count, 8000/$\mu$L; no crystals
C. Fluid, dark brown and viscous; white blood cell count, 1200/$\mu$L; crystals, needle-like and strongly negatively birefringent
D. Fluid, cloudy and watery; white blood cell count, 12,000/$\mu$L; crystals, needle-like and strongly negatively birefringent
E. Fluid, cloudy and watery; white blood cell count, 4800/$\mu$L; crystals, rhomboidal and weakly positively birefringent

**X-1. The answer is C.** *(Chap. 306)* Microscopic polyangiitis (MPA) is a small-vessel vasculitis associated with antineutrophil cytoplasmic antibodies (ANCAs) of the perinuclear type. MPA was recognized as a discrete entity in 1992, when it was distinguished from polyarteritis nodosa because of the involvement primarily of small vessels. Twelve percent of cases present primarily with diffuse alveolar hemorrhage. MPA is distinct from Wegener's granulomatosis because it does not induce granulomatous inflammation. The glomerulonephritis associated with MPA is pauci-immune, showing a lack of immunoglobulin deposition. p-ANCA staining is positive in 75% of patients with MPA, with antimyeloperoxidase antibodies being the target of the immunofluorescent staining pattern of the p-ANCA. Therapy begins with high-dose steroids and often requires the addition of cytotoxic therapy with cyclophosphamide. The 5-year survival rate is 74%; however, the disease tends to be chronic, with at least a 34% relapse rate.

**X-2. The answer is E.** *(Chap. 306)* This patient most likely has polyarteritis nodosa with a symptom complex consisting of abdominal pain, weight loss, hypertension, and mononeuritis. Polyarteritis nodosa (PAN) is an uncommon vasculitis that affects primarily medium-size arteries without the involvement of venules. There are no diagnostic serologic tests for PAN. Up to 30% of patients with PAN are positive for hepatitis B surface antigen. In cases of PAN associated with hepatitis B, the virus, IgM, and complement can be demonstrated in vessel walls on biopsy. In light of the patient's past history of injection drug use, the presence of hepatitis B should be evaluated. However, demonstration of hepatitis B surface antigen is not diagnostic of PAN. ANCA is rarely positive in PAN patients, and hepatitis C is associated with cryoglobulinemic vasculitis but not with PAN. With the patient's abdominal pain that is worsened with eating, mesenteric ischemia caused by vasculitis should be considered. On mesenteric angiography, one would expect to find aneurysmal dilatation of the arteries. Again, however, this is not pathognomonic for PAN. The most definitive way to diagnose PAN is by finding vasculitis on a biopsy of the affected nerve. Therefore, a radial nerve biopsy should be pursued.

**X-3. The answer is C.** *(Chap. 306)* Before the addition of cyclophosphamide to therapy for Wegener's granulomatosis (WG), the prognosis was poor, with untreated patients having 90% mortality at 5 years. The use of glucocorticoids alone led to some improvement in mortality but not to sustained improvement, with most patients developing renal failure. The addition of cyclophosphamide to the treatment regimen for WG has caused a dramatic improvement in survival to 80% at 8 years. Ninety percent of these patients will have improvement in symptoms, with 75% achieving a complete remission. Because of the toxicity of long-term cyclophosphamide, a patient may be switched to methotrexate or azathioprine once remission has been achieved.

**X-4. The answer is B.** *(Chap. 311)* This patient has degenerative arthritis. His obesity predisposes him to degenerative joint disease that will be worse in the large weight-bearing joints. The physical examination findings of decreased range of motion, crepitus, and varus deformity that is exacerbated on weight bearing are consistent with this diagnosis. The radiogram of the knee demonstrates narrowing of the joint space with osteophyte formation. Occasional effusions may be seen, especially after overuse injuries. The joint fluid analysis in patients with degenerative disease reveals a clear, viscous fluid with a white blood cell count less than 2000/$\mu$L. Positively birefringent crystals on polarizing light microscopy will be seen in pseudogout that most commonly affects the knee, whereas negatively birefringent crystals are characteristic of gout. Joint fluid in these inflammatory conditions would generally have a white blood cell count of less than 50,000/mm$^3$ and is yellow and turbid in character. Septic arthritis presents with fevers and a very warm and tender joint. The joint fluid can have the appearance of frank pus and is opaque. The white blood cell count is usually higher than 50,000/mm$^3$ and can have a positive Gram stain for organisms.

**X-5.  The answer is A.**  *(Chap. 369)*  Polymyositis is an inflammatory myopathy that presents as symmetric, progressive muscle weakness. The patient reports difficulty with everyday tasks requiring the use of proximal muscles, such as getting up from a chair and climbing steps. Distal muscle strength is usually preserved until late in the course. In addition to the musculoskeletal findings, there are numerous extramuscular manifestations. This patient may have systemic symptoms of fever, malaise, weight loss, and Raynaud's phenomenon. There may be "overlap" features with other autoimmune diseases, such as systemic lupus erythematosus (SLE) and scleroderma. Involvement of the striated muscles and the upper esophagus may lead to dysphagia. Conduction defects, arrhythmia, and dilated cardiomyopathy may occur. Interstitial lung disease may precede myopathy or occur early in the disease, often in association with the presence of antibodies to t-RNA synthetases. Although dermatomyositis is linked with an increased incidence of cancer, polymyositis does not seem to be associated with an increased incidence.

**X-6.  The answer is B.**  *(Chap. 304)*  Sjögren's syndrome may present in patients as a primary disease or as a secondary disease in association with other autoimmune disorders, such as rheumatoid arthritis, systemic lupus erythematosus, scleroderma, mixed connective tissue disease, and primary biliary cirrhosis. This patient is typical in that most persons affected by this disorder are middle-aged females with a female-to-male ratio of 9:1. Symptoms are related to diminished lacrimal and salivary gland function. Oral dryness, or xerostomia, is very common. Parotid enlargement occurs in 66% of these patients. Ocular involvement resulting in symptoms of a sandy or gritty feeling under the eyelids, burning, redness, itching, decreased tearing, and photosensitivity is due to destruction of corneal and bulbar conjunctival epithelium, defined as keratoconjunctivitis sicca. Diagnostic evaluation includes the measurement of tear flow by Schirmer's I test. Slit-lamp examination of the cornea after rose Bengal staining may show punctate corneal ulcerations and attached filaments of corneal epithelium. The most common extranodal manifestation of Sjögren's syndrome is arthralgias or arthritis (up to 60% of patients). Autoantibodies to Ro/SSA or La/SSB are very suggestive of this syndrome and are part of the classification criteria. Rheumatoid arthritis may be considered; however, the examination did not demonstrate inflammation, and the diffuse joint complaints without persistent morning stiffness make this less likely. Vitamin A deficiency may lead to dry eye but does not explain the patient's other symptoms.

**X-7.  The answer is D.**  *(Chap. 304)*  Lymphoma is well known to develop specifically in the late stage of Sjögren's syndrome. Common manifestations of this malignant condition include persistent parotid gland enlargement, purpura, leukopenia, cryoglobulinemia, and low C4 complement levels. Most of the lymphomas are extranodal, marginal zone B cell, and low-grade. Low-grade lymphomas may be detected incidentally during a labial biopsy. Mortality is higher in patients with concurrent B symptoms (fevers, night sweats, and weight loss), a lymph node mass >7 cm, and a high or intermediate histologic grade.

**X-8.  The answer is C.**  *(Chap. 15)*  In a patient with back pain, any symptoms of pain at rest or pain not associated with specific postures should raise suspicion for a serious underlying cause, such as fracture, infection, or spinal tumors. The examination includes inspection of the lower spine, the surrounding musculature, and both hips. Straight leg raising is performed with the patient lying flat with passive flexion of the extended leg at the hip, which stretches L5, S1, and the sciatic nerve. Flexion of up to 80° is normal. A positive maneuver occurs if the patient's usual pain is reproduced. This maneuver may also be performed in the sitting position to determine if the pain is indeed reproducible. The crossed straight leg raising sign is positive when flexion of one leg reproduces the pain in the opposite leg or buttocks. This sign is less sensitive than straight leg raising, but it is more specific for disk herniation. The nerve or nerve root lesion is always on the side of the pain. The reverse straight leg raising maneuver is performed by having the patient stand next to the examination table and passively extend each leg. This stretches the L2–L4 nerve roots and the femoral nerve.

**X-9 and X-10. The answers are B and E.** *(Chap. 308)* The figure shows an erythematous, swollen pinna characteristic of relapsing polychondritis. Relapsing polychondritis is an inflammatory disorder of the cartilage that predominantly affects the ears, nose, and respiratory tract. It typically affects patients 40 to 50 years of age, with no sex or race predominance. Diagnostic criteria include recurrent chondritis of both auricles (the earlobes are not involved), nonerosive arthritis, chondritis of the nasal cartilage, ocular inflammation, laryngeal or tracheal chondritis, and cochlear chondritis. Antibodies to type II collagen may be involved in the pathogenesis. The onset of inflammation is often acute but may be preceded by systemic symptoms of inflammation. Episodes often resolve spontaneously, but repeated episodes lead to cartilaginous destruction. There may also be an associated vasculitis. Laboratory findings are consistent with inflammation, but there are no diagnostic serologic tests. c-ANCA or p-ANCA may be positive. Complications include aortic regurgitation, respiratory failure from damage to the trachea or bronchi, stroke or seizures from vasculitis, and glomerulonephritis. The pancreas is not involved in relapsing polychondritis. Treatment is with prednisone 40 to 60 mg/d for acute episodes. Resistant disease may require the addition of an immunosuppressive agent such as cyclophosphamide, methotrexate, azathioprine, or cyclosporine. Options for maintenance therapy include lower-dose prednisone and dapsone. There have been no trials of etanercept or plasmapheresis in relapsing polychondritis. Patients with severe upper respiratory disease may require tracheostomy or stenting.

**X-11. The answer is B.** *(Chap. 299)* Type 1 diabetes mellitus is an autoimmune disease. Autoimmunity may result from exogenous factors (molecular mimicry, superantigen stimulation, microbial adjuvanticity) or endogenous mechanisms (altered antigen presentation, increased T cell help, increased B cell function, apoptotic defects, cytokine imbalance, altered immunoregulation). There is also evidence in humans of susceptibility genes for autoimmunity. The combination of these factors accounts for the 15 to 30% concordance in monozygotic twins for diseases such as type 1 diabetes, multiple sclerosis, and systemic lupus erythematosus. The disease concordance in dizygotic twins is less than 5%. Different autoimmune diseases also may cluster in families, suggesting an environmental trigger in patients with genetic susceptibility. Major histocompatibility complex, complement, apoptosis, and cytokine genes have been implicated as susceptibility factors for autoimmune diseases. Hormonal status is also a strong factor in autoimmunity, explaining the female sex bias of most autoimmune diseases.

**X-12. The answer is D.** *(Chap. 369)* The figure shows the classic heliotrope rash of dermatomyositis (DM). Other skin findings in DM include a flat red rash on the face or trunk and photosensitive erythema with a raised violaceous scaly eruption on the knuckles (Gottron rash), knees, elbows, neck, chest, or back. The skin findings typically precede the muscle weakness and distinguish DM from polymyositis (PM). The myositis is subacute, progressive, and symmetric. It typically involves the proximal muscles early in disease and the distal muscles late. Facial and ocular muscles are spared. Fever, malaise, and weight loss are common. DM, but not PM, is associated with an increased frequency of malignancy, particularly ovarian cancer, melanoma, breast cancer, colon cancer, and non-Hodgkin's lymphoma. Antinuclear antibodies are found in approximately 20% of patients with DM. Antisynthetase antibodies such as anti-Jo-1 are common and identify a subset of patients with a high frequency (80%) of interstitial lung disease.

**X-13.   The answer is C.**   *(Chap. 369)*   This patient presents with the classic symptoms, signs, and laboratory findings of polymyositis (PM) with antisynthetase antibodies. The differential diagnosis for a patient with proximal muscle weakness includes inclusion-body myositis, viral infections, denervating conditions such as amyotrophic lateral sclerosis (ALS), metabolic myopathies such as acid maltase deficiency, endocrine myopathies such as hypothyroidism, paraneoplastic myopathy, and drug-induced myopathies such as D-penicillamine, procainamide, statins, and glucocorticoids. PM is associated with an elevated creatine kinase, electromyography (EMG) showing irritability, and biopsy showing T cell infiltrates primarily in the muscle fascicles. Many patients with PM have autoantibodies targeted against the ribonucleoproteins involved in protein synthesis (antisynthetases). The antibody directed against histidyl-transfer RNA synthetase or anti-Jo-1 identifies a group of patients with PM who have a high likelihood (80%) of having interstitial lung disease. Antiglomerular antibodies are found in patients with Goodpasture's syndrome, antihistone antibodies in those with drug-induced lupus, and antimicrosomal antibodies in those with autoimmune hepatitis.

**X-14.   The answer is C.**   *(Chap. 15)*   Acute low back pain is defined as pain of less than 3 months' duration. Most patients with back pain have symptoms that are "mechanical," such as pain that is worsened by activity and relieved by rest. Initial assessment of all these patients must evaluate for serious causes of spine pathology, such as infection, malignant disease, and trauma. Risk factors include age over 50 years, prior diagnosis of cancer, intravenous drug use, chronic infection such as cystitis or pneumonia, a history of spine trauma, bed rest without relief, duration of pain of more than 1 month, urinary incontinence or nocturia, focal leg weakness or numbness, pain radiating into the leg or legs from the back, pain that increases with standing and is relieved by sitting, and chronic steroid use. Examination findings that raise concern for serious underlying disease include fever, weight loss, a positive straight leg raise, an abdominal or rectal mass, and neurologic examination abnormalities, either motor or sensory.

**X-15.   The answer is E.**   *(Chap. 15)*   This patient's symptoms are most consistent with abnormalities of the C8 or T1 nerve roots. The diagnosis of diabetes mellitus is possible, but his symptoms are not consistent with diabetic neuropathy, which would more commonly be symmetric in both hands. The patient does not have any other signs or symptoms of systemic vasculitis and does not describe risk factors or other findings consistent with cholesterol emboli. Cervical spondylosis is possible, but this is typically a disease process of C2–C4 nerve roots and presents with pain in the neck radiating into the back of the head, shoulders, and arms. The thoracic outlet contains the first rib, the subclavian artery and vein, the brachial plexus, the clavicle, and the lung apex. Neurogenic thoracic outlet syndrome results from compression of the lower brachial plexus. Signs may include weakness of the intrinsic muscles of the hand and diminished sensation on the palmar surface of the fourth and fifth digits. EMG testing and imaging with either contrast CT scan or magnetic resonance imaging (MRI) confirms the diagnosis. Treatment consists of surgical decompression of the brachial plexus. Other forms of thoracic outlet syndrome (TOS) include arterial TOS, which results in compression of the vasculature and subsequent thrombus formation, and disputed TOS, which is described in patients with chronic arm and shoulder pain with an unclear etiology.

**X-16 and X-17.   The answers are A and B.**   *(Chap. 307)*   Behçet's syndrome is a multisystem disorder of uncertain cause that is marked by oral and genital ulcerations and ocular involvement. This disorder affects males and females equally and is more common in persons of Mediterranean, Middle Eastern, and Far Eastern descent. Approximately 50% of these persons have circulating autoantibodies to human oral mucosa. The clinical features are quite varied. The presence of recurrent aphthous ulcerations is essential for the diagnosis. Most of these patients have primarily oral ulcerations, although genital ulcerations are more specific for the diagnosis. The ulcers are generally painful, can be shallow or deep, and last for 1 or 2 weeks. Other skin involvement may occur, including folliculitis, erythema nodosum, and vasculitis. Eye involvement is the most dreaded complication because it may progress rapidly to blindness. It often presents as panuveitis, iritis, retinal vessel occlusion, or optic neuritis. This patient also presents with superficial venous thrombosis. Superficial and deep venous thromboses are present in one-fourth of these patients. Neurologic involvement occurs in up to 10%. Laboratory findings are nonspecific with elevations in the erythrocyte sedimentation rate and the white blood cell count.

Treatment varies with the extent of the disease. Patients with mucous membrane involvement alone may respond to topical steroids. In more serious or refractory cases, thalidomide is effective. Other options for mucocutaneous disease include colchicines and intralesional interferon $\alpha$. Ophthalmologic or neurologic involvement requires systemic glucocorticoids and azathioprine or cyclosporine. Life span is usually normal unless neurologic disease is present. Ophthalmic disease frequently progresses to blindness.

**X-18 and X-19. The answers are B and B.** *(Chap. 305)* This young female is presenting with symptoms of inflammatory back pain and limited spinal flexion consistent with the diagnosis of ankylosing spondylitis (AS). This disorder of unknown cause preferentially affects males 3 to 1 compared with females. The median age at the onset of symptoms is 23 years. A striking association with HLA-B27 positivity is seen: more than 90% of patients with AS are HLA-B27-positive. In population surveys, however, only 1 to 6% of patients who inherit HLA-B27 develop AS, whereas this risk increases to 10 to 30% if a first-degree relative has AS. The pathology of AS is inflammation originating at the enthesis where ligaments attach to bone, with the pathology most apparent in the axial spine. Sacroiliitis is one of the earliest manifestations of AS. The MRI shows early sacroiliitis on the right side. The asterisks show areas of edema, the thin arrow shows an area of edema in the joint capsule, and the thick arrow shows edema in the interosseous ligaments. Limitation of flexion of the lumbar spine is decreased early in the disease out of proportion to the degree of ankylosis as a result of marked spasm in the paraspinal muscles. Bone mineral density is decreased early in the disease before the onset of marked immobility for reasons that are not clear.

The diagnosis of AS uses the modified New York criteria developed in 1984. To definitively diagnose AS, one must have evidence of sacroiliitis by radiography—either plain roentgenograms or magnetic resonance imaging—and any one of the following three criteria: (1) history of inflammatory back pain, (2) limitation of the motion of the lumbar spine in both the sagittal and the frontal planes, (3) limitation of chest expansion compared with age- and sex-matched controls. HLA-B27 positivity is neither necessary nor sufficient for a diagnosis of the disease.

**X-20. The answer is A.** *(Chap. 305)* Anterior uveitis occurs in up to 30% of AS patients and may antedate the onset of the spondylitis. Attacks usually occur unilaterally with pain, photophobia, and blurred vision. Recurrent attacks are common, and ultimately cataracts may result. Other commonly seen problems include inflammation in the colon and ileum in up to 60% of AS patients, but only rarely do these patients develop inflammatory bowel disease. Cardiac disease is present in only a few percent of these patients and most commonly presents as aortic regurgitation. Other cardiac manifestations include complete heart block and congestive heart failure. Rare complications are upper lobe pulmonary fibrosis and retroperitoneal fibrosis.

**X-21. The answer is B.** *(Chap. 305)* Before the introduction of anti-tumor necrosis factor (TNF) $\alpha$ therapy, the mainstay of treatment for ankylosing spondylitis was nonsteroidal anti-inflammatory drugs (NSAIDs) and exercise therapy. In 2000, infliximab and etanercept were introduced and since that time have been shown to confer a rapid, profound, and sustained reduction in all clinical and laboratory measures of disease activity. Even patients with long-standing disease and ankylosis show significant improvement in spinal mobility and pain relief. MRI findings in patients treated with these agents also show marked improvement in marrow edema, enthesitis, and joint effusions. The long-term effects of these agents are not known.

Other treatments for AS can be used, including NSAIDs and COX-2 inhibitors, to decrease pain, especially in mild cases. An ongoing exercise program is encouraged to maintain posture and range of motion. In patients with more severe pain, sulfasalazine or methotrexate may be added with modest benefit, especially in those with peripheral arthritis. Diverse other agents have been tried, including thalidomide, bisphosphonates, and radium-224. Glucocorticoids have no role in the treatment of this disease.

**X-22.** **The answer is E.** *(Chap. 305)* Anti-TNF-α therapy for rheumatoid arthritis has been used since 2000. Two agents are currently used. Infliximab is a chimeric human-mouse anti-TNF-α monoclonal antibody, and etanercept is a soluble p75 TNF-α monoclonal antibody. These agents are potent immunosuppressants, and six types of common side effects have been described. Serious infections are most frequently seen, with a marked increase in disseminated tuberculosis. Other side effects include pancytopenia, demyelinating disorders, exacerbations of congestive heart failure, hypersensitivity to the infusion or injection, and the development of drug-induced systemic lupus erythematosus. An increased incidence of malignancy is of theoretical concern, but this has not been borne out in the limited follow-up of patients treated with these drugs. Pulmonary fibrosis has not been reported.

**X-23.** **The answer is B.** *(Chap. 305)* The presence of arthritis after episodes of infectious diarrhea or urethritis has been recognized for centuries, with the symptoms of diarrhea or dysuria occurring 1 to 4 weeks before the onset of the arthritis. The most common organisms that are implicated are bacteria that cause acute infectious diarrhea. All four *Shigella* species have been reported to cause reactive arthritis, although *S. flexneri* is only rarely implicated. Other bacteria that have been identified as triggers include several *Salmonella* species, *Yersinia enterocolitica,* and *Campylobacter jejuni.* In addition, some organisms that cause urethritis are also causative; these include *Chlamydia trachomatis* and *Ureaplasma urealyticum.* Arthritis associated with disseminated gonococcal infection is directly related to an infectious cause and responds to antibiotics, unlike reactive arthritis.

**X-24.** **The answer is B.** *(Chap. 305)* *Enthesopathy* or *enthesitis* is the term used to describe inflammation at the site of tendinous or ligamentous insertion into bone. This type of inflammation is seen most frequently in patients with seronegative spondyloarthropathies and various infections, especially viral infections. The other definitions apply to other terms used in the orthopedic and rheumatic examination. *Subluxation* is the alteration of joint alignment so that articulating surfaces incompletely approximate each other. *Synovitis* refers to inflammation at the site of tendinous or ligamentous insertion into bone. Inflammation of a saclike cavity near a joint that decreases friction is the definition of *bursitis.* Finally, *crepitus* is a palpable vibratory or crackling sensation elicited with joint motion.

**X-25.** **The answer is A.** *(Chap. 310)* This patient presents with episodic serositis associated with fever and joint pain consistent with the diagnosis of familial Mediterranean fever (FMF). This autosomal recessive disease can be misdiagnosed and mistakenly treated as systemic lupus erythematosus. However, FMF does not respond to steroid therapy. Because of the chronic inflammatory process, patients with FMF have a high incidence of renal failure related to AA amyloidosis, which is also known as reactive or secondary amyloidosis. It occurs most frequently as a consequence of a chronic inflammatory disease. During inflammation, the inflammatory cytokines interleukin 1, interleukin 6, and tumor necrosis factor α cause increased production of serum amyloid A by the liver as an acute-phase reactant. Over time, these proteins accumulate as AA protein, commonly affecting the kidneys and peripheral nerves. The most common causes of AA amyloid are osteomyelitis, tuberculosis, and leprosy; however, AA amyloidosis is quite common with untreated FMF. In patients with FMF, the incidence of AA amyloidosis can be decreased with colchicines because this medication decreases inflammation and prevents attacks of serositis.

**X-26.  The answer is A.**  *(Chap. 310)*   This patient presents with a multisystem illness involving the heart, kidneys, and peripheral nervous system. The physical examination is suggestive of amyloidosis with classic waxy papules in the folds of his body. The laboratories are remarkable for renal failure of unclear etiology with significant proteinuria but no cellular casts. A possible etiology of the renal failure is suggested by the elevated gamma globulin fraction and low hematocrit, bringing to mind a monoclonal gammopathy perhaps leading to renal failure through amyloid AL deposition. This could also account for the enlarged heart seen on the echocardiogram and the peripheral neuropathy. The fat pad biopsy is generally reported to be 60 to 80% sensitive for amyloid; however, it would not allow a diagnosis of this patient's likely myeloma. A right heart catheterization probably would prove that the patient has restrictive cardiomyopathy secondary to amyloid deposition; however, it too would not diagnose the underlying plasma cell dyscrasia. Renal ultrasound, although warranted to rule out obstructive uropathy, would not be diagnostic. Similarly, the electromyogram and nerve conduction studies would not be diagnostic. The bone marrow biopsy is about 50 to 60% sensitive for amyloid, but it would allow evaluation of the percent of plasma cells in the bone marrow and allow the diagnosis of multiple myeloma to be made. Multiple myeloma is associated with amyloid AL in approximately 20% of cases. Light chains most commonly deposit systemically in the heart, kidneys, liver, and nervous system, causing organ dysfunction. In these organs, biopsy would show the classic eosinophilic material that, when exposed to Congo red stain, has a characteristic apple-green birefringence.

**X-27 and X-28.  The answers are D and B.**  *(Chap. 370; Sharpe et al, BMJ 312:22–26, 1996; Whiting et al, JAMA 286:1360–1368, 2001.)*   Chronic fatigue syndrome is characterized by the presence of persistent unexplained fatigue of new or definite onset that is not due to exertion. It causes a reduced capacity for occupation, education, and social and personal activities. CDC criteria require these findings with four or more of the following symptoms over 6 months: concentration and short-term memory impairment, sore throat, tender cervical or axillary lymph nodes, myalgia, arthralgia, headache, sleep disturbance, and postexertional malaise for more than 24 h. Arthritis would be distinctly atypical for chronic fatigue syndrome, and this symptom or finding should prompt a more thorough evaluation. Although a number of therapies have anecdotally been reported to be helpful in this disorder, only cognitive-behavioral therapy has been shown to provide improvement in controlled trials

CDC Criteria for Diagnosis of Chronic Fatigue Syndrome

A case of chronic fatigue syndrome is defined by the presence of:
1. Clinically evaluated, unexplained, persistent or relapsing fatigue that is of new or definite onset; is not the result of ongoing exertion; is not alleviated by rest; and results in substantial reduction of previous levels of occupational, educational, social, or personal activities; and
2. Four or more of the following symptoms that persist or recur during 6 or more consecutive months of illness and that do not predate the fatigue:
   • Self-reported impairment in short-term memory or concentration
   • Sore throat
   • Tender cervical or axillary nodes
   • Muscle pain
   • Multijoint pain without redness or swelling
   • Headaches of a new pattern or severity
   • Unrefreshing sleep
   • Postexertional malaise lasting ≥24 h

*Note*: CDC, U.S. Centers for Disease Control and Prevention.
*Source*: Adapted from K Fukuda et al: Ann Intern Med 121:953, 1994; with permission.

**X-29.  The answer is A.**  *(Chap. 316)*   This patient has a classic presentation for olecranon bursitis, with warmth, swelling, fluctuance, and tenderness over the posterior aspect of the elbow. Most often this is due to repeated trauma or pressure to the area that can occur through leaning on the elbow or through immobility with continuous pressure. Alternatively, infections, generally with gram-positive organisms, can cause olecranon bursitis, and crystalline disease, especially monosodium urate, can cause this picture. Initial evaluation involves aspiration of the fluid for Gram stain, culture, cell count and differential, and crystal evaluation. Empirical antibiotics would be warranted in this patient because of concern for infection with fevers and systemic illness. Incision and drainage should be reserved for bursitis of infectious etiology that is not responding to antibiotics and repeated aspirations.

**X-30.** **The answer is D.** *(Chap. 305)* The clinical symptoms of enthesitis and a uveitis or conjunctivitis should lead one to the diagnosis of reactive arthritis. Originally described in World Wars I and II, the term *Reiter's syndrome* was used to describe the triad of reactive arthritis, urethritis, and conjunctivitis that occurred in the context of antecedent sexually transmitted disease or diarrheal illness. The most commonly implicated organisms are *Yersinia, Campylobacter, Shigella,* and *Salmonella* species as well as *C. trachomatis.* A history of prior infectious illness should be elicited. Often a previous urethritis is asymptomatic; thus, the patient should be asked about new sexual partners. On clinical examination, an oligoarthritis is usually present, although the arthritis may involve only a single joint. Additional evidence of enthesitis with pain to palpation of tendinous and ligamentous insertion sites is seen. These symptoms are usually most prominent in the lower extremities. Dactylitis may be seen with diffuse swelling of a single joint. This gives the typical appearance of a "sausage digit." Other associated symptoms are fever, fatigue, and weight loss. Uveitis and conjunctivitis are common eye complications. A pustular skin rash, keratoderma blenorrhagica, is characteristic, although it is rarely seen.

Reactive arthritis is a clinical diagnosis. There are no diagnostic radiologic or laboratory tests. HLA-B27 positivity is seen in 85% of persons with reactive arthritis. Nonspecific elevations in white blood cell count, erythrocyte sedimentation rate, and C-reactive protein may be seen.

**X-31.** **The answer is C.** *(Chap. 305)* In long-term follow-up, 30 to 60% of patients with reactive arthritis develop chronic joint symptoms with episodes of acute recurrence. Up to 25% will become disabled to the extent that they can no longer work or are forced to change jobs. Chronic heel pain is the most common symptom. Patients who are HLA-B27-positive are more likely to develop chronic symptoms. *Yersinia*-associated arthritis has a better prognosis than does arthritis caused by *Shigella.*

**X-32.** **The answer is D.** *(Chap. 305)* This patient shows the typical features of psoriatic arthritis. Five to 10% of patients with psoriasis will develop an arthritis associated with the rash. In 60 to 70% of cases, the rash precedes the diagnosis. However, another 15 to 20% of patients will have joint complaints as the presenting symptom of their psoriasis. The disease typically begins in the fourth or fifth decade of life. Psoriatic arthritis has varied joint presentations with five commonly described patterns of joint involvement: (1) arthritis of the distal interphalangeal (DIP) joints, (2) asymmetric oligoarthritis, (3) symmetric polyarthritis similar to rheumatoid arthritis (RA), (4) axial involvement, and (5) arthritis mutilans with the typical "pencil in cup" deformity seen on hand radiography. Erosive joint disease ultimately develops in almost all these patients, and most of them become disabled. Nail changes are prominent in 90% of patients with psoriatic arthritis. Changes that are frequently seen include pitting, horizontal ridging, onycholysis, yellowish discoloration of the nail margins, and dystrophic hyperkeratosis. The diagnosis of psoriatic arthritis is primarily clinical. Thus, in patients with joint symptoms that precede the onset of rash, the diagnosis is frequently missed until dermatologic or nail changes develop. A family history of psoriasis is important to ascertain in any patient with an undiagnosed inflammatory polyarthropathy. The differential diagnosis of DIP arthritis is short; only osteoarthritis and gout are commonly seen in these joints. Radiography may show typical changes, particularly in patients with arthritis mutilans. Treatment is directed at both the rash and the joint disease simultaneously. Anti-TNF-$\alpha$ therapy has recently been shown to be helpful for both dermatologic and joint manifestations of disease. Other treatments include methotrexate, sulfasalazine, cyclosporine, retinoic acid derivatives, and psoralen plus ultraviolet light.

**X-33.  The answer is D.**  *(Chap. 306)*   Kawasaki disease is a vasculitis of medium-size vessels that occurs in children. Over 80% of cases are described in children under age 5 years. This disease is also known as mucocutaneous lymph node syndrome. The clinical manifestations include fevers; nonsuppurative cervical adenitis; erythema of the oral cavity, lips, and tongue (so-called strawberry tongue); and desquamation of the skin on the palms and soles. The most feared complication of this illness is aneurysmal dilation of the coronary arteries, which occurs in 25% of cases. This complication usually occurs in the recovery stage of the illness in the third and fourth weeks. High-dose intravenous immunoglobulin and aspirin have been shown to decrease the incidence of this complication markedly when initiated early in the disease. Histologically, the lesions of Kawasaki disease reveal vasculitis within the coronary arteries with intimal proliferation and mononuclear cell infiltration into the vessel wall.

**X-34.  The answer is B.**  *(Chap. 306)*   Much about the pathogenesis of vasculitis remains unknown. In general, most of the vasculitic syndromes are thought to be mediated by immune reactions to antigenic stimuli. Multiple mechanisms of immune reaction have been described, including immune-complex deposition, cellular immunity, and delayed-type hypersensitivity.

Tissue damage from circulating immune complexes resembles that seen in serum sickness. In this situation, immune complexes form in the setting of antigen excess and are deposited in tissue. For vasculitis, this deposition is specifically within the vessel wall. Deposition of complexes stimulates complement activation primarily through C5a. This protein is a strong chemoattractant for neutrophils, thus propagating the immune reaction further. This results in ongoing immune-mediated damage to the blood vessel wall, ultimately resulting in thrombosis and tissue ischemia.

Antineutrophil cytoplasmic antibodies (ANCAs) have been described in several vasculitic syndromes. The exact role of these antibodies in the disease process has not been fully elucidated. Two types of ANCAs are seen, based on the immunofluorescent staining pattern: perinuclear ANCA (p-ANCA) and cytoplasmic ANCA (c-ANCA). p-ANCA is seen in a multitude of vasculitic and nonvasculitic inflammatory syndromes. Multiple protein targets of these antibodies have been described, including myeloperoxidase, elastase, cathepsin G, and lysozyme. However, antibodies to myeloperoxidase are the only antibodies that have been shown to be associated with vasculitis. Other nonvasculitic entities that can cause positive p-ANCA include inflammatory bowel disease, certain drugs, and endocarditis. c-ANCA is seen in >90% of patients with Wegener's granulomatosis. Its protein target is proteinase-3. The degree to which these antibodies contribute to the immune-mediated damage is unclear. One mechanism by which these antibodies cause disease is by binding to receptors on the surface of neutrophils previously activated by TNF-$\alpha$ or IL-6. Once bound, the antibodies cause neutrophil degranulation and further tissue damage.

**X-35 and X-36.  The answers are D and E.**  *(Chap. 306)*   This patient has Wegener's granulomatosis (WG) as manifested by sinus, renal, pulmonary, and neurologic involvement. This disorder has an estimated prevalence of 3 per 100,000 with a predominance among white people. The mean age of onset is 40 years. WG is a small and medium-size vessel vasculitis with marked granulomatous inflammation. Involvement of the upper airway occurs in 95% of these patients and typically manifests as sinusitis and epistaxis. Nasal septal perforation and saddle nose deformity may occur. The next most common manifestation is lung disease, with cough, dyspnea, or hemoptysis occurring in up to 90% of these patients. The most serious common complication of WG is renal disease. The course of the renal disease usually dominates the clinical picture. Present in 75% of patients with

WG, glomerulonephritis and the associated renal dysfunction contribute most significantly to morbidity and mortality. Other manifestations may occur but are much rarer. The tinnitus and hearing loss this patient is exhibiting are consistent with a cranial nerve VIII neuritis.

The diagnosis of WG is made by demonstrating necrotizing granulomatous vasculitis on biopsy. The tissue with the highest yield on biopsy is lung tissue. Biopsy of the upper airway frequently shows granulomatous inflammation without vasculitis. Renal biopsy will demonstrate pauci-immune glomerulonephritis. More than 90% of patients with WG have evidence of a positive c-ANCA, but this is not considered sufficient for the diagnosis because false-positive ANCAs have been reported with certain infectious and neoplastic diseases.

The prognosis of WG patients was uniformly poor before the introduction of cyclophosphamide in addition to steroid therapy. The average survival from diagnosis was less than 3 years, with most patients dying from complications of renal disease within months. Currently, there is more than a 90% 5-year survival rate on a regimen of cyclophosphamide initially at a dose of 2 mg/kg and prednisone 1 mg/kg daily. More than 75% of these patients will have a complete remission, although half will have one or more relapses.

**X-37.   The answer is A.**   *(Chap. 306)*   Forty-eight to 60% of patients with Churg-Strauss syndrome will have positive antineutrophil cytoplasmic antibodies. These antibodies are more commonly directed against myeloperoxidase than against proteinase-3, thus giving these patients a perinuclear pattern of staining. Antinuclear, anti-Smith, and antihistone antibodies are seen most commonly in patients with systemic lupus erythematosus. Anti—tRNA synthetase antibodies are best known as anti-Jo-1 antibodies and are associated with dermatomyositis and polymyositis.

**X-38.   The answer is A.**   *(Chap. 316)*   Adhesive capsulitis is characterized by pain and restricted motion of the shoulder. Usually this occurs in the absence of intrinsic shoulder disease, including osteoarthritis and avascular necrosis. It is, however, more common in patients who have had bursitis or tendinitis previously as well as patients with other systemic illnesses, such as chronic pulmonary disease, ischemic heart disease, and diabetes mellitus. The etiology is not clear, but adhesive capsulitis appears to develop in the setting of prolonged immobility. Reflex sympathetic dystrophy may also occur in the setting of adhesive capsulitis. Clinically, this disorder is more commonly seen in females over age 50. Pain and stiffness develop over the course of months to years. On physical examination, the affected joint is tender to palpation, with a restricted range of motion. The gold standard for diagnosis is arthrography with limitation of the amount of injectable contrast to less than 15 mL. In most patients, adhesive capsulitis will regress spontaneously within 1 to 3 years. NSAIDs, glucocorticoid injections, physical therapy, and early mobilization of the arm are useful therapies.

**X-39.   The answer is C.**   *(Chaps. 305 and 315)*   This patient complains of symptoms consistent with a diagnosis of fibromyalgia. These patients frequently complain of diffuse body pain, stiffness, paresthesias, disturbed sleep, easy fatigability, and headache. The prevalence of fibromyalgia is approximately 3.4% of females and 0.5% of males. This disorder is thought to represent a disturbance of pain perception. Disturbed sleep with a loss of stage 4 sleep has been implicated as a factor in the pathogenesis of the disease. Serotonin levels in the cerebrospinal fluid have also commonly been seen and may play a role in the pathogenesis. A diagnosis of fibromyalgia is based on the American College of Rheumatology criteria, which combine symptoms and physical examination. The patient must exhibit diffuse pain in all areas of the body with tenderness to palpation at 11 of 18 designated tender point sites. These sites include the occiput, trapezius, cervical spine, lateral epicondyles, supraspinatus muscle, second rib, gluteus, greater trochanter, and knee. Digital palpation should be performed with a moderate degree of pressure. Examination of the joints shows no evidence of inflammatory arthropathy. There are no laboratory tests that are specific for the diagnosis. Positive antinuclear antibodies may be seen, but at the same frequency as in the normal population. HLA-B27 is found in 7% of the white population, but only 1 to 6% of people with HLA-B27 will develop ankylosing spondylitis. Radiograms are normal in these patients.

**X-40.** **The answer is C.** *(Chap. 315)* Multiple therapies have been tried in the treatment of fibromyalgia, including antidepressants, anxiolytics, glucocorticoids, and NSAIDs. Among these treatments, glucocorticoids have the least benefit and should not be used because of their significant side effects. Medications that improve sleep have been shown to be of benefit and include tricyclic antidepressants, cyclobenzaprine, trazodone, and zolpidem. These medications should be used 1 to 2 h before bedtime. If restless leg syndrome is also present, clonazepam may be useful as well. The selective serontonin reuptake inhibitors should be considered if depression or anxiety is present. Aerobic exercise and regular stretching should be encouraged once the pain is better controlled. Acetaminophen and tramadol are the pain medications of choice, and narcotic pain medications should be avoided. NSAIDs may be used but are of limited benefit. Psychological support is important in the care of these patients, and group or individual therapy with biofeedback can be considered.

**X-41.** **The answer is B.** *(Chap. 315)* Patients with diabetes mellitus are at increased risk of developing neuropathic joint disease, especially in the setting of poor glucose control and neuropathy. First described in 1868 by Jean-Martin Charcot, neuropathic joint disease is a destructive arthritis that is related to loss of pain perception, proprioception, or both. Commonly called Charcot joint, neuropathic joint disease is most commonly seen in patients with diabetes mellitus. Other associated disorders include leprosy, yaws, peroneal muscle atrophy, and amyloidosis. Pathologically, the development of Charcot joints is related to repeated trauma without appropriate pain responses. Clinically, the symptoms usually start with pain in a single joint, although multiple joints may become symptomatic over time. The involved joint progressively becomes enlarged from bony overgrowth and effusions. Loose bodies may be palpated, and joint laxity or subluxation may be present as the disease progresses. The estimated incidence of this disease in diabetes mellitus patients is 0.5%, with the foot and knee being the most frequently affected. When the foot is affected, there is often loss of the arch, and the patient may develop downward collapse of the tarsal bones, leading to convexity of the sole, or "rocker foot." Radiograms and magnetic resonance imaging are useful in confirming the diagnosis. Treatment is directed at improving joint stability with braces and splints. Care must be taken to avoid skin breakdown at sites of contact because these patients lack appropriate sensation of pressure or pain. When this is recognized early in a diabetic patient, maintenance of non-weight-bearing status for 8 weeks may prevent further joint destruction.

**X-42.** **The answer is B.** *(Chap. 314)* Bacteria may enter a joint, which is normally a sterile space, through multiple mechanisms; the majority of cases involve direct inoculation. There is no direct mechanism for lymphatic drainage to enter the joint space; thus, this is not a common way in which acute bacterial arthritis develops. In patients with hematogenous infection the bacteria enter the joint from synovial capillaries because they do not have an impermeable basement membrane. The bacteria adhere to articular cartilage, and this results in the degradation of the cartilage. Direct inoculation of the joint space by surgery or trauma is also a common mechanism. Bacterial factors also play an important role in the pathogenesis of infective arthritis. These factors include surface-associated adhesions in *Staphylococcus aureus* and endotoxins that promote the degradation of cartilage.

**X-43.** **The answer is D.** *(Chap. 314)* Patients with rheumatoid arthritis have the highest incidence of infective arthritis, usually from *Staphyllococcus aureus*. These patients are most at risk because of chronically inflamed joints, chronic steroid use, and often breakdown of the skin overlying deformed joints. Other immunosuppressant therapies used in patients with rheumatoid arthritis, such as etanercept and infliximab, also predispose to bacterial arthritis from mycobacterial organisms. Other risk factors for these patients include diabetes mellitus, end-stage renal disease (chronic kidney disease stage V), steroid therapy, alcohol dependence, deficiencies of humoral immunity, HIV, intravenous drug use, and malignancy.

**X-44.** **The answer is E.** *(Chap. 301)* This patient has typical signs and symptoms of rheumatoid arthritis, including symmetric polyarthritis, morning stiffness, generalized fatigue and malaise, and synovitis on physical examination. Most of these patients have symptoms for more than 9 months before the diagnosis. No laboratory or radiographic findings are specific for the diagnosis of rheumatoid arthritis. In 1987, the American College of Rheumatology developed diagnostic criteria for the diagnosis of rheumatoid arthritis. These criteria have been demonstrated to have a sensitivity of 91 to 94% and a specificity of 89% when used to classify patients with rheumatoid arthritis compared with patients with other rheumatic disorders. For a patient to be diagnosed with rheumatoid arthritis, four of seven criteria must be attained: (1) morning stiffness lasting 1 h; (2) arthritis of three or more joint areas as documented by a physician; (3) arthritis of hand joints; (4) symmetric arthritis; (5) positive rheumatoid factor; (6) typical radiographic changes with erosions; and (7) rheumatoid nodules.

**X-45.** **The answer is B.** *(Chap. 301)* The prevalence of rheumatoid arthritis (RA) is 0.8%, and females are three times more likely to be affected than are males. However, as the population ages, the prevalence increases and the sex difference diminishes. RA is found throughout the world and affects people of all races. Age of onset is most commonly 35 to 50 years. Family studies show a clear genetic predisposition. First-degree relatives have approximately four times the expected rate of RA. Other risk factors for RA include the class II major histocompatibility antigen HLA-DR4. Approximately 70% of patients with RA have HLA-DR4. However, this association is not true in Africans or African Americans, among whom 75% do not show this allele. The role of this allele in the pathogenesis of RA remains unknown because the cause of RA is unknown. The earliest lesion in RA is microvascular injury with an increase in the number of synovial lining cells. Increased numbers of mononuclear cells are seen in the synovial lining, and this is thought to be under the control of CD4+ T lymphocytes. As the inflammation continues, the articular matrix is degraded by collagenases and cathepsins produced by the inflammatory cells. Other cytokines produced by the inflammatory cells include IL-1 and TNF-$\alpha$. Over time, bone and cartilage are destroyed, leading to the end-stage clinical manifestations. Rheumatoid factor (RF) is an IgM molecule directed against the Fc portion of IgG and is found in two-thirds of patients with RA. However, this molecule is found in approximately 5% of healthy persons and more than 10% of persons older than age 60. It is not known to have a role in the pathogenesis of the disease, but titers of RF are shown to be predictive of the severity of clinical manifestations or the presence of extraarticular manifestations.

**X-46.** **The answer is D.** *(Chap. 301)* This patient most likely is experiencing pulmonary fibrosis and pneumonitis related to his treatment with methotrexate. This is an idiosyncratic reaction that occurs in 1% of patients receiving methotrexate. Pulmonary fibrosis can be associated with rheumatoid arthritis (RA), although it would be unlikely in this patient with mild disease that is controlled on medication. In addition, low titers of rheumatoid factor would argue against this patient developing extraarticular disease. Caplan's syndrome is a diffuse nodular and fibrotic process that occurs in individuals with RA and a preexisting pneumonconiosis. Cytomegalovirus and *Pneumocystis carinii* infections are opportunistic infections that are seen rarely in patients on immunosuppressive therapy but would be expected to present with fevers and cough. In addition, the presence of fibrosis on high-resolution CT imaging is not seen in patients with infectious causes of RA.

**X-47.** **The answer is D.** *(Chap. 301)* Felty's syndrome is a syndrome of chronic RA, splenomegaly, and neutropenia. Anemia and thrombocytopenia are also sometimes related. Patients who develop Felty's syndrome most commonly have more active disease with high titers of rheumatoid factor, subcutaneous nodules, and other systemic manifestations of disease. However, Felty's syndrome can develop when joint inflammation has regressed. The leukopenia is a selective neutropenia with polymorphonuclear leukocytes below 1500/mm$^3$. Bone marrow biopsy reveals hypercellularity with a lack of mature neutrophils. Hypersplenism has been proposed as a cause of Felty's syndrome, but splenectomy does not consistently correct the abnormality. Excessive margination of granulocytes caused by antibodies to these cells, complement activation, or binding of immune complexes may contribute to neutropenia.

**X-48.   The answer is B.**   *(Chap. 301)*   The course of rheumatoid arthritis (RA) is quite variable and difficult to predict in an individual patient. Most patients experience persistent but fluctuating disease activity, with fewer than 20% having no disability or joint destruction at 10 years. Additionally, approximately 50% of patients with RA have work disability at 10 years. Several factors have been shown to predict more severe disease with joint destruction and disability. They include the presence of >20 inflamed joints, a markedly elevated erythrocyte sedimentation rate, high titers of rheumatoid factor, the presence of rheumatoid nodules, advanced age at onset, and the presence of functional disability or persistent inflammation. Remissions of disease activity are most likely to occur within the first year. Sustained disease for more than 1 year has a worse prognosis. White females tend to have more persistent inflammation and joint destruction than do white males. The median life expectancy of patients with RA is shortened by 3 to 7 years. In the 2.5-fold increase in mortality rate, RA itself is a contributing factor in 15 to 30% of cases. Recent evidence has shown an increased cardiovascular risk in patients with RA, perhaps related to persistent inflammation. Other factors associated with early death include disability, disease duration or severity, glucocorticoid use, age at onset, and low socioeconomic or educational status.

**X-49.   The answer is A.**   *(Chap. 301)*   The principles of treatment of rheumatoid arthritis (RA) reflect the variability of the disease, the frequently persistent inflammation and its potential to cause disability, and the need for frequent reevaluation. At disease onset, it is difficult to predict the course of the disease in any individual. The usual approach is to initiate treatment with nonsteroidal anti-inflammatory drugs or cyclooxygenase-2 inhibitors. However, none of these therapies has been shown to be more effective than aspirin alone. However, because of the frequency of gastrointestinal side effects with aspirin, other NSAIDs are often chosen. Once NSAIDs are initiated, the patient must be followed very closely to assess the adequacy of the response. If significant disability persists, the addition of a disease-modifying antirheumatic drug (DMARD) and/or low-dose glucocorticoid therapy should be considered. Multiple DMARDs have been tried over the years and include methotrexate, gold, penicillamine, antimalarials, and sulfasalazine. No trials have shown a consistent advantage of any one DMARD over any other. However, methotrexate has become the DMARD of choice because of its relatively rapid onset of action. In addition, toxicities need to be considered. In this patient, methotrexate should not be used because of the presence of active hepatitis. High doses of glucocorticoids are not recommended, but prednisone at doses lower than 7.5 mg daily may be added to NSAIDs if needed. If the patient has ongoing disease activity, anticytokine therapy has newly been added to the treatment panel for RA. Options for anticytokine therapy include infliximab, etanercept, and adalimumab. Physical therapy is a useful adjunctive therapy but should not be used alone for the treatment of rheumatoid arthritis.

**X-50.   The answer is D.**   *(Chap. 49)*   Pemphigus vulgaris is a blistering skin disease that affects primarily elderly persons. It is marked by acantholysis with a loss of cohesion between epidermal cells with the formation of epidermal blisters. Clinically, pemphigus vulgaris presents as flaccid blisters that have either a normal or an erythematous base. These blisters rupture easily, leaving denuded skin. In severe cases, a large percentage of the body surface area may be affected. Mild pressure or trauma may elicit the development of new areas of blistering, a phenomenon known as the Nikolsky's sign. Lesions usually begin on the oral mucosa but advance to include the face, scalp, trunk, and axilla. Other mucosal surfaces, including vaginal and rectal mucosa, may become involved as well. The lesions heal without scarring unless they are complicated by secondary infection or mechanically induced dermal wounds. Pathologically, pemphigus vulgaris is marked by the presence of IgG on keratinocytes most commonly directed against desmogleins. Desmogleins are transmembrane desmosomal glycoproteins that are responsible for keratinocyte attachments. Before the use of glucocorticoids, mortality from pemphigus vulgaris was 60 to 90%. The current mortality rate is 5%. Death usually results from secondary infections. Treatment consists of glucocorticoids at a dose equivalent to prednisone 60 to 80 mg/d. If the disease fails to respond to steroids alone, the addition of azathioprine, mycophenolate mofetil, or cyclophosphamide should be considered.

By contrast, bullous pemphigoid is an autoimmune disease that creates tense blisters distributed over the lower abdomen, the groin, and the flexor surfaces of the extremities. The oral mucosa is affected in only 10 to 40% of patients. These lesions also heal without scarring unless the underlying dermis is affected through mechanical abrasion or infection. The pathology associated with bullous pemphigoid is IgG directed against the epidermal basement membrane. This disease tends to have multiple exacerbations and remissions. The mortality rate is relatively low.

**X-51.** **The answer is C.** *(Chap. 49)* This patient's skin disease is typical of dermatitis herpetiformis, an intensely pruritic papulovesicular skin disease that is frequently associated with celiac disease. Even without clinical malabsorption, biopsies of the small bowel usually reveal blunting of intestinal villi and a lymphocytic infiltrate in the lamina propria. Patients with dermatitis herpetiformis often describe intense burning or stinging pain in addition to the pruritus. On biopsy, typically granular IgA deposits are seen in papillary dermis and along the epidermal basement membrane. Recent studies have shown that the autoantibody in patients with dermatitis herpetiformis is an IgA directed against epidermal transglutaminase, similar to the autoantibodies in celiac disease. Dapsone in doses of 50 to 200 mg/d is the mainstay of therapy. Close follow-up is required to assess for hemolysis and methemoglobinemia. In addition, a gluten-free diet alone may control the skin disease.

**X-52.** **The answer is E.** *(Chap. 295; Frank, N Engl J Med 316:1525–1530, 1987.)* Complement activity, which results from the sequential interaction of a large number of plasma and cell-membrane proteins, plays an important role in the inflammatory response. The classic pathway of complement activation is initiated by an antibody-antigen interaction. The first complement component (C1, a complex composed of three proteins) binds to immune complexes with activation mediated by C1q. Active C1 then initiates the cleavage and concomitant activation of components C4 and C2. The activated C1 is destroyed by a plasma protease inhibitor termed *C1 esterase inhibitor*. This molecule also regulates clotting factor XI and kallikrein. Patients with a deficiency of C1 esterase inhibitor may develop angioedema, sometimes leading to death by asphyxia. Attacks may be precipitated by stress or trauma. In addition to low antigenic or functional levels of C1 esterase inhibitor, patients with this autosomal dominant condition may have normal levels of C1 and C3 but low levels of C4 and C2. Danazol therapy produces a striking increase in the level of this important inhibitor and alleviates the symptoms in many patients. An acquired form of angioedema caused by a deficiency of C1 esterase inhibitor has been described in patients with autoimmune or malignant disease.

**X-53.** **The answer is D.** *(Chap. 298)* Urticaria and angioedema are common disorders, affecting approximately 20% of the population. In acute urticarial angioedema, attacks of swelling are of less than 6 weeks' duration; chronic urticarial angioedema is by definition more long-standing. Urticaria usually is pruritic and affects the trunk and proximal extremities. Angioedema is generally less pruritic and affects the hands, feet, genitalia, and face. This female has chronic urticaria, which probably is due to a cutaneous necrotizing vasculitis. The clues to the diagnosis are the arthralgias, the presence of residual skin discoloration, and the elevated sedimentation rate, which would be uncharacteristic of other urticarial diseases. The diagnosis can be confirmed by skin biopsy. Chronic urticaria rarely has an allergic cause; hence, allergy skin tests and measurement of total IgE levels are not helpful. Measurement of C1 esterase inhibitor activity is useful in diagnosing hereditary angioedema, a disease that is not associated with urticaria. Patch tests are used to diagnose contact dermatitis.

**X-54.    The answer is D.**    *(Chap. 298; Naclerio, N Engl J Med 325:860–869, 1991.)*    Allergic rhinitis can be either seasonal as a result of pollen exposure or perennial as a result of exposure to dust or mold spores or both. In these IgE-mediated reactions to inhaled foreign substances, nasal eosinophilia is common. Vasomotor rhinitis is a chronic, nonallergic condition in which vasomotor control in the nasal membranes is altered. Irritating stimuli such as odors, fumes, and changes in humidity and barometric pressure can cause nasal obstruction and discharge in affected persons, and nasal eosinophilia is not noted. Because this male has either perennial allergic rhinitis that is due to dust or mold-spore allergy or eosinophilic nonallergic rhinitis, skin testing for responses to suspected allergens should be diagnostic. Although total serum IgE may be elevated, demonstration of specificity is critical. Specificity can be demonstrated by binding to a solid-phase antigen and can be detected by uptake of radiolabeled anti-IgE allergosorbent technique (RAST). RAST is more difficult than skin testing because of the requirement for defined antigens and stan-dardization. Pollen skin tests are unlikely to be helpful because of the perennial nature of the condition. An elimination diet can be used diagnostically or therapeutically in persons with suspected food allergy; however, food allergy rarely causes rhinitis. Sinus x-rays, whether positive or negative, would not reveal the underlying cause of the rhinitis.

**X-55.    The answer is C.**    *(Chap. 300)*    Renal disease is clinically evident in about half of persons with SLE. However, nearly all persons with SLE have some evidence of renal disease on renal biopsy. Renal disease associated with SLE includes both glomerulone-phritis and interstitial nephritis. Glomerular disease has been subdivided into membranous nephritis and mesangial, focal, and diffuse glomerulonephritis. Immune-complex intersti-tial nephritis occurs most commonly in persons who have diffuse glomerulonephritis. Urinalysis in persons with active renal disease usually reveals microscopic hematuria, red blood cell casts, and proteinuria; the exception is membranous lupus nephritis, in which proteinuria is the dominant finding. Drug-induced lupus rarely leads to renal disease. Anti-dsDNA antibodies at a high titer are associated with severe nephritis. Renal biopsy is not necessary in SLE patients whose renal function is rapidly deteriorating when they have an active sediment. If those patients fail to respond to the prompt initiation of glucocorticoid therapy demanded in such a situation, biopsy should be undertaken. Patients with mild clinical disease should have a biopsy to determine if they have active, severe, inflammatory lesions, which might respond to therapy.

**X-56.    The answer is C.**    *(Chap. 297; Sneller, Ann Intern Med 118:720–730, 1993.)*    Common variable immunodeficiency refers to a heterogeneous group of adults who have in common deficiencies of all major immunoglobulin classes. The defect is believed to be due to an abnormality in B cell maturation, though most of these patients tend to have normal levels of clonally diverse B lymphocytes. The B cells can recognize antigen and proliferate but fail to differentiate to the immunoglobulin-secreting stage. Associated with this abnor-mality is nodular lymphoid hyperplasia in various organs (including the gut) and spleno-megaly. This panhypogammaglobulinemic disorder should be suspected in adults with chronic pulmonary infections, unexplained bronchiectasis (as in this patient), chronic giar-diasis, malabsorption, and atrophic gastritis. These patients develop intestinal neoplasms with an increased frequency. They also develop autoimmune conditions such as Coombs-positive hemolytic anemia and idiopathic thrombocytopenic purpura. There is some sug-gestion that in addition to failure of B cells to secrete immunoglobulin, T cells have an impaired ability to release lymphokines. The mainstay of therapy for common variable immunodeficiency is to increase the antibody content by administering intravenous im-munoglobulin concentrates. The goal is to increase the IgG level to 5 g/L, which can generally be accomplished through monthly administration of 200 to 400 mg/kg of intravenous immunoglobulin. True anaphylactic reactions to immunoglobulin treatment are rare.

**X-57.** **The answer is D.** *(Chap. 307; Sakane et al, N Engl J Med 341:1284–1291, 1999.)* Behçet's disease is manifested by recurrent oral and genital ulcers, ulceration of the uvea, and skin lesions. The skin lesions are most commonly erythema nodosum (painful red nodules generally on the legs), but pseudofolliculitis, papulopustular lesions, and acneiform lesions can also occur. Ulcers may occur on the scrotum and penis in men or on the vulva in females. Ocular lesions can manifest as uveitis or involve the retina, which can lead to blindness. Arthritis occurs in about half these patients. Gastrointestinal involvement is much less common but can occasionally lead to perforation and be confused with inflammatory bowel disease. Small-vessel vasculitis, of unknown etiology, accounts for most of the pathologic lesions. This disease, which is more prevalent in Turkey, Japan, Korea, China, Iran, and Saudi Arabia, can usually be diagnosed clinically on the basis of recurrent oral ulceration and at least two of the following: genital ulceration, eye lesions, skin lesions, or a positive pathergy test. The pathergy test involves pricking a sterile needle into the patient's arm. A positive test occurs when an aseptic erythematous nodule or pustule develops 2 days after the induced trauma. The disease can be confused with inflammatory bowel disease, herpes simplex virus infection, and Sweet's syndrome (neutrophilic infiltration of the dermis). Behçet's disease generally responds to immunosuppressive agents such as glucocorticoids.

**X-58.** **The answer is C.** *(Chap. 306)* This patient has symptoms and laboratory values characteristic of temporal arteritis. The disease classically presents with fever, anemia, an elevated erythrocyte sedimentation rate (ESR), and headaches in an elderly patient. Other manifestations include fatigue, malaise, sweats, anorexia, weight loss, and arthralgias. Scalp tenderness and jaw claudication may occur as well. Laboratory findings include an elevated ESR and normochromic or slightly hypochromic anemia. Liver function abnormalities are common, particularly increased alkaline phosphatase levels. A catastrophic potential complication, particularly in untreated patients, is ocular involvement resulting from ischemic optic neuritis, which may lead to sudden and irreversible blindness. The diagnosis is often made clinically and confirmed by temporal artery biopsy. A temporal artery biopsy should be obtained as quickly as possible, and in the setting of ocular symptoms, therapy should not be delayed while waiting to do a biopsy. Therapy consists of high-dose glucocorticoids, to which the disease is quite responsive. MRI/MRA cannot establish the diagnosis and hence is not warranted. This patient's presentation is classic for temporal arteritis and would be unusual for either metastatic colon cancer or meningitis.

**X-59.** **The answer is A.** *(Chap. 298; Bochner, N Engl J Med 324:1785–1790, 1991.)* *Anaphylaxis* is the term used to describe the rapid and generalized immunologically mediated events characterized clinically by cutaneous wheals and upper or lower airway obstruction (or both) after exposure to a specific antigen. The angioedema and urticaria that occur during anaphylaxis are believed to be due to the release of mast cell (and possibly basophil) mediators (histamine and serum proteases from preformed granules, arachidonic acid metabolites such as leukotrienes, and cytokines, including but not limited to tumor necrosis factor $\alpha$, interferon $\gamma$, and interleukin 1). The mechanism of this release depends on the inciting agent. For example, anaphylaxis in response to bee stings, foods, and heterologous serum (e.g., tetanus antitoxin) is believed to occur on the basis of an IgE-mediated reaction against the relevant protein. In contrast, anaphylaxis to penicillin and other antibiotics is due to IgE recognition of protein-hapten conjugants. Dialysis-induced anaphylaxis is due to complement activation. Finally, radiocontrast media directly activate mast cells, basophils, or both to release the mediators of anaphylaxis.

**X-60.** **The answer is D.** *(Chap. 297; Burrows, Cooper, Adv Immunol 65:245–276, 1997.)* IgA deficiency is the most common primary immunodeficiency. It is more common in whites than in individuals of Asian or African origin. Patients with isolated IgA deficiency have a mild to moderate clinical syndrome consisting of recurrent respiratory infections, although some may progress to bronchiectasis, chronic diarrheal diseases, and eczema. These individuals are more likely to experience infections, drug allergies, and other immune disorders, such as lupus, vitiligo, thyroiditis, and rheumatoid arthritis, than are age-matched controls. Because of the development of significant levels of antibodies to IgA, affected individuals are susceptible to severe anaphylactic reactions when transfused with blood products, which may be contaminated with IgA. Chronic immunoglobulin therapy will not increase the low levels of IgA; moreover, such infusions carry the risk of anaphylaxis. Only the rare patient with IgA deficiency who is also deficient in IgG2 and IgG4 antibodies would benefit from immunoglobulin infusions.

**X-61.   The answer is E.**   *(Chap. 300)*   Patients with SLE may have a host of autoantibodies. Virtually all have antinuclear antibodies directed at multiple nuclear and cytoplasmic antigens. Approximately 50% have an anticardiolipin antibody, which is associated with a prolonged partial thromboplastin time and false-positive serologic tests for syphilis. This so-called lupus anticoagulant may be manifested by thrombocytopenia, venous or arterial clotting, recurrent fetal loss, and valvular heart disease. Although thrombotic problems are most common, if the antibody is associated with hypoprothrombinemia, severe thrombocytopenia, or an antibody to clotting factors (usually VIII or IX), bleeding may result. Confirmation that the partial thromboplastin time is prolonged on the basis of a lupus anticoagulant may be made by failure of normal plasma to correct the defect.

**X-62.   The answer is C.**   *(Chap. 303)*   Patients with the more malignant variant of systemic sclerosis (scleroderma) have diffuse cutaneous disease characterized by skin thickening in the extremities, face, and trunk. It is this subset of patients, in contrast to those with limited cutaneous disease who often have the CREST syndrome, who are at risk for developing kidney and other visceral disease. Hypertension heralds the onset of a renal crisis manifested by malignant hypertension, encephalopathy, retinopathy, seizures, and left ventricular failure. The renin-angiotensin system is markedly activated; therefore, angiotensin converting-enzyme inhibitors are particularly effective. Even patients who require dialysis may reverse course and have a slow return of renal function after the passage of several months. Patients with systemic sclerosis may also develop esophageal dysfunction, hypomotility of the small intestine (which can produce pain and malabsorption), pulmonary fibrosis sometimes progressing to pulmonary hypertension, and heart failure caused by myocardial fibrosis.

**X-63.   The answer is E.**   *(Chap. 303)*   MCTD is a syndrome characterized by high titers of circulating antibodies to the ribonucleoprotein component of extractable nuclear antigen in association with clinical features similar to those of SLE, systemic sclerosis, polymyositis, and rheumatoid arthritis. The average patient with MCTD is a middle-aged female with Raynaud's phenomenon who also has polyarthritis, sclerodactyly (including swollen hands), esophageal dysfunction, pulmonary fibrosis, and inflammatory myopathy. Cutaneous manifestations include telangiectasias on the face and hands, alopecia, a lupuslike heliotropic rash, and erythematous patches over the knuckles. The myopathy may involve severe weakness of proximal muscles associated with high levels of creatine phosphokinase and aldolase. Both pulmonary involvement and esophageal dysmotility are common but are frequently asymptomatic until quite advanced. Almost all these patients have high titers of rheumatoid factor and antinuclear antibodies. Such antibodies are directed toward the ribonuclease-sensitive ribonucleoprotein component of extractable nuclear antigen.

**X-64.   The answer is B.**   *(Chap. 313; Emmerson, N Engl J Med 334:445–451, 1996.)*   Monosodium urate gout (diagnosed on the basis of the presence of urate, birefringent needle-shaped intracellular crystals on an obligatory joint fluid examination) usually affects one joint initially, especially the great toe. Although abnormalities of uric acid metabolism (high serum or urinary levels) are often seen at some point, many patients present with normal or low serum uric acid. Treatment typically consists of a nonsteroidal anti-inflammatory agent or colchicine, but these agents are relatively contraindicated in this patient because of the comorbid conditions. Steroid injection is a simple and highly effective alternative. Urate-lowering drugs should not be initiated during acute attacks.

**X-65.   The answer is A.**   *(Chap. 303)*   Systemic sclerosis can be classified into two variants depending on whether scleroderma is present only in the fingers (sclerodactyly) or is also present proximal to the metacarpophalangeal joints. The former disorder is associated with a constellation of findings labeled the CREST syndrome: calcinosis, Raynaud's phenomenon, esophageal dysmotility, sclerodactyly, and telangiectasia. Although once thought not to be associated with significant internal organ involvement, the CREST variant of systemic sclerosis has occurred in association with the development of pulmonary arterial hypertension or biliary cirrhosis. The fluorescent antinuclear antibody (ANA) test is positive in 40 to 80% of persons with systemic sclerosis. Antibodies are produced to deoxyribonucleoprotein, nucleolar, centromere, and topoisomerase 1 antigens. MCTD is the overlap of three rheumatic disease syndromes: SLE, polymyositis, and the CREST variant of systemic sclerosis. It is associated with high titers of ANAs directed against the extractable nuclear antigen ribonucleoprotein. Arthritis and a positive ANA test are not sufficient to make a diagnosis of SLE. Overlap syndromes are diseases that fulfill the diagnostic criteria for two rheumatic diseases. In this case, symptoms and signs were insufficient to fulfill the diagnostic criteria for more than one rheumatic syndrome.

**X-66.   The answer is E.**   *(Chap. 300)*   Although most clinicians believe that females with SLE should not become pregnant if they have active disease or advanced renal or cardiac disease, the presence of SLE itself is not an absolute contraindication to pregnancy. The outcome of pregnancy is best for females who are in remission at the time of conception. Even in females with quiescent disease, exacerbations may occur (usually in the first trimester and the immediate postpartum period), and 25 to 40% of these pregnancies end in spontaneous abortion. Fetal loss rates are higher in patients with lupus anticoagulant or anticardiolipin antibodies. Flare-ups should be anticipated and vigorously treated with steroids. Steroids given throughout pregnancy also usually have no adverse effects on the child. In this case, the fact that the female had a life-threatening bout of disease a year ago would argue against stopping her drugs at this time. Neonatal lupus, which is manifested by thrombocytopenia, rash, and heart block, is rare but can occur when mothers have anti-Ro antibodies.

**X-67.   The answer is E.**   *(Chap. 304)*   Sjögren's syndrome, an autoimmune destruction of the exocrine glands, can be primary or can occur in association with rheumatoid arthritis, SLE, or systemic sclerosis. A mononuclear cell infiltrate that can be seen in virtually any organ is pathognomonic if found in the salivary gland in association with keratoconjunctivitis sicca (conjunctival and corneal dryness) and xerostomia (lack of salivation). Since minor salivary glands will be obtained in a lip biopsy, such a procedure can be diagnostic. Severe dryness of the mouth can lead to an increased incidence of dental caries. Corneal dryness may be severe enough to result in ulceration. The most common form of renal involvement (seen in 40% of patients with primary Sjögren's) is an interstitial nephritis that results in renal tubular acidosis. Hypersensitivity vasculitis, manifested by palpable purpura of the lower extremities, is not uncommon. Sensory neuropathies, interstitial pneumonitis, and autoimmune thyroid disease may also accompany primary Sjögren's syndrome. Finally, pseudolymphoma, characterized by lymphadenopathy and enlargement of the parotid gland, and frank non-Hodgkin's lymphoma may occur. Cardiac disease is very rare in patients with Sjögren's syndrome.

**X-68.   The answer is E.**   *(Chap. 309)*   Although 10 to 20% of patients with sarcoidosis present with asymptomatic disease found incidentally on chest x-ray and 40 to 70% have the characteristic insidious development of disease, the remainder present over the span of a few weeks. Constitutional and respiratory symptoms dominate the acute presentation. Two distinct patterns of acute sarcoidosis are recognized. Lofgren's syndrome, which is seen in Scandinavian, Irish, and Puerto Rican females, is characterized by erythema nodosum, arthralgias, and bilateral hilar lymphadenopathy. The constellation of findings in the Heerfordt-Waldenstrom syndrome consists of fever, parotid enlargement, anterior uveitis, and facial nerve palsy. Interstitial pulmonary involvement would be rare in patients with acute sarcoidosis. Myopathy and skin lesions are most consistent with dermatomyositis. Although 5% of patients with sarcoidosis have cardiac abnormalities, valvular heart disease other than occasional instances of papillary muscle dysfunction is rare.

**X-69.   The answer is E.**   *(Chaps. 311 and 314; Baker, N Engl J Med 329:1013–1020, 1993.)* The analysis of synovial fluid begins at the bedside. When fluid is withdrawn from a joint into a syringe, its clarity and color should be assessed. Cloudiness or turbidity is caused by the scattering of light as it is reflected off particles in the fluid; these particles are usually white blood cells, although crystals may also be present. The viscosity of synovial fluid is due to its hyaluronate content. In patients with inflammatory joint disease, synovial fluid contains enzymes that break down hyaluronate and reduce fluid viscosity. In contrast, synovial fluid taken from a joint in a person with a degenerative joint disease, a noninflammatory condition, would be expected to be clear and have good viscosity. The color of the fluid can indicate recent or old hemorrhage into the joint space. Pigmented villonodular synovitis is associated with noninflammatory fluid that is dark brown in color ("crankcase oil") as a result of repeated hemorrhage into the joint. Gout and calcium pyrophosphate deposition disease produce inflammatory synovial effusions, which are cloudy and watery. In addition, these disorders may be diagnosed by identification of crystals in the fluid: Sodium urate crystals of gout are needle-like and strongly negatively birefringent, whereas calcium pyrophosphate crystals are rhomboidal and weakly positively birefringent.

# XI. ENDOCRINOLOGY AND METABOLISM

## QUESTIONS

**DIRECTIONS:** Each question below contains five or six suggested responses. Choose the **one best** response to each question.

**XI-1.** A 31-year-old female complains of a 2-month history of a 15-lb unintentional weight loss, anxiety, and "feeling jittery." The neck examination is unremarkable. Physical examination shows tachycardia and increased deep tendon reflexes. Thyroid-stimulating hormone (TSH) is below 0.01. Total $T_4$ is elevated. Whole-body radionuclide iodine scan shows only low uptake in the region of the thyroid. Serum thyroglobulin levels are within the normal range. What is the most likely diagnosis?

A. Graves' disease
B. Struma ovarii
C. Subacute thyroiditis
D. Lymphocytic thyroiditis
E. Thyrotoxicosis factitia

**XI-2.** The World Health Organization (WHO) recently defined osteoporosis operationally as

A. a patient with a bone density less than the mean of age-, race-, and gender-matched controls
B. a patient with a bone density less than 1.0 standard deviation (SD) below the mean of race- and gender-matched controls
C. a patient with a bone density less than 1.0 SD below the mean of age-, race-, and gender-matched controls
D. a patient with a bone density less than 2.5 SD below the mean of race- and gender-matched controls
E. a patient with a bone density less than 2.5 SD below the mean of age-, race-, and gender-matched controls

**XI-3.** A 40-year-old female complains of low-grade fevers and anterior neck pain for 6 days. She denies tremor, weight loss, or visual changes. Examination shows a tender and slightly enlarged thyroid gland. There is no bruit. The rest of the examination is unremarkable. TSH is low. $T_4$ and $T_3$ are both elevated. A radionuclide scan shows low uptake. Anti-TPO antibodies are negative. What would be the most appropriate therapy at this point?

A. Radioiodine ablation
B. Methimazole
C. Prednisone
D. Levothyroxine
E. Surgery

**XI-4.** Which of the following statements regarding hypothyroidism is true?

A. Hashimoto's thyroiditis is the most common cause of hypothyroidism worldwide.
B. The annual risk of developing overt clinical hypothyroidism from subclinical hypothyroidism in patients with positive thyroid peroxidase (TPO) antibodies is 20%.
C. Histologically, Hashimoto's thyroiditis is characterized by marked infiltration of the thyroid with activated T cells and B cells.
D. A low TSH level excludes the diagnosis of hypothyroidism.
E. Thyroid peroxidase antibodies are present in less than 50% of patients with autoimmune hypothyroidism.

**XI-5.** A 40-year-old female with Graves' disease was recently started on methimazole. One month later she comes to the clinic for a routine follow-up. She notes some low-grade fevers, arthralgias, and general malaise. Laboratories are notable for a mild transaminitis and a glucose of 150 mg/dL. All the following are known side effects of methimazole *except*

A. agranulocytosis
B. rash
C. arthralgia
D. hepatitis
E. insulin resistance

**XI-6.** Which of the following is consistent with a diagnosis of subacute thyroiditis?

A. A 38-year-old female with a 2-week history of a painful thyroid, elevated $T_4$, elevated $T_3$, low TSH, and an elevated radioactive iodine uptake scan

**XI-6.** *(Continued)*

   B. A 42-year-old male with a history of a painful thyroid 4 months ago, fatigue, malaise, low free $T_4$, low $T_3$, and elevated TSH.
   C. A 31-year-old female with a painless enlarged thyroid, low TSH, elevated $T_4$, elevated free $T_4$, and an elevated radioiodine uptake scan
   D. A 50-year-old male with a painful thyroid, slightly elevated $T_4$, normal TSH, and an ultrasound showing a mass
   E. A 46-year-old female with 3 weeks of fatigue, low $T_4$, low $T_3$, and low TSH

**XI-7.** Which of the following is the most common site for a fracture associated with osteoporosis?

   A. Femur
   B. Hip
   C. Radius
   D. Vertebra
   E. Wrist

**XI-8.** All the following are risk factors for the development of osteoporotic fractures *except*

   A. African-American race
   B. current cigarette smoking
   C. female sex
   D. low body weight
   E. physical inactivity

**XI-9.** All the following drugs are associated with an increased risk of osteoporosis in adults *except*

   A. cyclosporine
   B. dilantin
   C. heparin
   D. prednisone
   E. ranitidine

**XI-10.** A 44-year-old male is involved in a motor vehicle collision. He sustains multiple injuries to the face, chest, and pelvis. He is unresponsive in the field and is intubated for airway protection. An intravenous line is placed. The patient is admitted to the intensive care unit (ICU) with multiple orthopedic injuries. He is stabilized medically and on hospital day 2 undergoes successful open reduction and internal fixation of the right femur and right humerus. After his return to the ICU, you review his laboratory values. TSH is is 0.3 mU/L, and the total $T_4$ level is normal. $T_3$ is 0.6 $\mu$g/dL. What is the most appropriate next management step?

   A. Initiation of levothyroxine
   B. A radioiodine uptake scan
   C. A thyroid ultrasound
   D. Observation

**XI-10.** *(Continued)*

   E. Initiation of prednisone

**XI-11.** A 23-year-old female nursing student is brought to the emergency room by her parents after being found unconscious at home. She is noted to have a fingerstick glucose of 29 mg/dL. After administration of intravenous D50, she rapidly regains consciousness. Her parents state that this is the fourth time in a month that this has occurred. She is not taking any medications. The medical history is unremarkable except for a history of depression and a mother with diabetes mellitus. Examination is unremarkable. During an observed period in the hospital, the patient is noted to have a symptomatic glucose level of 31 mg/dL. Plasma insulin levels are elevated, and C-peptide levels are low. Which of the following is the most likely cause of her hypoglycemia?

   A. Glipizide overdose
   B. Surreptitious insulin use
   C. Insulinoma
   D. Glucagonoma
   E. Diabetic ketoacidosis

**XI-12.** A 52-year-old female is admitted to the hospital for weight loss, diarrhea, and dehydration. She reports 1 to 2 months of watery diarrhea that is unrelated to food intake. Concurrent with the diarrhea she often has cramping abdominal pain and flushing of the neck and face. The onset of these symptoms is often sudden and is preceded by stress, alcohol intake, or eating cheese. Initially the flushing lasted approximately 5 min, but it now lasts up to an hour. The flushing episodes are usually followed by diarrhea. The symptoms have not improved despite the elimination of all dairy products from her diet. The physical examination is notable for a blood pressure of 90/70 mmHg and a heart rate of 95/min. The patient's blood pressure falls and her heart rate increases when she sits. The patient also has hepatomegaly, with a liver span of 15 cm. An ultrasound demonstrates lesions in the liver consistent with metastases. Which of the following tests is most likely to yield the diagnosis?

   A. Flow cytometry of a bone marrow aspirate
   B. Serum $\alpha$ fetoprotein
   C. Serum cortisol
   D. Serum glucose
   E. Urinary 5-HIAA

**XI-13.** This patient probably will demonstrate a neoplasm originating in the

   A. adrenal gland
   B. bone marrow
   C. bronchus

**XI-13.** *(Continued)*
D. ileum
E. pancreas

**XI-14.** A 25-year-old female notes increasing facial hair and acne for the last 4 months. She has noticed some deepening of her voice but denies changes in her libido or genitalia. She weighs 94 kg and is 5 feet 5 inches tall. Blood pressure is 126/70 mmHg. Examination is notable for moderate obesity. There is no evidence of abdominal striae or bruising. All the following would be important initial steps in the clinical assessment of this patient *except*

A. medication history
B. family history
C. serum testosterone level
D. serum dehydroepiandrosterone sulfate (DHEAS) level
E. abdominal ultrasound

**XI-15.** All the following are pharmacologic therapies for androgen excess *except*

A. glucocorticoids
B. oral contraceptives
C. spironolactone
D. cyproterone acetate
E. fludracortisone

**XI-16.** All the following biochemical markers are a measure of bone resorption *except*

A. serum alkaline phosphatase
B. serum cross-linked N-telopeptide
C. serum cross-linked C-telopeptide
D. urine hydroxyproline
E. urine total free deoxypyridonoline

**XI-17.** All but which of the following statements about osteoporosis and bone fractures are true?

A. Osteoporosis is defined as a bone density that is 1.5 standard deviations (SD) below the mean for young healthy adults of the same race and gender.
B. Up to 2 million men in the United States have osteoporosis.
C. The risk of hip fracture is higher in whites than in African Americans.
D. The incidence of deep venous thrombosis in patients with hip fractures is more than 20%.
E. More than 10% of white women over age 50 years will have a hip fracture.

**XI-18.** All the following are associated with bone loss *except*

A. vitamin D deficiency
B. menopause

**XI-18.** *(Continued)*
C. glucocorticoids
D. tobacco use
E. running

**XI-19.** A 51-year-old Asian female comes to your clinic for routine health screening. She is otherwise healthy and takes no medications. The family history is notable only for a mother with osteoporosis. A review of systems is notable for hot flashes and mood changes over the last year. The patient's last menstrual period was 3 months ago. The examination is unremarkable. You make arrangements for age-appropriate cancer screening, measure her cholesterol, and order a bone densitometry scan (DEXA). The DEXA shows multiple sites with *t*-scores more than −2.5 SD below the mean. All the following are reasonable treatment recommendations *except*

A. calcium supplementation
B. vitamin D supplementation
C. weekly alendronate
D. tamoxifen
E. exercise

**XI-20.** A 35-year-old male is referred to your clinic for evaluation of hypercalcemia noted during a health insurance medical screening. He has noted some fatigue, malaise, and a 4-lb weight loss over the last 2 months. He also has noted constipation and "heartburn." He is occasionally nauseated after large meals and has water brash and a sour taste in his mouth. The patient denies vomiting, dysphagia, or odynophagia. He also notes decreased libido and a depressed mood. Vital signs are unremarkable. Physical examination is notable for a clear oropharynx, no evidence of a thyroid mass, and no lymphadenopathy. Jugular venous pressure is normal. Heart sounds are regular with no murmurs or gallops. The chest is clear. The abdomen is soft with some mild epigastric tenderness. There is no rebound or organomegaly. Stool is guaiac-positive. Neurologic examination is nonfocal. Laboratory values are notable for a normal complete blood count. Calcium is 11.2 mg/dL, phosphate is 2.1 mg/dL, and magnesium is 1.8 meq/dL. Albumin is 3.7 g/dL, and total protein is 7.0 g/dL. TSH is 3 $\mu$IU/mL, prolactin is 250 $\mu$g/L, testosterone is 620 ng/dL, and serum insulin-like growth factor 1 (IGF-1) is normal. Serum intact parathyroid hormone level is 135 pg/dL. In light of the patient's abdominal discomfort and heme-positive stool, you perform an abdominal computed tomography (CT) scan that shows a lesion measuring 2 cm by 2 cm in the head of the pancreas. What is the diagnosis?

A. Multiple endocrine neoplasia (MEN) type 1
B. MEN type 2a
C. MEN type 2b

**XI-20.** *(Continued)*

    D.   Polyglandular autoimmune syndrome

    E.   Von–Hippel Lindau (VHL) syndrome

**XI-21.** Postmenopausal estrogen therapy has been shown to increase a female's risk of all the following clinical outcomes *except*

    A.   breast cancer

    B.   hip fracture

    C.   myocardial infarction

    D.   stroke

    E.   venous thromboembolism

**XI-22.** Using available data on morbidity and mortality, the most widely used definition threshold for obesity is

    A.   weight more than 2 standard deviations above the mean for age, sex, and race

    B.   a waist-to-hip ratio above 1.0 in men and 0.9 in women

    C.   a body mass index (BMI) higher than 30

    D.   weight more than 100 kg for women and 120 kg for men

    E.   electrical impedance more than 2 standard deviations above the mean for age, sex, and race

**XI-23.** Obesity is associated with an increased incidence of all the following *except*

    A.   diabetes mellitus

    B.   cancer

    C.   hypertension

    D.   biliary disease

    E.   chronic obstructive lung disease

**XI-24.** All but which of the following statements regarding diabetes mellitus (DM) are true?

    A.   Scandinavia has the highest incidence of type 1 DM.

    B.   Up to 60% of women with gestational diabetes mellitus (GDM) go on to develop overt diabetes mellitus.

    C.   Hispanic Americans are the ethnic group that has the highest prevalence of DM in the United States.

    D.   The prevalence of DM is rising worldwide.

    E.   The concordance of type 2 DM in identical twins is higher than the concordance of type 1 DM in identical twins.

**XI-25.** All the following are direct actions of parathyroid hormone (PTH) *except*

    A.   increased calcium resorption from bone

    B.   increased calcium resorption from the kidney

    C.   increased calcium resorption from the gastrointestinal tract

**XI-25.** *(Continued)*

    D.   increased synthesis of 1,25 dihydroxyvitamin D

    E.   decreased phosphate resorption from the kidney

**XI-26.** A 50-year-old male presents to the clinic for a routine health examination. A comprehensive metabolic panel shows a serum calcium level of 11.2 mg/dL. Serum phosphate is 3.0 mg/dL. Serum creatinine is normal. He denies bone pain, lethargy, weakness, or weight loss. What is the most common cause of hypercalcemia in outpatients?

    A.   Malignancy

    B.   Medications

    C.   Milk-alkali syndrome

    D.   Primary hyperparathyroidism

    E.   Granulomatous disease

**XI-27.** All the following are effects of hypercalcemia *except*

    A.   diarrhea

    B.   confusion

    C.   polyuria

    D.   a shortened QT interval

    E.   nephrolithiasis

**XI-28.** Which of the following statements is true about familial hypocalciuric hypercalcemia (FHH)?

    A.   It is inherited in an autosomal recessive pattern.

    B.   The cause is a defect in the parathyroid hormone receptor.

    C.   Clinical symptoms first manifest in the third and fourth decades of life.

    D.   Treatment is rarely necessary.

    E.   Renal calcium reabsorption is more than 99%.

**XI-29.** All the following are causes of hypocalcemia *except*

    A.   hypomagnesemia

    B.   sepsis

    C.   burn injury

    D.   tumor lysis syndrome

    E.   immobilization

**XI-30.** All but which of the following statements about pheochromocytoma are true?

    A.   The majority are malignant.

    B.   Up to 25% of cases are associated with an inherited form of the disease.

    C.   It occurs more frequently in patients under age 50.

    D.   Diagnosis is made by 24-h urine collection of catecholamines.

    E.   $\alpha$-Adrenergic blockade is mandatory before surgical excision.

**XI-31.** All the following are features of abetalipoprotein-emia *except*

A. autosomal recessive inheritance
B. spinocerebellar degeneration
C. retinopathy
D. childhood presentation
E. elevated cholesterol levels

**XI-32.** All the following are features of lipoprotein lipase deficiency *except*

A. low levels of plasma chylomicrons
B. acute pancreatitis
C. hepatosplenomegaly
D. xanthomas
E. autosomal recessive inheritance

**XI-33.** All the following are side effects of HMG-CoA reductase inhibitors (statins) *except*

A. hepatitis
B. myopathy
C. dyspepsia
D. headache
E. pulmonary fibrosis

**XI-34.** A 55-year-old male is admitted to the intensive care unit with 1 week of fever and cough. He was well until 1 week before admission, when he noted progressive shortness of breath, cough, and productive sputum. On the day of admission the patient was noted by his wife to be lethargic and unresponsive. 911 was called, and the patient was intubated in the field and then brought to the emergency department. His medications include insulin. The past medical history is notable for alcohol abuse, diabetes mellitus, and chronic renal insufficiency. Temperature is 38.9°C (102°F). He is hypotensive with a blood pressure of 76/40 mmHg. Oxygen saturation is 86% on room air. On examination, the patient is sedated and intubated. Jugular venous pressure is normal. There are decreased breath sounds at the right lung base with egophony. Heart sounds are normal. The abdomen is soft. There is no peripheral edema. Chest radiography shows a right lower lobe infiltrate with a moderate pleural effusion. An electrocardiogram is normal. Sputum Gram stain shows gram-positive diplococci. White blood cell count is $23 \times 10^3/\mu L$, with 70% polymorphonuclear cells and 6% bands. Blood urea nitrogen is 80 mg/dL, and creatinine is 6.1 mg/dL. Plasma glucose is 425 mg/dL. He is started on broad-spectrum antibiotics, intravenous fluids, omeprazole, and an insulin drip. A nasogastric tube is inserted, and tube feedings are started. On hospital day 2 plasma phosphate is 1.0 mg/dL. All of following are causes of hypophosphatemia *except*

A. sepsis
B. renal failure

**XI-34.** *(Continued)*

C. insulin
D. alcoholism
E. malnutrition

**XI-35.** A 21-year-old competitive runner is evaluated for irregular menstruation. She had menses at age 14 and normally has a 28-day cycle with 5 days of menses. Over the last 4 months she has noted irregularity in her cycles. Menses may last between 2 and 7 days, and she has not had a period for the last month. There is no change in cramping or abdominal symptoms. Pelvic examination is normal. Urine and blood tests for pregnancy are negative. What is the most appropriate management step?

A. Progesterone challenge
B. Hysterosalpingography
C. CT scan of the abdomen with contrast
D. Serum prolactin
E. Chromosome analysis

**XI-36.** A 48-year-old female is undergoing evaluation for flushing and diarrhea. Physical examination is normal except for nodular hepatomegaly. A CT scan of the abdomen demonstrates multiple nodules in both lobes of the liver consistent with metastases in the liver and a 2-cm mass in the ileum. The 24-h urinary 5-HIAA excretion is markedly elevated. All the following treatments are appropriate *except*

A. diphenhydramine
B. interferon-α
C. octreotide
D. odansetron
E. phenoxybenzamine

**XI-37.** While undergoing a physical examination during medical student clinical skills, this patient develops severe flushing, wheezing, nausea, and light-headedness. Vital signs are notable for a blood pressure of 70/30 mmHg and a heart rate of 135/min. Which of the following is the most appropriate therapy?

A. Albuterol
B. Atropine
C. Epinephrine
D. Hydrocortisone
E. Octreotide

**XI-38.** A 31-year-old female is evaluated for amenorrhea for the last 6 months. Her height is 170 cm, and her weight is 50 kg. Pelvic examination is unremarkable. A pregnancy test is negative. Serum LH and follicle-stimulating hormone (FSH) are elevated. Estradiol is low. What is the most likely diagnosis?

**XI-38.** *(Continued)*
  A. Polycystic ovarian disease
  B. Panhypopituitarism
  C. Asherman's syndrome
  D. Ovarian failure
  E. Turner syndrome

**XI-39.** A 21-year-old female with a history of type 1 diabetes mellitus is brought to the emergency room with nausea, vomiting, lethargy, and dehydration. Her mother notes that she stopped taking insulin 1 day before presentation. She is lethargic, has dry mucous membranes, and is obtunded. Blood pressure is 80/40 mmHg, and heart rate is 112 beats/min. Heart sounds are normal. Lungs are clear. The abdomen is soft, and there is no organomegaly. She is responsive and oriented ×3 but diffusely weak. Serum sodium is 126 meq/L, potassium is 4.3 meq/L, magnesium is 1.2 meq/L, blood urea nitrogen is 76 mg/dL, creatinine is 2.2 mg/dL, bicarbonate is 10 meq/L, and chloride is 88 meq/L. Serum glucose is 720 mg/dL. All the following are appropriate management steps *except*

  A. arterial blood gas
  B. intravenous insulin
  C. intravenous potassium
  D. 3% sodium solution
  E. intravenous fluids

**XI-40.** The Diabetes Control and Complications Trial (DCCT) provided definitive proof that reduction in chronic hyperglycemia

  A. improves microvascular complications in type 1 diabetes mellitus
  B. improves macrovascular complications in type 1 diabetes mellitus
  C. improves microvascular complications in type 2 diabetes mellitus
  D. improves macrovascular complications in type 2 diabetes mellitus
  E. improves both microvascular and macrovascular complications in type 2 diabetes mellitus

**XI-41.** All the following therapies have been shown to reduce the risk of hip fractures in postmenopausal women with osteoporosis *except*

  A. alendronate
  B. estrogen
  C. parathyroid hormone
  D. raloxifene
  E. risedronate
  F. vitamin D plus calcium

**XI-42.** A 64-year-old male with COPD has been treated frequently with prednisone for exacerbations. Bone densitometry reveals a *z*-score of −3.0. Which of the follow-

**XI-42.** *(Continued)*
ing is the most appropriate treatment to reduce the risk of fractures?

  A. Calcitonin
  B. Estrogen
  C. Hydrochlorothiazide
  D. Risedronate
  E. Vitamin D

**XI-43.** A 33-year-old male with end-stage renal disease who is on hemodialysis complains of decreased libido, inability to maintain erections, increasing fatigue, and mild weakness. He has been on a stable hemodialysis regimen for 8 years, and all his electrolytes are normal. Further evaluation reveals a reduced serum testosterone level. Measurement of which of the following will distinguish primary from secondary hypogonadism?

  A. Aldosterone
  B. Cortisol
  C. Estradiol
  D. Luteinizing hormone
  E. Thyroid-stimulating hormone

**XI-44.** All the following drugs may interfere with testicular function *except*

  A. cyclophosphamide
  B. ketoconazole
  C. metoprolol
  D. prednisone
  E. spironolactone

**XI-45.** A 55-year-old female comes to her primary care physician's office for evaluation of episodes of flushing. The symptoms started about 1 year ago when she noted occasional night sweats as well as daily facial flushing lasting 3 to 5 min and vaginal dryness. Her menses have become irregular, with the last menstrual period having occurred 6 months ago. Past medical history is notable for rheumatoid arthritis and frequent urinary tract infections since young adulthood. Current medications are etanercept and occasional ibuprofen. She quit smoking cigarettes 20 years ago and has no other habits. The following laboratory data are obtained:
  TSH   1.23 mIU/mg   normal 0.5 to 4.5
  FSH   35 mIU/mL   upper limit of normal 10
  She is interested in discussing the benefits of estrogen-progesterone replacement therapy. Her physician can tell her that there is scientific evidence that this therapy will decrease all the following *except*

  A. progression of bone loss
  B. incidence of urinary tract infections
  C. incidence of myocardial infarction
  D. vaginal dryness
  E. vasomotor symptoms

**XI-46.** A 25-year-old female visits her primary care physician after 3 years of intermittent abdominal pain, peripheral neuropathy, and increasing episodes of anxiety and hallucinations. The physician suspects acute intermittent porphyria. She can make this diagnosis by doing which of the following tests?

A. Sunlight administration with observation for rash
B. Urine porphyrobilinogen (PBG) level during an attack
C. Peripheral blood testing for an HFE C282Y mutation
D. Urine PBG level when the patient is well
E. Hypoglycemic provocation testing

**XI-47.** A 35-year-old male with no significant past medical history complains of 6 weeks of abdominal pain, watery diarrhea, and heartburn. These symptoms were not relieved by a 2-week course of omeprazole. He has no anorexia but has lost 10 lb. He is on no medications currently, does not smoke cigarettes, and does not use alcohol. Further investigation by endoscopy reveals prominent gastric folds and three duodenal ulcers. Fasting serum gastrin is elevated. Which of the following results is most likely to provide a diagnosis in this case?

A. An elevated serum chromogranin A
B. An increase in serum gastrin 15 min after intravenous infusion of secretin
C. A positive antigliadin antibody test
D. A positive gastric biopsy urease test
E. A positive periodic acid–Schiff (PAS) stain on duodenal biopsy

**XI-48.** A 47-year-old nurse complains of episodic confusion, headaches, disorientation, sweating, and tremors that occur approximately three times a week, usually at work. These episodes began about 4 months ago. She notes they occur more frequently during stressful times at work when she has to skip lunch. The episodes resolve after a few minutes, often after the patient drinks some juice. There is no past medical history except a history of irritable bowel syndrome. During a recent episode at work in the hospital, her serum glucose was found to be 40 mg/dL. Which of the following serum tests should be done during a hypoglycemic episode to determine the etiology of her symptoms?

A. Cortisol
B. C peptide
C. Glucagon
D. Hemoglobin $A_{1C}$
E. Serotonin

**XI-49.** A 49-year-old male is brought to the hospital by his family because of confusion and dehydration. The family reports that for the last 3 weeks he has had per-

**XI-49.** *(Continued)*
sistent copious watery diarrhea that has not abated with the use of over-the-counter medications. The diarrhea has been unrelated to food intake and has persisted during fasting. The stool does not appear fatty and is not malodorous. The patient works as an attorney, is a vegetarian, and has not traveled recently. No one in the household has had similar symptoms. Before the onset of diarrhea, he had mild anorexia and a 5-lb weight loss. Since the diarrhea began, he has lost at least 10 pounds. The physical examination is notable for blood pressure of 100/70, heart rate of 110/min, and temperature of 36.8°C (98.2°F). Other than poor skin turgor, confusion, and diffuse muscle weakness, the physical examination is unremarkable. Laboratory studies are notable for a normal complete blood count and the following chemistry results:

| | |
|---|---|
| $Na^+$ | 146 meq/L |
| $K^+$ | 3.0 meq/L |
| $Cl^-$ | 96 meq/L |
| $HCO_3^-$ | 36 meq/L |
| BUN | 32 mg/dL |
| Creatinine | 1.2 mg/dL |

A 24-h stool collection yields 3 L of tea-colored stool. Stool sodium is 50 meq/L, potassium is 25 meq/L, and stool osmolality is 170 mosmol/L. Which of the following diagnostic tests is most likely to yield the correct diagnosis?

A. Serum cortisol
B. Serum TSH
C. Serum VIP
D. Urinary 5-HIAA
E. Urinary metanephrine

**XI-50.** A 63-year-old male seeks medical attention for a 6-month history of lack of libido and generalized malaise. He has a history of mild obstructive sleep apnea and is trying to lose weight. After a complete evaluation, the patient is found to have a reduced serum testosterone of 150 ng/dL. Testosterone replacement therapy probably will have all the following effects *except*

A. improved libido
B. improved sleep apnea symptoms
C. increased bone density
D. increased energy
E. increased lean muscle mass

**XI-51.** A patient is seen in the clinic for routine follow-up for hypertension. A basic metabolic panel is ordered along with a lipid profile while the patient is fasting. The lipid profile is normal. Electrolytes, blood urea nitrogen (BUN), and creatinine are normal. Glucose is 111 mg/dL. On recheck, fasting glucose is 113 mg/dL. The patient can be told which of the following?

A. A hemoglobin $A_{1C}$ will need to be checked to ensure that he does not have diabetes mellitus.

**XI-51.** *(Continued)*
  B.  He has diabetes mellitus.
  C.  He has impaired fasting glucose.
  D.  His laboratory work is normal.
  E.  He will need an oral glucose tolerance test to evaluate for impaired glucose tolerance.

**XI-52.** Which of the following statements about the possible diagnosis of impaired fasting glucose is correct?

  A.  Impaired fasting glucose can be diagnosed when the fasting glucose ranges from 115 mg/dL to 125 mg/dL.
  B.  Patients with impaired fasting glucose are at increased risk for cardiovascular disease.
  C.  Patients with impaired fasting glucose have a minimally increased risk for developing diabetes mellitus over the next decade.
  D.  Patients with impaired fasting glucose should be tested for anti–islet cell antibodies to diagnose autoimmune diabetes mellitus early and prevent severe complications.
  E.  Patients with impaired fasting glucose should have regular checks of their hemoglobin $A_{1C}$.

**XI-53.** A 22-year-old male is referred to a physician after he is found to have an elevated serum calcium during a life insurance screening examination. The patient is asymptomatic and has no past medical history. Family history is positive for a father and two brothers with hypercalcemia. Repeat laboratory tests reveal a serum calcium of 11.2 mg/dL and are otherwise normal. Which of the following is the most useful next step in establishing a diagnosis?

  A.  24-h urinary calcium excretion
  B.  24-h urinary protein excretion
  C.  Serum intact parathyroid
  D.  Serum TSH
  E.  Serum vitamin D

**XI-54.** This patient is most likely to develop which of following clinical disorders?

  A.  Addison's disease
  B.  Crest syndrome
  C.  Graves' disease
  D.  Ehlers-Danlos syndrome
  E.  Zollinger-Ellison syndrome

**XI-55.** During an employment physical examination, an 18-year-old male is found to have a 1.5-cm nodule in the apex of the left lobe of the thyroid. A fine-needle aspiration reveals malignant C cells that stain positive for calcitonin. All but which of the following statements regarding this patient's condition are true?

**XI-55.** *(Continued)*
  A.  He is likely to have distant metastases.
  B.  He is at risk of developing hyperparathyroidism.
  C.  He is at risk of developing a pancreatic cell tumor.
  D.  He is at risk of developing a pheochromocytoma.
  E.  It is likely that other members of his family have the same malignancy.

**XI-56.** A 23-year-old female is admitted to the hospital with 1 day of diffuse abdominal pain. She has no past medical history and takes no medications. Physical examination shows tachycardia, mild hypotension, a fruity odor to her breath, and a mildly diffusely tender abdomen. Blood chemistries show a sodium of 136 meq/L, a potassium of 5.6 meq/L, a chloride of 101 meq/L, and an undetectable bicarbonate. The glucose is 551 mg/dL. Blood ketones are positive at a 1:8 dilution. Three hours after the initiation of intravenous insulin and normal saline, the laboratories are as follows: sodium 140 meq/L, potassium 4.1 meq/L, chloride 106 meq/L, bicarbonate 14 meq/L, and glucose 190 mg/dL. The most appropriate next step in management is to

  A.  discontinue intravenous fluids
  B.  discontinue insulin infusion and administer subcutaneous insulin
  C.  discontinue insulin infusion and begin 5% dextrose normal saline infusion
  D.  discontinue normal saline and begin 5% dextrose normal saline infusion
  E.  measure a follow-up serum ketone level before making decisions about insulin or fluid management

**XI-57.** A patient is seen in the clinic for follow-up of type 2 diabetes mellitus. Her hemoglobin $A_{1C}$ has been poorly controlled at 9.4% recently. The patient can be counseled to expect all the following improvements with improved glycemic control *except*

  A.  decreased microalbuminuria
  B.  decreased risk of nephropathy
  C.  decreased risk of neuropathy
  D.  decreased risk of peripheral vascular disease
  E.  decreased risk of retinopathy

**XI-58.** The patient's blood pressure is 163/94 mmHg. With improved blood pressure control, the patient can expect all the following *except*

  A.  Decreased risk of death
  B.  Decreased risk of neuropathy
  C.  Decreased risk of retinopathy
  D.  Decreased risk of stroke
  E.  All of the above

**XI-59.** Which of the following statements regarding dyslipidemia and diabetes mellitus is correct?

**XI-59.**   *(Continued)*

A.   In diabetic individuals, LDL cholesterol is structurally similar to LDL cholesterol in normal individuals.

B.   In diabetic individuals without coronary artery disease, the goal LDL level is below 120 mg/dL.

C.   LDL particles in type 2 diabetic patients are less susceptible to oxidation than they are in individuals without diabetes.

D.   Male patients with diabetes mellitus have a goal HDL of over 55 mg/dL.

E.   The most common forms of dyslipidemia in diabetic patients are elevated triglycerides and reduced HDL levels.

**XI-60.**   A 59-year-old female is seen in the clinic regarding her diagnosis of type 2 diabetes mellitus. She has attempted diet control and exercise for the last 6 months; however, her hemoglobin $A_{1C}$ is 8.6%, and it is now recommended that she begin medication for diabetes. The patient takes lisinopril and aspirin and has no allergies. Her other medical problems are mild congestive heart failure and hypertension. Blood work is notable for a creatinine of 1.5 mg/dL. Which of the following medications is it appropriate to start at this time?

A.   Metformin

B.   Glipizide

C.   Insulin

D.   Pioglitazone

E.   Metformin and glipizide

**XI-61.**   The use of repeated phlebotomy in the treatment of persons with symptomatic hemochromatosis may be expected to result in

A.   increased skin pigmentation

B.   improved cardiac function

C.   return of secondary sex characteristics

D.   decreased joint pain

E.   an unchanged 5-year survival rate

**XI-62.**   Which of the following studies is most sensitive for detecting diabetic nephropathy?

A.   Serum creatinine level

B.   Creatinine clearance

C.   Urine albumin

D.   Glucose tolerance test

E.   Ultrasonography

**XI-63.**   A 7-year-old girl is referred for evaluation of vaginal bleeding for the last 2 months. The girl's mother says that she has not been exposed to exogenous estrogens. Physical examination reveals height at the 98th percentile, Tanner stage III breast development, and no axillary or pubic hair. No abdominal or pelvic masses are palpated.

**XI-63.**   *(Continued)*

Neurologic examination is normal. Radiographic and laboratory evaluations reveal the following:

Brain MRI: normal pituitary and hypothalamus
Bone age: 10 years
Urinary 17-ketosteroids: 1.7 $\mu$mol (0.5 mg)/g creatinine per 24 h
Urinary gonadotropins: undetectable

The appropriate next step in the management of this girl would be

A.   exploratory laparotomy

B.   treatment with medroxyprogesterone acetate

C.   measurement of the plasma androstenedione level

D.   abdominal CT scanning and/or pelvic sonography

E.   karyotype analysis

**XI-64.**   A 40-year-old male presents with an insidious onset of fatigue, headaches, muscle weakness, and paresthesia. Physical examination reveals hypertension, an enlarged tongue, wide spacing of the teeth, and a doughy appearance to the skin. Which of the following laboratory results would be consistent with the expected diagnosis?

A.   Elevated serum thyroxine level

B.   Fasting serum glucose of 3.3 mmol/L (60 mg/dL)

C.   Elevated insulin-like growth factor 1 (IGF-1)

D.   Growth hormone concentration of 0.2 $\mu$g/L (0.2 ng/mL) 1 h after oral administration of 100 g glucose

E.   Decreased IGF binding protein 3

**XI-65.**   A female patient arrives in your clinic with a serum calcium of 2.7 mmol/L (10.8 mg/dL). The patient is asymptomatic, and this abnormality is found on routine laboratory analysis. A workup includes a normal complete blood count (CBC), normal liver function tests, and a normal serum protein electrophoresis. A serum parathyroid hormone level is 136 ng/L (136 pg/mL), a 24-h urinary calcium is 268 mg, and a serum alkaline phosphatase level is 106 U/L. The patient has no history of orthopedic fractures or nephrolithiasis. A bone densitometry study is performed that reveals a lumbar spine $z$-score of $-0.86$, a femoral neck $z$-score of $-1.34$, and a radius $z$-score of $-1.42$. A parathyroidectomy is likely to result in which of the following?

A.   Normalization of the serum calcium level, improvement of the bone densitometry studies, and a decreased incidence of nephrolithiasis

B.   Normalization of the serum calcium level, improvement of the bone densitometry studies, and a decreased incidence of renal failure

C.   Normalization of the serum calcium level, improvement of the bone densitometry studies, and a decrease in the incidence of pelvic and hip fractures

**XI-65.** *(Continued)*

   D.   Normalization of the serum calcium level, improvement of the bone densitometry studies, and a decrease in the incidence of radial fractures

   E.   Normalization of the serum calcium level and improvement of the bone densitometry studies only

**XI-66.**   A person with hypercalcemia caused by sarcoidosis would have which of the following findings?

   A.   A normal chest x-ray

   B.   Increased absorption of calcium from the gastrointestinal tract

   C.   Normal urine calcium excretion

   D.   Increased serum parathyroid hormone level

   E.   Hypogammaglobulinemia

**XI-67.**   An obese female has hypertriglyceridemia without hypercholesterolemia. The most appropriate first step in the treatment of this female would be

   A.   weight reduction

   B.   nicotinic acid

   C.   gemfibrozil

   D.   clofibrate therapy

   E.   bile acid–binding resin therapy

**XI-68.**   A 30-year-old female is seen in your clinic during her first pregnancy. She is 26 weeks pregnant and has had an uncomplicated pregnancy so far. There is no family history for diabetes mellitus. She has no other significant past medical history. On physical examination she has normal vital signs, including a normal blood pressure. She is not obese. A 50-g oral glucose challenge is given to the patient. One hour later a serum glucose level of 8.3 mmol/L (150 mg/dL) is obtained. Which of the following statements is correct?

   A.   The patient has gestational diabetes mellitus.

   B.   The test is valid only if it is performed during the morning after an overnight fast.

   C.   The test should be repeated and a serum glucose level should be obtained 2 h after the oral glucose challenge.

   D.   The test should be repeated with a 100-g glucose challenge and serum glucose levels measured 1, 2, and 3 h after the test.

   E.   The test should be repeated using a 75-g oral glucose challenge and measuring the serum glucose 2 h after the test.

**XI-69.**   A 55-year-old female presents to her physician with mild fatigue. Past medical history is unremarkable. She is taking no medication. No abnormalities are detected on physical examination. The only abnormality detected on routine blood testing is an elevated calcium [2.96 mmol/L (11.9 mg/dL)] and a serum inorganic phosphorus of

**XI-69.** *(Continued)*
0.65 mmol/L (2 mg/dL). An immunoreactive parathyroid hormone level is undetectable. The most likely etiology for this patient's high serum calcium is

   A.   primary hyperparathyroidism

   B.   malignancy

   C.   hypervitaminosis

   D.   hyperthyroidism

   E.   familial hypocalciuric hypercalcemia

**XI-70.**   During a routine checkup, a 67-year-old male is found to have a level of serum alkaline phosphatase three times the upper limit of normal. Serum calcium and phosphorus concentrations and liver function test results are normal. He is asymptomatic. The most likely diagnosis is

   A.   metastatic bone disease

   B.   primary hyperparathyroidism

   C.   occult plasmacytoma

   D.   Paget's disease of bone

   E.   osteomalacia

**XI-71.**   A 34-year-old female has had three hospital admissions in the last year because of nephrolithiasis. The rate of 24-h urinary calcium excretion has been above the normal range on all three occasions, and serum calcium concentrations were between 2.5 and 2.8 mmol/L (10.2 and 11.5 mg/dL). The serum phosphorus concentration was 0.77 mmol/L (2.4 mg/dL), and the parathyroid hormone level was 229 nL eq/mL (normal, less than 150 nL eq/mL). The most appropriate management at this time would be

   A.   to begin administration of prednisone 40 mg daily and taper the dose over a period of 4 weeks

   B.   to administer thiazide diuretics to decrease calcium excretion

   C.   symptomatic treatment of renal lithiasis only

   D.   calcium supplementation to prevent progressive bone loss

   E.   surgical exploration of the neck

**XI-72.**   Which of the following conditions is characteristic of the presentation of osteomalacia in adults?

   A.   Bowing of the tibia

   B.   Pseudofractures

   C.   Increased thickness of the epiphyseal growth plate

   D.   Hypocalcemia

   E.   Hyperphosphatemia

**XI-73.**   A 61-year-old female noticed severe sharp pain in her back after lifting a suitcase. A compression fracture of the T11 vertebral body is identified on x-ray examination. Routine laboratory evaluation discloses a serum calcium concentration of 2 mmol/L (8.0 mg/dL), a serum phosphorus concentration of 0.77 mmol/L (2.4 mg/dL),

**XI-73.** *(Continued)*

and increased serum alkaline phosphatase activity. The serum parathyroid hormone level subsequently is found to be elevated as well. The most likely diagnosis is

A. Paget's disease of bone
B. ectopic parathyroid hormone secretion
C. primary hyperparathyroidism
D. postmenopausal osteoporosis
E. vitamin D deficiency

**XI-74.** Which of the following conditions is most likely to be associated with a normal serum 25(OH) vitamin D level?

A. Dietary deficiency of vitamin D
B. Chronic severe cholestatic liver disease
C. Chronic renal failure
D. Anticonvulsant therapy with phenobarbital or phenytoin
E. High-dose glucocorticoid therapy

**XI-75.** Four weeks postpartum, a 32-year-old female develops palpitations, heat intolerance, and nervousness. She is diagnosed with hyperthyroidism. Her thyroid is not enlarged or tender. The 24-h uptake of radioactive iodine is 1%. The most appropriate treatment for this patient is

A. radioactive iodine ablation of the thyroid gland
B. methimazole
C. prednisone 60 mg a day followed by a rapid taper
D. a beta blocker
E. iodine drops (SSKI)

**XI-76.** Which of the following statements concerning patients with polyglandular autoimmune syndrome type II (Schmidt's syndrome) is true?

A. The onset of this disease typically occurs during childhood.
B. It has an autosomal recessive mode of inheritance.
C. After Addison's disease, the second most common endocrine abnormality is hypothyroidism.
D. Mucocutaneous candidiasis is a typical hallmark of this syndrome.
E. Hypoparathyroidism is a common feature.

**XI-77.** Which of the following statements regarding erectile dysfunction is correct?

**XI-77.** *(Continued)*

A. Patients with testosterone deficiency are able to achieve erections with visual stimuli.
B. Patients with psychogenic erectile dysfunction have excess parasympathetic stimulation that decreases penile smooth muscle tone.
C. Both beta blockers and $\alpha$-adrenergic blockers are commonly implicated in erectile dysfunction.
D. Individuals with diabetes mellitus have normal levels of nitric oxide synthase in both endothelial and neural tissues.
E. Increased prolactin levels cause erectile dysfunction by directly reducing testicular androgen synthesis.

**XI-78.** Which of the following statements concerning the use of sildenafil for the treatment of erectile dysfunction is correct?

A. Sildenafil inhibits phosphodiesterase isoenzyme type V levels, thus increasing the concentration of cyclic AMP.
B. Sildenafil may cause a transient alteration in color vision.
C. Sildenafil may increase a patient's libido.
D. Sildenafil is hepatically cleared, and therefore no dose reduction is required for patients with impaired renal function.
E. Sildenafil is ineffective in the treatment of patients with diabetes mellitus who also have erectile dysfunction.

**XI-79.** A 30-year-old male, the father of three children, has had progressive breast enlargement during the last 6 months. He does not use any drugs. Laboratory evaluation reveals that both LH and testosterone are low. Further evaluation of this patient should include which of the following?

A. Blood sampling for serum glutamic-oxaloacetic transaminase (SGOT) and serum alkaline phosphatase and bilirubin levels
B. Measurement of estradiol and human chorionic gonadotropin (hCG) levels
C. A 24-h urine collection for the measurement of 17-ketosteroids
D. Karyotype analysis to exclude Klinefelter syndrome
E. Breast biopsy

# XI. ENDOCRINOLOGY AND METABOLISM

## *ANSWERS*

**XI-1.** **The answer is E.** *(Chap. 320)* Thyrotoxicosis factitia is characterized by exogenous of thyroid hormone. Radionuclide scans show low uptake. Unlike the situation in cases of thyroiditis, serum thyroglobulin levels are low or normal. Stuma ovarii and ectopic thyroid tissue are identified by evidence of uptake on whole-body radionuclide scans. Graves' disease is characterized by diffuse thyroid enlargement and increased uptake on uptake scanning.

**XI-2.** **The answer is D.** *(Chap. 333)* Osteoporosis is defined as a reduction of bone mass or density or the presence of a fragility fracture. Operationally, the WHO defines osteoporosis as a bone density more than 2.5 SD less than the mean for young healthy adults of the same race and sex. Dual-energy x-ray absorptiometry (DXA) is the most widely used study to determine bone density. Bone density is expressed as a *t*-score, that is, the SD below the mean of young adults of the same race and gender. A *t*-score higher than 2.5 characterizes osteoporosis, and a *t*-score less than 1 identifies patients at risk of osteoporosis. The *z*-score compares individuals with those in an age-, race-, and gender-matched population. The figure shows the relationship between *z*-scores and *t*-scores.

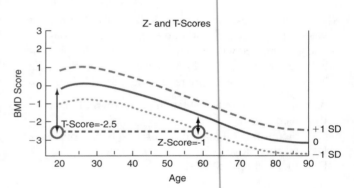

**XI-3.** **The answer is C.** *(Chap. 320)* This patient's history is most consistent with the thyrotoxic phase of subacute thyroiditis. The peak incidence occurs between ages 30 and 50. The etiology is usually viral. There is a significant female predominance. The low uptake on a radionuclide scan in the setting of a recent onset of a painful thyroid clearly points to subacute thyroiditis. Elevation in $T_4$ and $T_3$ points to the thyrotoxic phase rather than the hypothyroid phase. The patient would be expected to improve over the course of months, and so permanent ablation with radioiodine or surgery is inappropriate. Antithyroid medications such as methimazole and propylthiouracil (PTU) have no role because the pathophysiology of thyroiditis relates to destruction of the gland and hormonal release, not hyperactivity, as in the case of Graves' disease and multinodular goiter. Levothyroxine may play a role in the hypothyroid phase, but not while the patient is acutely thyrotoxic. Anti-inflammatory medications such as nonsteroidal anti-inflammatory drugs (NSAIDs) and steroids are most appropriate. Beta blockers would be appropriate if the patient were having more symptoms of thyrotoxicosis.

**XI-4.** **The answer is C.** *(Chap. 320)* Iodine deficiency is the most common worldwide cause of hypothyroidism. Autoimmune, or Hashimoto's, thyroiditis is a common cause in developed countries with dietary iodine supplementation. Histologically, it is characterized by lymphocytic infiltration of the thyroid with activated T cells and B cells. Thyroid cell destruction is thought to be mediated by cytotoxic CD8+ T lymphocytes. Primary hypothyroidism is characterized by an elevation in TSH as the feedback inhibition of the anterior pituitary is diminished. However, patients with hypothyroidism may have low TSH in the setting of secondary hypothyroidism. In this case, a clinical and radiologic evaluation of the pituitary is required. Subclinical hypothyroidism is characterized by abnormalities in the serum levels of TSH but minimal symptoms and often minimal change in the free $T_4$ level. The rate of development of overt, symptomatic hypothyroidism is about 4% per year, especially in the case of positive TPO antibodies, which are present in 90 to 95% of patients with autoimmune hypothyroidism.

**XI-5. The answer is E.** *(Chap. 320)* The thionamides propylthiouracil (PTU), carbimazole, and methimazole are the main antithyroid medications used for the treatment of hyperthyroidism. They all inhibit the function of thyroid peroxidase, reducing oxidation and organification of iodide. PTU also inhibits the deiodination of $T_4$ to $T_3$. PTU has a half-life much shorter than that of methimazole. Rash, urticaria, fever, and arthralgias are common side effects, occurring in up to 5% of these patients. They may resolve spontaneously. Major side effects are rare but include hepatitis, agranulocytosis, and a systemic lupus erythematosus (SLE)-like syndrome. If major side effects are noted, it is essential that antithyroid medications be stopped.

**XI-6. The answer is B.** *(Chap. 320)* Subacute thyroiditis, also known as de Quervain's thyroiditis, granulomatous thyroiditis, and viral thyroiditis, is characterized clinically by fever, constitutional symptoms, and a painful enlarged thyroid. The etiology is thought to be a viral infection. The peak incidence is between 30 and 50 years of age, and women are affected more frequently than are men. The symptoms depend on the phase of the illness. During the initial phase of follicular destruction, there is a release of thyroglobulin and thyroid hormones. As a result, there is increased circulating $T_4$ and $T_3$, with concomitant suppression of TSH. Symptoms of thyrotoxicosis predominate at this point. Radioiodine uptake is low or undetectable. After several weeks, thyroid hormone is depleted and a phase of hypothyroidism ensues, with low unbound $T_4$ levels and moderate elevations of TSH. Radioiodine uptake returns to normal. Finally, after 4 to 6 months, thyroid hormone and TSH levels return to normal as the disease subsides. Patient A is consistent with the thyrotoxic phase of subacute thyroiditis except for the increased radioiodine uptake scan. Patient C is more consistent with Graves' disease with suppression of TSH, an elevated uptake scan, and elevated thyroid hormones as a result of stimulating immunoglobulin. Patient D is consistent with a neoplasm. Patient E is consistent with central hypothyroidism.

**XI-7. The answer is D.** *(Chap. 333)* The epidemiology of fractures follows trends similar to those for loss of bone density. Fractures of the radius increase until age 50 and then plateau by age 60. There are approximately 250,000 wrist fractures each year in the United States. However, there are approximately 300,000 hip fractures annually, with incidence rates doubling every 5 years after age 70. The shift from arm and wrist fractures to hip fractures may be related to the way elderly people fall, with less frequent landing on the hands and more frequent direct hip trauma with increasing age. There are approximately 700,000 vertebral fractures each year in the United States. Most are clinically silent and rarely require hospitalization. They may lead to height loss, kyphosis, and pain secondary to altered biomechanics.

**XI-8 and XI-9. The answers are A and E.** *(Chap. 333)* Nonmodifiable risk factors for the development of osteoporosis include a personal history of fracture or a history of fracture in a first-degree relative, female sex, advanced age, and white race. African Americans have approximately one-half the risk of osteoporotic fractures as whites. Diseases that increase the risk of falls or frailty, such as dementia and Parkinson's disease, also increase fracture risk. Cigarette smoking, low body weight, low calcium intake, alcoholism, and lack of physical activity are all associated with increased bone loss and fractures. Multiple drugs are associated with an increased risk of osteoporosis. In addition to those listed, other anticonvulsants, cytotoxic drugs, excessive thyroxine, aluminum, gonadotropin-releasing hormone agonists, and lithium are associated with decreased bone mass and osteoporosis. Histamine antagonists are not associated with osteoporosis.

**XI-10. The answer is D.** *(Chap. 320)* Sick-euthyroid syndrome, or nonthyroidal illness, can occur in the setting of any acute, severe illness. Abnormalities in the levels of circulating TSH and thyroid hormone are thought to result from the release of cytokines in response to severe stress. Multiple abnormalities may occur. The most common hormone pattern is a decrease in total and unbound $T_3$ levels as peripheral conversion of $T_4$ to $T_3$ is impaired. Teleologically, the fall in $T_3$, the most active thyroid hormone, is thought to limit catabolism in starved or ill patients. TSH levels may vary dramatically, from 0.1 to >20 mU/L, depending on when they are measured during the course of illness. Very sick patients may have a decrease in $T_4$ levels. This patient undoubtedly has abnormal thyroid function tests as a result of his injuries from the motor vehicle accident. Administration of thyroid hormone replacement has been shown to improve outcomes in patients with nonthyroidal illness. There is no indication for obtaining further imaging in this case. Steroids have no role. The most appropriate management consists of simple observation. Over the course of weeks to months, as the patient recovers, thyroid function will return to normal.

**XI-11. The answer is B.** *(Chap. 324)* Factitious hypoglycemia from self-administration of insulin or ingestion of a sulfonylurea shares clinical and laboratory features with insulinoma. The absence of an elevated C peptide distinguishes exogenous insulin use from insulinoma. An undetectable sulfonylurea level works against a diagnosis of sulfonylurea toxicity. Factitious hypoglycemia is more common in health care workers, patients with diabetes and their relatives, and patients with psychiatric histories.

**XI-12 and XI-13. The answers are E and D.** *(Chap. 329)* The cardinal features of the carcinoid syndrome include diarrhea, flushing, and abdominal pain (see table). Other features, such as wheezing, pellagra, and heart failure, are less common. These patients are typically in their fifties, but the range of presentation spans adulthood to old age. Carcinoid tumors may secrete a variety of substances, including gastrointestinal (GI) peptides [gastrin, insulin, vasoactive intestinal peptide (VIP), glucagons], other peptides (ACTH, calcitonin), and bioactive amines (serotonin). Cardiac involvement is present in up to 40% of cases during the course of disease. Endocardial fibrosis, predominantly on the right side, is most common. This can result in pulmonic stenosis, tricuspid regurgitation, and right-sided heart failure. The carcinoid syndrome occurs when a sufficient concentration of secreted substance reaches the systemic circulation. This most commonly occurs (over 90% of cases) once there are metastases to the liver. Serotonin is a major product of carcinoid tumors that causes the typical carcinoid syndrome. In these patients increased amounts of the serotonin metabolite 5-HIAA is excreted in the urine and is the most frequently used diagnostic test. False positives may occur if the patient is eating serotonin-rich foods such as bananas, pineapple, and walnuts or is taking a medication such as guaifenesin, salicylates, acetaminophen, or L-dopa. Chronic myelogenous leukemia or systemic mastocytosis should be included in the differential diagnosis of typical carcinoid syndrome. The most common origin of liver metastases in the carcinoid syndrome is the ileum. Overall, carcinoid most commonly originates in the bronchi or lung, and this site may cause the carcinoid syndrome; however, bronchial/lung carcinoid does not usually cause metastatic disease (see table).

Clinical Characteristics in Patients with Carcinoid Syndrome

|  | At Presentation | During Course of Disease |
|---|---|---|
| Symptoms/signs |  |  |
| Diarrhea | 32–73% | 68–84% |
| Flushing | 23–65% | 63–74% |
| Pain | 10% | 34% |
| Asthma/wheezing | 4–8% | 3–18% |
| Pellagra | 2% | 5% |
| None | 12% | 22% |
| Carcinoid heart disease present | 11% | 14–41% |
| Demographics |  |  |
| Male | 46–59% | 46–61% |
| Age |  |  |
| Mean | 57 yr | 52–54 yr |
| Range | 25–79 yr | 9–91 yr |
| Tumor location |  |  |
| Foregut | 5–9% | 2–33% |
| Midgut | 78–87% | 60–87% |
| Hindgut | 1–5% | 1–8% |
| Unknown | 2–11% | 2–15% |

Carcinoid Tumor Location, Frequency of Metastases, and Association with the Carcinoid Syndrome

| | Location (% of Total) | Incidence of Metastases | Incidence of Carcinoid Syndrome |
|---|---|---|---|
| Foregut | | | |
| Esophagus | <0.1 | — | — |
| Stomach | 4.6 | 10 | 9.5 |
| Duodenum | 2.0 | — | 3.4 |
| Pancreas | 0.7 | 71.9 | 20 |
| Gallbladder | 0.3 | 17.8 | 5 |
| Bronchus, lung, trachea | 27.9 | 5.7 | 13 |
| Midgut | | | |
| Jejunum | 1.8 | }58.4 | 9 |
| Ileum | 14.9 | | 9 |
| Meckel's diverticulum | 0.5 | — | 13 |
| Appendix | 4.8 | 38.8 | <1 |
| Colon | 8.6 | 51 | 5 |
| Liver | 0.4 | 32.2 | — |
| Ovary | 1.0 | 32 | 50 |
| Testis | <0.1 | — | 50 |
| Hindgut | | | |
| Rectum | 13.6 | 3.9 | — |

*Source*: Location is from the PAN-SEER data (1973–1999), and incidence of metastases from the SEER data (1992–1999), reported by IM Modlin et al: Cancer 97:934, 2003. Incidence of carcinoid syndrome is from 4349 cases studied from 1950–1971, reported by JD Godwin: Cancer 36: 560, 1975.

**XI-14.** **The answer is E.** *(Chap. 44)* Hirsutism is defined as excessive male-pattern hair growth. It may represent a variation on the norm or be a prelude to a more serious underlying condition. Virilization refers to the state in which androgen levels are elevated enough to cause signs and symptoms of changes in voice, enlargement of genitalia, and increased libido. Virilization is a concerning sign for an ovarian or adrenal cause of excess androgen production. This patient's change in voice and body habitus heightens one's concern about a virilizing process. A thorough medication history is indicated because drugs such as phenytoin, minoxidil, and cyclosporine have been associated with androgen-dependent hair growth. Family history is critical in that some families have a higher incidence of hirsutism than others do. Congenital conditions such as congenital adrenal hyperplasia can show distinct patterns of inheritance. Androgens are secreted by both the ovaries and the adrenal glands. An elevation in plasma total testosterone above 12 nmol/L usually indicates a virilizing tumor. A basal DHEAS level above 18.5 $\mu$mol/L suggests an adrenal source. Therefore, checking both levels is a useful initial hormonal screen in evaluating virilization. Although polycystic ovarian syndrome is by far the most common cause of ovarian androgen excess, initial screening with ultrasound is not recommended. Polycystic ovaries may be found in females without any evidence of excess androgen secretion. Likewise, females may have an ovarian source of androgen secretion with only slightly enlarged ovaries on ultrasound. Therefore, ultrasound is an insensitive and nonspecific test.

**XI-15.** **The answer is E.** *(Chaps. 321 and 328)* Virilization secondary to androgen excess typically has an ovarian or adrenal source in response to the respective tropic hormones, luteinizing hormone (LH) and adrenocorticotropic hormone (ACTH). Optimal pharmacologic treatment depends on the source of excess androgens. In the case of congenital adrenal hyperplasia, an enzymatic defect impedes the ability of the adrenal glands to secrete glucocorticoids efficiently. This results in decreased negative feedback inhibition of ACTH and subsequent adrenal hyperplasia. Therefore, replacement with a glucocorticoid such as prednisone or dexamethasone is the mainstay of treatment for congenital adrenal hyperplasia (CAH). Oral contraceptives suppress the secretion of LH and are the mainstay of treatment for polycystic ovarian syndrome. In patients with a contraindication to oral contraceptive therapy, such as thromboembolic disease or breast cancer, direct antiandrogen therapy may be indicated. Cyproterone acetate directly inhibits the binding of testosterone and dihydrotestosterone to the androgen receptor. Spironolactone has weak antiandrogen properties but is effective at elevated doses. Fludracortisone is a direct mineralocorticoid and has no role in the treatment of androgen excess.

**XI-16. The answer is A.** *(Chap. 333)* A number of biochemical tests are used to assess the rate of bone remodeling. Bone remodeling is related to the rate of formation and resorption. Remodeling markers do not predict bone loss well enough to be applied clinically. However, measures of bone resorption may help in the prediction of risk of fracture in older patients. In women over 65 years old, even in the presence of normal bone density, a high index of bone resorption should prompt consideration for treatment. Measures of bone resortion fall quickly after the initiation of antiresorptive therapy (bisphosphonates, estrogen, raloxifene, calcitonin) and provide an earlier measure of response than does bone densitometry. Serum alkaline phosphatase is a measure of bone formation, not resorption, as are serum osteocalcin and serum propeptide of type I procollagen.

Biochemical Markers of Bone Metabolism in Clinical Use

Bone formation
  Serum bone-specific alkaline phosphatase
  Serum osteocalcin
  Serum propeptide of type I procollagen
Bone resorption
  Urine and serum cross-linked N-telopeptide
  Urine and serum cross-linked C-telopeptide
  Urine total free deoxypyridinoline
  Urine hydroxyproline
  Serum tartrate-resistant acid phosphatase
  Serum bone sialoprotein
  Urine hydroxylysine glycosides

**XI-17. The answer is A.** *(Chap. 333)* Osteoporosis is defined as a reduction of bone mass or the presence of a fragility fracture. A more specific definition is a bone density that is 2.5 SD below the mean for young healthy adults of the same race and gender. This is referred to as the *t*-score. Individuals with *t*-scores below 1 SD are at increased risk of osteoporosis. As many as 8 million to 10 million women and 2 million men in the United States have osteoporosis. Another 15 million to 20 million people are at risk (*t*-score more than 1 SD below the mean). Increasing age, white race, and female sex are the main predictors. Hip fracture is a common occurrence in the elderly. Up to 300,000 hip fractures occur yearly in the United States. The probability that a 50-year-old white female will have a hip fracture during her lifetime is up to 14%. Infection and thromboembolism are major causes of morbidity and mortality in patients with hip fractures, with between 20 and 50% of these patients having a deep venous thrombosis or pulmonary embolism.

**XI-18. The answer is E.** *(Chap. 333)* Osteoporosis results from bone loss caused by normal age-related changes in bone remodeling as well as extrinsic and intrinsic factors. Bone remodeling is regulated by several circulating hormones, including estrogens, androgens, vitamin D, and parathyroid hormone. Bone loss decreases calcium intake. The recommended daily intake is 1000 to 1200 mg for adults. Daily calcium intakes below 400 mg are associated with decreases in bone density. Vitamin D causes increased bone absorption in the intestine. It also promotes the hydroxylation of parathyroid hormone. Deficiency of vitamin D causes rickets in children and osteomalacia in adults. There is evidence that vitamin D deficiency may be more prevalent than previously was thought. Estrogen regulates the activation of bone remodeling sites and affects the balance between osteoblast and osteoclast activity. Deficiency secondary to ovarian failure promotes rapid bone loss and is responsible for the increased incidence of osteoporosis in women relative to men. Replacement is associated with bone remodeling, but recent studies have indicated a negative effect on cardiovascular health. Many medications result in bone loss. Glucocorticoids, anticonvulsants, and immunosuppressants are thought to contribute significantly to early bone loss. Physical activity is associated with higher bone mass than is inactivity. Fracture risk is lower in rural communities and in countries where physical activity is maintained into old age. Tobacco use is associated with bone loss.

**XI-19. The answer is D.** *(Chap. 333)* A large body of evidence shows that optimal calcium intake reduces bone loss and suppresses bone turnover. The preferred source of calcium is dairy products and other foods, but many patients require supplementation. Supplementation should be in doses of less than 600 mg at a time because absorption decreases at higher doses. The addition of vitamin D is beneficial, as has been shown in multiple trials. Exercise in younger individuals promotes the achievement of maximal bone mass. Although in older individuals exercise does not promote a large increase in bone mass, there probably is an improvement in neuromuscular function that aids in the prevention of falls and subsequent fractures. Although estrogen is effective in promoting bone mass and formation, multiple trials have suggested an adverse effect on cardiovascular morbidity and mortality, and there is considerable debate about the indications for estrogen replacement therapy. Selective estrogen receptor modulators (SERMs) have been shown to be useful in the prevention and treatment of osteoporosis. Raloxifene and tamoxifen have beneficial effects on bone density and help prevent bone loss. Raloxifene reduces the risk of vertebral fractures in certain populations and may not have the adverse cardiovascular effects of estrogen. It increases the occurrence of hot flashes and may not be optimal in women with significant menopausal symptoms. Its cardiovascular effects are being evaluated in a large pivotal study, Raloxifene Use for the Heart (RUTH), that should be available in the next few years. Tamoxifen also has beneficial effects on bone density. However, its use is restricted to patients with breast cancer. It has stimulating effects on the uterus and increases the risk of endometrial cancer. It has no role in the routine treatment of osteoporosis. Bisphosphonates are emerging as the first-line therapy for osteoporosis. They act to stabilize osteoclast activity and reduce bone resorption. Weekly alendronate has been shown to be equivalent to daily alendronate. Bisphosphonates must be given with a full glass of water and on an empty stomach to improve absorption. Some patients may experience esophageal irritation from reflux esophagitis. Other formulations of bisphosphonates are also effective (risidronate, zolendronate, etc.).

**XI-20. The answer is A.** *(Chap. 330)* This patient's clinical scenario is most consistent with MEN 1, or the "3 Ps": parathyroid, pituitary, and pancreas. MEN 1 is an autosomal dominant genetic syndrome characterized by neoplasia of the parathyroid, pituitary, and pancreatic islet cells. Hyperparathyroidism is the most common manifestation of MEN 1. The neoplastic changes affect multiple parathyroid glands, making surgical care difficult. Pancreatic islet cell neoplasia is the second most common manifestation of MEN 1. Increased pancreatic islet cell hormones include pancreatic polypeptide, gastrin, insulin, vasoactive intestinal peptide, glucagons, and somatostatin. Pancreatic tumors may be multicentric, and up to 30% are malignant, with the liver being the first site of metastases. The symptoms depend on the type of hormone secreted. Elevations of gastrin result in the Zollinger-Ellison syndrome (ZES). Gastrin levels are elevated, resulting in an ulcer diathesis. Conservative therapy is often unsuccessful. Insulinoma results in documented hypoglycemia with elevated insulin and C-peptide levels. Glucagonoma results in hyperglycemia, skin rash, anorexia, glossitis, and diarrhea. Elevations in vasoactive intestinal peptide result in profuse watery diarrhea. Pituitary tumors occur in up to half of patients with MEN 1. Prolactinomas are the most common. The multicentricity of the tumors makes resection difficult. Growth hormone–secreting tumors are the next most common, with ACTH- and corticotropin-releasing hormone (CRH)-secreting tumors being more rare. Carcinoid tumors may also occur in the thymus, lung, stomach, and duodenum.

**XI-21. The answer is B.** *(Chap. 333)* The Women's Health Initiative (WHI) demonstrated that estrogen-progestin therapy can reduce the risk of hip fractures by 34%. Other clinical trials have shown a decrease in all osteoporotic fractures, including vertebral compression fractures. The beneficial effect of estrogen appears to be maximal in those who start therapy early and continue taking the medication. The benefit declines after discontinuation, and there is no net benefit by 10 years after discontinuation. These effects are present for oral and transdermal formulations. However, the WHI also demonstrated that estrogens are associated with a 30% increase in myocardial infarction, a 40% increase in stroke, a 100% increase in venous thromboembolism, and a 25% increase in breast cancer. In the WHI study there was no overall effect of estrogen-progestin therapy on mortality, probably because of the balance between the detrimental cardiovascular effects and the beneficial effects (in addition to fractures, there was a beneficial effect on the development of colon cancer).

**XI-22.   The answer is C.**   *(Chap. 64)*   Obesity is a state of excess adipose tissue mass. Although body weight is often viewed as equivalent to adipose tissue mass, this is not always the case. Therefore, more objective measurements linked to morbidity and mortality have been formulated to provide a more accurate and practical guideline for physicians and patients. Body mass index is the most commonly used index to gauge obesity. It is equal to weight/height$^2$. Other methods, such as skin-fold measurements, underwater weighing, and electrical impedance, are used to varying degrees; however, because of its usefulness, ease of calculation, and correlation with outcome, BMI is the most widely used method to measure obesity. A BMI above 25 is associated with a substantially increased risk of all-cause, metabolic, cancer, and cardiovascular mortality. A BMI more than 30 is the formal definition of obesity. At this threshold, the risk of a poor outcome dramatically rises. A BMI between 25 and 30 is termed *overweight* by some authorities, although there is a movement to change the definition of obesity to a BMI over 25.

**XI-23.   The answer is E.**   *(Chap. 64)*   Obesity leads to a major increase in morbidity and mortality. Individuals who are more than 150% of their ideal body weight have as much as a 12-fold increase in mortality. Insulin resistance leading to diabetes mellitus is one of the most prominent features of obesity. The vast majority of patients with type 2 diabetes are obese. Weight loss to a moderate degree may be associated with improvements in insulin sensitivity. Obesity is an independent risk factor for cardiovascular disease. Obesity is associated with hypertension. The impact of obesity on cardiovascular mortality may be seen in persons with BMIs above 25. Obesity is associated with an increased incidence of cholesterol stones. Periodic fasting may increase the supersaturation of bile by decreasing the phospholipid component. Multiple studies have indicated increased mortality from cancer in obese individuals. Some of this increase may result from the increased conversion of androstenedione to estrone in adipose tissue. Obesity decreases chest wall compliance. Restrictive lung defects may occur in these individuals. Sleep apnea and obesity hypoventilation syndrome may occur. Although obesity may be associated with obstructive sleep apnea, it is not typically associated with other forms of chronic obstructive lung disease (COPD).

**XI-24.   The answer is C.**   *(Chap. 323)*   Diabetes mellitus is classified on the basis of the pathogenic process that leads to hyperglycemia. Type 1 DM results from destruction of the pancreas and impaired insulin secretion, typically through autoimmune processes. This usually occurs early in life and may be associated with certain autoantibodies. Type 2 DM is a heterogeneous group of disorders characterized by variable degrees of insulin resistance, impaired insulin secretion, and increased glucose production. Other etiologies for DM include specific genetic defects in insulin secretion or action, metabolic abnormalities, mitochondrial diseases, and other rare conditions that affect glucose tolerance. DM is increasing worldwide. Most of this increase is due to a rise in the prevalence of type 2 DM. There is significant geographic diversity in the prevalence of cases, with regions such as Scandinavia having the highest incidence of type 1 DM and the Pacific islands having the highest incidence of type 2 DM. There is clearly an interplay between genetic and environmental factors. The concordance of type 2 DM in identical twins ranges from 70 to 90%. The concordance of type 1 DM in identical twins is 30 to 70%. The reasons are unclear. In the United States, certain ethnic groups have a high prevalence of DM. African Americans and Hispanic Americans have high rates, but Native Americans have the highest, with a prevalence of nearly 15%. Similarly, although only a small percentage of females develop gestational diabetes during pregnancy, those females are at a much higher risk of developing overt DM.

**XI-25.   The answer is C.**   *(Chap. 332)*   The four parathyroid glands are located posterior to the thyroid gland. Parathyroid hormone is the primary regulator of calcium. PTH acts directly on bone and the kidney and indirectly, through the action of vitamin D, on the GI tract. Calcium induces calcium absorption from the kidney and bone. It stimulates hydroxylation of 25-hydroxyvitamin D, resulting in the more active form. Vitamin D stimulates calcium resorption from the GI tract. Calcium and vitamin D are part of a feedback loop that inhibits PTH release and synthesis. PTH prevents resorption of phosphate from the kidney.

**XI-26.   The answer is D.**   *(Chap. 332)*   Primary hyperparathyroidism and malignancy account for over 90% of cases of hypercalcemia. In asymptomatic patients, primary hyperparathyroidism is the most common cause. In patients admitted to the hospital with symptomatic hypercalcemia, malignancy is the most common cause. Calcium is regulated in bone, the gastrointestinal tract, and the kidney. Other causes of increased bone turnover include Paget's disease, immobilization, hyperthyroidism, hypervitaminosis A, and adrenal insufficiency. Causes of increased GI absorption include vitamin D intoxication and milk-alkali syndrome. Hypercalcemia from thiazide diuretics and familial hypocalciuric hypercalcemia result from disordered regulation of calcium in the kidney.

**XI-27.   The answer is A.**   *(Chap. 332)*   Hypercalcemia manifests in a variety of ways. "Stones, bones, groans, and psychiatric overtones" often is used on rounds as a way to remember the clinical symptoms and signs. Neurologic changes may range from depression to confusion and frank coma. These patients often are constipated and may have nausea, vomiting, and abdominal pain. Increased calcium may affect the genitourinary tract with nephrolithiasis, renal tubular acidosis, and polyuria. A shortened QT interval may result in cardiac arrhythmias.

**XI-28.   The answer is D.**   *(Chap. 332)*   FHH is inherited as an autosomal dominant trait. It results from a defect in serum calcium sensing by the parathyroid gland and renal tubule, causing inappropriate secretion of PTH and excessive renal reabsorption of calcium. The calcium-sensing receptor is sensitive to extracellular calcium concentration, suppressing PTH secretion and therefore resulting in negative-feedback regulation. Many different mutations in the calcium-sensing receptor have been described in patients with FHH. These mutations lower the ability of the sensor to bind calcium, resulting in excessive secretion of PTH and subsequent hypercalcemia. Urinary excretion of calcium is very low, with reabsorption more than 99%. The hypercalcemia is often detected in the first decade of life. This contrasts with primary hyperparathyroidism, which rarely occurs before age 10. Few clinical signs or symptoms are present in patients with FHH. These patients have excellent outcomes, and surgery or medical therapy is rarely necessary. Jansen's disease refers to mutations in the PTH receptor.

**XI-29.   The answer is E.**   *(Chap. 332)*   Causes of hypocalcemia may be classified on the basis of the action of parathyroid hormone (PTH). PTH is the primary regulator of calcium; therefore, for hypocalcemia to occur, the action of PTH must be ineffective. PTH may be absent in hereditary forms of hypoparathyroidism, acquired hypoparathyroidism, and hypomagnesemia. Magnesium affects the secretion of PTH, and correction of hypomagnesemia results in the return of plasma PTH levels to normal. Hereditary hypoparathyroidism may occur as an isolated entity or result from congenital malformations such as diGeorge syndrome. The action of PTH may be ineffective in cases of chronic renal failure, lack of dietary vitamin D, and receptor defects that cause pseudohypoparathyroidism. In cases of massive cell injury such as rhabdomyolysis and tumor lysis syndrome, the action of PTH may be overwhelmed.

**XI-30.   The answer is A.**   *(Chap. 322)*   Pheochromocytomas are derived from the adrenal medulla or the chromaffin cells in or about sympathetic ganglia. They produce, store, and

secrete catecholamines. Therefore, the symptoms and signs result from the excessive release of catecholamines. The symptoms include hypertension, headache, anxiety, tachycardia, and an increased metabolic rate. Symptoms may be episodic. In adults, the majority
of pheochromocytomas (more than 80%) are unilateral, solitary, and benign. There is an
inexplicable predominance of right-sided lesions. Occurrence is more common in women
and younger adults. Rarely, extraadrenal pheochromocytomas occur, usually in the abdomen in association with celiac, superior mesenteric, and inferior mesenteric ganglia.
Pheochromocytomas produce both norepinephrine and epinephirine. Diagnosis is made by
measuring urinary catecholamine metabolites such as vanillylmandelic acid, metanephrines, and other unconjugated catecholamines. Up to one-fourth of cases are associated
with familial syndromes such as multiple endocrine neoplasia, von Hippel–Lindau syndrome, and neurofibromatosis. Features that suggest familial disease include bilaterality,
multicentricity, and age of onset over 30 years. The treatment is primarily surgical. Surgery
or mechanical manipulation can result in a hypertensive crisis. $\alpha$-Adrenergic blockade is
essential before successful surgical treatment. Phenoxybenzamine is the most useful long-
lasting, noncompetitive $\alpha$-receptor blocker. Phenoxybenzamine should be administered up
to 2 weeks before surgery. Beta blockers should be administered only after alpha blockade
has been achieved because unopposed alpha stimulation and subsequent hypertensive
emergency may occur. Malignant pheochromocytoma frequently recurs in the retroperi-
toneum and commonly metastasizes to the lung and bone. It is typically resistant to radiotherapy. Combination chemotherapy may be beneficial.

**XI-31.**  **The answer is E.**  *(Chap. 335)*  Abetalipoproteinemia results from a mutation in the
gene that encodes microsomal transfer protein (MTP). MTP is essential for the packaging
of hepatic triglycerides with other major components of very low density lipoproteins
(VLDLs). This autosomal recessive disease results in extremely low cholesterol and triglyceride levels and an absence of chylomicrons, VLDL, and low-density lipoproteins
(LDLs). The clinical manifestations stem from defects in the absorption and transport of
fat-soluble vitamins. Lack of vitamin E results in spinocerebellar degeneration, which is
clinically manifested by decreased vibratory and proprioceptive sense, dysmetria, ataxia,
and the development of a spastic gait. Other clinical features include diarrhea, fat malabsorption, failure to thrive, pigmented retinopathy, and acanthocytosis. Symptoms and signs
develop in childhood. Treatment consists of low-fat, high-calorie diets that are enriched
with large supplemental doses of fat-soluble vitamins.

**XI-32.**  **The answer is A.**  *(Chap. 335)*  Lipoprotein lipase (LPL) and its cofactor apo CII are
required for the hydrolysis of triglycerides in chylomicrons and very low density lipoproteins (VLDLs). A genetic deficiency of either protein impairs lypolysis and results in an
elevation in plasma chylomicrons. VLDL is also elevated. The triglyceride-rich proteins
persist for days in the circulation, causing fasting levels higher than 1000 mg/dL. The
inheritance pattern is autosomal recessive. Heterozygotes have normal or mildly elevated
plasma triglyceride levels. Clinically, these patients may have repeated episodes of pancreatitis secondary to hypertriglyceridemia. Eruptive xanthomas may appear on the back,
the buttocks, and the extensor surfaces of the arms and legs. Hepatosplenomegaly may
result from the uptake of circulating chylomicrons by the reticuloendothelial cells. The
diagnosis is made by assaying triglyceride lipolytic activity in plasma. Dietary fat restriction is the treatment of choice.

**XI-33.**  **The answer is E.**  *(Chap. 335)*  Statins have emerged over the last decade as one of the
most clinically important classes of medications. Numerous studies have indicated important benefits in both primary and secondary prevention of cardiovascular disease. Statins
act by inhibiting HMG-CoA reductase, the rate-limiting step in cholesterol biosynthesis.
Statins are generally well tolerated, with an excellent safety profile over the years. However, attention must be paid to the side effects, which may be severe. Dyspepsia, headache,
fatigue, and myalgias may occur and are generally well tolerated. Myopathy and rhabdomyolysis are rare but serious side effects. The risk of myopathy is increased in the presence

of renal insufficiency and with concomitant use of certain medications, including some antibiotics, antifungal agents, some immunosuppressive drugs, and fibric acid derivatives. Hepatitis is another side effect. Liver transaminases should be checked before therapy is started and 4 to 8 weeks afterward. Elevations more than three times the normal range may mandate stopping therapy.

**XI-34. The answer is B.** *(Chap. 331)*    Hypophosphatemia results from one of three mechanisms: inadequate intestinal phosphate absorption, excessive renal phosphate excretion, and rapid redistribution of phosphate from the extracellular space into bone or soft tissue. Inadequate intestinal absorption is rare. Malnutrition from fasting or starvation may result in depletion of phosphate, causing hypophosphatemia during refeeding. In hospitalized patients, redistribution is the main cause. Insulin drives phosphate into cells. Sepsis may cause destruction of cells and metabolic acidosis, resulting in a net shift of phosphate from the extracellular space into cells. Renal failure is associated with hyperphosphatemia, not hypophosphatemia.

**XI-35. The answer is A.** *(Chap. 326)*    This patient has dysfunctional uterine bleeding. The most likely cause in a woman with a prior history of normal menses is anovulatory cycles. This is not due to a structural abnormality in the uterus or cervix but instead to an interruption in the normal sequence of the follicular and luteal phases of the menstrual cycle. Primary dysfunctional uterine bleeding may result from one of three disorders: estrogen withdrawal bleeding, estrogen breakthrough bleeding, and progesterone breakthrough bleeding. Estrogen withdrawal bleeding occurs when estrogen is given to a castrate or postmenopausal female and then withdrawn. Estrogen breakthrough bleeding occurs when there is continuous estrogen stimulation of the endometrium without interruption by cyclic progesterone secretion and withdrawal. This is the most common presentation and usually results from anovulatory cycles. This patient's running may be the etiology. Polycystic ovarian syndrome is another common cause in young females. Other causes include estrogen-secreting tumors and chronic estrogen replacement therapy. Progesterone withdrawal bleeding may occur in patients taking chronic low-dose oral contraceptives. In this case, administration of progesterone or oral contraceptives may serve to regulate the cycle and stimulate proper ovulation and menses. Withdrawal of progesterone will cause menstrual bleeding and confirm that anovulation with estrogen present is the cause. Evaluation for a structural defect, pituitary tumor, or genetic abnormality is not warranted in the initial workup.

**XI-36 and XI-37. The answers are E and E.** *(Chap. 329)*    In patients with a nonmetastatic carcinoid, surgery is the only potentially curative therapy. The extent of surgical resection depends on the size of the primary tumor because the risk of metastasis is related to the size of the tumor. Symptomatic treatment is aimed at decreasing the amount and effect of circulating substances. Drugs that inhibit the serotonin 5-$HT_1$ and 5-$HT_2$ receptors (methysergide, cyproheptadine, ketanserin) may control diarrhea but not flushing. 5-$HT_3$ receptor antagonists (odansetron, tropisetron, alosetron) control nausea and diarrhea in up to 100% of these patients and may alleviate flushing. A combination of histamine $H_1$ and $H_2$ receptor antagonists may control flushing, particularly in patients with foregut carcinoid tumors. Somatostatin analogues (octreotide, lanreotide) are the most effective and widely used agents to control the symptoms of carcinoid syndrome, decreasing urinary 5-HIAA excretion and symptoms in 70 to 80% of patients. Interferon $\alpha$, alone or combined with hepatic artery embolization, controls flushing and diarrhea in 40 to 85% of these patients. Phenoxybenzamine is an $\alpha_1$-adrenergic receptor blocker that is used in the treatment of pheochromocytoma.

Carcinoid crisis is a life-threatening complication of carcinoid syndrome. It is most common in patients with intense symptoms from foregut tumors or markedly high levels of urinary 5-HIAA. The crisis may be provoked by surgery, stress, anesthesia, chemotherapy, or physical trauma to the tumor (biopsy or, in this case, physical compression of liver lesions). These patients develop severe typical symptoms plus systemic symptoms such as hypotension and hypertension with tachycardia. Synthetic analogues of somato-statin (octreotide, lanreotide) are the treatment of choice for carcinoid crisis. They are also effective in preventing crises when administered before a known inciting event. Octreotide 150 to 250 $\mu$g subcutaneously every 6 to 8 h should be started 24 to 48 h before a procedure that is likely to precipitate a carcinoid crisis.

**XI-38. The answer is D.** *(Chap. 326)* Premature ovarian failure is used to describe women who cease menstruating before age 40. The ovaries in those women contain few or no follicles as a result of accelerated atresia. This may also result from autoimmune processes either alone or as part of a polyglandular failure. Low output of estrogens from the ovary results in increased FSH and LH levels from the pituitary. The elevated FSH and LH are not consistent with a pituitary process. Asherman's syndrome results from destruction and fibrosis of the endometrium and does not cause a hormone imbalance. A genetic cause such as Turner syndrome typically has a characteristic body habitus. Patients with poly-cystic ovarian syndrome typically have menstrual abnormalities from childhood, have elevated estrogen levels, and have an increased ratio of LH to FSH because of positive feedback on LH secretion and negative feedback on FSH secretion.

**XI-39. The answer is D.** *(Chap. 323)* Diabetic ketoacidosis is an acute complication of dia-betes mellitus. It results from a relative or absolute deficiency of insulin combined with a counterregulatory hormone excess. In particular, a decrease in the ratio of insulin to glu-cagons promotes gluconeogenesis, glycogenolysis, and the formation of ketone bodies in the liver. Ketosis results from an increase in the release of free fatty acids from adipocytes, with a resultant shift toward ketone body synthesis in the liver. This is mediated by the relationship between insulin and the enzyme carnitine palmitoyltransferase I. At physio-logic pH, ketone bodies exist as ketoacids, which are neutralized by bicarbonate. As bi-carbonate stores are depleted, acidosis develops. Clinically, these patients have nausea, vomiting, and abdominal pain. They are dehydrated and may be hypotensive. Lethargy and severe central nervous system depression may occur. The treatment centers on re-placement of the body's insulin, which will result in cessation of the formation of ketoacids and improvement of the acidotic state. Assessment of the level of acidosis may be done with an arterial blood gas. These patients have an anion gap acidosis and often a concom-itant metabolic alkalosis resulting from volume depletion. Volume resuscitation with in-travenous fluids is critical. Many electrolyte abnormalities may occur. Patients are total body sodium-, potassium-, and magnesium-depleted. As a result of the acidosis, intracel-lular potassium may shift out of cells and cause a normal or even elevated potassium level. However, with improvement in the acidosis, the serum potassium rapidly falls. Therefore, potassium repletion is critical despite the presence of a "normal" level. Because of the osmolar effects of glucose, fluid is drawn into the intravascular space. This results in a drop in the measured serum sodium. There is a drop of 1.6 meq/L in serum sodium for each rise of 100 mg/dL in serum glucose. In this case, the serum sodium will improve with hydration alone. The use of 3% saline is not indicated because the patient has no neurologic deficits, and the expectation is for rapid resolution with intravenous fluids alone.

**XI-40. The answer is A.** *(Chap. 323)* The DCCT found definitive proof that reduction in chronic hyperglycemia can prevent many of the early complications of type 1 DM. This multicenter randomized trial enrolled over 1400 patients with type 1 DM to either intensive or conventional diabetes management and prospectively evaluated the development of retinopathy, nephropathy, and neuropathy. The intensive group received multiple admin-istrations of insulin daily along with education and psychological counseling. The intensive group achieved a mean hemoglobin $A_{1C}$ of 7.3% versus 9.1% in the conventional group. Improvement in glycemic control resulted in a 47% reduction in retinopathy, a 54% re-duction in nephropathy, and a 60% reduction in neuropathy. There was a nonsignificant trend toward improvement in macrovascular complications. The results of the DCCT showed that individuals in the intensive group would attain up to 7 more years of intact vision and up to 5 more years free from lower limb amputation. Later, the United Kingdom

Prospective Diabetes Study (UKPDS) studied over 5000 individuals with type 2 DM. Individuals receiving intensive glycemic control had a reduction in microvascular events but no significant change in macrovascular complications. These two trials were pivotal in showing a benefit of glycemic control in reducing microvascular complications in patients with type 1 and type 2 DM, respectively. Another result from the UKPDS was that strict blood pressure control resulted in an improvement in macrovascular complications.

**XI-41. The answer is D.** *(Chap. 333)* The selective estrogen receptor modulators (SERMs) tamoxifen and raloxifene act in a fashion similar to that of estrogen in decreasing bone turnover and bone loss in postmenopausal women. These agents have been shown to decrease the risk of invasive breast cancer. Raloxifene, which is approved for the prevention of osteoporosis, reduces the risk of vertebral fractures by 30 to 50%. There are no data confirming a similar effect on nonvertebral fractures. Optimal calcium intake reduces bone loss and suppresses bone turnover. Vitamin D plus calcium supplements have been shown to reduce the risk of hip fractures by 20 to 30%. The bisphosphonates alendronate and risedronate are structurally related to pyrophosphate and are incorporated into bone matrix. They reduce the number of osteoclasts and impair the function of those already present. Both have been shown to reduce the risk of vertebral and hip fractures by 40 to 50%. One trial found that risedronate reduced hip fractures in osteoporotic women in their seventies but not in older women without osteoporosis. Risedronate may be administered weekly. The newer bisphosphonates zoledronate and ibandronate may be dosed yearly or monthly. An daily injection of exogenous parathyroid hormone analogue superimposed on estrogen therapy produced increases in bone mass and decreased vertebral and nonvertebral fractures by 45 to 65%. There are no published studies of combinations of parathyroid hormone and SERMs or bisphosphonates.

**XI-42. The answer is D.** *(Chap. 333)* Glucocorticoid-induced osteoporosis and subsequent fractures are among the most devastating complications of long-term steroid therapy. Glucocorticoids increase bone loss through inhibition of osteoblast function, inhibition of osteoblast apoptosis, stimulation of bone resorption, impairment of intestinal absorption of calcium, increases in urinary excretion of calcium, suppression of normal estrogen and androgen secretion, and induction of steroid myopathy that decreases physical activity. It is important that patients receiving glucocorticoids have adequate calcium and vitamin D intake. Patients receiving long-term (more than 6 months) glucocorticoids should have measurements of bone density. Only bisphosphonates have reduced the risk of fractures in patients receiving glucocorticoids. Calcitonin has some beneficial effect on spine density. Thiazide diuretics reduce urinary calcium excretion but do not have a proven role in reducing fractures. Estrogen is not advised for use in men simply to reduce bone loss.

**XI-43. The answer is D.** *(Chap. 325)* Measurement of luteinizing hormone (LH) or follicle-stimulating hormone (FSH) will distinguish primary from secondary hypogonadism in men with reduced serum testosterone levels. Elevations in LH and FSH suggest primary gonadal dysfunction, whereas normal or reduced LH and FSH suggest a central hypothalamic-pituitary defect. Patients with chronic illness such as HIV, end-stage renal disease, COPD, and cancer and patients receiving chronic corticosteroids have a high frequency of hypogonadism that is associated with muscle wasting. There are some reports of reversal of hypogonadism in patients with end-stage renal disease on hemodialysis after a renal transplant.

**XI-44. The answer is C.** *(Chap. 325)* Many drugs may interfere with testicular function through a variety of mechanisms. Cyclophosphamide damages the seminiferous tubules in a dose- and time-dependent fashion and causes azospermia within a few weeks of initiation. This effect is reversible in approximately half these patients. Ketoconazole inhibits testosterone synthesis. Spironolactone causes a blockade of androgen action. Glucocorticoids lead to hypogonadism predominantly through inhibition of hypothalamic-pituitary function. Sexual dysfunction has been described as a side effect of therapy with beta blockers. However, there is no evidence of an effect on testicular function. Most reports of sexual dysfunction were in patients receiving older beta blockers such as propranolol and timolol.

**XI-45.  The answer is C.**  *(Chap. 327)*   Menopause is characterized by several symptoms, including hot flashes, vaginal dryness, depression, and cessation of menstrual cycles for 12 months. Laboratory evaluation is imperfect; however, in general, a high FSH level coupled with a low estradiol level predicts ovarian failure and menopause. LH also rises in menopause, but it can be elevated during the preovulatory gonadotropin surge during a normal menstrual cycle. Symptoms of menopause can be debilitating for some women. Furthermore, hormone replacement therapy (HRT), which reduces symptoms, including hot flashes and vaginal dryness, has been said to offer many benefits to postmenopausal women other than symptom relief. Data from randomized clinical trials support the statement that HRT reduces symptoms of menopause, including vasomotor symptoms and genitourinary symptoms. The Women's Health Initiative study demonstrated significantly fewer hip and total fractures among patients randomly assigned to continuous combination therapy versus placebo. Similar randomized controlled trials have shown decreased urinary tract infections in HRT-treated women versus those receiving placebo. Decreased cardiovascular mortality was touted as a benefit of HRT for many years. However, recent data derived from the HERS trial, in which women were randomized to estrogen-progestin therapy or placebo and followed prospectively for 4 years, showed a 50% increase in the risk of coronary events in the first year in the treatment arm of the cohort. Other trials in both primary and secondary prevention of cardiovascular disease suggest that HRT may cause an increased risk of cardiovascular events and certainly is not better than placebo. Thus, HRT can no longer be recommended to decrease the incidence or progression of cardiovascular disease.

**XI-46.  The answer is B.**  *(Chap. 337)*   Acute intermittent porphyria (AIP) is one of a collection of disorders characterized by enzyme dysfunction in the heme biosynthetic pathway. Heme is synthesized in the bone marrow and liver, and mutations in the gene generally affect one organ system or the other. For instance, the erythropoietic porphyrias, including porphyria cutanea tarda (PCT), have primarily dermatologic manifestations, whereas AIP is a hepatic porphyria that presents with intermittent abdominal pain, peripheral neuropathy caused by axonal degeneration, and psychiatric symptoms that include paranoia, depression, anxiety, and hallucinations. During an attack of AIP, the precursors to heme build up. The diagnosis is made by demonstrating elevated levels of these precursors, most commonly porphyrobilinogen, during the episode. The porphyrobilinogen level will drop in the recovery phase and can be normal when the patient is well. These patients often have triggers of attacks, including menstruation, steroids, calorie restriction, alcohol, and numerous drugs. PCT, in contrast, is triggered by sunlight, with the development of the classic vesicular rash in exposed areas. PCT is closely associated with mild iron overload, and many of these patients also have hemochromatosis-causing mutations such as HFE C282Y. This mutation, however, is not associated with AIP.

**XI-47.  The answer is B.**  *(Chap. 329)*   The Zollinger-Ellison syndrome (ZES) is caused by a neuroendocrine tumor that secretes gastrin. Chronic hypergastrinemia causes acid hypersecretion, growth of gastric mucosa, an increased number of parietal cells, and proliferation of gastric enterochromaffin-like (ECL) cells. The acid hypersecretion usually causes severe peptic ulcer disease that is often refractory to treatment. At endoscopy, the ulcers are usually duodenal but may be multiple and in unusual locations. Prominent gastric folds are also a typical feature of gastrinoma. Diarrhea is common in patients with gastrinoma, and the combination of duodenal ulcer and diarrhea should raise the suspicion of this diagnosis. Approximately 20 to 25% of patients with gastrinoma have the multiple endocrine neoplasia syndrome type 1 (MEN 1). *Helicobacter pylori* is present in less than 50% of patients with peptic ulcer disease caused by gastrinoma in contrast to its presence in more than 90% of patients with typical peptic ulcer disease. The diagnosis of ZES requires demonstration of fasting hypergastrinemia and increased basal acid output. The differential diagnosis includes *H. pylori* infection, antral G cell hyperplasia, gastric outlet obstruction, and renal failure. The secretin provocative test can confirm the diagnosis of gastrinoma. Normally, an intravenous infusion of secretin causes a decrease in serum gastrin concentration; however, gastrinoma cells respond paradoxically with an increase in serum gastrin. Serum chromogranin A may be elevated in any GI neuroendocrine tumor and is not specific for gastrinoma. Antigliadin antibodies are present in gluten-sensitive enteropathy. The urease test on gastric biopsies is used to detect the presence of *H. pylori*. A positive PAS stain on duodenal biopsy is diagnostic of Whipple disease.

**XI-48. The answer is B.** *(Chap. 329)* The differential diagnosis of a patient with symptomatic hypoglycemia during fasting includes insulinoma and surreptitious insulin (or oral hypoglycemic agents) use. Insulinomas occur typically in patients 40 to 50 years old and present with neuropsychiatric symptoms consistent with hypoglycemia. Coma may occur in severe cases. Symptoms caused by the appropriate catecholamine response are also usually present. The catecholamine response is responsible for the ability of the symptoms to resolve without therapy. Insulinomas arise in the pancreas and are usually small, solitary, and not malignant (85 to 95%). They may be associated with MEN 1. Insulin is synthesized as proinsulin with $\alpha$ and $\beta$ chains connected by C peptide. In insulinomas, during episodes of hypoglycemia (usually provoked by a monitored fast), serum insulin and C-peptide levels are elevated. Exogenous insulin does not include the C-peptide fraction. Surreptitious insulin use is characterized by hypoglycemia, elevated serum insulin, and low C peptide. It most commonly occurs as a component of psychiatric illness in health care workers who have access to insulin or oral hypoglycemic agents.

**XI-49. The answer is C.** *(Chap. 329)* This patient presents with the classic findings of a VIPoma, including large-volume watery diarrhea, hypokalemia, dehydration, and hypochlorhydria (WDHA, or Verner-Morrison, syndrome). Abdominal pain is unusual. The presence of a secretory diarrhea is confirmed by a stool osmolal gap [2(stool Na + stool K) − (stool osmolality)] < 35 and persistence during fasting. In osmotic or laxative-induced diarrhea, the stool osmolal gap is over 100. In adults, over 80% of VIPomas are solitary pancreatic masses that usually are larger than 3 cm at diagnosis. Metastases to the liver are common and preclude curative surgical resection. The differential diagnosis includes gastrinoma, laxative abuse, carcinoid syndrome, and systemic mastocytosis. Diagnosis requires the demonstration of large-volume secretory diarrhea (over 700 mL/d) and elevated serum VIP. CT scan of the abdomen will often demonstrate the pancreatic mass and liver metastases.

---

Contraindications for Androgen Replacement

- The presence or history of prostate cancer
- Baseline PSA $\geq$ 4 ng/mL or a palpable abnormality of the prostate without urologic evaluation to rule out prostate cancer
- Severe symptoms of lower urinary tract obstruction as indicated by IPSS or AUA symptom score of $\geq$22
- Baseline hematocrit >52%
- Severe sleep apnea
- Class IV congestive heart failure

---

*Note*: PSA, prostate-specific antigen; IPSS, International Prostate Symptom Score; AUA, American Urological Association.

**XI-50. The answer is B.** *(Chap. 325)* Testosterone replacement therapy is indicated in men with testosterone levels below 250 ng/dL. This treatment can improve libido, increase bone density, increase energy and well-being, and increase lean muscle mass. These effects have been found only in men with documented androgen deficiency. The aim of therapy is to restore testosterone levels to the midnormal range. Oral agents do not provide adequate sustained levels for chronic replacement. Transdermal patches, gel formulations, and injectable formulations provide sustained adequate levels. Testosterone replacement is contraindicated in patients with prostate carcinoma because the androgens may promote tumor growth. Other adverse effects and potential contraindications (see table) include worsening of prostatic hypertrophy, increased hematocrit (3 to 5%), and worsening of sleep apnea symptoms.

**XI-51 and XI-52. The answers are C and B.** *(Chap. 323)* Screening for diabetes mellitus with fasting plasma glucose measurement is indicated in all adults over 45 years old every 3 years and earlier in individuals with additional risk factors. Once the results are obtained, they can be interpreted in light of the revised diagnostic criteria issued by the National Diabetes Data Group and the World Health Organization. Currently, normal fasting plasma glucose is less than 110 mg/dL. Impaired fasting glucose is defined by values greater than 110 mg/dL but less than 126 mg/dL. Diabetes mellitus is diagnosed when fasting plasma glucose is 126 mg/dL or higher. In addition, any individual with symptoms of hyperglycemia and a random glucose >200 mg/dL can be diagnosed as having diabetes mellitus. Hemoglobin $A_{1C}$, though a useful marker of glycemic control in individuals who have a diagnosis of diabetes, is not used in screening or diagnosing diabetes mellitus. This patient meets the criteria for impaired fasting glucose. The diagnosis of impaired fasting glucose is important to make, as it is associated with an increased risk of cardiovascular disease. Furthermore, 40% of individuals with impaired fasting glucose levels will develop frank diabetes in the next decade; thus, close observation is indicated. It is important to note that screening for diabetes mellitus is aimed at identifying persons with type 2 disease. Patients with type 1 diabetes mellitus have a relatively short time delay between pancreatic pathology and the development of symptoms and thus have early presentations. Screening is not indicated for this population. However, many patients with type 2 diabetes mellitus have a long period of asymptomatic hyperglycemia. It is preferable to identify these patients earlier to prevent microvascular complications in the future.

**XI-53 and XI-54.   The answers are C and E.**   *(Chaps. 330 and 332)*   Asymptomatic hypercalcemia in a young person with a positive family history should raise the suspicion of multiple endocrine neoplasia type 1 (MEN 1). MEN 1 is inherited in an autosomal dominant fashion and is characterized by hyperplasia/neoplasia of the parathyroid, pancreatic islet, pituitary, and other neuroendocrine cell types. It does not involve the thyroid or cause Graves' disease. The disease has variable penetrance of the neoplastic components, making the diagnosis difficult at times. These patients may be asymptomatic or develop typical symptoms of hypercalcemia. Hypercalcemia of MEN 1 may be due to multicentric parathyroid hyperplasia (more common in younger patients) or multicentric parathyroid adenomas (more common in older patients). The diagnosis of hyperparathyroidism requires a normal or high intact parathyroid hormone level concurrent with an elevated total and/or ionized calcium. Vitamin D intoxication is also a cause of hypercalcemia, but in the absence of oral intake or granulomatous disease and with a positive family history this is less likely. Pancreatic islet tumors related to MEN 1 secrete hormones such as pancreatic polypeptide (75 to 85%); gastrin (60%), the cause of Zollinger-Ellison syndrome; insulin (25 to 35%); glucagons (5 to 10%); and VIP (3 to 5%). Approximately 25% of all patients with Zollinger-Ellison syndrome have MEN 1. 30 to 35% of pancreatic tumors are malignant and may metastasize to the liver. Patients suspected of having MEN 1 should be screened regularly for the development of pancreatic islet tumors. Pituitary adenomas occur in >50% of patients with MEN 1. Prolactinomas are the most common, followed by adenomas that secrete growth hormone (acromegaly) and ACTH (Cushing's disease). Carcinoid tumors also may develop in MEN 1 patients and occur in the lung, thymus, stomach, or duodenum (foregut origin). These tumors may be locally invasive or may metastasize. Mutations in the *MEN1* gene are found in >90% of these patients. Genetic screening to identify carriers and persons at risk of disease is commercially available.

**XI-55.   The answer is C.**   *(Chap. 330)*   A thyroid nodule containing malignant C cells that stain positive for calcitonin is diagnostic of medullary thyroid carcinoma (MTC). These tumors typically arise in the upper regions of the thyroid where most C cells are located and metastasize early to regional lymph nodes in the neck. Most (80%) MTCs occur sporadically, typically in patients 40 to 50 years old. Occurrence in a young patient makes MEN 2A or MEN 2B likely. MEN 2A is an autosomal dominant syndrome characterized by MTC, hyperparathyroidism, and pheochromocytoma (see table). Pheochromocytoma occurs in approximately 50% of patients with MEN 2A, and half of those pheochromocytomas are bilateral. Hyperparathyroidism occurs in 15 to 20% of these patients and clinically is indistinguishable from primary hyperparathyroidism. Familial MTC is a subvariant of MEN 2A without pheochromocytoma. MEN 2B is also autosomal dominant and is characterized by MTC, pheochromocytoma, mucosal neuromas, intestinal ganglioneuro-matosis, and marfanoid features. MEN 2B develops at a younger age and is more aggres-sive than MEN 2A. Death from MTC can be prevented with early thyroidectomy, and so early diagnosis and screening of family members is indicated. MEN 2 is associated with mutations in the *RET* protooncogene. Screening for pheochromocytoma in asymptomatic patients with known MEN 2 is also indicated because of the risk of morbidity during surgery. Children with identified *RET* mutations characteristic for MEN 2B should be considered for early thyroidectomy. In patients with extensive metastatic disease, radiation or chemotherapy may provide palliative, not curative, relief.

Disease Associations in the Multiple Endocrine Neoplasia (MEN) Syndromes

| MEN 1 | MEN 2 | Mixed Syndromes |
|---|---|---|
| Parathyroid hyperplasia or ad-enoma | MEN 2A | von Hippel–Lindau syndrome, pheochromocytoma, islet cell tumor, renal cell carcinoma, hemangioblastoma of central nervous system, retinal angi-oma |
| Islet cell hyperplasia, ade-noma, or carcinoma | MTC | |
| | Pheochromocytoma | |
| Pituitary hyperplasia or ade-noma | Parathyroid hyperplasia or adenoma | |
| | Cutaneous lichen amyloidosis | |
| Other less common manifesta-tions: foregut carcinoid, pheochromocytoma, subcuta-neous or visceral lipomas | Hirschsprung disease | Neurofibromatosis with fea-tures of MEN 1 or 2 |
| | Familial MTC | Carney complex |
| | MEN 2B | Myxomas of heart, skin, and breast |
| | MTC | |
| | Pheochromocytoma | Spotty cutaneous pigmentation |
| | Mucosal and gastrointestinal neuromas | Testicular, adrenal, and GH-producing pituitary tumors |
| | Marfanoid features | Peripheral nerve schwannoma |

*Note*: MTC, medullary thyroid carcinoma.

**XI-56. The answer is D.** *(Chap. 323)* The patient is admitted with diabetic ketoacidosis as manifest by an anion gap acidosis that features positive serum ketones and hyperglycemia. Insulin is administered to allow cells to take up glucose and, perhaps more important, interrupt the process of fatty acid breakdown in the liver that results in ketogenesis. In addition, hyperglycemia results in an osmotic diuresis, and patients with this disorder are generally profoundly dehydrated and require intravenous hydration. Concomitant electro-lyte disorders are common. Appropriately, this patient is given both intravenous insulin and normal saline. Decisions regarding further management of diabetic ketoacidosis are guided by blood chemistries. The insulin infusion, which disrupts ketogenesis, must not be discontinued until the anion gap has been closed. In this case, the anion gap persists at the time of the second blood chemistries. As the patient's glucose is approaching normal levels and the anion gap is still open, requiring insulin infusion, the most appropriate next step is to stop normal saline infusion and begin infusion of 5% dextrose normal saline. In this way, hypoglycemia will be prevented and the insulin drip can continue. Once the diagnosis of ketoacidosis is made and ketones are initially demonstrated in the blood, it is not necessary to check repeat measurements. In fact, the primary ketone, $\beta$-hydroxybu-tyrate, is synthesized at three times the rate of the synthesis of acetoacetate, which is preferentially detected by commonly available assays. During its degradation process, $\beta$-hydroxybutyrate is converted to acetoacetate; thus, measured ketone levels may actually rise when diabetic ketoacidosis has been interrupted and is resolving.

**XI-57 and XI-58. The answers are D and E.** *(Chap. 323)* Tight glycemic control with a hemoglobin $A_{1C}$ of 7% or less has been shown in the Diabetes Control and Complications Trial (DCCT) in type 1 diabetic patients and the United Kingdom Prospective Diabetes Study (UKPDS) in type 2 diabetic patients to lead to improvements in microvascular disease. Notably, a decreased incidence of neuropathy, retinopathy, microalbuminuria, and nephropathy was shown in individuals with tight glycemic control. Interestingly, glycemic control had no effect on macrovascular outcomes. Instead, it was blood pressure control to at least moderate goals (142/88 mmHg) in the UKPDS that resulted in a decreased incidence of macrovascular outcomes, namely, DM-related death, stroke, and heart failure. Improved blood pressure control also resulted in improved microvascular outcomes.

**XI-59. The answer is E.** *(Chap. 323)*   Dyslipidemia is common among diabetic patients, and current recommendations are to screen aggressively for and treat abnormalities that are identified. The most common forms of dyslipidemia in diabetic patients are hypertriglyceridemia and reduced high-density lipoprotein (HDL) levels. Elevated levels of LDL cholesterol are not more common among diabetic patients; however, they are more atherogenic and are noted to be smaller and denser. LDL particles are more easily glycated and are more susceptible to oxidation in diabetic patients. This finding has led to the recommendation of many organizations, including the American Heart Association and the National Cholesterol Education Program, that patients with diabetes mellitus, regardless of their history of cardiovascular disease, have a goal LDL of less than 100 mg/dL. The American Heart Association also recommends the following targets: HDL >45 mg/dL in men and >55 mg/dL in women and triglycerides <150 mg/dL.

**XI-60. The answer is B.** *(Chap. 323)*   In the initial decision about which hypoglycemic agent to use, one must take into account the comorbidities of the patient and relative contraindications. Insulin secretagogues, $\alpha$-glucosidase inhibitors, thiazolidinediones, biguanides, and insulin are all approved for monotherapy for diabetes. In light of the extensive clinical experience and generally acceptable safety profile, most patients are initially started on either a sulfonylurea or metformin. Although this regimen is generally very well tolerated, it is important to note that sulfonylureas are contraindicated for those with significant hepatic and liver dysfunction. Glipizide is primarily cleared by the liver and should be used preferentially in patients with mild to moderate renal dysfunction. Hypoglycemia is more common with sulfonylureas than it is with metformin. Metformin often causes gastrointestinal side effects with nausea, vomiting, and diarrhea. The most feared complication of metformin therapy is lactic acidosis. The risk of lactic acidosis is increased in patients with heart failure, liver disease, severe hypoxia, any form of acidosis, intravenous contrast administration, and renal insufficiency. Current recommendations are to avoid metformin in men with creatinine higher than 1.5 mg/dL and women with creatinine higher than 1.4 mg/dL. Thiazolidinediones reduce insulin resistance, and older generations of this class of drugs are associated with liver toxicity. The association of hepatotoxicity with rosiglitazone and pioglitazone is less well established; however, currently the U.S. Food and Drug Administration (FDA) recommends avoiding the use of these drugs in patients with liver disease and frequent monitoring of liver function testing in patients who are taking them. They are associated with exacerbations of congestive heart failure and peripheral edema. Of note, this class of drugs has been shown to induce ovulation in women with polycystic ovarian syndrome, and premenopausal women should be warned about an increased incidence of pregnancy.

**XI-61. The answer is B.** *(Chap. 336)*   In persons with symptomatic hemochromatosis, repeated phlebotomy, by removing excessive iron stores, results in marked clinical improvement. Specifically, the liver and spleen decrease in size, liver function improves, cardiac failure is reversed, and skin pigmentation ("bronzing") diminishes. Carbohydrate intolerance may abate in up to half of all affected persons. For unknown reasons, there is no improvement in the arthropathy or hypogonadism (resulting from pituitary deposition of iron) associated with hemochromatosis. The 5-year survival rate increases from 33 to 90% with treatment; prolonged survival actually may increase the risk of hepatocellular carcinoma, which affects one-third of persons treated for hemochromatosis. However, if phlebotomy is begun in the precirrhotic stage, which is possible with effective genetic screening, liver cancer will not develop.

**XI-62.** **The answer is C.** *(Chap. 323; Nathan, N Engl J Med 328:1676–1685, 1993.)* Nephropathy is a leading cause of death in diabetic patients. Diabetic nephropathy may be functionally silent for 10 to 15 years. Clinically detectable diabetic nephropathy begins with the development of microalbuminuria (30 to 300 mg of albumin per 24 h). The glomerular filtration rate actually may be elevated at this stage. Only after the passage of additional time will the proteinuria be overt enough (0.5 g/L) to be detectable on standard urine dipsticks. Microalbuminuria precedes nephropathy in patients with both non-insulin-dependent and insulin-dependent diabetes. An increase in kidney size also may accompany the initial hyperfiltration stage. Once the proteinuria becomes significant enough to be detected by dipstick, a steady decline in renal function occurs, with the glomerular filtration rate falling an average of 1 mL/min per month. Therefore, azotemia begins about 12 years after the diagnosis of diabetes. Hypertension clearly is an exacerbating factor for diabetic nephropathy.

**XI-63.** **The answer is D.** *(Chap. 326)* In a 7-year-old girl, isosexual precocity that is associated with undetectable levels of gonadotropins and urinary 17-ketosteroid levels appropriate for her chronologic age most likely is due to an estrogen-secreting tumor. Tumor localization procedures such as abdominal CT and pelvic sonography should be performed before laparotomy. Plasma androstenedione measurement is unlikely to be helpful if urinary 17-ketosteroid excretion is low or normal. In idiopathic precocious puberty, a diagnosis of exclusion, urinary gonadotropins are normal for chronologic age or are elevated; in addition, if plasma gonadotropins are measured frequently during a 24-h period, the characteristic pubertal nocturnal surge should be seen in patients with idiopathic precocious puberty.

**XI-64.** **The answer is C.** *(Chap. 318)* Growth hormone excess in adults results in a clinical syndrome known as *acromegaly*, an insidious disease characterized by bony and soft tissue overgrowth, enlargement of the jaw and tongue, wide spacing of the teeth, and coarsened facial features. Hypertension may result from expansion of plasma volume and total body sodium. Laryngeal hypertrophy leads to a hollow-sounding voice. A moist, oily, doughy handshake is also characteristic. Because of the slow onset, relatives and friends who see the patient daily may not notice these changes. The diagnosis is more likely to be made by those who have not seen the patient before or for many years.

Laboratory abnormalities include abnormal glucose tolerance and mild hyperprolactinemia. The reason for growth hormone excess in virtually all patients with acromegaly is a pituitary adenoma. Useful screening tests for the diagnosis of acromegaly include measurements of glucose-suppressed growth hormone concentrations (60 min after the oral administration of 100 g glucose, growth hormone normally should be suppressed to a value <1 $\mu$g/L) and IGF binding protein 3. IGF-1 concentrations are elevated secondary to the high levels of growth hormone. Once a laboratory test has confirmed the clinical suspicion of acromegaly, magnetic resonance imaging (MRI) or CT should be done to define the presumptive pituitary adenoma. Thyroid function, gonadotropins, and sex steroids may be decreased because of tumor mass effect.

**XI-65.** **The answer is E.** *(Chaps. 332 and 333; Silverberg et al, N Engl J Med 341:1249–1254, 1999.)* Primary hyperparathyroidism is diagnosed commonly in asymptomatic patients. Patients who present with symptoms of bone disease typically have the triad of painful arthralgias, abdominal discomfort, and nephrolithiasis. These patients should undergo a definitive parathyroidectomy. The appropriate treatment for patients with asymptomatic hyperparathyroidism is unclear; many of these patients have a benign clinical course without significant progression. Most asymptomatic patients who undergo parathyroidectomy have normalization of the biochemical values as well as increased bone marrow density studies. Most asymptomatic patients who do not undergo parathyroidectomy do not have progression of the disease. For patients choosing a wait-and-watch approach who subsequently develop symptomatic hyperparathyroidism, a parathyroidectomy should be performed.

**XI-66.   The answer is B.**   *(Chap. 331)*   The hypercalcemia of sarcoidosis usually is associated with disseminated disease. Therefore, almost all persons with sarcoidosis who have hypercalcemia also have an abnormal chest x-ray (diffuse fibronodular infiltration, marked enlargement of hilar nodes, or both). This is an important point in the differential diagnosis of hypercalcemia—sarcoidosis is unlikely as a cause of hypercalcemia if the chest x-ray is normal. Hypergammaglobulinemia is another helpful clue to the presence of sarcoidosis. The hypercalcemia of sarcoidosis is thought to be a consequence of increased synthesis of $1,25(OH)_2$ vitamin $D_3$ and the subsequent increased intestinal absorption of calcium. The elevated serum calcium concentration in patients with sarcoidosis causes a decreased level of serum parathyroid hormone, resulting in marked hypercalciuria.

**XI-67.   The answer is A.**   *(Chaps. 64 and 335)*   Whether hypertriglyceridemia in an overweight person is due to familial hypertriglyceridemia, multiple lipoprotein-type hyperlipidemia, or sporadic hypertriglyceridemia, the primary mode of therapy should be weight reduction. Dietary saturated fats should be restricted as part of the weight reduction regimen. Hypothyroidism and diabetes mellitus, if present, should be treated, and the use of alcohol and oral contraceptives should be avoided. If these measures are inadequate, drug therapy with nicotinic acid or gemfibrozil should be tried. Bile acid–binding resins such as cholestyramine and colestipol are used in the treatment of hypercholesterolemia but are not useful for treating hypertriglyceridemia.

**XI-68.   The answer is D.**   *(Chap. 323; Kjos, Buchanan, N Engl J Med 341:1749–1756, 1999.)*   At 24 to 28 weeks, women with low-risk clinical characteristics may not need further testing. The risk in these women is low. Although the effect of not performing glucose screening has never been evaluated, women with any clinical characteristic that places them at risk should undergo glucose testing. In most populations a two-step testing procedure will limit the number of full glucose tolerance tests performed. The screening test typically is given as a 50-g 1-h glucose challenge test. The 50-g oral glucose challenge test is meant as a screening test. A serum glucose cut-off point of 7.7 mmol/L (140 mg/dL) has a sensitivity of ~80%. A more stringent cut-off at 7.2 mmol/L (130 mg/dL) is associated with a sensitivity of 90%. In patients who test positive, a full glucose tolerance test should be performed. The diagnosis of gestational diabetes is based on the results of the oral glucose tolerance test. Although there is no specific agreement about the conduct or interpretation of the oral glucose tolerance test in pregnant women, the approach that was recommended in 1979 by the National Diabetes Data Group is based on a 3-h, 100-g test. This typically is performed after an overnight fast, and values at 1 h of 10.0 mmol/L (180 mg/dL), at 2 h of >8.6 mmol/L (155 mg/dL), or at 3 h of 7.7 mmol/L (140 mg/dL) are thought to be associated with gestational diabetes mellitus. The World Health Organization has proposed different criteria for interpreting the results of a 75-g 2-h glucose tolerance test in pregnant women, but there are no data on perinatal or maternal outcomes to support the use of these criteria.

**XI-69.   The answer is B.**   *(Chap. 332; Burtis, N Engl J Med 322:1106–1112, 1990.)*   Patients who present with hypercalcemia and hypophosphatemia should be thought of as having an excess of parathyroid hormone activity. Patients with nonparathyroid hormone–like mediated hypercalcemia, such as those with excessive levels of vitamin D caused by intoxication or sarcoidosis or by increased bone turnover as in hyperthyroidism, would not be expected to have a low serum phosphate. Patients with familial hypocalciuric hypercalcemia, an autosomal dominant trait, often have normal or slightly low levels of immunoreactive parathyroid hormone. Thus, those with hypercalcemia and hypophosphatemia without elevated levels of parathyroid hormone are likely to have the hypercalcemia of malignancy. The clinical setting usually but not invariably makes this diagnosis obvious. It is clearly recognized that many solid tumors, including carcinomas of the lung and kidney, may produce a parathyroid hormone–related protein that will not be identified by the currently available assays that detect true parathyroid hormone elaborated from the parathyroid gland. This parathyroid-related protein synthesized by tumors bears striking amino acid homology to that of native parathyroid hormone with regard to amino acids 1 through 13 but is thereafter unique. In fact, it is recognized that the majority of patients with cancer and hypercalcemia have humoral hypercalcemia, as determined by elevated urinary cyclic AMP excretion.

**XI-70.** **The answer is D.** *(Chap. 334)* Paget's disease of bone is relatively common, and the incidence increases with age. An estimated prevalence of 3% in persons over age 40 years is a generally accepted figure. Most frequently, the disease is asymptomatic and is diagnosed only when the typical sclerotic bones are incidentally detected on x-ray examinations done for other reasons or when increased alkaline phosphatase activity is recognized during routine laboratory measurements. The etiology is unknown, but increased bone resorption followed by intensive bone repair is thought to be the mechanism that causes increased bone density and increased serum alkaline phosphatase activity as a marker of osteoblast activity. Because increased mineralization of bone takes place (although in an abnormal pattern), hypercalcemia is not present unless a severely affected patient becomes immobilized. Hypercalcemia in fact would be an expected finding in a patient with primary hyperparathyroidism, bone metastases, or plasmacytoma, with plasmacytoma typically producing no increase in alkaline phosphatase activity. Osteomalacia resulting from vitamin D deficiency is associated with bone pain and hypophosphatemia; normal or decreased serum calcium concentration produces secondary hyperparathyroidism, further aggravating the defective bone mineralization.

**XI-71.** **The answer is E.** *(Chaps. 268 and 332)* Patients with primary hyperparathyroidism are usually asymptomatic, and mild degrees of hypercalcemia in such patients usually can be managed with adequate hydration. Whether observation alone is appropriate in these patients is controversial, especially when the diagnosis is made at a young age, since surveillance of renal function and bone status is lifelong and cumbersome. However, definitive treatment is clearly indicated when complications arise. In this patient, hypercalcemia and nephrolithiasis constitute a clear-cut indication for surgical treatment of the hyperparathyroidism. An additional reason would be to prevent bone loss in this young female that would place her at increased risk for the later development of skeletal complications. Glucocorticoids are usually ineffective in the management of primary hyperparathyroidism and would affect bone metabolism negatively, besides producing other serious side effects when administered on a long-term basis. Thiazide diuretics and calcium supplementation are contraindicated in this patient because of the risk of inducing hypercalcemia.

**XI-72.** **The answer is B.** *(Chap. 334)* Osteomalacia and rickets are both characterized by defective mineralization of bone; osteomalacia affects the adult skeleton, and rickets impairs the developing skeleton. Muscle weakness, hypocalcemia, hypophosphatemia, skeletal pain, and pseudofractures are cardinal features of both forms of osteomalacia. Although common in children who have rickets, bowing of the tibia and increased thickness of the epiphyseal growth plates are not prominent in affected adults.

**XI-73.** **The answer is E.** *(Chaps. 61, 331, 332, and 334)* The combination of hypocalcemia, hypophosphatemia, elevated serum parathyroid hormone levels, and bone fractures is consistent with a diagnosis of osteomalacia in this patient. In the absence of other gastrointestinal or renal abnormalities leading to malabsorption or increased renal loss of calcium or phosphorus, vitamin D deficiency is likely to be present. Inadequate intake of vitamin D and calcium together and limited exposure to the sun are common in this age group. Postmenopausal osteoporosis also is associated with vertebral and hip fractures, but laboratory abnormalities are not present. Primary hyperparathyroidism is associated with increased serum calcium concentration, as is ectopic parathyroid hormone secretion (although the existence of the latter has been questioned). Paget's disease of bone does not produce hypocalcemia, and it causes typical sclerotic changes on x-ray examination.

**XI-74.   The answer is C.** *(Chaps. 331 and 332)*   Measurement of the serum concentration of 25(OH) vitamin D, the major circulating form of vitamin D, can be used to assess the adequacy of dietary intake and absorption of the vitamin. (Vitamin D also is made in the skin in the presence of sunlight.) Once ingested or synthesized, vitamin D is metabolized to 25(OH) vitamin D in the liver. This reaction is not tightly regulated, and an increase in dietary intake or endogenous production of vitamin D is reflected by linear elevations of serum 25(OH) vitamin D levels. Levels are reduced in patients with severe chronic parenchymal and cholestatic liver disease but usually are normal in patients with renal failure. Anticonvulsant drugs and glucocorticoids induce hepatic microsomal enzymes, which metabolize vitamin D and 25(OH) vitamin D into inactive products; this phenomenon, along with other complex effects on calcium metabolism, helps explain why these drugs cause osteopenia.

**XI-75.   The answer is D.** *(Chap. 320)*   This patient has postpartum thyroiditis, which occurs in 5 to 9% of all postpartum women. Appropriate treatment is symptomatic because the hyperthyroidism is caused by the release of preformed thyroid hormone from a damaged thyroid gland. Therefore, therapies aimed at decreasing the formation of thyroid hormone, such as methimazole, or at inhibiting its release, such as SSKI, are ineffective. Radioactive iodine also is ineffective because it will not be taken up by the damaged thyroid gland (reflected in the 1% 24-h iodine uptake). In addition, the hyperthyroidism will resolve spontaneously. Steroids are effective in treating subacute thyroiditis, which is characterized by a tender thyroid and often is preceded by a viral illness, but are not used for postpartum thyroiditis. Therapies, such as beta blockers, aimed at treating symptoms are the most effective treatment.

    Postpartum thyroiditis is a form of lymphocytic thyroiditis, a painless inflammation of the thyroid that is thought to be autoimmune in etiology. About one-third of these patients enter a hypothyroid phase after experiencing hyperthyroidism. Eighty percent of these females recover normal thyroid function, but 20% remain hypothyroid and require indefinite replacement therapy. Therefore, serial thyroid function testing is indicated.

**XI-76.   The answer is C.** *(Chap. 330; Neufeld et al, Medicine 60:355–362, 1981.)*   Polyglandular autoimmune syndrome type II (Schmidt's syndrome) is characterized by lymphocytic infiltration of the adrenal and thyroid glands along with type 1 diabetes mellitus in about half of affected families. Hypogonadism is also common. A few patients develop transient hypoparathyroidism caused by antibodies that compete with parathyroid hormone for binding to the parathyroid receptor. Mucocutaneous candidiasis does not occur as part of this syndrome. Instead, it occurs in most patients with polyglandular autoimmune syndrome type I. Patients who are found to have hypothyroidism should be checked for adrenal insufficiency before the initiation of thyroid replacement medication.

**XI-77.   The answer is A.** *(Chap. 43; Lue, N Engl J Med 342:1802–1813, 2000.)*   Androgens increase libido, but their exact role in erectile dysfunction is unclear. Individuals with castrate levels of testosterone can still achieve erections from visual or sexual stimuli. Increased prolactin levels decrease libido by suppressing gonadotropin-releasing hormone (GnRH), which indirectly leads to a decreased serum testosterone level. Patients with diabetes mellitus have reduced amounts of nitric oxide synthase in both endothelial and neural tissues. Psychogenic erectile dysfunction is caused by a psychogenic stimulus to the sacral cord that inhibits reflexogenic responses. In addition, excess sympathetic stimulation may cause increased penile smooth muscle tone. Among the antihypertensive agents, the thiazide diuretics and beta blockers have been implicated most frequently. Calcium channel blockers and angiotensin converting-enzyme inhibitors are cited less frequently. Alpha blockers are less likely to be associated with erectile dysfunction.

**XI-78.   The answer is B.** *(Chap. 43; Lue, N Engl J Med 342:1802–1813, 2000; Goldstein et al, Sildenafil Study Group, N Engl J Med 338:1397–1404, 1998.)*   Sildenafil has been proved to be effective in the treatment of erectile dysfunction. Sildenafil is a selective inhibitor of cyclic GMP–specific phosphodiesterase type V. This is the predominant iso-enzyme that metabolizes cyclic GMP in the corpus cavernosum. The mechanism by which cyclic GMP stimulates relaxation in the smooth muscles has not been elucidated. Sildenafil has no effect on libido or sexual performance. Sildenafil is effective in the management of erectile dysfunction from a broad range of causes. These causes include psychogenic, diabetic, vasculogenic, postradical prostatectomy, and spinal cord injury. The onset of action is ~60 to 90 min; reduced initial doses should be considered for patients who are elderly or who have renal insufficiency. In addition, patients taking nitrates for coronary disease should avoid sildenafil. Side effects associated with sildenafil include headaches, facial flushing, dyspepsia, and nasal congestion. In addition, about 7% of men may ex-perience a transient altered color vision (blue halo effect).

**XI-79. The answer is B.** *(Chap. 326)* Pathologic gynecomastia develops when the effective ratio of testosterone to estrogen ratio is decreased owing to diminished testosterone pro-duction (as in primary testicular failure) or increased estrogen production. The latter may arise from direct estradiol secretion by a testis stimulated by LH or hCG or from an increase in peripheral aromatization of precursor steroids, most notably androstenedione. Elevated androstenedione levels may result from increased secretion by an adrenal tumor (leading to an elevated level of urinary 17-ketosteroids) or decreased hepatic clearance in patients with chronic liver disease. A variety of drugs, including diethylstilbestrol, heroin, digitalis, spironolactone, cimetidine, isoniazid, and tricyclic antidepressants, also can cause gyne-comastia. In this patient, the history of paternity and the otherwise normal physical ex-amination indicate that a karyotype is unnecessary, and the bilateral breast enlargement essentially excludes the presence of carcinoma and thus the need for biopsy. The presence of a low LH and testosterone suggests either estrogen or hCG production. Because of the normal testicular examination, a primary testicular tumor is not suspected. Carcinoma of the lung and germ cell tumors both can produce hCG, causing gynecomastia.

# XII. NEUROLOGIC DISORDERS

## QUESTIONS

**DIRECTIONS:** Each question below contains five suggested responses. Choose the **one best** response to each question.

**XII-1.** A 56-year-old male is admitted to the intensive care unit with a hypertensive crisis after cocaine use. Initial blood pressure is 245/132. On physical examination the patient is unresponsive except to painful stimuli. He has been intubated for airway protection and is being mechanically ventilated, with a respiratory rate of 14. His pupils are reactive to light, and there are normal corneal, cough, and gag reflexes. The patient has a dense left hemiparesis. When presented with painful stimuli, the patient responds with flexure posturing on the right side. Computed tomography (CT) reveals a large area of intracranial bleeding in the right frontoparietal area. Over the next several hours the patient deteriorates. The most recent examination reveals a blood pressure of 189/100. The patient now has a dilated pupil on the right side. The patient continues to have corneal reflexes. You suspect rising intracranial pressure related to the intracranial bleed. All but which of the following can be done to decrease the patient's intracranial pressure?

A. Administer intravenous mannitol at a dose of 1 g/kg body weight.
B. Administer hypertonic fluids to achieve a goal sodium level of 155 to 160 meq/L.
C. Consult neurosurgery for an urgent ventriculostomy.
D. Initiate intravenous nitroprusside to decrease the mean arterial pressure to a goal of 100 mmHg.
E. Increase the respiratory rate to 30.

**XII-2.** All the following are associated with a decreased sense of smell *except*

A. head trauma
B. HIV infection
C. influenza B infection
D. Kallmann syndrome
E. parainfluenza virus type 3 infection

**XII-3.** A 56-year-old male presents to your clinic complaining of hearing loss in the right ear. On examination,

**XII-3.** *(Continued)*
the Rinne test at 256 Hz reveals louder conduction through placement on the mastoid process and the Weber test best localizes the sound to the right ear. The otologic examination is shown below. What is the diagnosis?

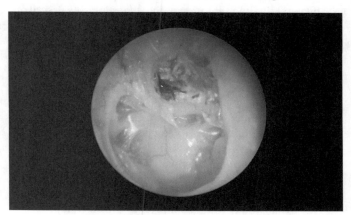

A. Otitis externa
B. Otosclerosis
C. Cholesteatoma
D. Acoustic neuroma
E. Presbycusis

**XII-4.** A 66-year-old male seeks evaluation of difficulty walking. He first noticed this problem 1 week ago. There is no back pain or noticeable weakness. The patient describes his problem as a feeling that he frequently trips. He has no difficult arising from a chair but has tripped while climbing the stairs at home. Past history is notable for adult-onset diabetes mellitus that does not require insulin therapy. The most recent hemoglobin A1$_C$ is 6.8%. His only medication is metformin 500 mg twice daily. On physical examination the patient appears comfortable. He has no tenderness or deformity in the back. The left patellar reflex is decreased compared with the right, and there has been a loss of dorsiflexion in the left foot. When walking, the patient has been noted to swing the left leg higher than the right. What term is used to describe this gait?

**XII-4.** *(Continued)*

    A.   Cerebellar ataxic

    B.   Parkinsonian

    C.   Sensory ataxic

    D.   Steppage

    E.   Waddling

**XII-5.** What is the most likely cause of the patient's abnormality?

    A.   Diabetic neuropathy

    B.   Herniated L5 disc

    C.   Lumbar spinal stenosis

    D.   Middle cerebral artery thrombotic cerebrovascular accident

    E.   Vitamin $B_{12}$ deficiency

**XII-6.** You are a physician practicing in a small community in the Rocky Mountains near Aspen, Colorado. A 33-year-old female comes to your office for evaluation of a bilateral tingling sensation in the fingertips. She describes the sensation as affecting all the fingers on both hands. She has no medical problems and takes no medications. She is a vegetarian and is visiting the area from San Diego, California. She denies any other symptoms, including headache, nausea, vomiting, shortness of breath, and urinary frequency. On physical examination the patient has a normal sensory examination, including reaction to light touch and pinprick and vibratory sensation. She is able to stand normally with the arms extended and the eyes closed. A cerebellar examination reveals normal finger-to-nose testing and no dysdiadochokinesis. Her gait is normal, including tandem gait, toe walking, and heel walking. What would you recommend as the next step?

    A.   Blood tests for serum vitamin $B_{12}$

    B.   Fasting blood glucose level

    C.   Reassurance

    D.   Serologic testing for syphilis

    E.   Treatment with acetazolamide for altitude sickness

**XII-7.** A 78-year-old female with a long history of vascular disease presents after an embolic cerebrovascular accident (CVA) with severe and unrelenting pain on the right side. She describes the pain as burning as if she had been bathed in acid. Where is the most likely site of the recent embolic CVA?

    A.   Frontal lobe

    B.   Hypothalamus

    C.   Pons

    D.   Temporal lobe

    E.   Thalamus

**XII-8.** A 33-year-old male is brought to your clinic by his family. His sister states that "he has not been himself" for

**XII-8.** *(Continued)*

4 months. He has been slurring his words and has had short-term memory loss. The past medical history is unremarkable. His sister notes only a "crazy" uncle on his mother's side. On neurologic examination there is dysmetria on finger-to-nose testing bilaterally. He has a slight resting tremor. Gait is normal. Sensory examination and reflexes are normal. The rest of the physical examination is unremarkable. Laboratories are unremarkable except for a slight transaminitis. You suspect Wilson's disease. All the following are helpful in making a diagnosis of Wilson's disease *except*

    A.   24-h urine copper assay

    B.   A trial of penicillamine

    C.   Liver biopsy

    D.   Magnetic resonance imaging (MRI) of the brain

    E.   Ophthalmologic examination

**XII-9.** A 34-year-old female complains of lower extremity weakness for the last 3 days. She has noted progressive weakness in the lower extremities with loss of sensation "below the belly button" and incontinence. She had had some low-grade fevers for the last week. She denies recent travel. Past medical history is unremarkable. Physical examination is notable for a sensory level at the level of the umbilicus. The lower extremities show +3/5 strength bilaterally proximally and distally. Reflexes, cerebellar examination, and mental status are normal. All the following are appropriate steps in evaluating this patient *except*

    A.   antinuclear antibodies

    B.   electromyography

    C.   lumbar puncture

    D.   MRI of the spine

    E.   viral serologies

**XII-10.** Which of the following statements about syringomyelia is true?

    A.   More than half the cases are associated with Chiari malformations.

    B.   Symptoms typically begin in middle age.

    C.   Vibration and position sensation are usually diminished.

    D.   Syrinx cavities are always congenital.

    E.   Neurosurgical decompression is usually effective in relieving the symptoms.

**XII-11.** A 50-year-old male complains of weakness and numbness in the hands for the last month. He describes paresthesias in the thumb and the index and middle fingers. The symptoms are worse at night. He also describes decreased grip strength bilaterally. He works as a mechanical engineer. The patient denies fevers, chills, or weight loss. The examination is notable for atrophy of the thenar eminences bilaterally and decreased sensation in a

**XII-11.** *(Continued)*
median nerve distribution. All the following are causes of carpal tunnel syndrome *except*

A. amyloidosis
B. chronic lymphocytic leukemia
C. diabetes mellitus
D. hypothyroidism
E. rheumatoid arthritis

**XII-12.** A 62-year-old male with a history of hypertension and diabetes presents to the emergency department with a left facial droop and left-sided hemiparesis. He is not sure when the symptoms began. His wife noted that 4 h before he arrived at the hospital he was "normal" but did not see him again until 20 min before presentation. Past medical history is significant for reflux esophagitis seen on endoscopy 1 year ago. His medications include hydrochlorothiazide and omeprazole. Family history is noncontributory. Physical examination is notable for a blood pressure of 152/74 mmHg and an oxygen saturation of 98% on room air. He has an obvious left facial droop and has left-sided hemiparesis. Sensation is intact. The patient's stool is heme-negative. A complete blood count is normal, and coagulation studies are within normal limits. A computed tomography scan of the head shows a right middle cerebral artery territory infarct. There is no hemorrhage. What is the most appropriate next management step?

A. Aspirin
B. Clopidogrel
C. Intraarterial catheter-based thrombolytic therapy
D. Intravenous thrombolytic therapy
E. Intravenous heparin

**XII-13.** The most common cause of a cerebral embolism is

A. cardiac prosthetic valves
B. rheumatic heart disease
C. dilated cardiomyopathy
D. endocarditis
E. atrial fibrillation

**XII-14.** A 54-year-old male is referred to your clinic for evaluation of atrial fibrillation. He first noted the irregular heartbeat 2 weeks ago and presented to his primary care physician. He denies chest pain, shortness of breath, nausea, or gastrointestinal symptoms. Past medical history is unremarkable. There is no history of hypertension, diabetes, or tobacco use. His medications include metoprolol. The examination is notable for a blood pressure of 126/74 mmHg and a pulse of 64 beats/min. The jugular venous pressure is not elevated. His heart is irregularly irregular, with normal $S_1$ and $S_2$. The lungs are clear, and there is no peripheral edema. An echocardiogram shows a left

**XII-14.** *(Continued)*
atrial size of 3.6 cm. Left ventricular ejection fraction is 60%. There are no valvular or structural abnormalities. Which of the following statements regarding his atrial fibrillation and stroke risk is true?

A. He requires no antiplatelet therapy or anticoagulation because the risk of embolism is low.
B. Lifetime warfarin therapy is indicated for atrial fibrillation in this situation to reduce the risk of stroke.
C. He should be admitted to the hospital for intravenous heparin and undergo electrical cardioversion; afterward there is no need for anticoagulation.
D. His risk of an embolic stroke is less than 1%, and he should take a daily aspirin.
E. He should be started on subcutaneous low-molecular-weight heparin and transitioned to warfarin.

**XII-15.** All but which of the following statements regarding amyotrophic lateral sclerosis (ALS) are true?

A. Dementia occurs in the late stages of the disease.
B. The main cause of death is respiratory failure.
C. Familial ALS is inherited in an autosomal dominant fashion.
D. Glutamate plays a key role in the death of motor neurons in patients with ALS.
E. Riluzole improves survival in patients with ALS.

**XII-16.** All but which of the following statements about Becker's muscular dystrophy are true?

A. The inheritance is X-linked.
B. Serum creatinine kinase levels are elevated.
C. The underlying genetic defect is in the myosin gene.
D. Survival is better than it is in patients with Duchenne's muscular dystrophy (DMD).
E. Cardiomyopathy may occur, resulting in heart failure.

**XII-17.** A 16-year-old female is referred to your clinic for evaluation of an elevated creatinine kinase. For the last 2 months she has noted pain and weakness in the legs and thighs while jogging. During these episodes her urine becomes darker. She has had to quit the high school volleyball team as a result of these symptoms. A week before this visit the patient presented to a local emergency room after suffering an episode while rearranging her room. Laboratories were normal except for an elevated creatinine kinase of 9000 IU/L. Serum creatinine was normal. She was given intravenous fluids over the course of a day and discharged to follow-up in your clinic. On examination you notice some stiff and painful muscles in the thighs and lower legs. Sensation is normal. Reflexes and cerebellar examination are also normal. Serum CK is now

**XII-17.** *(Continued)*

600 IU/L. The rest of the examination is unremarkable. You are suspicious of a glycolytic defect. What is the most appropriate next test?

 A. Dystrophin gene analysis
 B. Electrodiagnostic testing
 C. Forearm exercise test
 D. Muscle biopsy
 E. Serum aldolase

**XII-18.** The most common cause of recurrent myoglobinuria is

 A. acid maltase deficiency
 B. carnitine palmitoyltransferase (CPT) deficiency
 C. McArdle's disease
 D. mitochondrial myopathy
 E. phosphofructokinase deficiency

**XII-19.** A 71-year-old male presents to your clinic to receive routine medical care. On examination you notice a left carotid bruit. You order a carotid ultrasound that shows a 60% stenosis of the left internal carotid artery. All but which of the following statements are true?

 A. If this patient has symptoms of transient ischemic attacks (TIAs), he will receive a significant benefit from a carotid endarterectomy.
 B. Without symptoms, his risk of stroke is approximately 2% a year.
 C. Balloon angioplasty with stenting has been shown to be equivalent to carotid endarterectomy.
 D. There is evidence that this patient will benefit from carotid endarterectomy (CEA) even in the absence of symptoms.
 E. Surgery is recommended only in centers with perioperative complication rates under 6%.

**XII-20.** All the following have been shown to reduce the risk of atherothrombotic stroke in primary or secondary prevention *except*

 A. aspirin
 B. blood pressure control
 C. clopidogrel
 D. statin therapy
 E. warfarin

**XII-21.** All the following cause primarily a sensory neuropathy except

 A. acromegaly
 B. critical illness
 C. HIV infection
 D. hypothyroidism
 E. vitamin $B_{12}$ deficiency

**XII-22.** All but which of the following statements about Guillain-Barré syndrome are true?

 A. Up to 30% of cases are associated with *Escherichia coli* infection.
 B. Ascending areflexic motor paralysis is the typical clinical pattern.
 C. Cerebrospinal fluid protein is often elevated.
 D. The effectiveness of treatment diminishes if it is initiated more than 2 weeks after the onset of symptoms.
 E. The main cause of mortality is pulmonary complications.

**XII-23.** All but which of the following statements regarding neuropathy are true?

 A. Neurologic symptoms often precede the diagnosis of small-cell lung cancer in patients with anti-Hu paraneoplastic neuropathy.
 B. Twenty-five percent of patients with chronic inflammatory demyelinating polyradiculoneuropathy (CIDP) have a monoclonal gammopathy of undetermined significance (MGUS).
 C. Polyneuropathy is associated with less than 5% of cases of myeloma with osteosclerotic features.
 D. Multifocal motor neuropathy (MMN) is associated with polyclonal anti-GM1 antibodies in a majority of cases.
 E. The most common pattern of neuropathy in patients with vasculitis is a mononeuritis multiplex.

**XII-24.** All but which of the following statements regarding prion diseases are true?

 A. Prions are the only known infectious agent that is devoid of DNA or RNA.
 B. The majority of human cases are familial and have an autosomal dominant pattern.
 C. Variant Creutzfeldt-Jakob (vCJD) disease has been associated with bovine spongiform encephalopathy (BSE) infection in cattle.
 D. The median age of presentation for sporadic CJD (sCJD) is 50 to 70 years of age.
 E. Histologically, the brain of a patient with CJD is characterized by spongiform degeneration and astrocytic gliosis with an absence of inflammation.

**XII-25.** A 21-year-old man presents to your clinic complaining of progressive weakness in the feet for the last 2 years. He describes slowly progressive difficulty in lifting his feet off the ground when walking. The legs have "gotten smaller" in bulk. Past medical history is unremarkable. The family history is significant for his father, brother, and paternal grandmother all having similar "weaknesses." The examination is notable for distal atrophy be-

**XII-25.** *(Continued)*
low the mid-calves and for prominent high arches. There is obvious footdrop, and dorsiflexion of the foot is severely diminished bilaterally. You suspect a form of Charcot-Marie-Tooth disease and order nerve conduction studies. Which of the following statements about CMT disease is true?

A. CMT disease is usually a motor neuropathy; sensory features are rare and should prompt an alternative diagnosis.
B. Immunotherapy with intravenous immune globulin and/or plasmapheresis may slow the progression of CMT disease.
C. CMT disease affects approximately 1 in 100,000 individuals.
D. Transmission is most commonly autosomal dominant but may be autosomal recessive or X-linked.
E. The age of this patient at presentation is atypical; patients usually present in the fourth and fifth decades of life.

**XII-26.** An 18-year-old male is brought to your clinic by his mother for evaluation of his "strange behavior." Over the last week he has had four witnessed episodes of "staring spells," with each one preceded by the smell of lemons. A few seconds after the strange smell the patient is noted to appear dazed and unresponsive, but with his eyes open. These episodes typically last 20 to 30 s; afterward he is noted to make lip-smacking movements and remain confused. The confusion lasts up to an hour. The patient has no recollection of these events, and they are described in detail only by his mother. This presentation is consistent with which of the following diagnoses?

A. Absence seizure
B. Atonic seizure
C. Complex partial seizure
D. Grand mal seizure
E. Simple partial seizure

**XII-27.** All the following are common causes of seizures in adults older than 50 years of age *except*

A. cerebrovascular disease
B. central nervous system (CNS) neoplasia
C. degenerative disease
D. mesial temporal sclerosis
E. subdural hematoma

**XII-28.** All but which of the following statements regarding epilepsy are true?

A. The incidence of suicide is higher in epileptic patients than it is in the general population.
B. Mortality is no different in patients with epilepsy than it is in age-matched controls.
C. A majority of patients with epilepsy that is completely controlled with medication eventually will

**XII-28.** *(Continued)*
be able to discontinue therapy and remain seizure-free.
D. Surgery for mesial temporal lobe epilepsy (MTLE) decreases the number of seizures in over 70% of patients.
E. Tricyclic antidepressants lower the seizure threshold and may precipitate seizures.

**XII-29.** All the following are side effects of phenytoin *except*

A. ataxia
B. gum hyperplasia
C. hirsutism
D. leukopenia
E. lymphadenopathy

**XII-30.** A 34-year-old female complains of weakness and double vision for the last 3 weeks. She has also noted a change in her speech, and her friends tell her that she is "more nasal." She has noticed decreased exercise tolerance and difficulty lifting objects and getting out of a chair. The patient denies pain. The symptoms are worse at the end of the day and with repeated muscle use. You suspect myasthenia gravis. All the following are useful in the diagnosis of myasthenia gravis *except*

A. acetylcholine receptor (AChR) antibodies
B. edrophonium
C. electrodiagnostic testing
D. muscle-specific kinase (MuSK) antibodies
E. voltage-gated calcium channel antibodies

**XII-31.** In the patient described in Question XII-30 you confirm the diagnosis of myasthenia gravis. The patient's symptoms improve markedly after an initial dose of glucocorticoids and pyridostigmine. What is the best next treatment option for this patient?

A. Surgical consultation
B. Glucocorticoids
C. Glucocorticoids and azathioprine
D. Intravenous immunoglobulin
E. Cyclosporine

**XII-32.** For the last 5 weeks a 35-year-old female has had episodes of intense vertigo that last several hours. Each episode is associated with tinnitus and a sense of fullness in the right ear; during the attacks she prefers to lie on the left side. Examination during an attack shows that she has fine rotary nystagmus that is maximal on gaze to the left. There are no ocular palsies, cranial nerve signs, or long-tract signs. An audiogram shows high-tone hearing loss in the right ear, with recruitment but no tone decay. The most likely diagnosis in this case is

**XII-32.** *(Continued)*
  A.  labyrinthitis
  B.  Ménière's disease
  C.  vertebral-basilar insufficiency
  D.  acoustic neuroma
  E.  multiple sclerosis

**XII-33.**   A 29-year-old female who uses oral contraceptives comes to the emergency room because when she looked in the mirror this morning, her face was twisted. It felt numb and swollen. While eating breakfast, she found that the food tasted different and that she drooled out of the right side of her mouth when swallowing. Neurologic examination discloses only a dense right facial paresis equally involving the frontalis, orbicularis oculi, and orbicularis oris. Finger rubbing is appreciated as louder in the right ear than in the left. The physician should

  A.  instruct the patient in using a patch over the right eye during sleep
  B.  recommend that she discontinue oral contraceptives
  C.  order brainstem auditory evoked potentials to assess the hearing asymmetry
  D.  inform her that her chances of substantial improvement within several weeks are only about 40%
  E.  order an echocardiogram to rule out mitral valve prolapse as a source of emboli

**XII-34.**   A 45-year-old male presents with a daily headache. He describes two attacks per day over the last 3 weeks. Each attack lasts about an hour and awakens the patient from sleep. The patient has noted associated tearing and reddening of the right eye as well as nasal stuffiness. The pain is deep, excruciating, and limited to the right side of the head. The neurologic examination is nonfocal. The most likely diagnosis of this patient's headache is

  A.  migraine headache
  B.  cluster headache
  C.  tension headache
  D.  brain tumor
  E.  giant cell arteritis

**XII-35.**   A 65-year-old male presents with severe right-sided eye and facial pain, nausea, vomiting, colored halos around lights, and loss of visual acuity. His right eye is quite red, and that pupil is dilated and fixed. Which of the following diagnostic tests would confirm the diagnosis?

  A.  CT of the head
  B.  MRI of the head
  C.  Cerebral angiography
  D.  Tonometry
  E.  Slit-lamp examination

**XII-36.**   The most common presenting finding or symptom of multiple sclerosis is

  A.  internuclear ophthalmoplegia
  B.  transverse myelitis
  C.  cerebellar ataxia
  D.  optic neuritis
  E.  urinary retention

**XII-37.**   A 68-year-old female presents with an 18-month history of progressive loss of recent memory and inattentiveness. At this time she is having difficulty speaking, her judgment appears to be impaired, and she occasionally evidences paranoid behavior. In addition to neurofibrillary tangles, the neuropathologic findings in this condition include plaques made of

  A.  low-density lipoprotein
  B.  unesterified cholesterol
  C.  $\beta$-amyloid protein
  D.  immunoglobulin proteins
  E.  protease inhibitor

**XII-38.**   A previously active 25-year-old female presents with profound fatigue. She had an upper respiratory infection about 6 months ago from which she has never recovered. She now complains of intermittent headaches, sore throat, muscle and joint aches, and occasional feverishness. The fatigue is so severe that she is unable to work. She now complains of excessive irritability, confusion, and inability to concentrate. Her physician has documented the presence of fever to 38.6°C (101.5°F) orally and the presence of palpable anterior cervical adenopathy both now and approximately 2 months ago. The patient has undergone an extensive workup, including complete blood count, serum chemistry analysis, HIV serology, Epstein-Barr virus serology, cytomegalovirus serology, and CT scan of the head, all of which were negative or not consistent with an acute infection. The patient has had no psychiatric or medical problems. Appropriate therapy at this time would consist of

  A.  acyclovir
  B.  glucocorticoids
  C.  vitamin $B_{12}$ injections
  D.  intravenous immunoglobulin
  E.  ibuprofen

**XII-39.**   A 72-year-old female presents with brief, intermittent excruciating episodes of lancinating pain in the lips, gums, and cheek. These intense spasms of pain may be initiated by touching the lips or moving the tongue. The results of a physical examination are normal. MRI of the head is also normal. The most likely cause of this patient's pain is

  A.  acoustic neuroma
  B.  meningioma

**XII-39.** *(Continued)*
   C.   temporal lobe epilepsy
   D.   trigeminal neuralgia
   E.   facial nerve palsy

**XII-40.**   A 45-year-old male complains of severe right arm pain. He gives a history of having slipped on the ice and severely contusing his right shoulder approximately 1 month ago. At this time he has sharp knifelike pain in the right arm and forearm. Physical examination reveals a right arm that is more moist and hairy than the left arm. There is no specific weakness or sensory change. However, the right arm is clearly more edematous than the left, and the skin appears somewhat atrophic in the affected limb. The patient's pain most likely is due to

   A.   subclavian vein thrombosis
   B.   brachial plexus injury
   C.   reflex sympathetic dystrophy
   D.   acromioclavicular separation
   E.   cervical radiculopathy

**XII-41.**   A 72-year-old right-handed male with a history of atrial fibrillation and chronic alcoholism is evaluated for dementia. His son gives a history of a stepwise decline in

**XII-41.** *(Continued)*
the patient's function over the last 5 years with the accumulation of mild focal neurologic deficits. On examination he is found to have a pseudobulbar affect, mildly increased muscle tone, and brisk deep tendon reflexes in the right upper extremity and an extensor plantar response on the left. The history and examination are most consistent with which of the following?

   A.   Binswanger's disease
   B.   Alzheimer's disease
   C.   Creutzfeldt-Jakob disease
   D.   Vitamin B$_{12}$ deficiency
   E.   Multi-infarct dementia

**XII-42.**   In addition to progressive memory loss, which of the following clinical findings is helpful in suggesting the diagnosis of Alzheimer's disease?

   A.   Onset of symptoms before age 40
   B.   Episodes of altered consciousness
   C.   Neurofibrillary tangles
   D.   Diminished independence in activities of daily living
   E.   Absence of a family history of a similar disorder

**XII-1.** **The answer is D.** *(Chap. 258)* This patient has evidence of increased intracranial pressure and needs to be managed urgently. A variety of maneuvers may decrease intracranial pressure acutely. Hyperventilation causes vasoconstriction, reducing cerebral blood volume and decreasing intracranial pressure. However, this can be used only for a short period as the decrease in cerebral blood flow is of limited duration. Mannitol, an osmotic diuretic, is recommended in cases of increased intracranial pressure resulting from cytotoxic edema. Hypotonic fluids should be avoided. Instead, hypertonic saline is given to elevate sodium levels and prevent worsening of edema. A more definitive treatment to decrease intracranial pressure is to have a ventriculostomy placed by which excessive pressure can be relieved by draining cerebrospinal fluid (CSF). Further decreases in mean arterial pressure may worsen the patient's clinical status. The patient already has had more than a 20% reduction in mean arterial pressure, which is the recommended reduction in cases of hypertensive emergency. In addition, the patient is exhibiting signs of increased intracranial pressure, which indicates that cerebral perfusion pressure [mean arterial pressure (MAP) − intracranial pressure (ICP)] has been lowered. Paradoxically, the patient may need a vasopressor agent to increase MAP and thus improve cerebral perfusion. Finally, in cases of increased intracranial pressure, nitroprusside is not a recommended intravenous antihypertensive agent because it causes arterial vasodilation and may decrease cerebral perfusion pressure and worsen neurologic function.

**XII-2.** **The answer is C.** *(Chap. 26)* Head trauma is the most common etiology of a decreased sense of smell in young adults and children. In most cases this is permanent, with only 10% of these patients experiencing recovery. In older adults viral infections predominate. Parainfluenza virus type 3 is the most common associated virus. Patients with HIV also frequently have a distorted sense of smell, and this is associated with HIV wasting syndrome. Although rare, genetic defects such as Kallmann syndrome and albinism are also causes of anosmia. Influenza virus is not a cause of anosmia.

**XII-3.** **The answer is C.** *(Chap. 26)* This patient exhibits conductive hearing loss as manifested by the Rinne and Weber tests. In the Rinne test, the vibrating tines of a 256- or 512-Hz tuning fork are placed near the opening of the external auditory canal, and then the stem is placed on either the mastoid process or the teeth. If the sound is heard loudest when the fork is placed on bone, this is evidence of conductive hearing loss. The Weber test is performed by placing a vibrating tuning fork on the midline of the forehead. The sound is heard loudest in the affected ear if conductive hearing loss is present and in the unaffected ear if sensorineural hearing loss is present. This patient thus has evidence of conductive hearing loss. The picture reveals a rupture of the tympanic membrane filled with cheesy white squamous debris that is typical of cholesteatoma. The pathogenesis of this lesion is unclear but pathologically is defined by the presence of stratified squamous epithelium in the middle ear or mastoid. Surgery is required to prevent further hearing loss from erosion of the ossicles. Otosclerosis would have a normal appearance on examination. Otitis externa should not cause hearing loss and would be associated with pain on examination. Both presbycusis and acoustic neuroma cause sensorineural hearing loss.

**XII-4 and XII-5.** **The answers are D and B.** *(Chap. 21)* The patient has a steppage gait, which is caused by weakness of ankle dorsiflexion. Because of the footdrop, the leg must be lifted higher than usual to avoid dragging of the toe when he steps forward. As the condition described in this case is unilateral, the finding of left ankle weakness is most consistent with an L5 radiculopathy. Diabetic neuropathy and vitamin $B_{12}$ would be expected to cause bilateral sensory neuropathies. The weakness after a cerebrovascular accident is not localized to a single nerve root. The gait associated with this is described as hemiparetic and is notable for elevation and circumduction at the hip with contralateral tilt of the trunk. Finally, lumbar spinal stenosis should cause a paraparetic gait with scissoring related to bilateral lower limb spasticity.

**XII-6.** **The answer is C.** *(Chap. 22)* The patient's nonspecific dysesthesia is related to hyperventilation in response to the patient's change in altitude from sea level to a mountainous area. The normal respiratory response to decreased atmospheric oxygen tension is to increase the respiratory rate. This hyperventilation causes a mild respiratory alkalosis and is experienced as acral and periorbital dysesthesias. Acetazolamide is often given to patients who have a past history of altitude sickness manifested as headache, nausea with vomiting, and in severe cases pulmonary edema. This patient is experiencing none of those symptoms, and in fact, dysesthesias are a common side effect related to treatment with acetazolamide. No further blood testing is necessary as the symptoms are not associated with any neurologic abnormalities. Diabetes mellitus, vitamin $B_{12}$ deficiency, and tertiary syphilis are all associated with a sensory neuropathy, which this patient does not demonstrate.

**XII-7.** **The answer is E.** *(Chap. 22)* Thalamic pain syndrome may follow an embolic or lacunar thalamic infarct if it affects the ventral posterolateral (VPL) nucleus or the adjacent white matter. The pain is persistent and severe, affecting only the contralateral side of the body. Other symptoms that may be associated with thalamic infarcts include hemianesthesia, hemiataxia, choreoathetoid movements, and athetoid posture. The eponym applied to this syndrome is Dejerine-Roussy syndrome.

**XII-8.** **The answer is B.** *(Chaps. 290 and 346)* Although chelators are useful in therapy for established Wilson's disease, they have no role in the diagnosis. An MRI of the brain in a patient with suspected neuropsychiatric Wilson's disease may show deposits in the basal ganglia and occasionally in the pons, medulla, thalamus, and cerebellum. An examination for Kayser-Fleischer rings is essential as they are present in over 99% of patients with neurologic/psychiatric forms of the disease. An elevated 24-h urine copper level is suggestive of impaired copper metabolism, which is associated with Wilson's disease. Liver biopsy is the gold standard for establishing excessive copper deposition.

**XII-9.** **The answer is B.** *(Chap. 356)* This patient has a history and examination consistent with a myelopathy. The rapidity of onset and the lack of other antecedent symptoms (e.g., pain) make a noncompressive etiology most likely. An MRI is the initial test of choice and will easily identify a structural lesion such as a neoplasm or subluxation. Noncompressive myelopathies result from five basic causes: spinal cord infarction; systemic disorders such as vasculitis, systemic lupus erythematosus (SLE), and sarcoidosis; infections (particularly viral); demyelinating disease such as multiple sclerosis; and idiopathic. Therefore, serologies for antinuclear antibodies, viral serologies such as HIV and HTLV-I, and lumbar puncture are all indicated. Because the clinical scenario is consistent with a myelopathy, an electromyogram is not indicated.

**XII-10.** **The answer is A.** *(Chap. 356)* Syringomyelia is a developmental, slowly enlarging cavitary expansion of the cervical cord that produces a progressive myelopathy. Symptoms typically begin in adolescence or early adulthood. They may undergo spontaneous arrest after several years. More than half are associated with Chiari malformations. Acquired cavitations of the spinal cord are referred to as syrinx cavities. They may result from trauma, myelitis, infection, or tumor. The classic presentation is that of a central cord syndrome with sensory loss of pain and temperature sensation and weakness of the upper extremities. Vibration and position sensation are typically preserved. Muscle wasting in the lower neck, shoulders, arms, and hands with asymmetric or absent reflexes reflects extension of the cavity to the anterior horns. With progression, spasticity and weakness of the lower extremities and bladder and bowel dysfunction may occur. MRI scans are the diagnostic modality of choice. Surgical therapy is generally unsatisfactory. Syringomyelia associated with Chiari malformations may require extensive decompressions of the posterior fossa. Direct decompression of the cavity is of debatable benefit. Syringomyelia secondary to trauma or infection is treated with decompression and a drainage procedure, with a shunt often inserted that drains into the subarachnoid space. Although relief may occur, recurrence is common.

**XII-11.  The answer is B.**  *(Chap. 363)*   Carpal tunnel syndrome is caused by entrapment of the median nerve at the wrist. Symptoms begin with paresthesias in the median nerve distribution. With worsening, atrophy and weakness may develop. This condition is most commonly caused by excessive use of the wrist. Rarely, systemic disease may result in carpal tunnel syndrome. This may be suspected when bilateral disease is apparent. Tenosynovitis with arthritis as in the case of rheumatoid arthritis and thickening of the connective tissue as in the case of amyloid or acromegaly are also causes. Other systemic diseases, such as hypothyroidism and diabetes mellitus, are also possible etiologies. Leukemia is not typically associated with carpal tunnel syndrome.

**XII-12.  The answer is C.**  *(Chap. 349)*   Cerebrovascular diseases account for up to 200,000 deaths a year in the United States and are a major cause of morbidity. Acute ischemic stroke results from an acute occlusion of an intracranial vessel from in situ thrombosis or an embolic source. The magnitude of the flow reduction is a function of the collateral blood flow, and this depends largely on the vascular anatomy of the individual patient. Brain tissue dies within minutes of a fall in cerebral blood flow. Therefore, reestablishment of flow and prevention of widening of the territory of infarction are two of the major goals of stroke therapy. A pivotal National Institute of Neurological Disorders and Stroke (NINDS) study showed that patients who received intravenous recombinant tissue plasminogen activator (rTPA) within 3 h of the onset of symptoms had a significant clinical benefit. This was the case despite a 6.4% risk of intracerebral hemorrhage. Other, more recent trials have looked at intraarterial delivery of rTPA by a catheter-based approach within a 6-h time frame for middle cerebral artery (MCA) territory infarctions, and there appears to be a significant benefit. Although this has not been approved by the U.S. Food and Drug Administration, based on early clinical trials, it is rapidly becoming the standard of care for patients with MCA strokes that fall out of the 3-h window for intravenous rTPA. Numerous studies have shown the benefit of aspirin administered within 48 h of stroke onset. Aspirin offers a modest benefit in regard to further stroke recurrence. Some literature supports a benefit of clopidogrel in ischemic stroke patients as a means of secondary prevention. Although frequently used, heparin remains unproven as a beneficial agent in the treatment of acute stroke. Because this patient has no contraindication to thrombolytic therapy but falls outside the 3-h window for intravenous rTPA, catheter-delivered rTPA is the next best option if the support facilities exist and should be recommended for this patient.

**XII-13.  The answer is E.**  *(Chap. 349)*   Cardioembolism accounts for up to 20% of all ischemic strokes. Stroke caused by heart disease is due to thrombotic material forming on the atrial or ventricular wall or the left heart valves. If the thrombus lyses quickly, only a transient ischemic attack may develop. If the arterial occlusion lasts longer, brain tissue may die and a stroke will occur. Emboli from the heart most often lodge in the middle cerebral artery (MCA), the posterior cerebral artery (PCA), or one of their branches. Atrial fibrillation is the most common cause of cerebral embolism overall. Other significant causes of cardioembolic stroke include myocardial infarction, prosthetic valves, rheumatic heart disease, and dilated cardiomyopathy. Furthermore, paradoxical embolization may occur when an atrial septal defect or a patent foramen ovale exists. This may be detected by bubble-contrast echocardiography. Bacterial endocarditis may cause septic emboli if the vegetation is on the left side of the heart or if there is a paradoxical source.

**XII-14. The answer is D.** *(Chap. 349)* Nonrheumatic atrial fibrillation is the most common cause of cerebral embolism overall. The presumed stroke mechanism is thrombus formation in the fibrillating atrium or atrial appendage. The average annual risk of stroke is around 5%. However, the risk varies with certain factors: age, hypertension, left ventricular function, prior embolism, diabetes, and thyroid function. Patients younger than 60 years of age without structural heart disease or without one of these risk factors have a very low annual risk of cardioembolism: less than 0.5%. Therefore, it is recommended that these patients only take aspirin daily for stroke prevention. Older patients with numerous risk factors may have annual stroke risks of 10 to 15% and must take warfarin indefinitely. Cardioversion is indicated for symptomatic patients who want an initial opportunity to remain in sinus rhythm. However, studies have shown that there is an increased stroke risk for weeks to months after a successful cardioversion, and these patients must remain on anticoagulation for a long period. Similarly, recent studies have shown that patients who do not respond to cardioversion and do not want catheter ablation have mortality and morbidity with rate control and anticoagulation similar to those of patients who opt for cardioversion. Low-molecular-weight heparin may be used as a bridge to warfarin therapy and may facilitate outpatient anticoagulation in selected patients.

**XII-15. The answer is A.** *(Chap. 353)* ALS is the most common form of progressive motor neuron disease. It is characterized by degeneration of both upper and lower motor neurons. Destruction of peripheral motor neurons results in denervation and consequent atrophy of the corresponding muscle fibers. This results in the "amyotrophy" seen on muscle biopsy. The loss of cortical motor neurons results in thinning of the corticospinal tracts that travel via the internal capsule and brainstem to the lateral and anterior white matter columns of the spinal cord. The loss of fibers in these lateral columns results in the "lateral sclerosis." The etiology is thought to be related to the excitotoxicity of glutamate, which may accumulate as a result of certain transporter defects or as a result of defective superoxide dismutase. Most cases are sporadic, but a small percentage are familial and are inherited in an autosomal dominant fashion. Clinically, these patients may present with weakness in any muscle group. The initial phase is usually asymmetric and starts in the limbs. Denervation results in spontaneous twitching of motor units, or fasciculations. Involvement of the bulbar muscles results in difficulty swallowing. Eventually these patients develop respiratory failure. This is the eventual cause of death in ALS patients. One hallmark of sporadic disease is the preservation of cognitive function. There is no cure for this disease. Riluzole was recently approved for ALS secondary to evidence that it improves survival by an average of approximately 3 months. The mechanism is unclear and may be related to a reduction in excitotoxicity by diminishing glutamate release.

**XII-16. The answer is C.** *(Chap. 368)* The muscular dystrophies are hereditary progressive diseases. Becker's muscular dystrophy is a less severe form of X-linked recessive muscular dystrophy than Duchenne's muscular dystrophy. It occurs 10 times less frequently than DMD. The underlying defect is in the same protein, dystrophin, which is part of a large complex of sarcolemmal proteins and glycoproteins. Clinically, Becker's muscular dystrophy (BMD) shows a similar pattern of proximal muscle weakness. Weakness becomes generalized with progression of the disease. Hypertrophy of muscles, particularly the calves, is an early feature. Most patients experience the initial symptoms in the first and second decades of life, but a later onset may occur. These patients have reduced life expectancy but are significantly more functional than are patients with DMD. Mental retardation may also occur in patients with BMD, and cardiac involvement may result in congestive heart failure. Serum creatinine kinase (CK) levels are elevated, and electrodiagnostic findings are similar to those seen in DMD. The diagnosis is made by demonstrating a reduced amount of dystrophin on Western blot analysis.

**XII-17.   The answer is C.**   *(Chaps. 367 and 368)*   Glycogen storage diseases and glycolytic defects may be suspected in patients who present with painful rhabdomyolysis and myoglobinuria without a compelling history for dehydration, trauma, or excessive exertion. Five glycolytic defects are associated with recurrent myoglobinuria. These defects are characterized clinically by symptoms of pain and muscle stiffness that occur during brief bursts of high-intensity exercise. The symptoms often begin in adolescence. Myoglobinuria and even renal failure may occur. By far the most common of these glycolytic defects is myophosphorylase deficiency, which is known as McArdle's disease. CK levels may vary widely, depending on the clinical scenario. All patients suspected of having glycolytic defects should undergo a forearm exercise test. In this test patients are asked to perform grip exercises repeatedly. Meanwhile, venous lactate and ammonia are measured. In normal individuals both levels rise, indicating metabolic activity. An impaired rise in lactate with a normal rise in ammonia is highly suggestive of a glycolytic defect. A lack of rise in either level indicates insufficient exercise. Aldolase is not helpful as there already is evidence of muscle damage in this patient. Electrodiagnostic studies may be suggestive of muscle defect but would not specifically aid in the diagnosis. Muscle biopsy would help in the definitive diagnosis but is premature at this point because of the level of evidence. Dystrophin gene analysis is useful in the diagnosis of Duchenne's muscular dystrophy or Becker's muscular dystrophy but has no role in this patient.

**XII-18.   The answer is B.**   *(Chap. 368)*   CPT II deficiency is the most common recognizable cause of recurrent myoglobinuria. Onset usually occurs in the second and third decades of life. Unlike the glycolytic defects, muscle pain in CPT II deficiency does not occur until the limits of utilization have been exceeded and muscle breakdown has begun. Levels of creatinine kinase are normal between episodes. Forearm exercise testing shows a normal rise in venous lactate, distinguishing this condition from glycolytic defects, particularly myophosphorylase deficiency, or McArdle's disease. Muscle biopsy is often not helpful. The diagnosis is made by direct measurement of muscle CPT. There is no proven treatment, although low-fat, high-carbohydrate diets are recommended by some experts.

**XII-19.   The answer is C.**   *(Chap. 349)*   Carotid atherosclerosis frequently occurs in the common carotid bifurcation and the proximal internal carotid artery. Five percent of ischemic strokes result from carotid atherosclerosis. The decision to perform surgery in a patient with carotid disease depends on the presence of symptoms and the degree of stenosis. In symptomatic patients two large trials—the North American Symptomatic Carotid Endarterectomy Trial (NASCET) and the European Carotid Surgery Trial—showed a substantial benefit from surgery in patients with stenosis greater than 70%. There was a 17% absolute reduction in ipsilateral stroke in the NASCET trial. That trial also showed benefit in the group with 50 to 70% stenosis. Neither study showed a benefit for patients with symptomatic stenosis less than 50%. Another finding of the studies was that the outcome was heavily dependent on institutional experience with the procedure. Institutions with perioperative complication rates above or equal to 6% did not have the benefits of the CEA procedure. Therefore, the recommendation is that in symptomatic patients with carotid stenosis, CEA is the procedure of choice provided that it is done at an experienced center. In asymptomatic patients the situation is a bit more controversial. A recent study—the Asymptomatic Carotid Atherosclerosis Study (ACAS)—randomized asymptomatic patients with stenosis greater than 60% to surgery versus medical therapy. Although there was a relative risk reduction of ipsilateral stroke of 53% over 5 years in the surgical group, the absolute risk reduction ended up being only 1.2% per year. It is unclear whether newer medical therapies with statins and antiplatelet agents will change this situation in favor of medical therapy. Asymptomatic patients have a stroke risk of about 2% per year, and aspirin and statin therapy are recommended for those patients. Interest in balloon angioplasty with stenting has increased. Although distal embolization has been a concern, newer devices designed to reduce this complication make this procedure an exciting potential alternative to surgery.

**XII-20. The answer is E.** *(Chap. 349)* Numerous studies have identified key risk factors for ischemic stroke. Old age, family history, diabetes, hypertension, tobacco smoking, and cholesterol are all risk factors for atherosclerosis and therefore stroke. Hypertension is the most significant among these risk factors. All cases of hypertension must be controlled in the setting of stroke prevention. Antiplatelet therapy has been shown to reduce the risk of vascular atherothrombotic events. The overall relative risk reduction of nonfatal stroke is about 25 to 30% across most large clinical trials. The "true" absolute benefit is dependent on the individual patient's risk; therefore, patients with a low risk for stroke (e.g., younger, with minimal cardiovascular risk factors) may have a relative risk reduction with antiplatelet therapy but a meaningless "benefit." Numerous studies have shown the benefit of statin therapy in the reduction of stroke risk even in the absence of hypercholesterolemia. Although anticoagulation is the treatment of choice for atrial fibrillation and cardioembolic causes of stroke, there is no proven benefit in regard to the prevention of atherothrombotic stroke; therefore, warfarin cannot be recommended.

**XII-21. The answer is B.** *(Chap. 363)* Peripheral neuropathy is a general term indicating peripheral nerve disorders of any cause. The causes are legion, but peripheral neuropathy can be classified by a number of means: axonal versus demyelinating, mononeuropathy versus polyneuropathy versus mononeuritis multiplex, sensory versus motor, and the tempo of the onset of symptoms. Mononeuropathy typically results from local compression, trauma, or entrapment of a nerve. Polyneuropathy often results from a more systemic process. The distinction between axonal and demyelinating can often be made only with nerve conduction studies. HIV infection causes a common, distal, symmetric, mainly sensory polyneuropathy. Vitamin $B_{12}$ deficiency typically causes a sensory neuropathy that predominantly involves the dorsal columns. Hypothyroidism and acromegaly may both cause compression and swelling of nerve fibers, resulting first in sensory symptoms and later in disease with motor symptoms. Critical illness polyneuropathy is predominantly motor in presentation. These patients may recover over the course of weeks to months. The etiology is unknown, but an association may exist with neuromuscular blockade and corticosteroids.

**XII-22. The answer is A.** *(Chap. 365)* Guillain-Barré syndrome (GBS) is a rare acute fulminant polyradiculoneuropathy that is autoimmune in etiology. Approximately 3500 cases occur per year in the United States and Canada. The majority of cases are preceded by an acute infectious process, usually respiratory or gastrointestinal in origin. *Campylobacter jejuni* is associated with up to 30% of cases in North America, Europe, and Australia. Other etiologic agents include cytomegalovirus and Epstein-Barr virus, mycoplasma, and vaccination. GBS occurs more frequently in patients with lymphoma and HIV infection. Clinically, patients develop a rapidly evolving areflexic motor paralysis with or without sensory disturbance. It is classically ascending in nature. Patients may notice rubbery legs first. Symptoms may evolve over the course of hours to a few days. The legs are usually more involved than are the arms, and facial paresis is present in 50% of these patients. Involvement of lower cranial nerves may cause difficulty with handling secretions and maintaining an airway. Thirty percent of these patients require mechanical ventilation at some point during their illness. Autonomic involvement is common in severe cases. Pain is also a common feature of GBS, ranging from a deep aching pain in the muscles to a shocklike paresthesia. Subtypes of GBS include the Miller Fisher variant, pure sensory forms, ophthalmoplegia with anti-GQ1b antibodies, and bulbar and facial paralysis. CSF findings are distinctive, consisting of an elevated CSF protein level without pleocytosis. Electrodiagnostic features vary, depending on the stage of clinical symptoms. Treatment includes immunotherapy with intravenous immune globulin or plasmapheresis. Treatment must be initiated as soon as possible as the effectiveness diminishes the later it is after the onset of symptoms. Outcomes are good, with the majority of patients having a good recovery within a year. However, many will have persistent minor neurologic sequelae. The main cause of morbidity and mortality is infection, often from pulmonary complications that result from mechanical ventilation. Enteropathic strains of *E. coli* have been associated with hemolytic-uremic syndrome, not with GBS.

**XII-23.  The answer is C.**  *(Chap. 365)*  In addition to Guillain-Barré syndrome, there are many other immune-mediated neuropathies. CIDP is distinguished from GBS by its chronic course. Symptoms may be asymmetric and may show considerable variability from case to case. CSF protein may be elevated as it is in GBS. Electrodiagnostically, there are variable degrees of conduction slowing, prolonged distal latencies, and conduction block. This is consistent with a demyelinating process. The etiology is unknown, and collagen vascular disease, HIV infection, and other systemic diseases must be ruled out. Approximately 25% of these patients have an MGUS present. MMN is an uncommon neuropathy that involves a slowly progressive motor weakness and atrophy in the distribution of selected nerve trunks. This occurs slowly over the course of years. Sensory fibers are relatively spared. Most of these patients are male, and the upper extremities are affected more than the lower extremities are. Fifty percent of these patients have a high titer of IgM antibodies to ganglioside GM1. Electrodiagnostic studies and pathology are consistent with an inflammatory demyelinating process. Polyneuropathy occurs in a minority of patients with multiple myeloma except in the rare case of those with osteosclerotic myeloma. This entity is associated with polyneuropathy in half the cases. In addition to polyneuropathy, other systemic findings may include thickening of the skin, hyperpigmentation, hypertrichosis, organomegaly, endocrinopathy, anasarca, and clubbing of the fingers. This constitutes the POEMS syndrome (polyneuropathy, organomegaly, endocrinopathy, M protein, and skin changes). Peripheral nerve involvement is common in some types of vasculitis, particularly polyarteritis nodosa. The most common pattern is mononeuritis multiplex caused by ischemic lesions of nerve trunks and roots. However, some types of vasculitic neuropathy present as a distal, symmetric motor-sensory neuropathy. Anti-Hu antibodies are associated with an autoimmune neuronopathy, resulting in an asymmetric sensory loss in the limbs, torso, and face. Marked sensory ataxia, pseudoathetosis, and inability to walk or stand are common features. Most cases are idiopathic, but in 25% of cases an underlying cancer, particularly small-cell lung cancer, is detected. Interestingly, the neurologic symptoms often precede the diagnosis of cancer by approximately 1 year.

**XII-24.  The answer is B.**  *(Chap. 362)*  Prions are the only known infectious agent that is devoid of DNA or RNA. They are infectious proteins that cause degeneration of the central nervous system. Prions reproduce by binding to the normal cellular isotype of the prion protein and causing a conformational change to a pathogenic isoform of the prion protein. The mechanism is unknown. Patients may have sporadic disease or may have a familial form. Sporadic cases account for the vast majority, with sCJD accounting for 85% of human cases. The median age of presentation is the sixth decade. Variant CJD is associated with BSE infection epidemiologically and may present at any age. Histologically, these patients have spongiform degeneration without inflammation. Clinically, CJD patients may have nonspecific prodromal symptoms, including fatigue, sleep disturbance, weight loss, headache, malaise, and pain. Most of these patients develop higher cortical deficits. These deficits progress over the course of weeks to months to a state of profound dementia characterized by memory loss, impaired judgment, and a total decline in intellectual function. There is no known treatment.

**XII-25.  The answer is D.**  *(Chap. 364)*  CMT disease is a heterogeneous group of inherited peripheral neuropathies. Transmission is usually autosomal dominant but may be recessive or X-linked. Numerous genetic defects are associated with CMT disease. It is very common, affecting up to 1 in 2500 persons. Clinically, patients usually present in the first or second decade of life, but later presentations may occur. The neuropathy affects both motor and sensory nerves. Symptoms may vary, ranging from distal muscle weakness and severe atrophy and disability to only pes cavus and minimal weakness. Although sensory findings and involvement are common, these patients often do not have dominant sensory complaints. However, if patients have no evidence of sensory involvement on detailed neurologic examination or electrodiagnostic studies, an alternative diagnosis should be considered. There is no known effective therapy for CMT disease. Orthotics and physical therapy are mainstays for preserving function.

**XII-26. The answer is C.** *(Chap. 348)* The classification of a seizure is important in determining the etiology and potential treatment options. The main characteristic that distinguishes the different categories of seizures is whether a seizure is partial or generalized. Partial seizures are seizures in which the activity is restricted to discrete regions of the brain. Generalized seizures involve diffuse regions of the brain simultaneously. Partial seizures are usually associated with structural abnormalities of the brain, whereas generalized seizures may result from cellular, biochemical, or structural abnormalities that have a more widespread distribution. With simple partial seizures, consciousness is maintained. With complex partial seizures, consciousness is impaired. Simple partial seizures may cause motor, sensory, autonomic, or psychic symptoms without an obvious impairment in consciousness. Motor seizures may include typical clonic activity that corresponds to a particular part of the brain on electroencephalography (EEG). Other forms may involve somatic sensation, equilibrium, and impairment in olfaction, hearing, or higher cortical functions (e.g., emotions). When these symptoms precede a complex partial or secondarily generalized seizure, these simple partial seizures are termed auras. Complex partial seizures are characterized by focal seizure activity accompanied by a transient impairment of the ability to maintain normal contact with the environment. The behavioral arrest is often accompanied by automatisms, which are involuntary automatic behaviors that may include chewing, lip smacking, swallowing, or more elaborate movements. Absence seizures often start in childhood. They are characterized by sudden brief lapses of consciousness without loss of postural control. There is no postictal confusion, and the episodes usually last only seconds. Generalized tonic-clonic, or grand mal, seizures involve generalized motor activity with loss of consciousness and a postictal phase. Atonic seizures are characterized by a sudden loss of postural muscle tone that lasts 1 to 2 s. There is no postictal confusion, and the loss of consciousness is brief. Myoclonic seizures involve sudden and brief muscle contraction. They usually coexist with other forms of generalized seizure disorders but are the predominant feature in juvenile myoclonic epilepsy.

**XII-27. The answer is D.** *(Chap. 348)* The causes of seizures vary with the age at presentation. In neonates, prepartum and peripartum factors predominate. Perinatal hypoxia or trauma, acute infection, maternal use of cocaine or opiates, and genetic disorders are the most common causes of seizure in that age group. In children older than 1 year through early adolescence (10 to 12 years of age), febrile seizures, genetic disorders, developmental disorders, trauma, and infection are common. In older patients (over 35 years of age), cerebrovascular disease, neoplasia, trauma (particularly subdural hematoma or intracranial hemorrhage), and degenerative diseases (e.g., Alzheimer's dementia) predominate. Mesial temporal lobe epilepsy (MTLE) is the syndrome most commonly associated with complex partial seizures. It is characterized by hippocampal sclerosis that is best seen on magnetic resonance imaging. Anticonvulsants are usually ineffective, but surgery may be curative. It usually presents in childhood or adolescence. It is uncommon for it to present in late adulthood.

**XII-28. The answer is B.** *(Chap. 348)* Optimal medical therapy for epilepsy depends on the underlying cause, type of seizure, and patient factors. The goal is to prevent seizures and minimize the side effects of therapy. The minimal effective dose is determined by trial and error. In choosing medical therapies, drug interactions are a key consideration. Certain medications, such as tricyclic antidepressants, may lower the seizure threshold and should be avoided. Patients who respond well to medical therapy and have completely controlled seizures are good candidates for the discontinuation of therapy, with about 70% of children and 60% of adults being able to discontinue therapy eventually. Patient factors that aid in this include complete medical control of seizures for 1 to 5 years, a normal neurologic examination, a normal EEG, and single seizure type. On the other end of the spectrum, about 20% of these patients are completely refractory to medical therapy and should be considered for surgical therapy. In the best examples, such as mesial temporal sclerosis, resection of the temporal lobe may result in about 70% of these patients becoming seizure-free and an additional 15 to 25% having a significant reduction in the incidence of seizures. In patients with epilepsy other considerations are critical. Psychosocial sequelae such as depression, anxiety, and behavior problems may occur. Approximately 20% of epileptic patients have depression, with their suicide rate being higher than that of age-matched controls. There is an impact on the ability to drive, perform certain jobs, and function in social situations. Furthermore, there is a twofold to threefold increase in mortality for patients with epilepsy compared with age-matched controls. Although most of the increased mortality results from the underlying etiology of epilepsy, a significant number of these patients die from accidents, status epilepticus, and a syndrome known as sudden unexpected death in epileptic patients (SUDEP). The cause is unknown, but research has centered on brainstem-mediated effects of seizures on cardiopulmonary function.

**XII-29.  The answer is D.**  *(Chap. 348)*   Phenytoin is a commonly used anticonvulsant. Its principal use is in patients with tonic-clonic seizures. It may be given either orally or intravenously. Typical dosing is about 300 to 400 mg/d in adults. The therapeutic range is between 10 and 20 $\mu$g/mL. Neurologic side effects include dizziness, ataxia, diplopia, and confusion. Systemic side effects include gum hyperplasia, hirsutism, facial coarsening, and osteomalacia. These patients may develop lymphadenopathy and Stevens-Johnson syndrome. Toxicity may be enhanced by liver disease and competition with other medications. Phenytoin alters folate metabolism and is teratogenic. Leukopenia is not a typical side effect and is seen more often with carbamazepine.

**XII-30.  The answer is E.**  *(Chap. 366)*   Myasthenia gravis (MG) is a neuromuscular disorder characterized by weakness and fatigability of skeletal muscles. The primary defect is a decrease in the number of acetylcholine receptors at the neuromuscular junction secondary to autoimmune antibodies. MG is not rare, affecting at least 1 in 7500 individuals. Women are affected more frequently than are men. Women present typically in the second and third decades of life, and men present in the fifth and sixth decades. The key features of MG are weakness and fatigability. Clinical features include weakness of the cranial muscles, particularly the lids and extraocular muscles. Diplopia and ptosis are common initial complaints. Weakness in chewing is noticeable after prolonged effort. Speech may be affected secondary to weakness of the palate or tongue weakness. Swallowing may result from weakness of the palate, tongue, or pharynx. In the majority of patients the weakness becomes generalized. The diagnosis is suspected after the appearance of the characteristic symptoms and signs. Edrophonium is an acetylcholinesterase inhibitor that allows ACh to interact repeatedly with the limited number of AChRs, producing improvement in the strength of myasthenic muscles. False-positive tests may occur in patients with other neurologic diseases. Electrodiagnostic testing may show evidence of reduction in the amplitude of the evoked muscle action potentials with repeated stimulation. Testing for the specific antibodies to AChR are diagnostic. In addition to anti-AChR antibodies, antibodies to MuSK have been found in some patients with clinical MG. Antibodies to voltage-gated calcium channels are found in patients with the Lambert-Eaton syndrome.

**XII-31.  The answer is A.**  *(Chap. 366)*   The pathophysiology of myasthenia gravis is thought to be autoimmune in nature, with the thymus playing a central role. Patients with MG often have an abnormal thymus. The incidence of thymoma is markedly increased in patients with MG. Although all the other treatment options are useful at varying points in the treatment of MG, clinical trials show that 85% of patients exhibit benefit from removal of the thymus as part of the treatment of myasthenia gravis. Up to 35% of these patients may attain long-term drug-free remission of disease. Therefore, all patients with MG between the ages of puberty and 55 years should undergo thymectomy as a possibly definitive treatment. There is concern that very young patients may experience long-term immunologic dysfunction as a result of early thymectomy. The benefit in older patients is less clear.

**XII-32.** **The answer is B.** *(Chap. 20)* The symptoms and signs described in this question are most consistent with Ménière's disease. In this disorder paroxysmal vertigo resulting from labyrinthine lesions is associated with nausea, vomiting, rotary nystagmus, tinnitus, high-tone hearing loss with recruitment, and, most characteristically, fullness in the ear. Labyrinthitis would be an unlikely diagnosis in this case because of the hearing loss and multiple episodes. Vertebral-basilar insufficiency and multiple sclerosis typically are associated with brainstem signs. Acoustic neuroma only rarely causes vertigo as the initial symptom, and the vertigo it does cause is mild and intermittent.

**XII-33.** **The answer is A.** *(Chap. 355)* The abrupt appearance of an isolated peripheral facial palsy, which may include ipsilateral hyperacusis resulting from involvement of fibers to the stapedius and loss of taste on the anterior two-thirds of the tongue resulting from involvement of the fibers of the chorda tympani, is most often idiopathic, as in patients with Bell's palsy. If the patient is unable to close the eye, artificial tears may be helpful during the day to prevent drying, and the eye should be patched at night to prevent corneal abrasion. Excellent recovery occurs in 80% of these cases. Oral contraceptives and mitral valve prolapse are not associated with the causes of this clinical picture. Evoked potentials are not helpful diagnostically.

**XII-34.** **The answer is B.** *(Chap. 14)* Cluster headaches, which can cause excruciating hemi-cranial pain, are notable for their occurrence during characteristic episodes. Usually attacks occur during a 4- to 8-week period in which the patient experiences one to three severe brief headaches daily. There may then be a prolonged pain-free interval before the next episode. Men between ages 20 and 50 are most commonly affected. The unilateral pain is usually associated with lacrimation, eye reddening, nasal stuffiness, ptosis, and nausea. During episodes alcohol may provoke the attacks. Even though the pain caused by brain tumors may awaken a patient from sleep, the typical history and normal neurologic examination do not mandate evaluation for a neoplasm of the central nervous system. Acute therapy for a cluster headache attack consists of oxygen inhalation, although intranasal lidocaine and subcutaneous sumatriptan may also be effective. Prophylactic therapy with prednisone, lithium, methysergide, ergotamine, or verapamil can be administered during an episode to prevent further cluster headache attacks.

**XII-35.** **The answer is D.** *(Chap. 25)* This patient has acute angle-closure glaucoma resulting from obstruction of the outflow of aqueous humor at the iris. The buildup of intraocular pressure can be confirmed by measurement and requires urgent treatment with hyperosmotic agents. Permanent treatment requires laser or surgical iridotomy. Angle-closure glaucoma is less common than is primary open-angle glaucoma, which is asymptomatic and is usually detectable only through measurements of intraocular pressure at a routine eye examination.

**XII-36.** **The answer is D.** *(Chap. 359)* Optic neuritis is the initial symptom in approximately 40% of persons who are eventually diagnosed with multiple sclerosis. This rapidly developing ophthalmologic disorder is associated with partial or total loss of vision, pain on motion of the involved eye, scotoma affecting macular vision, and a variety of other visual field defects. Ophthalmoscopically visible optic papillitis occurs in about half these patients.

**XII-37.** **The answer is C.** *(Chap. 350; Yankner, N Engl J Med 325:1849–1857, 1991.)* Alzheimer's disease is the most common cause of dementia in the elderly. It is highly prevalent, affecting up to 45% of those over age 85. In a relatively small percentage of cases the disease occurs in a familial pattern; this is thought to be due to autosomal dominant inheritance with linkage to chromosome 21 or 19. The clinical beginnings of the disease tend to be subtle. The initial symptoms are usually limited to loss of recent memory. Psychiatric symptoms may then supervene and can include depression, anxiety, delusions, and paranoid behavior. An extrapyramidal component exists so that patients walk in a shuffling manner with short steps. Radiographic evaluation usually reveals neuronal atrophy. Neuropathologically, the disease is characterized by neurofibrillary tangles, which may contain an abnormally phosphorylated form of a microtubular protein known as *tau* as well as spherical deposits known as *senile plaques*. A protein known as $\beta$-amyloid can be found in these plaques. Certain families with inherited Alzheimer's disease have been found to have a point mutation in the amyloid precursor protein. From a neurotransmitter standpoint, acetylcholine, a neurotransmitter that is important in memory formation, is synthesized at abnormally low levels. The current model for the pathogenesis of Alzheimer's disease is that altered cleavage of the amyloid precursor protein generates the so-called $\beta$-amyloid protein, which then binds to a protease inhibitor–enzyme complex, in turn preventing the normal inactivation of extracellular proteases. It is these abnormally activated extracellular proteases that may mediate the neuronal degeneration characteristic of Alzheimer's disease. Therapeutic strategies that could inhibit the generation of $\beta$-amyloid are of potential therapeutic interest.

**XII-38.  The answer is E.**  *(Chap. 370)*    Although a viral cause has been postulated, no clear-cut etiology has been demonstrated for chronic fatigue syndrome. Furthermore, while several subtle immunologic abnormalities have been documented in certain patients with this syndrome, there is no definitive diagnostic test. The diagnosis of chronic fatigue syndrome relies on the Centers for Disease Control and Prevention's working definition. A definitive diagnosis is based on the presence of both of the major criteria: persistent or relapsing fatigue that does not resolve with bed rest and is severe enough to reduce average daily activity by 50% and exclusion of other chronic conditions, including preexisting psychiatric diseases. The physical examination must include two of the following three physical findings by a doctor on at least two occasions 1 month apart: low-grade fever, pharyngitis, and palpable lymphadenopathy. Finally, at least six of the common symptoms must be present; these symptoms include mild fever or chills, sore throat, painful lymph nodes in the cervical chains, muscle weakness, muscle discomfort, fatigue after minimal exercise, new headaches, arthralgias, neuropsychological symptoms, and sleep disturbance. Patients who do not have the required physical findings have to fulfill eight of the symptom criteria. Because there is no specific therapy for this disease, treatment requires an understanding of the patient and the avoidance of unproven therapies such as acyclovir, vitamin $B_{12}$, intravenous gamma globulin, and steroids. Treatment should be symptom-directed. Thus, nonsteroidal anti-inflammatory drugs (NSAIDs), decongestants, and antidepressants may be helpful, depending on the symptoms. Finally, lifestyle modification, including a graded exercise program, minimal caffeine intake, and avoidance of complete rest, is advisable.

**XII-39.  The answer is D.**  *(Chap. 355)*    Brief paroxysms of severe, sharp pains in the face without demonstrable lesions in the jaw, teeth, or sinuses are called tic douloureux, or trigeminal neuralgia. The pain may be brought on by stimuli applied to the face, lips, or tongue or by certain movements of those structures. Aneurysms, neurofibromas, and meningiomas impinging on the fifth cranial nerve at any point during its course typically present with trigeminal neuropathy, which will cause sensory loss on the face, weakness of the jaw muscles, or both; neither symptom is demonstrable in this patient. The treatment for this idiopathic condition is carbamazepine or phenytoin if carbamazepine is not tolerated. When drug treatment is not successful, surgical therapy, including the commonly applied percutaneous retrogasserian rhizotomy, may be effective. A possible complication of this procedure is partial facial numbness with a risk of corneal anesthesia, which increases the potential for ulceration.

**XII-40.  The answer is C.**  *(Chap. 355)*    Pain, loss of function (without clear-cut sensory or motor deficits), and a localized autonomic impairment are called reflex sympathetic dystrophy (also known as shoulder-hand syndrome or causalgia). Precipitating events in this unusual syndrome include myocardial infarction, shoulder trauma, and limb paralysis. In addition to the neuropathic-type pain, autonomic dysfunction, possibly resulting from neuroadrenergic and cholinergic hypersensitivity, produces localized sweating, changes in blood flow, and abnormal hair and nail growth as well as edema or atrophy of the affected limb. Treatment is difficult; however, anticonvulsants such as phenytoin and carbamazepine may be effective, as they are in other conditions in which neuropathic pain is a major problem.

**XII-41.   The answer is E.**   *(Chaps. 23 and 350)*   All the choices given in the question are causes of or may be associated with dementia. Binswanger's disease, the cause of which is unknown, often occurs in patients with long-standing hypertension and/or atherosclerosis; it is associated with diffuse subcortical white matter damage and has a subacute insidious course. Alzheimer's disease, the most common cause of dementia, is also slowly progressive and can be confirmed at autopsy by the presence of amyloid plaques and neurofibrillary tangles. Creutzfeldt-Jakob disease, a prion disease, is associated with a rapidly progressive dementia, myoclonus, rigidity, a characteristic EEG pattern, and death within 1 to 2 years of onset. Vitamin $B_{12}$ deficiency, which often is seen in the setting of chronic alcoholism, most commonly produces a myelopathy that results in loss of vibration and joint position sense and brisk deep tendon reflexes (dorsal column and lateral corticospinal tract dysfunction). This combination of pathologic abnormalities in the setting of vitamin $B_{12}$ deficiency is also called subacute combined degeneration. Vitamin $B_{12}$ deficiency may also lead to a subcortical type of dementia. Multi-infarct dementia, as in this case, presents with a history of sudden stepwise declines in function associated with the accumulation of bilateral focal neurologic deficits. Brain imaging demonstrates multiple areas of stroke.

**XII-42.   The answer is D.**   *(Chap. 350; Mayeux, Sano, N Engl J Med 341:1670–1679, 1999.)* The definitive diagnosis of Alzheimer's disease remains elusive. Dementia is established by examination as well as by documentation of subjective testing. All patients with Alzheimer's disease have memory impairment and have at least one other cognitive function that is impaired, such as language or perception. These patients typically have worsening of their memory loss. Patients should not have an alteration of consciousness. The onset of Alzheimer's disease occurs between ages 40 and 90, and the absence of other brain disorders or systemic disease that may cause dementia should be established. In addition, the diagnosis of Alzheimer's disease is supported by the loss of motor skills, diminished independence and activities of daily living, altered patterns of behavior, a positive family history, and cerebral atrophy on CT. The presence of neurofibrillary tangles and senile plaques is made at postmortem examination; it confirms the diagnosis of clinical Alzheimer's disease but is not part of the clinical diagnostic criteria.

# REFERENCES

The Acute Respiratory Distress Syndrome Network: Ventilation with lower tidal volumes as compared with traditional tidal volumes for acute lung injury and the acute respiratory distress syndrome. *N Engl J Med* 342:1301–1208, 2000.

Adrogue HJ, Madias NE: Management of life-threatening acid-base disorders. First of two parts. *N Engl J Med* 338:26–34, 1998.

Annane D, Sebille V, Charpentier C, et al.: Effect of treatment with low doses of hydrocortisone and fludrocortisone on mortality in patients with septic shock. *JAMA* 288:862–871, 2002.

Baker DG, Schumacher HR Jr: Acute monoarthritis. *N Engl J Med* 329:1013–1020, 1993.

Bernard GR, Vincent JL, Laterre PF, et al.: Recombinant human protein C Worldwide Evaluation in Severe Sepsis (PROWESS) study group: Efficacy and safety of recombinant human activated protein C for severe sepsis. *N Engl J Med* 344:699–709, 2001.

Bick RL, Strauss JF, Frenkel EP: Thrombosis and hemorrhage in oncology patients. *Hematol Oncol Clin North Am* 10:875, 1996.

Bochner BS, Lichtenstein LM: *Anaphylaxis. N Engl J Med* 324:1785–1790, 1991.

Brickner ME, Hillis LD, Lange RA: Congenital heart disease in adults. *N Engl J Med* 342:256–263, 988, 2000.

Brochard L, Mancebo J, Wysocki M, et al.: Noninvasive ventilation for acute exacerbations of chronic obstructive pulmonary disease. *N Engl J Med* 333:817–822, 1995.

Buller HR, Davidson BL, Decousus H, et al.; Matisse Investigators: Subcutaneous fondaparinux versus intravenous unfractionated heparin in the initial treatment of pulmonary embolism. *N Engl J Med* 349:1695–1702, 2003.

Burrows PD, Cooper MD: *IgA deficiency. Adv Immunol* 65:245–276, 1997.

Burtis WJ, Brady TG, Orloff JJ, et al.: Immunochemical characterization of circulating parathyroid hormone-related protein in patients with humoral hypercalcemia of cancer. *N Engl J Med* 322:1106–1112, 1990.

The Bypass Angioplasty Revascularization Investigation (BARI) Investigators: Comparison of coronary bypass surgery with angioplasty in patients with multivessel disease. *N Engl J Med* 335:217–225, 1996.

Camm AJ, Garratt CJ: Adenosine and supraventricular tachycardia. *N Engl J Med* 325:1621–1629, 1991.

Caroff SN, Mann SC: Neuroleptic malignant syndrome. *Med Clin North Am* 77:185–202, 1993.

CAPRIE Steering Committee: A randomised, blinded trial of clopidogrel versus aspirin in patients at risk of ischemic events (CAPRIE). *Lancet* 348(9038):1329–1339, 1996.

Carter HB, Landis PK, Metter EJ, Fleisher LA, Pearson JD: Prostate-specific antigen testing of older men. *J Natl Cancer Inst* 91:1733–1737, 1999.

Catalina G, Navarro V: Hepatitis C: A challenge for the generalist. *Hosp Pract (Off Ed)* 35:97–108, 2000.

Chobanian AV, Bakris GL, Black HR, et al.: National Heart, Lung, and Blood Institute Joint National Committee on Prevention, Detection, Evaluation, and Treatment of High Blood Pressure; National High Blood Pressure Education Program Coordinating Committee: The Seventh Report of the Joint National Committee on Prevention, Detection, Evaluation, and Treatment of High Blood Pressure: the JNC 7 report. *JAMA* 289:2560–2572, 2003.

Collaborative Group on Hormonal Factors in Breast Cancer: Breast cancer and breastfeeding: collaborative reanalysis of individual data from 47 epidemiological studies in 30 countries, including 50302 women with breast cancer and 96973 women without the disease. *Lancet* 360:187–195, 2002.

Collard HR, Saint S, Matthay MA: Prevention of ventilator-associated pneumonia: An evidence-based systematic review. *Ann Intern Med* 138:494–501, 2003.

Dixon TC, Meselson M, Guillemin J, Hanna PC: Anthrax. *N Engl J Med* 341:815–826, 1999.

Duggan C, Marriott K, Edwards R, Cuzick J: Inherited and acquired risk factors for venous thromboembolic disease among women taking tamoxifen to prevent breast cancer. *J Clin Oncol* 21:3588–3593, 2003.

Eggimann P, Garbino J, Pittet D: Management of *Candida* species infections in critically ill patients. *Lancet Infect Dis* 3:772–785, 2003.

Emmerson BT *The management of gout. N Engl J Med* 334:445–451, 1996.

Fine KD, Schiller LR: AGA technical review on the evaluation and management of chronic diarrhea. *Gastroenterology* 116:1464–1486, 1999.

Fishbein DB, Robinson LE: Rabies. *N Engl J Med* 329:1632–1638, 1993.

Frank MM: *Complement in the pathophysiology of human disease. N Engl J Med* 316:1525–1530, 1987.

Furrer H, Egger M, Opravil M, et al.: Discontinuation of primary prophylaxis against *Pneumocystis carinii* pneumonia in HIV-1-infected adults treated with combination antiretroviral therapy. Swiss HIV Cohort Study. *N Engl J Med* 340:1301, 1999.

Fudala PJ, Bridge TP, Herbert S, et al.: Buprenorphine/Naloxone Collaborative Study Group: Office-based treatment of opiate addiction with a sublingual-tablet formulation of buprenorphine and naloxone. *N Engl J Med* 349:949–958, 2003.

Goldstein I, Lue TF, Padma-Nathan H, et al.: Sildenafil Study Group: Oral sildenafil in the treatment of erectile dysfunction. *N Engl J Med* 338:1397–1404, 1998.

Goldstein RA, Paul WE, Metcalfe DD, Busse WW, Reece ER: NIH conference. Asthma. *Ann Intern Med* 121:698–708, 1994.

Gregoratos G, Abrams J, Epstein AE, et al.: American College of Cardiology/American Heart Association Task Force on Practice Guidelines/North American Society for Pacing and Electrophysiology Committee to Update the 1998 Pacemaker Guidelines: ACC/AHA/NASPE 2002 guideline update for implantation of cardiac pacemakers and antiarrhythmia devices: summary article: a report of the American College of Cardiology/American Heart Association Task Force on Practice Guidelines (ACC/AHA/NASPE Committee to Update the 1998 Pacemaker Guidelines). *Circulation* 106:2145–2161, 2002.

Hall J, Schmidt G, Wood L (eds): *Principles of Critical Care*, 2d ed. New York, McGraw-Hill, 1998.

Heyland DK, MacDonald S, Keefe L, Drover JW: Total parenteral nutrition in the critically ill patient: a meta-analysis. *JAMA* 280:2013–2019, 1998.

Ifudu O: Care of patients undergoing hemodialysis. *N Engl J Med* 339:1054–1062, 1998.

International Perinatal HIV Group: The mode of delivery and the risk of vertical transmission of human immunodeficiency virus type 1—a meta-analysis of 15 prospective cohort studies. *N Engl J Med* 340:977–987, 1999.

Janicic N, Verbalis JG: Evaluation and management of hypo-osmolality in hospitalized patients. *Endocrinol Metab Clin North Am* 32:459–481, 2003

Jeu L, Piacenti FJ, Lyakhovetskiy AG, Fung HB: Voriconazole. *Clin Ther* 25:1321–1381, 2003.

Kjos SL, Buchanan TA: Gestational diabetes mellitus. *N Engl J Med* 341:1749–1756, 1999.

Koutsky LA, Ault KA, Wheeler CM, et al.; Proof of Principle Study Investigators: A controlled trial of a human papillomavirus type 16 vaccine. *N Engl J Med* 347:1645–1651, 2002.

Larsen GL: Asthma in children. *N Engl J Med* 326:1540–1542, 1992.

Lawn ND, Fletcher DD, Henderson RD, Wolter TD, Wijdicks EF: Anticipating mechanical ventilation in Guillain-Barre syndrome. *Arch Neurol* 58:893–898, 2001.

Lenzi R, Hess KR, Abbruzzese MC, et al.: Poorly differentiated carcinoma and poorly differentiated adenocarcinoma of unknown origin: Favorable subsets of patients with unknown-primary carcinoma? *J Clin Oncol* 15:2056–2066, 1997.

Light RW: Clinical practice. Pleural effusion. *N Engl J Med* 346:1971–1977, 2002.

Loftus EV: Microscopic colitis: Epidemiology and treatment. *Am J Gastroenterol* 98(12 Suppl): S31–S36, 2003.

Lowy FD: *Staphylococcus aureus* infections. *N Engl J Med* 339:520–532, 1998.

Lue TF: Erectile dysfunction. *N Engl J Med* 342:1802–1813, 2000.

Mangano DT, Layug EL, Wallace A, Tateo I: Effect of atenolol on mortality and cardiovascular morbidity after noncardiac surgery. Multicenter Study of Perioperative Ischemia Research Group. *N Engl J Med* 335:1713–1720, 1996.

Mangano DT, Goldman L: Preoperative assessment of patients with known or suspected coronary disease. *N Engl J Med* 333:1750–1756, 1995.

Mayeux R, Sano M: Treatment of Alzheimer's disease. *N Engl J Med* 341:1670–1679, 1999.

McFadden ER Jr, Elsanadi N, Dixon L, et al.: Protocol therapy for acute asthma: Therapeutic benefits and cost savings. *Am J Med* 99:651, 1995.

Morris MJ, Scher HI: Novel strategies and therapeutics for the treatment of prostate carcinoma. *Cancer* 89:1329–1348, 2000.

Moss AJ, Zareba W, Hall WJ, et al.; Multicenter Automatic Defibrillator Implantation Trial II Investigators: Prophylactic implantation of a defibrillator in patients with myocardial infarction and reduced ejection fraction. *N Engl J Med* 346:877–883, 2002.

Naclerio RM: *Allergic rhinitis. N Engl J Med* 325:860–869, 1991.

Nathan DM: *Long-term complications of diabetes mellitus. N Engl J Med* 328:1676–1685, 1993.

National Institutes of Health: Endoscopic Retrograde Cholangiopancreatography (ERCP) for Diagnosis and Therapy. Kensington, MD, National Institutes of Health, 2002. Available at: *http://consensus.nih.gov/ta/020/020sos_intro.htm*

*Neufeld M, Maclaren NK, Blizzard RM: Two types of autoimmune Addison's disease associated with different polyglandular autoimmune (PGA) syndromes. Medicine* 60:355–362, 1981.

Ney L, Kuebler WM: Ventilation with lower tidal volumes as compared with traditional tidal volumes for acute lung injury. *N Engl J Med* 343:812–814, 2000.

Ost D, Fein AM, Feinsilver SH: Clinical practice. The solitary pulmonary nodule. *N Engl J Med* 348:2535–2542, 2003.

Pappas PG, Rex JH, Sobel JD, et al.; Infectious Diseases Society of America: Guidelines for treatment of candidiasis. *Clin Infect Dis* 38:161–189, 2004.

Pettitt AR, Zuzel M, Cawley JC: Hairy-cell leukaemia: biology and management. *Br J Haematol* 106:2–8, 1999.

Piscitelli SC, Gallicano KD: Interactions among drugs for HIV and opportunistic infections. *N Engl J Med* 344:984–996, 2001.

Raghu G, Brown KK, Bradford WZ, et al.; Idiopathic Pulmonary Fibrosis Study Group: A placebo-controlled trial of interferon gamma-1b in patients with idiopathic pulmonary fibrosis. *N Engl J Med* 350:125–133, 2004.

Rubin LJ: Pulmonary hypertension, in *Hurst's The Heart*, 10th edition, V Fuster, RW Alexander, RA O'Rourke et al. (eds). New York, McGraw-Hill, Chap. 52, pp 1607–1623, 2001.

Ridker PM, Hennekens CH, Lindpaintner K, et al.: Mutation in the gene coding for coagulation factor V and the risk of myocardial infarction, stroke, and venous thrombosis in apparently healthy men. *N Engl J Med* 332:912, 1995.

Rossouw JE, Anderson GL, Prentice RL, et al.: Writing Group for the Women's Health Initiative Investigators: Risks and benefits of estrogen plus progestin in healthy postmenopausal women: principal results From the Women's Health Initiative randomized controlled trial. *JAMA* 288:321–333, 2002.

Rubin HR, Fink NE, Plantinga LC, et al.: Patient ratings of dialysis care with peritoneal dialysis vs hemodialysis. *JAMA* 291:697–703, 2004.

Ryan KJ, Ray CG: *Sherris' Medical Microbiology,* 4th edition. New York, McGraw-Hill, Chap. 39, pg. 581, 2004.

Sakane T, Takeno M, Suzuki N, Inaba G: Behcet's disease. *N Engl J Med* 341:1284–1291, 1999.

Sharpe M, Hawton K, Simkin S, et al.: Cognitive behaviour therapy for the chronic fatigue syndrome: a randomized controlled trial. *BMJ* 312:22–26, 1996.

Sillevis Smitt P, Kinoshita A, De Leeuw B, et al.: Paraneoplastic cerebellar ataxia due to autoantibodies against a glutamate receptor. IN Engl J Med 342:21–27, 2000.

Silverberg SJ, Shane E, Jacobs TP, Siris E, Bilezikian JP: A 10-year prospective study of primary hyperparathyroidism with or without parathyroid surgery. *N Engl J Med* 341:1249–1255, 1999.

Smith RA, Cokkinides V, Eyre HJ; American Cancer Society: American Cancer Society guidelines for the early detection of cancer, 2004. *CA Cancer J Clin* 54:41–52, 2004.

Sneller MC, Strober W, Eisenstein E, Jaffe JS, Cunningham-Rundles C: NIH conference. New insights into common variable immunodeficiency. *Ann Intern Med* 118:720–730, 1993.

Solomon R: Contrast-medium-induced acute renal failure. *Kidney Int* 53:230–242, 1998.

Takahashi Y, Murai C, Shibata S, et al.: Human parvovirus B19 as a causative agent for rheumatoid arthritis. *Proc Natl Acad Sci USA* 95:8227–8232, 1998.

Tenaglia AN, Califf RM, Candela RJ, et al.: Thrombolytic therapy in patients requiring cardiopulmonary resuscitation. *Am J Cardiol* 68:1015–1019, 1991.

Varon J, Marik PE: The diagnosis and management of hypertensive crises. *Chest* 118:214–227, 2000.

Vollmer WM, Sacks FM, Ard J, et al.: DASH-Sodium Trial Collaborative Research Group: Effects of diet and sodium intake on blood pressure: subgroup analysis of the DASH-sodium trial. *Ann Intern Med* 135:1019–1028, 2001.

Weverling GJ, Mocroft A, Ledergerber B, et al.: Discontinuation of Pneumocystis carinii pneumonia prophylaxis after start of highly active antiretroviral therapy in HIV-1 infection. EuroSIDA Study Group. *Lancet* 353:1293, 1999.

Wheeler AP, Bernard GR: Treating patients with severe sepsis. *N Engl J Med* 240:207–214, 1999.

Whiting P, Bagnall AM, Sowden AJ, et al.: Interventions for the treatment and management of chronic fatigue syndrome: a systematic review. *JAMA* 286:1360–1368, 2001.

Wilson WR, Karchmer AW, Dajani AS, et al.: Antibiotic treatment of adults with infective endocarditis due to streptococci, enterococci, staphylococci, and HACEK microorganisms. American Heart Association. *JAMA* 274:1706, 1995.

Wilt TJ, Ishani A, Stark G, et al.: Saw palmetto extracts for treatment of benign prostatic hyperplasia: a systematic review. *JAMA* 280:1604–1609, 1998.

Yankner BA, Mesulam MM: Seminars in medicine of the Beth Israel Hospital, Boston. beta-Amyloid and the pathogenesis of Alzheimer's disease. *N Engl J Med* 325:1849–1857, 1991.

# Color Atlas

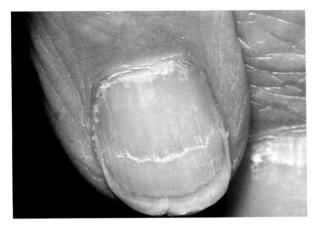

**Figure I-10**

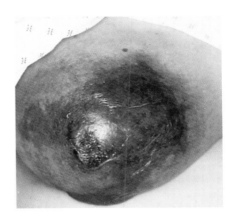

**Figure I-46**

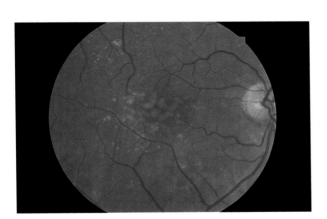

**Figure I-55**

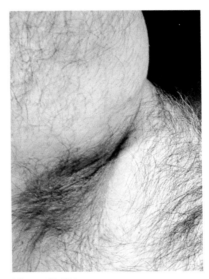

**Figure III-101**

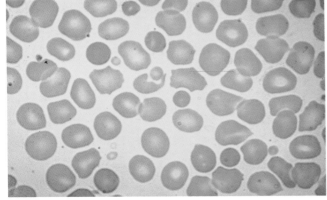

**Figure III-70**

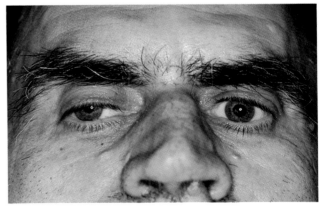

**Figure III-77**

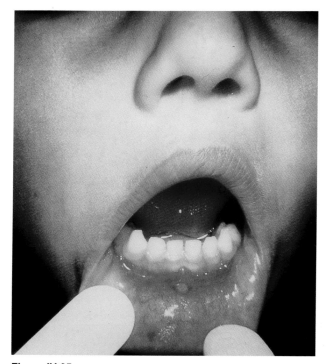

Figure IV-25

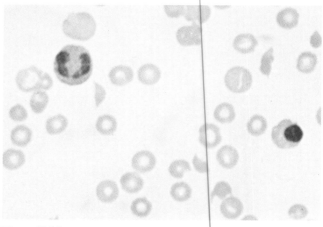

Figure III-81

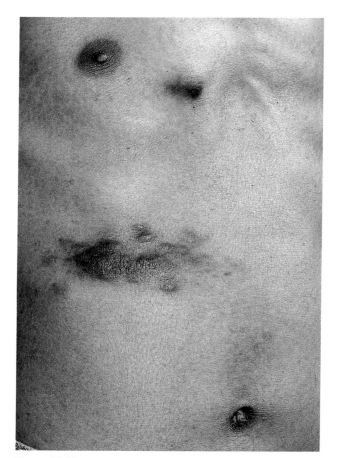

Figure IV-32

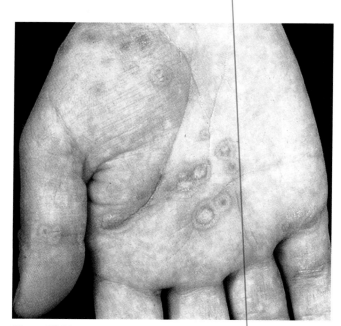

Figure IV-38

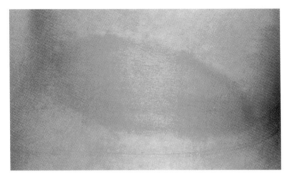

**Figure IV-73**

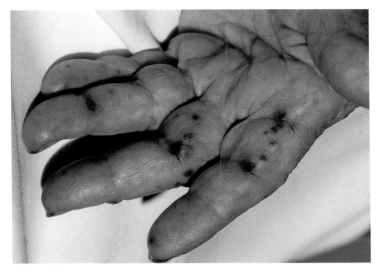

**Figure IV-94**

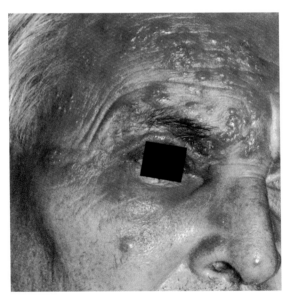

**Figure IV-74**

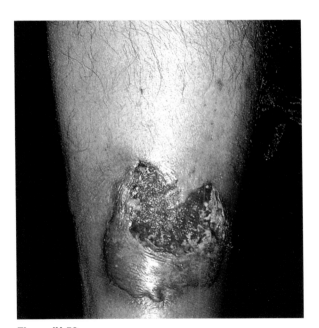

**Figure IX-53**

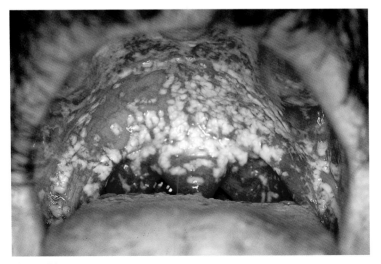

**Figure IV-78**

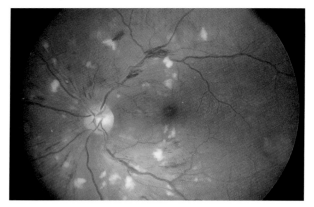

Figure V-79

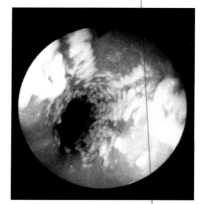

Figure IX-87

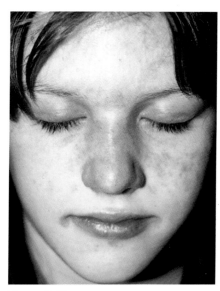

Figure X-12

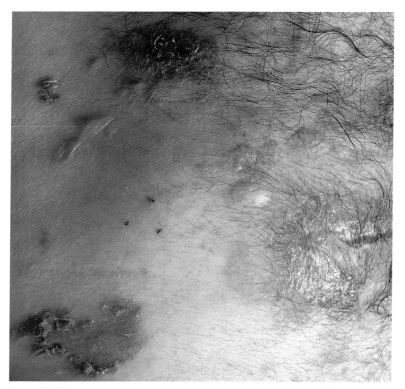

Figure X-50